THE ENCYCLOPEDIA OF

TRAUMA AND TRAUMATIC STRESS DISORDERS

THE ENCYCLOPEDIA OF

TRAUMA AND TRAUMATIC STRESS DISORDERS

Ronald M. Doctor, Ph.D.
and
Frank N. Shiromoto, Ph.D.

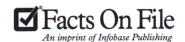

✓ Facts On File
An imprint of Infobase Publishing

The Encyclopedia of Trauma and Traumatic Stress Disorders

Facts On File
An imprint of Infobase Publishing
132 West 31st Street
New York, NY 10001

Library of Congress Cataloging-in-Publication Data

Doctor, Ronald M. (Ronald Manual)
The encyclopedia of trauma and traumatic stress disorders / Ronald M. Doctor and Frank N. Shiromoto.
p. ; cm.
Includes bibliographical references and index.
ISBN-13: 978-0-8160-6764-0 (hardcover : alk, paper)
ISBN-10: 0-8160-6764-3 (hardcover : alk. paper)
1. Psychic trauma—Encyclopedias. 2. Post-traumatic stress disorder—Encyclopedias.
I. Shiromoto, Frank. N. II. Title.
[DNLM: 1. Stress Disorders, Traumatic. 2. Encyclopedia. 3. Mental Disorders. WM 13 D637et 2009]
BF175.5.P75D63 2009
616.85'21003—dc22   2008053541

Facts On File books are available at special discounts when purchased in bulk quantities for businesses, associations, institutions or sales promotions. Please call our Special Sales Department in New York at
(212) 967-8800 or (800) 322-8755.

You can find Facts On File on the World Wide Web at http://www.factsonfile.com

Text and cover design by Cathy Rincon

Printed and bound in United States of America

MV Hermitage 10 9 8 7 6 5 4 3 2 1

This book is printed on acid-free paper and contains 30 percent post-consumer recycled content.

CONTENTS

PREFACE

The Encyclopedia of Trauma and Traumatic Stress Disorders is a compilation of trauma and stress-related terminology in the field of traumatic stress, where posttraumatic stress disorder (PTSD) has become a common headline in media and television reporting of soldiers' experiences in the Vietnam and Gulf Wars. Although PTSD has existed for millennia, it did not become a recognized diagnosis in the *Diagnostic and Statistical Manual of Mental Disorders* until 1980, when introduced by the American Psychiatric Association.

Since September 11, 2001, a new awareness dawned around the world. Terrorists had put fear into everyday lives. No longer could people just jump on an airplane without wondering if this would be their last flight. Terms such as *terrorism*, *9/11*, and *fear* became everyday topics of discussion as bombings continued around the world from Madrid to London to India.

With so many undefined words now leading major discussions, a need arose to define trauma and stress-related concepts in one volume—hence *The Encyclopedia of Trauma and Traumatic Stress Disorders*.

The uniqueness of PTSD as a psychiatric disorder is its emphasis of exposure to a traumatic event or stressor and how each individual responds to and copes with such extreme events. While some individuals cope effectively through appraisal, thereby coming to acceptance of the catastrophic event, others go on to develop full-blown PTSD. We include links to related diagnoses such as depression, anxiety and panic disorders, alcoholism, and drug abuse as possible co-diagnoses of PTSD.

Research into the etiology, nosology, and treatment of traumatic stress disorder has jumped dramatically since 2001. Research is expanding the understanding of trauma's impact on the brain through brain mapping and recognizing the neurobiochemical changes in both the central and autonomous nervous systems. We know that flashback trauma memories, increased sensitivity to startle response, and avoidance behaviors are more than psychological and behavioral mechanisms at work as brain research reveals further complexities of this disorder.

We hope the entries in this encyclopedia address all areas of extreme stress and trauma and innovative treatment approaches, as well as everyday definitions in a clear, nontechnical language, and that we succeed in answering readers' questions. The encyclopedia is aimed at educators, health-care providers, and researchers. In addition, individuals who have endured horrible events and their family members trying to better understand how they survived and how to lend support will find valuable information in this encyclopedia.

We hope this reference book can be a guide to a better understanding of the many medical and psychological effects trauma has on individuals and that traumatic experiences are not just labeled and put aside, but rather folded into the myriad of other health and psychologically related problems.

We value survivors' stories—your unique experience of how you have managed to move on with your life or if you are still struggling. Perhaps the information in this book will provide you with a starting point in your recovery.

We hope you find your peace.

—Frank N. Shiromoto, Ph.D.

ACKNOWLEDGMENTS

Many people contribute to the writing and production of a book. However, our wives, Lisa Lieberman Doctor and Jocelyne Shiromoto, have supported and encouraged this book in every aspect of its development and writing. We love them and are grateful for their support, grace, and love. Christine Adamec has been instrumental in guiding us to completion, and we wish to acknowledge her unwaivering encouragment, skill, and fortitude on our behalf. We also acknowledge the efforts of several CSUN students in compiling lists of terms: Megan McCoy, Ani Mgerdichians, and Sandra Viggiani. Finally, we have been supported throughout by the quiet presence and guidance of James Chambers at Facts On File.

INTRODUCTION

Bob Dylan once noted some years ago, "The Times They Are A-Changin'." It appears that in the 21st century, they *are* a-changin' rapidly and drastically in relation to many core beliefs about mental health and illness. In fact, society seems to be moving from what has been termed the "Age of Anxiety" into what might now be called the "Age of Trauma."

It is not that trauma itself is new, because it is not new at all—think of Noah and the great flood, or Moses killing all the worshippers of the Golden Calf. However, what *is* new is that the eyes of both science and humanity have begun to focus attention on the specific topic of trauma and to employ observational tools that are more sophisticated than ever. The results of analysis to date have been astonishing and staggering.

Already the artificial distinction between "mind" and "body" has been thrown out the window as experts have come to view the mind and the body as one and the same phenomenon. For example, the role and function of the central nervous system, neurology, and the endocrine system are being intimately and slowly unraveled to reveal their role in human development and behavior. *Traumatic stress* is now a source term for most studies of emotional and behavioral development, deviation, and pathology.

Traumatic experience has been made more real to many people because now most of the pathways within the brain, the nervous system, and the endocrine system can be traced. Powerful conceptual models have been developed that explain memory, posttraumatic stress, emotional modula-tion, concentration, and interpersonal behavior. As a result, new therapies have been developed to access the frontal and lower brain centers and the right hemisphere functions because these structures are intimately involved in traumatic reactions.

Somatically-based therapies are also merging, and these therapies help to release constrictions and the *body memory* of the stored traumatic events in a person's life. Such therapies can relieve pain that is directly or indirectly associated with past traumatic events, such as pain induced by physical, sexual, or emotional abuse that occurred in child-hood or adulthood.

Electronic biomeasurements provide some measure of autonomic nervous system activity. For example, using heart rate variability measures, it is now possible to monitor the individual's arousal (sympathetic) responses as well as relaxation (parasympathetic) responses, thereby capturing the relationship between these two ends of the scale. Likewise, measurements of carbon dioxide utilization and cortisol levels can provide other measures of autonomic variability and set points.

Finally, understanding of the concepts of trau-matic experience, which chronically affects 5 percent of men and 10 percent of women, can free individuals from the shameful shackles of being viewed as personally responsible for their condi-tion or considered defective. The reason for this is that traumatic stress—unlike any other psychiatric condition—is caused by events that occur out-side the individual, even though its effects linger within the person.

The study of traumatic stress has also gained depth and breadth because far more subtle forms of trauma (sometimes known as "small t traumas") are being extensively studied by researchers, in contrast to horrific single trauma events. Small *t*'s bring the study of trauma into the arena of abusive homes and physically and sexually abusive or neglectful environments and caretakers. Likewise, areas of concern toward those who are being bullied, criticized, and rejected are viewed as linked to traumatic reactivation.

Early maternal experience is also being studied by experts as it relates to traumatic reactions, poor interpersonal and intra self-evaluations, and the development of chronic diseases. Small *t*, or "complex trauma" as it is coming to be known, tends to tune up the physiology, leading to significant difficulties in the individual's concentration, affect modulation, self-regulation, bonding, and self-esteem.

Many addictive problems undoubtedly stem from developmental or complex trauma, as well as the individual's efforts to control affect (mood) and to find pleasure and function in the world. Recent evidence suggests that many psychiatric conditions are associated with complex trauma. Dissociative disorders, obsessive compulsive disorder (OCD), depression, personality disorders, and borderline personality disorder have all been linked to a past traumatic experience.

The presence and prevalence of trauma is pervasive in society. The National Comorbidity Survey (NCS) consisted of individual interviews with a representative group of Americans between the ages of 15 to 54. The study showed that 5 percent of the men and 10.4 percent of the women had experienced posttraumatic stress disorder (PTSD) at some point in their lives. In addition, 60.7 percent of the men and 51.2 percent of the women had experienced at least one traumatic event in their lifetime. In many cases these trauma sufferers are common citizens. However, this type of trauma statistic is much greater among individuals who are combat veterans, police and fire personnel, emergency paramedics, and others who are frequently exposed to violence and suffering.

Little data is available on trauma that is linked to children and adolescents, but some research indicates high levels (in the 30 to 40 percent range) of exposure to traumatic events, and as high as 21 percent of traumatized children and adolescents have developed diagnosable PTSD symptoms. At-risk samples of children (for example, those who were present where there were school shootings, gang violence, sexual abuse, and so on) bring the rate of PTSD in children up further, to above 50 percent, and some estimates are as high as 100 percent of children in these samples.

A History of Posttraumatic Stress Disorder (PTSD)

Historical literature has chronicled the exposure to terror, war, torture, natural disasters, and life-threatening events leading to psychological after-effects of trauma since the third century B.C., but only since 1980 has posttraumatic stress disorder (PTSD) been formally sanctioned by the psychiatric community in the *Diagnostic and Statistical Manual of Mental Disorders, Third Edition* (*DSM-III*). The significance of naming the disorder and validating the experiences of those who are exposed to traumatic events cannot be overstated. The concept of PTSD endorsed the notion that an external event, rather than an internal weakness, caused the disorder, and it set the framework for systematic study of trauma and the effects upon human experiences.

Nineteenth-Century Observations on the Effects of Trauma

Some of the earliest clinical observations on the effects of trauma on the mind and body date back to the 1870s. The diagnosis of "railway spine" was popularized in lawsuits of passengers involved in railroad accidents who presented with symptoms of postconcussion syndrome (whiplash or soft tissue injury), including nightmares about collisions, sleep disturbance, and intolerance of railway travel. Debates about railway spine promoted the question as to whether this disorder was organic or psychological. By the end of the 19th century, railway spine also became known as traumatic neurosis, the first time the word *trauma* was applied in psychiatry.

Other references in the late 19th century, following debates about railway spine, point to the works of the French neurologist Jean-Martin

Charcot, Sigmund Freud, and Pierre Janet on the similarities of the symptoms of railway spine to hysteria. Hysteria had an array of symptoms, including paralysis, tremors, disorders of sensation, and altered states of consciousness when the individual was reminded of past traumatic memories. Janet later called this "dissociation." Both Freud's and Janet's group of collaborators found that many of the symptoms of hysteria subsided when the trauma memory and emotions were integrated and put into words.

War and PTSD

Most experts agree that war leaves a lasting horrific memory for soldiers, and the physicians working with these soldiers observe the frequent distress of arousal and fatigue. Various terms, such as *soldier's heart, shell shock, war neurosis, combat fatigue, combat stress reaction,* or *combat trauma,* were used to describe a disorder of extreme fatigue, tremors, cardiovascular arousal, and the loss of will to fight. During the American Civil War, soldiers with overwhelming mental fatigue were diagnosed with soldier's heart, which included symptoms of startle response and arrhythmia.

In World War I, physicians described soldiers as shell-shocked when they presented neurological symptoms but no physical injury. From World War II emerged the term *battle fatigue*. During both world wars, developing knowledge of the condition grew slowly at best and was fraught with misunderstanding as military leaders were highly skeptical and unsympathetic to the sufferer. Later, the long-term traumatic effects of the Holocaust would haunt the developers of the *DSM* and contribute to the eventual inclusion of PTSD.

The Vietnam War inflicted severe psychological effects on returning veterans suffering from combat trauma, and research on this group provided a key catalyst for the inclusion of specific reactions to trauma for PTSD in *DSM-III*. The term *combat stress reaction* was mandated by the U.S. Department of Defense in 1999 and is currently used to describe the PTSD symptoms of veterans of the Gulf Wars and Afghanistan and Iraq conflicts. The diagnostic criteria of PTSD were based on Abram Kardiner's work on war neurosis derived from his treatment and observations of World War I veterans.

Kardiner encompassed Freud's psychoanalytic theory to explain why the soldier often developed amnesia for the traumatic event, even while reliving the experience. He viewed this as the individual protecting the integrity of his ego. In his works *Traumatic Neuroses of War* and *War Stress and Neurotic Illness,* Kardiner provided great insights into the phenomenology and treatment of war-related stress.

Kardiner's observations of war veterans did not affect his view of peacetime trauma, which he noted has the same structure as the wartime version. The *DSM-III* inclusion of PTSD fully recognized his contribution to understanding the nature of this syndrome.

War in Iraq and Afghanistan

Since the invasion of Iraq in March 2003 through 2008, it is estimated that the rate of posttraumatic stress disorder (PTSD) in veterans returning from the Gulf War region ranges from 12 to 20 percent. From the first 100,000 troops that have returned from Iraq and Afghanistan and treated at VA hospitals, 25 percent were given mental health diagnosis of PTSD, drug or alcohol abuse, or depression. Also the younger the soldier, the more prevalent these symptoms were reported.

The high rates of PTSD are thought to be a result of an undefined war front, battles within civilian city populations, the difficulty of discerning who is the enemy, frequent unpredictable suicide bombings, and no real "safe zones." During the Vietnam War, soldiers could rest and recuperate in safe areas, whereas in Iraq every place is a war zone. Not only are buddies maimed and killed, but also innocent civilian women and children are killed in public view, and it takes a toll. Another important factor to the risk of PTSD is multiple deployments to combat zones, each deployment lasting up to 15 months.

There is much debate about the nature of trauma. Does trauma result from directly experiencing or witnessing death in direct combat? Or does the constant fear of death in a protected Green Zone in Iraq create problems for those within the compound as well as those who patrol and engage the enemy in battle. Because there is no front line, there are constant threats of mortar, artillery, and improvised explosive devices (IED) targeting those within so-called safe zones. Some professionals have argued that being in a war zone does not constitute exposure to trauma, just that it is extremely stressful. However, most helping professionals agree to treat problems first and not minimize reasons to seek help.

The toughest part for any veteran is to step into a veteran center and ask for help. Although the Department of Veterans Affairs continues to publicly state it spends more than $3 billion a year on mental health care, many veterans never ask for help. There is a stigma about PTSD, and veterans distrust the system for fear of a mental health diagnosis that could end their military careers. In most cases veterans try to avoid the flashbacks, nightmares, and intrusive thoughts that disrupt daily work and home life. It is estimated that two-thirds of Iraq veterans who were screened positive for PTSD and other psychiatric disorders are not receiving treatment. Unfortunately, many veterans say to themselves, "I can handle it," while increasingly they succumb to drug and alcohol abuse, failed relationships and marriages, loss of jobs, and even suicide.

U.S. military psychiatrists are urging returning soldiers to get assistance for broader issues of postdeployment stress, as well as readjustment and reintegration into civilian life. This type of help includes career counseling to find a job, relationship counseling to help families adjust, substance abuse interventions to avoid addictive lifestyles, and efforts to address stressful or emotional concerns that fall short of PTSD.

Hope for greater understanding of PTSD must start with knowledge about trauma, its effect on deployment to combat areas such as Iraq and Afghanistan, and the provision of high-quality mental health care. With public advocacy from the American Psychiatric Association and the Gulf War Resource Center, veterans are now the focus of medical problems ranging from traumatic brain injury to posttraumatic stress disorder. The motto of military physicians is "Urge them to get help."

The Women's Movement

While traumatic disorders are common in combat situations, the greater influence in establishing the category of posttraumatic stress disorders in the American Psychiatric Association's *Diagnostic and Statistical Manual* (*DSM*) was the social awareness that came from the women's movement of the 1970s. A new awareness of three major social problems emerged from this movement. The first was rape. The psychological study of survivors found that for a vast majority there was severe damage to relationships and sexual behavior following this violent act. New laws were instituted against perpetrators, and victims began to receive follow-up counseling and improved examination and reporting procedures. The effects of rape were known as the "rape syndrome." The second, violence against women, was also publicized as what came to be called the "battered woman syndrome." Women beaten by boyfriends or husbands had recourse under new laws and could escape to safe homes where they and their children could stay in protected and secret housing havens. The third social problem was initially called the "battered child syndrome." Today it is called "child abuse," and it includes developmental trauma in the form of neglect and physical, sexual, and emotional abuse. These medical, psychological, and legal streams helped lead in 1980 to the inclusion of posttraumatic stress disorder as a new diagnostic category in the *DSM*.

—Ronald M. Doctor, Ph.D.

Birmes, P., L. Hatton, A. Brunet, and L. Schmitt. "Early Historical Literature for Post-Traumatic Symptomatology." *Stress and Health* 19, no. 1 (2003): 17–26.
Lasiuk, G. C., and K. M. Hegadoren. "Posttraumatic Stress Disorder Part I: Historical Development of the Concept." *Perspective in Psychiatric Care* 42, no. 1 (February 2006).

ENTRIES A to Z

abreaction An emotional release that occurs when an individual reexperiences a TRAUMATIC EVENT that he or she had repressed or suppressed from memory. Repression keeps information out of consciousness, and suppression consciously keeps information out of awareness. The individual feels as if he or she is reliving the particular traumatic event and experiencing the same or similar physical and emotional reactions as he or she felt when the trauma occurred. Some experts, such as the well-known psychoanalyst Sigmund Freud, believed that abreaction that occurs while under therapy was nearly always a major breakthrough for traumatized patients and was also a pathway to a cure. However, other experts do *not* see abreaction as therapeutic beyond the emotional release, nor do they believe that insight into the meaning of the past experience is always gained with abreaction.

In the trauma treatment area, abreaction is thought to resensitize the person and therefore is of little value or possibly delays effective treatment. Even Freud found that many of his classic patients on whom he based abreaction as curative actually regressed over time and had to be hospitalized. The tendency to reexperience a traumatic event was called by Freud "repetition compulsion." In EYE MOVEMENT DESENSITIZATION AND REPROCESSING (EMDR) based trauma treatment, *LOOPING* is a term for a stuck point in the process of desensitizing a traumatic experience. This is somewhat similar to the blocks associated with repetition compulsions.

See also CHILD ABUSE AND NEGLECT; CHILD PHYSICAL ABUSE; CHILDREN AND TRAUMA; CHILD SEXUAL ABUSE; FLASHBACK; THERAPY, TYPES OF; TRAUMATIC MEMORY; TREATMENT: PSYCHOTHERAPY, PSYCHOPHARMACOLOGY, AND ALTERNATIVE MEDICINE.

Acceptance and Commitment Therapy (ACT) Part of the "third wave" of behavioral therapies rooted in contextualism, or the behavior or ongoing action within a context. Acceptance and Commitment Therapy (ACT) targets experiential avoidance. This is the attempt to escape or avoid private experiences that are aversive. Experiential avoidance usually does not work, or it works only in the short term, and eventually, heightened reexperiencing or numbing, denial, and dissociation must be engaged by the individual over the long run.

While it is still in its developmental and empirical testing stage as of this writing, ACT does seem to offer an approach to trauma-based experience such as POSTTRAUMATIC STRESS DISORDER (PTSD). For example, in PTSD there are many avoidance networks in thought, memory, and perception of environmental stimuli. ACT advocates point out that uncontrollable intrusive thoughts, NIGHTMARES, and hyperarousal are the by-products of the individual's attempts to avoid aversive private stimulation. By using "defusion," mindfulness, and acceptance exercises to face these aversive private events, by-products are dealt with. Another aspect of ACT is the commitment to behavior change in support of the client's personal values, rather than devoting energies to avoidance.

See also THERAPY, TYPES OF.

acetylcholine A NEUROTRANSMITTER that stimulates both the peripheral and central nervous system nerves in humans and in most organisms. In the peripheral system, acetylcholine's presence stimulates muscle contractions and tension. In the brain, it causes excitatory actions. Glands that receive impulses from the PARASYMPATHETIC NERVOUS SYSTEM are also stimulated by this chemical.

Nerve gas agents (such as Sarin) inhibit the enzyme that breaks down acetylcholine, resulting in the continuous stimulation of muscles, glands, and the central nervous system.

Acetylcholine is important in mediating parasympathetic responses in the body, resulting in calming effects.

Acetylcholine was discovered by Henry Hallett Dale in 1914 and later (1921) confirmed by Otto Loewi, who initially gave it the name *vagusstoff* because it was released by the vagus nerve. Both Dale and Loewi received the Nobel Prize for their work in the areas of physiology and medicine.

See also BRAIN; CENTRAL NERVOUS SYSTEM; SYMPATHETIC NERVOUS SYSTEM.

ACTH See ADRENOCORTICOTROPHIC HORMONE; BRAIN.

acute stress disorder (ASD) Immediate traumatic reaction of people that may or may not lead to POSTTRAUMATIC STRESS DISORDER (PTSD). According to the fourth edition of the *Diagnostic and Statistical Manual of Mental Disorders (DSM-IV)* published in 1994, the category of acute stress disorder assumes the presence of a traumatic stressor (e.g., a life-threatening event to oneself or others and a sense of helplessness) such as a severe motor vehicle accident, a violent attack, or a natural disaster. ASD is classified as an ANXIETY DISORDER IN *DSM-IV-TR*, published in 2000.

Acute stress disorder, while a clinical problem itself, is thought to be a precursor to the development of PTSD. In fact, empirical research has established a link between ASD and subsequent PTSD. Harvey and Bryant (1998), for example, found that 78 percent of auto accident survivors who exhibited symptoms of ASD also developed PTSD (although only 13 percent of those in accidents reported ASD symptoms and another 21 percent had "subclinical" but ASD-like symptoms). These authors also concluded that the "dissociative and arousal clusters" may be less important than first thought. The term *clusters* refers to sets of symptoms or groups of symptoms within a disorder.

Symptoms and Diagnostic Path

The symptoms of acute stress disorder are similar to those of PTSD and include reexperiencing the event, increased arousal, FLASHBACKS, anxiety, and significant distress in social and/or occupational functioning. In addition, a diagnosis of ASD must also include three dissociative responses. The five types of dissociative symptoms are: (1) a subjective sense of numbing, detachment, or an absence of emotional responsiveness; (2) a reduction in one's awareness of one's surroundings (e.g., a "daze"); (3) derealization or a temporary feeling of sadness or low affect; (4) depersonalization or feeling detached from one's body or environment; and (5) dissociative AMNESIA or the inability to recall important aspects of the trauma. These dissociative features represent coping mechanisms for the adverse effects of the traumatic experience.

Another diagnostic requirement is that the disturbance in an acute stress disorder must last for two or more days and can persist for up to four weeks, beyond which it would be classified as PTSD. An example of a tool used to help diagnose ASD is the Acute Stress Disorder Scale, which is a 19-item self-report inventory based on the 1994 diagnostic criteria of *DSM-IV.*

Treatment Options and Outlook

Individuals with acute stress disorder may need and may benefit from psychotherapy. Many therapists, however, wait to see if the acute symptoms abate within the one-month period before diagnosing PTSD. Acute stress disorders are treated by somatic therapy and EYE MOVEMENT DESENSITIZATION AND REPROCESSING (EMDR). Talking about the incident usually just stimulates and coalesces the reaction, thereby prolonging healing. Cognitive behavioral therapies have also proven helpful with acute traumas, as has SSRIs medications such as paroxetine (Paxil), fluoxetine (Prozac), citalopram (Celexa) and anti-anxiety medications such as alprazolam (Xanax), lorazepam (Ativan) and diazepam (Valium), as well as the beta-blocker medication propranolol (Inderal), which some think may have some effects in preventing the eventual development of PTSD. The outlook for ASD depends on many factors, such as the severity of the stressor, the presence of risk factors for developing PTSD, and existing social support.

Risk Factors and Preventive Measures

Exposure to an acute traumatic event is usually impossible to predict or prevent. They are often sudden and unpredictable, such as motor vehicle accidents, violence, and reactions to medical procedures. The major risk factors associated with posttraumatic stress disorder also apply to ASD. These include prior individual or family psychological pathology, prior trauma, and lack of social support

See also DISORDERS OF TRAUMA; TRAUMA, COMBAT VERSUS CIVILIAN.

Harvey, A. G. and R. A. Bryant. "The Relationship between Acute Stress Disorder and Posttraumatic Stress Disorder: A Prospective Evaluation of Motor Vehicle Accident Survivors." *Journal of Consulting and Clinical Psychology* 66, no. 3 (1998): 507–512.

acute traumatic stress disorder (ATSD)   See ACUTE STRESS DISORDER.

addiction   Usually refers to a physical and psychological dependence on illegal drugs, misused prescription drugs, and sometimes to alcohol (alcoholism). Individuals who have undergone a traumatic experience may turn to substance abuse or dependence to try to numb themselves or to keep their painful memories from resurfacing; for example, adults who were abused as children have a greater risk than others who were not abused to become dependent on alcohol and/or drugs. Likewise, combat veterans frequently become drug or alcohol addicted in order to sustain themselves through their tour of duty. In addition, adolescents who are exposed to current extreme trauma may turn to alcohol or drugs to provide relief, including such trauma as abuse, extreme illness in the family (such as cancer), natural disasters, and other traumas.

The individual with an addiction has a physical tolerance to the drug, which means that he or she needs increasingly greater amounts of the substance to achieve the same level of effects. There is also a psychological dependence on the substance, such that the individual believes that he or she needs it in order to function normally. In addition, the substance is central to the individual's life, and a great deal of time is devoted to acquiring or using drugs or alcohol. Attempting to give up the substance is a traumatic event to the addicted person.

Another central aspect of addiction is that if the substance is withheld, either voluntarily or involuntarily, the addicted individual will experience withdrawal symptoms, which may range from relatively minor symptoms, such as nausea and vomiting, to extremely severe symptoms, such as seizures, delusions, or hallucinations. Some medications help ease these withdrawal symptoms; for example, BENZODIAZEPINES may ease the withdrawal symptoms from alcohol.

A common problem among addicts is the intense craving for the substance even after they have undergone rehabilitation and no longer have any of the substance remaining in their bodies. This craving must be dealt with in therapy, or the individual will usually resume abusing the substance and will become readdicted. Any people, places, or activities previously associated with alcohol use can trigger cravings and thereby increase the temptation to drink. The craving is automatically conditioned to those previously associated triggers and is "extinguished" only after years of practicing abstinence and developing alternative coping mechanisms.

Many addicts also find support in dealing with their intense cravings through such groups as Alcoholics Anonymous or Cocaine Anonymous, depending on the substance to which they are addicted. In these groups, other members have direct personal experience with the substance and can understand the problems that addicted individuals face and can help them stay off substances.

Some drugs counteract the craving for alcohol or drugs; for example, naltrexone (ReVia) and acamprosate (Campral) may diminish the craving for alcohol, while buprenorphine may decrease the craving for narcotics.

Methadone, a synthetic narcotic, is sometimes used to treat individuals who are addicted to heroin. It stops the craving for heroin and does not provide the euphoria that is seen with heroin use.

In addition, methadone is approved by the Food and Drug Administration (FDA) as a treatment for heroin addiction (as well as a medication to treat moderate to severe pain). Methadone is available as an oral medication, and thus it does not require needles. Many heroin addicts share needles when they use the drug illicitly, which increases the risk of spreading the human immunodeficiency virus (HIV), hepatitis, and other blood-borne diseases. As a result, eliminating this problem of shared needles is a benefit to society. However, some experts strongly disapprove of methadone maintenance, which they perceive as merely substituting one drug for another.

A further problem faced by most addicts is that even after they successfully complete an outpatient or inpatient rehabilitation program, often they return to the same environment where their addiction began. They frequently associate with former friends or relatives who abuse substances and may quickly become readdicted. This issue is another problem that therapists discuss with patients, offering workable strategies to help them refuse substances if the individual must return to his or her old neighborhood.

See also AMPHETAMINES.

Gwinnell, Esther, M.D., and Christine Adamec. *The Encyclopedia of Drug Abuse.* New York: Facts On File, 2008.

adrenocorticotropic hormone (ACTH) A hormone that is secreted by the pituitary gland. Stress or trauma causes elevated levels of adrenocorticotropic hormone (ACTH) to be released, and anxiety or DEPRESSION can also raise an individual's ACTH levels. ACTH is triggered in the pituitary by corticotrophin-releasing hormone (CRH), which is secreted by the hypothalamus. The secretion of CRH starts a well-defined hormonal stress cycle. Once ACTH is released, it activates the adrenal glands that release adrenaline and noradrenaline for activation, and CORTISOL, which at first sustains the arousal reaction and then prepares the body for action. Cortisol eventually helps restore the body to a calmer state by counteracting the effects of adrenaline. This hormone cycle is called the HYPO-THALAMIC-PITUITARY-ADRENAL (HPA) AXIS and acts in stress and traumatic stress.

See also BRAIN; PHYSIOLOGY OF TRAUMA.

Adult Attachment Projective (AAP) A classification system that was developed by Carol George and Malcolm West in the 1990s, and which uses the responses of individuals to eight pictures. The first picture is a neutral one of children playing ball, and the next seven pictures show scenes of attachment.

The responses are used to categorize individuals into four groups, including secure, dismissing, preoccupied, and unresolved. For example, one picture depicts a child looking out a window, with her back to the viewer. Another picture, called "departure," depicts a man and woman with suitcases who are facing each other. A third picture shows a child sitting alone on a bench. In a fourth picture, a child and a woman are facing each other at opposite ends of a bed. The fifth picture shows a woman and a child observing someone being placed on a stretcher into an ambulance. The sixth picture shows an adult male in front of a gravestone. The final picture shows a child standing in a corner, slightly turned.

These drawings were purposely chosen to depict events such as illness, death, solitude, separation, and threat. The therapist who is administering the test asks the respondent to make up a story about each picture, including what has led up to the scene, what the characters are thinking, and what could happen later. The responses are evaluated to determine the adult's type of attachment.

For example, according to George, West, and Petterm in their chapter in *Attachment Disorganization,* the following response to being asked to tell a story about the cemetery picture is an example of an unresolved attachment:

> [The respondent said] "Let me see, the anniversary of someone's death, and this man came to the graveyard to pay his respects, remember whoever passed away. Um, the outcome will be that he'll pay his respects and leave." When asked what the man may be thinking, the respondent said, "Probably sadness and emptiness and missing the person who isn't there anymore."

Here the therapist can see the lack of attachment or incompleteness of attachment for this individual by the fact that there is little grieving and almost no description of the dead person. The focus is on the "emptiness" felt by the respondent. This experience is typical for those with a lack of attachment or bonding with a significant other and coupled with the anonymity of the deceased, and these responses are indicative of an attachment disorder.

See also ATTACHMENT STYLES/DISORDERS.

George, C., M. West, and O. Petterm. "The Adult Attachment Projective: Disorganization of Adult Attachment at the Level of Representation." In *Attachment Disorganization,* edited by J. Solomon and C. George, 462–507. New York: Guilford Press, 1999.

affective disorders   Sustained extremes of mood. Affective disorders are also known as mood disorders. Affective disorders, particularly depressive disorders, are often associated with traumatic experiences and/or the presence of ANXIETY DISORDERS.

The primary affective disorders are depressive disorders (DEPRESSION) or mania and manic-depression (bipolar). Dysthymia is a form of depression that is not severe enough to meet the criteria for a major depressive disorder. Depressive disorders are more common than BIPOLAR DISORDER. Depression is a prolonged feeling of severely unhappy mood. Individuals with bipolar disorder may experience periods of euphoria and/or mania alternating with depression, while individuals with depression do not experience euphoria or mania.

Bipolar disorder, also known as manic-depressive illness, is a severe persistent mental illness characterized by periods of deep depression that alternates with periods of extreme elevated mood and energy known as mania. Mania can be mild (hypomania) to full-blown mania with psychotic features that include hallucinations and delusions.

Different from the normal ups and downs people normally feel, bipolar disorder distorts moods and thoughts to severe extremes, and in some people it results in SUICIDE. The manic and depressive episodes cycle throughout the life span. With proper mood-stabilizing medications, most people with bipolar disorder can remain symptom free between episodes.

A depressive disorder is significantly more than a feeling of sadness for one or several days, and instead, it lasts for at least two weeks, and symptoms occur daily. Some individuals experience depressive disorders that are related to severely distressing life events, such as bereavement, disasters, and other experiences, while others experience depression that is seemingly unrelated to the events of their lives. In general, women are more likely to suffer from depressive disorders than men, although men are at risk as well.

Symptoms and Diagnostic Path
Symptoms of a depressive disorder include

- a significant change in weight (loss or gain)
- loss of interest in normal activities that have given pleasure in the past
- an inability to concentrate
- sleep disturbance
- feelings of worthlessness and hopelessness
- inappropriate guilt
- recurrent thoughts of death or suicide (Some individuals talk of a suicide plan; these expressions should be taken seriously, and the individual should be referred immediately to a mental health professional.)

In contrast to depression, symptoms of the mania of bipolar disorder include

- an inflated self-esteem
- decreased need for sleep
- very rapid speech that is hard for others to follow
- grandiose delusions
- extreme distractibility
- irrational behaviors (such as spending very large sums of money for items the person would not normally purchase)

In diagnosing individuals, mental health professionals consider the individual's current mental state and behavior as well as take a psychiatric history. The clinician will also want to know whether others in the family have experienced similar symptoms, since affective disorders are often present in other family members, and there is a genetic risk for these disorders.

A physician may order laboratory tests, such as a thyroid-stimulating hormone (TSH) test to rule out hypothyroidism, which may cause lethargy and simulate a low level of depression. A complete blood count (CBC) can rule out anemia, which could cause similar symptoms.

Treatment Options and Outlook

If an individual is severely depressed or extremely manic and is at risk for suicide or other extreme actions that would harm him or her, the clinician may recommend hospitalization. Otherwise, the patient is treated on an outpatient basis with medications and psychotherapy. Depressed patients are treated with antidepressants, while patients with bipolar disorder are treated with mood stabilizers, such as lithium carbonate or valproate (Depakote, Depakene). Patients with bipolar disorder may also need antidepressants. Psychotherapy can help patients by educating them about their disorder and helping them identify possible triggers to their symptoms.

Patients with depression may need treatment for several months, several years, or for their lifetimes depending on the decision of the clinician. Patients with bipolar disorder often require treatment for years.

Risk Factors and Preventive Measures

Individuals with family members with depressive disorders or bipolar disorder are at risk for the development of an affective disorder. There is no way to prevent such disorders; however, should they occur, treatment can enable most individuals to lead successful lives.

See also AFFECT MODULATION; ASSOCIATED DISORDERS; BENZODIAZEPINES; BORDERLINE PERSONALITY DISORDER; SELECTIVE SEROTONIN REUPTAKE INHIBITOR (SSRI); THERAPY, TYPES OF.

affect modulation A clinical term that is used to describe the ability of a person to control his or her emotional and behavioral responses within an acceptable range of intensity, appropriateness, and duration. Although quite subjective and bound by observer bias, situational expectations, and values, the term *affect modulation* is used frequently with sufferers of POSTTRAUMATIC STRESS DISORDER (PTSD) as a summary label for critical PTSD-related symptoms. Another use of the term is *affect dysregulation*.

The major behavioral categories that are affected by affect modulation or dysregulation problems are concentration, memory recall, sustained focus, anger management, self-destructive behaviors, suicidal behaviors, and unmodulated (risky and frequent) sexual behavior. People with PTSD, and those who no longer display symptoms but have had PTSD in the past, report significantly more problems modulating their affective reactions than do non-PTSD people. Furthermore, the earlier that abuse or trauma takes place in one's life, the more likely the individual will demonstrate dysregulation of affect and behavior.

Two opposing poles of dysregulation caused by traumatic experiences are possible. At one end are highly repressed people who show "blunted" or little affect (mood) in their lives. They seem bland, unresponsive, cold, and disinterested, even though they appear to be intelligent and perceptive individuals.

At the other end are individuals at the reactive extreme side; they display emotional volatility and quick intense reactions to many situations in their lives. These people might be called the "screamer," the "bully," the "hysteric," or the "exploder."

Trauma is only one factor that can lead to affective regulation problems. Individual differences or variability in emotional control and regulation are certainly factors. Genetic variability combined with an early developmental environment that reinforced extreme behaviors, such as yelling, bullying, quietness. and nonresponsiveness are some of the behaviors that can follow an individual into adulthood, particularly if these behaviors appear to have some value to the adult.

Trauma leads to chronic activation, which, in turn, makes the modulation of affect more difficult and can lead to dysregulation. For example, some experts believe that the anger volatility seen in individuals with BORDERLINE PERSONALITY DISORDER may be related to early traumatic experiences.

See also AFFECTIVE DISORDERS; "BULLYCIDE" AND BULLYING.

Van der Kolk, B. A., et al. "Dissociation, Affect Dysregulation and Somatization: The Complex Nature of Adaptation to Trauma." *American Journal of Psychiatry* 153, no. 7 (1996), 83–93.

alexithymia   A condition in which a person has great difficulty in identifying his or her own emotions and is unable to communicate how he or she feels to others. The term was first coined by Peter Sifneos in 1972. Said Sifneos in a later article in 2000:

Alexithymia, a term I introduced for better or for worse in 1972, involves a marked difficulty to use appropriate language to express and describe feelings and to differentiate them from bodily sensations, a striking paucity of fantasies and a utilitarian way of thinking.

Symptoms and Diagnostic Path

When patients with alexithymia present to their doctor, they frequently report somatic complaints, such as headaches or stomach pain, although there are no identified underlying medical problems. Obviously, the emotion involved is not stated, and it is represented in these general and usually vague bodily complaints. Diagnosis is based on thorough interview with the patient and administering psychological tests such as the Toronto Alexithymia Scale, Bermond-Vorst Alexithymia Questionnaire, or the Observer Alexithymia Scale.

In an article in *Psychiatric Times,* René J. Muller described a teenager who engaged in cutting herself, burning herself, and other similar acts, yet described herself as "fine." When asked why she had jumped out of a window, she responded that she had no idea why she had done so. However, at the time of the window-jumping incident, the girl was having difficulties with her boyfriend. The teenager's mother told the clinician that the girl kept everything to herself.

The clinician determined that the girl had emotions that she did not understand, nor could she communicate her feelings to others. He considered and rejected a diagnosis of BORDERLINE PERSONAL-ITY DISORDER. Instead, the teenager was referred to experts at a psychiatric hospital for outpatient help in learning how to identify and express her emotions. According to Muller:

Identifying a patient as alexithymic opens a door to that person's pathological world and creates a fertile field for exploration in therapy. A workable identity can develop only after the elements of a person's life coalesce into a minimally satisfactory story.

In 2006 Burba et al. reported on their study of 120 adolescents diagnosed with SOMATOFORM DISORDER and compared them to a healthy control group of 60 subjects. Using the Toronto Alexithymia Scale, they found that 59 percent of the adolescents with somatoform disorder had alexithymia, compared to 1 percent of the subjects in the control group. Interestingly, the researchers also used the Hospital Anxiety and Depression Scale to compare the rates of anxiety and depression in the two groups. The patient group had a much higher rate of anxiety (62 percent) than the control group (15 percent); however, the rate of depression was low and not significantly different in both groups.

In his 2000 article, Sifneos said that alexithymia is associated with both politics and crime, and he pointed to criminals serving life sentences or even sentenced to death but who expressed no emotion at their sentencing. In addition, he cited historical figures such as Rudolf Hess, the commandant of Auschwitz, the deplorable concentration camp, as well as Adolf Eichmann, an SS officer, and Adolf Hitler himself as exhibiting symptoms of alexithymia in that they were devoid of emotion.

Treatment Options and Outlook

Alexithymia is treated by helping individuals learn to discriminate and identify their own emotional reactions. Often this includes asking them where in the body they feel some sensation (a perceptible but often slight bodily experience usually quite a bit less intense than a "feeling"). Then the therapist may ask the individual to describe the quality of that sensation (i.e., good or bad, pleasant or unpleasant, tingly, tight, achy, and so on). Gradually, through trial and error, discrimination and awareness of sensations develops. The next step is to help the individual focus on feelings or emotions as represented by more intense and usually more generalized sensations. For example, the individual may say, "I feel something in my stomach." The therapist may respond by asking if the sensation is strong enough to call it "fear." Gradually labels are applied to these strong sensations, and parts of the body are seen as reflecting different emotions or feelings to the individual. Often this approach is supplemented outside the therapy session with body massage performed by a certified massage therapist. This helps to identify areas of the body and sensations that the person experiences and can be very helpful in the training for learning to identify emotional reactions.

Risks and Preventive Measures

In many alexithymic individuals, the "numbing" that they experience could also be a form of DISSOCIATION that has developed in reaction to early traumatic experiences. In these cases, which form the vast majority of alexithymic individuals, introduction of trauma work usually occurs once discrimination develops and the patient is sufficiently contained to handle emotional arousal.

See also PSYCHIC NUMBING; THERAPY, TYPES OF.

Burba, Benjaminas, M.D., et al. "A Controlled Study of Alexithymia in Adolescent Patients with Persistent Somatoform Pain Disorder." *Canadian Journal of Psychiatry* 51, no. 7 (June 2006): 468–471.

Muller, René J. "When a Patient Has No Story to Tell: Alexithymia." *Psychiatric Times* 17, no. 7 (July 2000). Available online. URL: http://psychiatrictimes.com/p000771.html. Downloaded September 12, 2006.

Sifneos, Peter E. "Alexithymia, Clinical Issues, Politics and Crime." *Psychotherapy and Psychosomatics* 69 (2000): 113–116.

alienation from self Feeling of isolation from the self. Traumatic experiences have a global impact, and they affect the biological, emotional, cognitive, and spiritual dimensions of life for the traumatized victim. Trauma leads to DYSREGULATION or dysfunction within each of these dimensions and, in turn, produces an even more pervasive and subtle problem for individuals in that their sense of the self and of the world around them feels alienated, unsafe, and scared. They feel all alone.

In cases of extreme or chronic traumatic stimulation, the sense of self may be so alienated from the experience that several different identities or personalities may prevail and may subconsciously alternate in the person's experience. This is called dissociative identity disorder (DID), formerly known as a multiple personality. Most often, however, the effects are not as dramatic. Usually traumatized people experience a sense of alienation from others and from their own inner experience. They find it difficult to read other people, to know how they feel emotionally, or to trust their own experiences as authentic and valid. Both their inner and outer worlds seem unsafe and scary to them, and a deep sense of aloneness pervades their lives.

Most trauma therapists see that awareness, integration, and restoration of the sense of self are essential outcomes of successful trauma therapy.

See also DISSOCIATION DISSOCIATIVE DISORDERS; DISSOCIATIVE EXPERIENCES SCALE.

McLaren, K. *Emotional Genius: Discovering the Deepest Language of the Soul.* Columbia, Calif.: Laughing Tree Press, 2001.

alienists An old original term for psychiatrists that preceded World War I. At that time, psychiatry was basically an asylum-based discipline. Alienists tried to legitimize their work (since it was considered nonmedical, but they were medical doctors), first by adopting phrenology (determining problems based on bumps in the head) and later by advocating humanistic treatment centers that used what was called "moral" treatment: essentially, positive reinforcement and group influence in a kindly atmosphere.

With the advent of the Civil War and later World War I, and the influx of huge numbers of soldiers with SHELL SHOCK, treatment changed to a more outpatient and group form that emphasized custodial care. After World War I, the influence of Freudian psychoanalysis guided treatment toward more individualized care and relational therapy, but many psychiatrists still held on to the constitutional deficiencies theory. *Constitutional deficiencies* refers to genetic deficiencies. Many, if not most, forms of mental illness were thought to be the inheritance of weak genes that lead to a particular disorder. This kept psychiatry within the realm of medicine because medicine saw psychiatry as one step removed from witchcraft. Freud introduced "psychological" causes but also believed that there were inherent genetic weaknesses that produced the neuroses, so his theories kept psychiatry within the medical view of disorders.

See also ABREACTION; THERAPY, TYPES OF.

Healy, David. *Images of Trauma: From Hysteria to Post-Traumatic Stress Disorder.* London: Faber and Faber, 1993.

altered body image See DISSOCIATION DISSOCIATIVE DISORDERS.

altered pain perception An abnormal perception of pain, either pain is felt too acutely, or it is not experienced sufficiently. Pain is very important to the sustenance of life. When pain is not felt appropriately, as when pain is not experienced at all or is experienced only minimally, the individual will not seek assistance for an injury or medical problem. For example, the person with advanced diabetes may not experience pain in the feet and thus may not notice and thus not treat a cut or abrasion that steadily worsens to the point that the foot or even the leg itself may have to be amputated. In the case where an altered pain perception causes pain to be experienced very acutely, the individual may seek constant medical attention and be frequently dissatisfied with the treatment received.

Victims of trauma often experience altered body senses as well as an altered pain perception. NUMBING is a common outcome of trauma, and it is one of five criteria for POSTTRAUMATIC STRESS DISORDER diagnosis. In this case, numbing can occur within the body as well as at a psychic level.

See also SOMATOFORM DISSOCIATION.

alternative treatments Nontraditional treatments for serious trauma. There are a variety of treatment options for POSTTRAUMATIC STRESS DISORDER (PTSD), and many individuals find a combination of treatments to be the most effective. Alternative treatments can help manage the symptoms of PTSD as well as any additional symptoms of ANXIETY DISORDERS and DEPRESSION.

There are medical systems throughout the world in addition to Western medicine. Cultures vary in their healing practices, but they generally address human suffering as part of rebalancing the human body. Some of these systems are described in this entry.

Traditional Chinese medicine is based on 4,000 years of practice and looks at health as the balance of the yin and yang (negative and positive energies). The use of herbs, acupuncture, nutrition, and forms of exercise (such as tai chi) help restore balance to the diseased state, both physical and mental.

Native American Indian healing practices combine spiritual practices, herbal medicine, and purifying ceremonies that have been in use by hundreds of tribes for thousands of years for treating trauma, addictions, and medical illness.

Ayurveda, traditional medicine within India, is the oldest medical system that is based on energy and balance to restore wholeness to the mind-body system. In this system, all individuals have their own distinct bioenergetic type (*doshas*), known as Vata, Pitta, and Kapha, and it is this harmony of the three *doshas* that determines health and illness. The emphasis is on the mind, body, and spirit, using such techniques as meditation, aromatherapy, yoga, nutrition, and exercise to trigger the body's own natural healing processes.

Other Treatment Alternatives

There are many treatment alternatives that have few empirical studies but much anecdotal evidence of support, and several key alternatives are described here.

Creative arts therapies use dance, music, drawings, and creative writing to reduce the symptoms of emotional distress. These activities address the right brain neurons, which can be difficult to reach using traditional behavioral talk therapy, such as COGNITIVE BEHAVIORAL THERAPY.

Walking the labyrinth is a procedure that occurs primarily in Central American countries and involves a slow meditative walk through a labyrinth (maze) laid out on the ground. The psychology of the labyrinth is that it gradually brings the individual inside himself or herself and into deeper and deeper levels until early traumas are brought into the individual's awareness.

Energy therapies are based on the belief that energy fields surround and penetrate the body and that they can be manipulated by movement, meditation, prayer, or by another person who places a hand over the body, without touching it. This form of therapy is also known as *bioenergetic therapy.*

Nutritional approaches involve the use of a broad array of vitamins, herbs, and other supplements and have been shown to balance moods and overcome anxieties.

Aromatherapy has been in use for more than 6,000 years, since the days of ancient Rome and Egypt and uses oils extracted from flowers, herbs, and plants to treat distress. The olfactory nerves send messages directly into the LIMBIC SYSTEM of the brain. Research has shown that different scents can affect different brainwave patterns. Aromatherapy is used for many disorders, including stress, anxiety, and pain.

Mind-body techniques incorporate both the mind and the body, and key examples include yoga, exercise, visualization, and deep breathing. Mind-body approaches have become commonplace and are often integrated into a comprehensive treatment approach for trauma survivors. Meditation, hypnosis, biofeedback, and acupuncture, along with massage therapy and chiropractic body-touch forms of manipulations, are used extensively today with trauma victims.

Other nontraditional therapies include the many alternatives to mainstream therapeutic approaches, such as cognitive behavioral therapy or EYE MOVEMENT DESENSITIZATION AND REPROCESSING (EMDR) to treat PTSD. EMDR has garnered the most research of any alternative treatment. By having the individual engage in or experience "bi-lateral" stimulation (therapist-guided eye movements back and forth on the horizontal plane, or the therapist tapping on the client's left- and right-side knees or hands, etc.) it is thought that both hemispheres of the brain are activated, and this state seems to facilitate problem solving and desensitization of traumatic memories. EMDR is based on an information-processing model in which new associations are formed between the traumatic memory and more adaptive views of the traumatic event.

Four therapies have been studied in the literature for their effectiveness in reducing posttraumatic symptoms. They are Thought Field Therapy (TFT), the Trauma Recovery Institute (TRI) method, TRAUMATIC INCIDENT REDUCTION (TIR), and VISUAL/ KINESTHETIC DISASSOCIATION (V/KD).

Thought Field Therapy was developed by psychologist Roger Callahan, Ph.D., in the early 1980s. It taps various energy areas of the body to relieve anxiety, depression, phobias, and psychological trauma. TFT is a mind/body treatment based on energy fields or acupuncture meridians. To date there are no controlled studies on TFT. The Trauma Recovery Institute (TRI) method was developed by Louis Tinnin in 1991. TRI uses several procedures such as hypnosis, narration, video-therapy, and voluntary dissociation to stabilize and resolve intrusive traumatic symptoms. Traumatic incident reduction (TIR) is a regressive desensitization procedure and was developed by Frank Gerbode. Visual/Kinesthetic Disassociation (V/KD) is a three-point displacement exposure approach imagining observing themselves watching themselves view their traumatic experiences. It is used by Richard Bandler and John Grinder and adapted from Eric Fromm. Another therapy being explored empirically as of this writing is TESTIMONY THERAPY, a form of psychotherapy in which the survivor tells his or her story of the traumatic life-shattering experiences to a psychiatrist who records it and makes it known to others so it is never forgotten. For example, the psychiatrist may read or tell of the account from the patient to the patient's family so they have a clear understanding of what happened to the patient and the patient's reaction to these events.

See also ART THERAPY; THERAPY, TYPES OF; TREATMENT: PSYCHOTHERAPY, PSYCHOPHARMACOLOGY, AND ALTERNATIVE MEDICINE.

amnesia A serious loss of MEMORY that is unrelated to the normal forgetting of information and that is not organically based. Organic diseases involve dysfunctions or physiological abnormality of bodily organs, such as the BRAIN, which are produced by external events (such as injury) or internal events (such as high fever or disease processes), as with Alzheimer's disease or other forms of dementia. Amnesia may result from a severe physical trauma, such as from a TRAUMATIC BRAIN INJURY. It may also be caused by extreme sustained psychological stress or an unusually stressful situation.

Symptoms and Diagnostic Path

Retrograde amnesia refers to the loss of memories of the past, while anterograde amnesia refers to amnesia that occurs after the precipitating event that led to the amnesia. Dissociative amnesia, formerly known as psychogenic amnesia, is a form of amnesia that occurs directly after the distressing event, and which includes a loss of personal identity. It is not, however, comparable to the repressed memories of individuals who have experienced CHILD PHYSICAL ABUSE or CHILD SEXUAL ABUSE. In general, dissociative amnesia resolves itself within several weeks. Other forms of amnesia may be more long lasting. Amnesia is diagnosed by first obtaining a detailed medical history, a physical examination including blood tests, and MRI if the brain has been damaged. Detailed interviews with the patient and family members are also necessary. For the diagnosis of dissociative amnesia there are several questionnaires such as the DISSOCIATIVE EXPERIENCES SCALE and the STRUCTURED CLINICAL INTERVIEW (SCID-D).

Treatment Options and Outlook

Amnesia is somewhat responsive to hypnosis and the use of sodium pentothal (truth serum). Some forms of amnesia remit spontaneously with time. Reconstructing stressful or traumatic situations and bringing the patient into them can also activate lost memories. However, no one method of treatment is guaranteed, and much depends on the personal strength of the patient and his or her motivation and willingness to remember.

Risk Factors and Preventive Measures

Often memory loss is a form of DISSOCIATION, and as the tendency to dissociate is treated, the memory may return. Amnesia can also be a function of drug states in which memory occurs only when the individual returns to the state that he or she was in when the events occurred. Memory loss is a by-product of dissociation, stress, and altered states, and as such is difficult to prevent because it is usually seen only after the fact.

See also FALSE MEMORY SYNDROME; POSTTRAUMATIC AMNESIA; THERAPY, TYPES OF.

amphetamine   A sympathetic nervous system stimulant drug that, if abused, can cause extreme anxiety and even psychosis, inducing a traumatic state. Some individuals begin abusing amphetamines when they are under severe stress, such as soldiers in combat situations. Note that amphetamine can be used legally if prescribed by a physician, such as for a patient with attention-deficit/hyperactivity disorder (ADHD).

Amphetamine psychosis, caused by the severe abuse of amphetamines, can be extremely difficult to distinguish from the symptoms of schizophrenia and is characterized by hallucinations, paranoia, picking at the skin, and sometimes by aggressive behavior. Amphetamine psychosis may persist for months or years, even when use of the drug is discontinued.

According to the World Health Organization in 2004, after marijuana (which was and still is the most abused substance in the world), the next most abused drug was amphetamine, which is used by 35 million people globally.

Common Side Effects of Amphetamines

Common side effects that may occur with the lawful use of amphetamine (and that may be amplified with the high dosages used by abusers) may include

- constipation
- insomnia
- headache
- dry mouth
- weight loss
- dizziness
- paranoia

Some individuals develop a dependence on methamphetamine, a form of amphetamine that can increase aggression and cause individuals to behave in ways that they would not normally act. Individuals may abuse methamphetamine to gain an illegal high; they may also abuse the drug to deal with stress or past traumatic events.

Methamphetamine is rarely legally used to treat ADHD, and most methamphetamine is produced illegally in clandestine laboratories and then sold illicitly. Methamphetamine has been associated with all forms of CHILD ABUSE as well as with sexual assaults and other violent acts. It can also cause rapid aging and an extreme and unhealthy weight loss. Abuse may also lead to seizures and hyperthermia (extremely high body temperature). It also heightens sexual arousal and the frequency of sex.

Federal laws in the United States limit the amount of specific precursor chemicals that are used to make methamphetamine, such as ephedrine and pseudoephedrine, which can be purchased by individuals. Such laws were created to attempt to limit the private production of illicit methamphetamine.

Withdrawal from Amphetamines

The withdrawal from amphetamine should occur in a treatment center that is experienced with amphetamine treatment. Withdrawal may take from six to 18 weeks. The withdrawal is usually quite severe and traumatizing to the individual with such symptoms as moderate to severe depression, anxiety, fear, irritability, exhaustion, and increased sleep as well as an intense craving for the drug.

See also ADDICTION; CHILD PHYSICAL ABUSE; CHILD SEXUAL ABUSE; TREATMENT: PSYCHOTHERAPY, PSYCHO-PHARMACOLOGY, AND ALTERNATIVE MEDICINE.

Department of Mental Health and Substance Abuse. *Global Status Report on Alcohol 2004.* Geneva: Switzerland: World Health Organization, 2004. Available online. URL: http://www.who.int/substance_abuse/publications/global_status_report_2004_overview.pdf. Downloaded July 31, 2006.

Gwinnell, Esther, M.D., and Christine Adamec. *The Encyclopedia of Drug Abuse.* New York: Facts On File, 2008.

Johnston, Lloyd D., et al. *Monitoring the Future: National Survey Results on Drug Use, 1975–2004. Volume II: College Students & Adults Ages 19–45.* Bethesda, Md.: National Institute on Drug Abuse, National Institutes of Health, 2005.

amygdala   At the tip of each temporal lobe in the BRAIN lies the almond-shaped amygdala, the Greek word for almond. As part of the LIMBIC SYSTEM, the amygdala is the center for basic emotions, primarily fear, aggression, and sexual responses and is connected to the frontal cortex for visual, auditory, and sensory inputs. The amygdala can signal the body to full alertness in times of perceived danger as it puts emotional meaning to incoming stimuli from the environment, such as the sound of an explosion. The amygdala is also involved in both conscious and subconscious emotional memory.

In a study of patients with POSTTRAUMATIC STRESS DISORDER (PTSD), experiences of their trauma were written in detailed narratives and then read back to the patients. This reading triggered flashbacks and marked autonomic responses. Positron emission tomography (PET) scans of the patients' brains showed heightened activity in the right hemisphere, the parts of the limbic system connected to the amygdala, and the amygdala itself. The amygdala appears to be at the center of the brain associated with traumatic emotional memory.

See also AUTONOMIC NERVOUS SYSTEM; CORPUS COLLUSCUM; HIPPOCAMPUS; LOCUS COERULUS; PHYSIOLOGY OF TRAUMA; SYMPATHETIC NERVOUS SYSTEM.

Rauch, S. L., B. A. van der Kolk, R. E. Fisher, N. M. Alpert, S. P. Orr, C. R. Savage, A. J. Fischman, M. A. Jenike, and R. K. Pitman. "A Symptom Provocation Study of Posttraumatic Stress Disorder Using Positron Emission Tomography and Script-driven Imagery." *Archives of General Psychiatry* 53, no. 5 (May 1996): 380–387.

anhedonia   The inability to take pleasure in activities that an individual formerly enjoyed or to take pleasure in any aspect of life. It is a state of emotional numbness. Anhedonia may be related to the development of DEPRESSION. It is also a common symptom of POSTTRAUMATIC STRESS DISORDER (PTSD). Anhedonia is a serious problem that requires therapy. The individual may also benefit from taking antidepressants. Successful processing of a traumatic experience frees individuals to enjoy life and to be more like themselves.

Anhedonia is distinguished from psychological NUMBING in that it is usually a lifelong condition with no real onset. In contrast, numbing is a symptom of severe trauma in which the body shuts down in order to cope with arousal and feelings. Numbing can also be seen as a form of depression or suppression, but it usually has an onset centered on traumatic experiences and is not a lifelong condition.

See also THERAPY, TYPES OF.

antianxiety medication Medications that are used to treat ANXIETY DISORDERS. Anxiety is usually manageable by the individual, but sometimes it can become serious, and medication is required in order for the individual to sustain functioning and perform daily activities. Both antidepressant and antianxiety medications are used and approved for managing anxiety reactions. Probably the most commonly used antianxiety drug is alcohol, which is frequently used as a form of self-medication, but the use of this drug can lead to alcoholism and the severely problematic effects of this disease.

The main antianxiety medications are BENZODI-AZEPINES, also known as minor tranquilizers. These medications relieve anxiety quickly, but they also have many short- and long-term side effects. The primary benzodiazepines used to treat anxiety disorders as of this writing are alprazolam (Xanax), diazepam (Valium), lorazepam (Ativan), and clonazepam (Klonopin).

Some non-benzodiazepines are also approved to treat anxiety, including buspirone (BuSpar) and propranolol (Inderal). Propranolol is a beta-blocker medication that is commonly used to treat high blood pressure (hypertension).

The benzodiazepines act quickly (usually within 20 minutes) to quiet anxiety, but often multiple daily doses are required, since the medication can wear off within three to five hours. Benzodiazepines are not toxic, and therefore in most cases a dose can be added to another dose without the risk of dangerous effects. However, sedation levels (drowsiness, fatigue, etc.) are easily achieved. In addition, these drugs interact with alcohol to produce multiplicative effects.

Benzodiazepines can cause side effects, such as dry mouth, fatigue, confusion, and nervousness. The continued use of benzodiazepines over time diminishes short-term memory. Furthermore, withdrawal from these drugs is often very difficult because there is a flood of overwhelming anxiety that occurs with the termination of the drug, and thus causes concern, fear, and added anxiety. Seizures are also possible. For these reasons, physicians carefully prescribe and monitor the use of benzodiazepines.

Antidepressants have broad-spectrum effects and often make the person feel better and thus provide an anxiety deterrent. The first antidepressant approved for anxiety use was clomipramine (Anafranil), a tricyclic antidepressant. Almost any dose of this drug seemed to help anxiety patients. Subsequently, the SELECTIVE SEROTONIN REUPTAKE INHIBITORS (SSRIs) were developed, and they have largely replaced the tricyclics as antidepressant agents for anxiety. The SSRIs include fluoxetine (Prozac), fluvoxamine (Luvox), and paroxetine (Paxil). The SSRIs generally are not as effective in reducing anxiety as are the benzodiazepines, but they have far fewer side effects and withdrawal is also easier. However, they are slow acting; their buildup time is weeks, and SSRIs effectively help only a small percentage of anxiety patients.

The general empirical and clinical consensus is that medication is most effective when it is combined with talk therapy and exposure work. The idea that medication calms the individual down and then he or she can build exposure experiences works for only a very small minority of clients. Generally, the stressors that activate and actuate the anxiety must be addressed and faced before the individual can make significant progress.

See also THERAPY, TYPES OF; TREATMENT: PSYCHO-THERAPY, PSYCHOPHARMACOLOGY, AND ALTERNATIVE MEDICINE.

anxiety disorders A group of diagnostic categories in which anxiety is the main component or symptom. The anxiety disorders are among the most prevalent psychological disorders, and they affect almost 19 million American adults. Most people with anxiety disorders live productive lives but at the cost of poor self-esteem, doubt, worry, avoidance, and struggles with overpowering arousal/anxiety in their lives.

There are six major types of anxiety disorders, including PANIC DISORDER, OBSESSIVE-COMPULSIVE DISORDER (OCD), POSTTRAUMATIC STRESS DISORDER (PTSD), SOCIAL ANXIETY DISORDER, SPECIFIC PHOBIAS, and GENERALIZED ANXIETY DISORDER (GAD). Each disorder is defined by a particular set of symptoms or problems of behavior. It is important to remember that clinical levels of these symptoms are at the extremes of frequency or intensity, and they involve some degree of limitation or restriction of behavior.

Panic Disorder

Panic disorder affects about 2.4 million adults in the United States and is characterized by panic attacks. Panic attacks are usually described as a sudden terror response with exaggerated heartbeat, difficulty breathing, dizziness, disorientation and DISSOCIATION, weakness and feelings of helplessness, and tingling. The individual may have a fear of losing control and/or of having a heart attack, a brain stroke, "going crazy," or dying. The individual usually wants to run or escape to a safe place during these attacks. One panic attack by itself does not constitute a diagnosis of panic disorder. Several panic attacks within a brief period of time (usually two weeks) are necessary before a diagnosis of panic disorder is offered. Medications such as BENZODIAZEPINES may help as may cognitive-behavioral therapy and exposure therapy.

Women are about twice as likely to suffer from panic disorder as males. There is an inherited tendency toward panic disorder, and if a first-degree relative has panic disorder, others in the family have an eight times greater risk of developing it. Patients with some syndromes, such as irritable bowel syndrome, interstitial cystitis, and chronic fatigue syndrome, have higher rates of panic disorder than others. There are no known preventive measures for panic disorder.

Obsessive-Compulsive Disorder (OCD)

Patients with obsessive-compulsive disorder (OCD) experience persistent worried thoughts, anxiety, and often develop rituals to undo or diminish this anxiety. *Obsessions* may revolve around contamination, sexual ideas, religious preoccupations, medical worries or diseases, or thoughts of harming oneself or others. These thoughts or images are persistent, worrisome, and unwelcome. *Compulsions* are rituals patients feel compelled to act out in order to reduce or eliminate their anxiety. A combination of medication, response prevention, and exposure therapy can be used to treat OCD. The disorder may begin in childhood and occurs at similar rates in men and women.

Posttraumatic Stress Disorder (PTSD)

Posttraumatic stress disorder (PTSD) is a major life-altering disorder that occurs after a person has experienced a traumatic event. PTSD is a debilitating condition that affects an estimated 5.2 million adults in the United States, most of them women. It develops in some people after a terrifying event but can even fully develop years afterward.

The core symptoms of PTSD are intrusive thoughts, avoidance, and hyperarousal. The most well known intrusions are FLASHBACKS, making the survivor relive the traumatic experience, placing him or her back in the past. DEPRESSION and anxiety are common side effects of the debilitation caused by the symptoms of PTSD. Unfortunately, depression and anxiety responses can disguise the underlying traumatic roots to these reactions.

PTSD was thought to be untreatable until therapists began to focus on treatment using bodily responses, exposure, and modifying catastrophic cognitions. These therapies seem to speed recovery and restoration. Medications are also used, but seem to work best when combined with active behavioral therapy.

NATURAL DISASTERS, such as earthquakes, tornados, or hurricanes, usually result in an overall increase in PTSD, but human-against-human incidents (rape, assault, physical and sexual abuse, terrorism, medical procedures, robberies, kidnappings, and so on) seem to produce the most long lasting and the highest incidence of PTSD symptoms. Even nondirect or vicarious exposure to these events can lead to PTSD in some people. Reminders and anniversaries can trigger relapses and flashbacks.

Social Anxiety Disorder

This disorder involves a fear or phobia of general situations, such as being in a crowd, or specific situations, such as urinating in public restrooms, signing one's name in public, or public speaking. It is also called social phobia,

People with social anxiety disorder usually experience persistent and intense fear of being observed and judged by others or feeling embarrassed or humiliated. The most common form of social anxiety is fear of public speaking In its general form, social anxiety disorder can involve anxiety about almost any situation.

Antidepressant medications may be used to treat social anxiety disorder, but recent understanding of the disorder indicates that treatment must also address gaps in the patient's social skills. Individuals with social phobias often have difficulty starting conversations, communicating their needs, or meeting the needs of others, so these skills must be taught. A combination of medication and cognitive-behavioral skill building are often effective.

Social phobias of a narrow or generalized nature usually begin in late childhood or adolescence and continue into adulthood and may be preceded by shyness early in life.

Specific Phobias

Many people have *aversions* to particular things, such as snakes or insects, but when such an aversion interferes with one's life, it becomes a *phobia*. Specific phobias involve an intense fear to a particular triggering stimuli. Common stimuli are heights, edges, deep water, highway driving, closed spaces, flying, small animals, snakes, and blood.

Many fears that people share are prepared, or genetically transmitted, tendencies of certain stimuli to evoke fear responses in humans. They are survival mechanisms that may explain why almost 90 percent of people who fear snakes have never actually seen a snake.

The most effective treatment for phobias are exposure-based desensitization approaches, which involve both the gradual exposure (approach) to the feared stimulus while working with triggering cognitions. Flooding, or extreme exposure at a full intensity, has also been used, but it is a distressing form of treatment, and its effect does not seem to last for long.

Generalized Anxiety Disorder (GAD)

Patients suffering from generalized anxiety disorder (GAD) live in a chronic state of varying degrees of anxiety, seemingly without specific triggers. However, empirical studies have shown that GAD sufferers are chronic and exaggerated worriers, which causes them high degrees of tension and anticipation. About 6.8 million American adults have GAD on a lifetime basis, or 2.2 percent of the general population.

People with GAD cannot seem to eliminate or diminish their worries and, consequently, they experience the side effects fatigue, muscle tension, headaches, irritability, sweating, and trembling. They tend to hyperventilate, feel light-headed, out of breath, and nauseated, and they may urinate frequently. They find it difficult to relax, have trouble concentrating, and may experience sleep difficulties. Unlike people with the other anxiety disorders, people with GAD usually do not avoid situations that cause anxiety unless the disorder is severe.

Medications such as antianxiety drugs (benzodiazepines) and antidepressants such as selective serotonin reuptake inhibitors (SSRIs) are often used by individuals with GAD. The disorder tends to run in families, but it is more of a learned than genetic behavior. It is commonly comorbid with depression, other anxiety disorders, and substance abuse.

Treatment of Anxiety Disorders

The AMYGDALA is a key BRAIN structure in anxiety disorder. The amygdala is a limbic or midbrain structure that serves as a communications hub among different parts of the brain. Along with the adjacent HIPPOCAMPUS, the amygdala interprets incoming sensory signals, and it can trigger fear responses to threatening emotional memories that are stored in these areas of the brain. The hippocampus plays a key role in helping to encode information into memories.

Studies of combat veterans and abused children have discovered reductions in the size of their hippocampus, suggesting a greater reactivity to less-threatening stimuli in these groups. This also has implications for PTSD, in which flashbacks and deficits in MEMORY are also features of the disorder.

Treatment of anxiety disorders has been highly successful. Medications are frequently used to treat the various anxiety disorders, and certain drugs are favored for different anxiety disorders. For example, medications in the selective serotonin reuptake inhibitors (SRRIs) class are commonly prescribed for panic disorder, OCD, PTSD and social phobia. However, many people have difficulty taking or staying on SSRIs due to their side effects.

Benzodiazepines are another category of medications given to treat anxiety disorders. They are generally given for short periods of time because they have an immediate anxiety-reducing effect. A drug tolerance often develops with benzodiazepines, requiring greater doses over time, and withdrawal from these medications can be long and very difficult with prolonged and intense usage. The benzodiazepines are frequently used to treat social anxiety disorder, GAD, and panic disorder.

COGNITIVE BEHAVIORAL THERAPY (CBT) has proven to be the most effective form of treatment (particularly when combined with medications) for anxiety disorders. The *cognitive* component is aimed at changing the thinking that produces anxiety and fear. For example, people with panic disorder usually misinterpret their body sensations by assuming that they are having heart attacks or undergoing disabling and catastrophic physical events, rather than experiencing a state of temporary anxiety.

Individuals who suffer from social phobia also can benefit from more rational and reasonable beliefs, moving away from thinking that they are being watched and judged. The *behavioral* component of CBT usually involves some form of gradual exposure to the feared situation or object while the therapist encourages more rational, adaptive, and less fear-provoking thinking. Those with social phobia need to use what they have learned in therapy in real-life social situations.

Behavior therapy or exposure therapy carefully introduces tolerable degrees of the critical anxiety-evoking stimuli, starting with the lowest levels of arousal and gradually exposing the individual to more intense levels as desensitization occurs to less intense exposure elements. Relaxation training and exercise combined with exposure has been very successful in reducing anxiety and improving functioning. In addition, relaxation training and exercise seem to be necessary activities in any treatment approach for anxiety.

Cognitive support may or may not be necessary. People afraid of heights might start their exposure at only one or two feet off the ground and gradually proceed to higher heights, as calmness is connected with distance from the ground. Cognitive work may also be introduced to change irrational anxiety-producing thoughts in the situation. These therapies are highly individualized to the sufferer's reactions and cognitions. Overall, behavioral and cognitive behavior therapies for anxiety can help an estimated 75 to 90 percent of sufferers live less restricted lives with less anxiety and greater freedom and productivity.

See also ANTIANXIETY MEDICATION; ANXIETY DISORDERS SCHEDULE; ANXIETY MANAGEMENT TRAINING; ASSOCIATED DISORDERS; THERAPY, TYPES OF; TREATMENT: PSYCHOTHERAPY, PSYCHOPHARMACOLOGY, AND ALTERNATIVE MEDICINE.

Doctor, Ronald M., Ada P. Kahn, and Christine Adamec. *The Encyclopedia of Phobias, Fears, and Anxieties.* 3rd ed. New York: Facts On File, 2008.

Anxiety Disorders Schedule   The purpose of this schedule or interview is to reach a differential diagnosis among the various ANXIETY DISORDERS described in the *Diagnostic and Statistical Manual* of the American Psychiatric Association. It is also called the Anxiety Disorders Interview Schedule or ADIS-IV. The interview schedule is structured with a specific flow of questions and branch or side questions on topics. It is usually administered by a professional psychologist or diagnostician trained in its administration and purpose. Hospitals, clinics, and research programs are the most common users of the Anxiety Disorders Schedule.

Along with an adult version, there is also a child interview schedule and a parent interview schedule for use in diagnosing anxiety disorders in children. The child version includes sections on mood and externalization disorders to permit a fuller differential diagnosis assessment, particularly around issues of comorbidity (one or more additional psychiatric problems). The child and parent versions are also sensitive to the age of the child.

The Anxiety Disorders Schedule is also structured to assist in treatment planning for the child's problem. There are screening sections to assess possible external factors, such as SUBSTANCE ABUSE, psychosis, and eating and learning disorders. The school refusal section is comprehensive and attempts to assess components that are associated with this serious problem. The two developers of the child and parent versions are Wendy Silverman, Ph.D. and Anne Marie Albano, Ph.D. two psychologists.

See also ASSESSMENT AND DIAGNOSIS; INSTRUMENTS/SURVEYS THAT EVALUATE POSTTRAUMATIC STRESS DISORDER (PTSD).

Anxiety Management Training (AMT) A program that combines relaxation therapy with cognitive awareness. AMT is meant to provide control over anxiety within about eight sessions by enabling patients to decrease their levels of arousal and also become aware of the onset of signs of stress in themselves. The program was first developed by psychologist Richard M. Suinn in 1990.

Since its inception, AMT has compared more favorably to other behavioral treatments, such as SYSTEMATIC DESENSITIZATION, COGNITIVE BEHAVIORAL THERAPY, psychoanalytic therapies, and so forth, and AMT also seems to maintain long-term improvements.

See also ANXIETY DISORDERS; THERAPY, TYPES OF; TREATMENT: PSYCHOTHERAPY, PSYCHOPHARMACOLOGY, AND ALTERNATIVE MEDICINE.

approach-avoidance conflict A term that describes the conflict in which the further an individual is from making a choice, the more attractive the choice appears; however, the nearer to when the choice must be made, the less attractive it appears. The concept of the approach-avoidance conflict was originally developed in the 1950s by the learning theorist Neil Miller. An example of an approach-avoidance conflict is the decision to get married or to have a child. In the abstract, future marriage or having a family may appear an attractive choice; however, when the individual believes the decision must be made soon, it may cause great

anxiety and even trauma. This is also true in the case of an unexpected pregnancy. The individual may have wished to have children in the future but feel unready and unprepared should an unplanned pregnancy occur.

It can be extremely difficult for individuals to resolve such conflicts, and some individuals do not make such a choice and let time take its course. If the decision is whether to get married and no plans are made, then the marriage will not occur. In the case of a pregnancy, if the choice is to continue or terminate the pregnancy and no action is taken, the pregnancy will be continued.

art therapy The use of drawing, painting, modeling of clay, and other expressive methods in an attempt to help traumatized children or adults "talk" about themselves and express their experiences in a nonverbal manner. Sometimes emotions that cannot be orally articulated can be expressed more adequately as well as more creatively through art therapy.

In a study of 41 college students published in 2004 in *Art Therapy: Journal of the American Art Therapy Association*, the researchers analyzed whether the students responded more positively to writing about their stressful experiences or by using art therapy to express themselves.

The researchers found that art therapy was significantly more enjoyable for the participants and that they were also more likely to continue with therapy than were those engaged in writing therapy. Said the researchers:

> Participants who engaged in writing therapy found it less enjoyable, were less likely to continue with therapy, were less likely to recommend treatment to a friend or family member, felt more stressed, and were less likely to share the experience with other than were participants [in art therapy].

As the researchers pointed out, writing therapy has little value if participants discontinue treatment after one session.

Some authors have provided specific examples of how individuals have used art therapy for their self-healing. For example, according to another article in *Art Therapy*, published in 2005, an abused child known as Tammy entered the foster care system at age four. She had been severely abused and neglected. Over the next three years, she was placed in three foster homes, one residential treatment center, and four day-care centers, and Tammy had four different caseworkers. Tammy was unable to talk about the abuse she suffered at the hands of her biological mother. Tammy was moved to a preadoptive home, but she struggled with this relationship.

One day Tammy announced that she wanted to make a "sister" (although she had neither a biological or preadoptive sister), and she proceeded to create a life-size doll. According to the author, Tammy used her doll "Tina" to assume those roles that she was not yet comfortable with and that she feared would betray her biological mother. Thus, Tammy had the doll Tina "sleep" with the foster parents. Tina, the doll, also "watched" the foster mother cook dinner and work on the computer. Through Tammy, Tina was able to tell the foster mother that she loved her. According to the author:

> Tammy could not betray her own mother by showing love to her foster parents even though she loved them. She was able to work toward some resolution of this dilemma through her art making. She had created a self who could be affectionate without betraying, a self who could express feelings that were too difficult for her to consciously acknowledge, a self who could say and do the things that she could not. Tammy was able to practice with Tina, try on a different role, and see what it felt like to be a full member of a family.
>
> Tammy was later adopted and was doing well with her family.

See also ALTERNATIVE TREATMENTS; CHILD ABUSE AND NEGLECT; CHILD SEXUAL ABUSE; THERAPY, TYPES OF.

Klorer, P. Gussie, "Expressive Therapy with Severely Maltreated Children: Neuroscience Contributions." *Art Therapy: Journal of the American Art Therapy Association* 22, no. 4 (2005): 213–220.

Pizarro, Judith, "The Efficacy of Art and Writing Therapy: Increasing Positive Mental Health Outcomes and Participant Retention After Exposure to Traumatic Experience." *Art Therapy: Journal of the American Art Therapy Association* 21, no. 1 (2004): 5–12.

assessment and diagnosis There are a broad array of instruments designed to help mental health professionals with the diagnosis of traumatic stress disorders as well as with diagnosing various psychiatric problems that often accompany traumatic experiences. An instrument is a written tool used to help assess whether a condition exists and/or to measure the severity of the condition. The key diagnostic classification manual used by mental health professionals to diagnose ACUTE STRESS DISORDER (ASD) or POSTTRAUMATIC STRESS DISORDER (PTSD) (as well as many other disorders) is the *DIAGNOSTIC AND STATISTICAL MANUAL OF MENTAL DISORDERS-*4TH EDITION, TEXT REVISION (*DSM-IV-TR*), most recently published by the American Psychiatric Association in 2000. It provides specific examples of symptoms and criteria that are common to individuals with many different disorders.

There are many assessment instruments that are useful to mental health professionals; for example, the Harvard Trauma Questionnaire helps with the measure of posttraumatic stress (PTS). Other helpful instruments include the TRAUMA AND ATTACHMENT BELIEF SCALES, the Trauma Symptom Inventory, the Trauma Symptom Checklist/Trauma Symptom Checklist for Children, the TRAUMATIC STRESS SCHEDULE, the Trauma-Related Guilt Inventory, and the TRAUMATIC MEMORY INVENTORY (TMI).

There are also some tests that are meant specifically for individuals with posttraumatic stress disorder (PTSD), such as the Davidson Trauma Scale, the Clinician-Administered PTSD Scale (CAPS), the PTSD Checklist, and the Posttraumatic Stress Diagnostic Scale (PSDS). In addition, the STROOP TEST has been shown to be predictive for individuals with PTSD. Other tests that measure issues associated with trauma are the Brief Betrayal Trauma Survey, the DISSOCIATIVE EXPERIENCES SCALE, and the SOMATOFORM DISSOCIATION QUESTIONNAIRE.

Some instruments measure the overall impact of events on an individual, such as the Impact of Event Scale and the Impact of Event Scale-Revised, as well as the LIFE EVENTS CHECKLIST and the GLOBAL ASSESSMENT OF FUNCTIONING. Other instruments, such as the ROSENBERG SELF-ESTEEM SCALE, the SOCIAL ADJUSTMENT SCALE, and the COPE INVENTORY/BRIEF COPE INVENTORY, provide very helpful supplementary information to mental health professionals about traumatized individuals.

In the case of individuals who may be suffering from secondary traumatization, also called COMPASSION FATIGUE, mental health professionals may decide to avail themselves of the COMPASSION SATISFACTION AND FATIGUE TEST or the PROFESSIONAL QUALITY OF LIFE SCALE.

Trauma Instruments

There are many different trauma instruments based on the need of the traumatized individual; for example, sometimes a rapid assessment is needed, while other times an instrument may need to be adapted into other languages to treat people from other countries. Some tests measure childhood trauma, while others assess specific types of trauma or reactions to trauma such as guilt.

The Harvard Trauma Questionnaire is an interview checklist to assess a variety of trauma events cross-culturally. Developed by the Harvard Program in Refugee Trauma, the Harvard Trauma Questionnaire was first used with Indochinese refugees speaking three different languages: Laotian, Cambodian, and Vietnamese. Later versions added a checklist in Japanese after the 1995 Kobe earthquake, as well as a Croatian veteran's version and a Bosnian version for civilian survivors of the various wars fought in the Balkans in the 1990s.

The Trauma and Attachment Belief Scale (TABS) is a brief self-report and easily understood tool that is used by clinicians to assess the needs and expectations of trauma survivors in 15 minutes, based on their self-assumptions in relation to others. The therapist uses this information to help plan a treatment goal for the client. The TABS has 10 subscales measuring each psychological need area in relation to the self and others, such as self-trust and others-trust (trust of others). TABS items focus on the individual's relationship history and is useful even if the client does not meet the full diagnostic criteria for posttraumatic stress disorder (PTSD).

The Trauma Symptom Inventory (TSI) is a 100-item test used to evaluate acute and chronic symptoms of the psychological effects of rape, spousal abuse, childhood trauma and abuse, combat and war experiences, and natural disasters. It has 10 clinical subscales to assess the broad symptoms related to posttraumatic stress disorder and ACUTE STRESS DISORDER and additional intra- and interpersonal difficulties associated with chronic psychological trauma that has occurred over a six-month period.

The Trauma Symptom Checklist/Trauma Symptom Checklist for Children/Traumatic Stress Schedule are administered to determine the presence of traumatic reactions in adults who experienced trauma in childhood or adulthood. The Trauma Symptom Checklist-40 (TSC-40) was developed by John Briere and Marsha Runtz as a research instrument to evaluate symptoms in adults with childhood or adult traumatic experiences. The TSC-40 is a 40-item self-report instrument with six subscales: anxiety, DEPRESSION, DISSOCIATION, sexual abuse trauma index (SATI), sexual problems, and sleep disturbance. The TSC-40 should not be used to validate a psychological diagnosis of posttraumatic stress disorder (PTSD) since it does not measure all the 17 criteria of PTSD. The TSC-40 requires only 10 to 15 minutes to complete and five to 10 minutes to score.

The Trauma Symptom Checklist for Children (TSCC) is a self-report instrument measuring posttraumatic stress and related psychological symptoms in children ages eight to 16 years old who experienced TRAUMATIC EVENTS such as physical abuse, sexual abuse, witnessing a violent act, or natural disasters. The 54-item measure can be given individually or in a group in 15 to 20 minutes. The TSCC was developed by John Briere and is standardized on a large sample of diverse children in urban and suburban environments.

The Traumatic Stress Schedule (TSS) is a short instrument for measuring the occurrence and impact of traumatic events, and it can be administered by a lay interviewer. The event categories of traumatic events assessed by the TSS are: robbery, physical assault, sexual assault, the tragic death of a friend or family member, a motor vehicle accident, military combat, loss through fire, natural disaster, or hazard or danger. There is also a category for other unspecified traumatic events.

Another instrument, the Trauma-Related Guilt Inventory (TGRI), assesses the individual's feeling of guilt related to specific traumatic events, such as in the cases of combat or physical and sexual abuse. Since the TRGI assesses 22 specific trauma-related beliefs, it may also be useful for the mental health professional to use as a treatment outcome measure in cognitive-behavioral interventions that are used to modify guilt/survivor beliefs about the patient's roles in trauma. (Many individuals feel guilty about what they could have done or should have done during a traumatic event, even when it is clear to others that they could not have done more than they actually did.)

The Traumatic Memory Inventory (TMI) was developed to investigate the nature of traumatic and nontraumatic memories in detail. The Traumatic Memory Inventory (TMI) attempts to capture the complexities of how traumatic memories are retrieved by people experiencing a traumatic event, and discover how this event differs from nontraumatic, yet highly emotional events. The TMI is a 60-item structured interview that collects data to assess the characteristics of traumatic memories, beginning with the nature and the duration of trauma, as well as whether subjects had always remembered the trauma and under what circumstances subjects first experienced intrusive memories.

Posttraumatic Stress Disorder Instruments

There are many instruments designed to help mental health professionals determine the presence and the severity of PTSD, as well as to help in treating specific aspects of PTSD.

The Davidson Trauma Scale (DTS) is a 17-item self-report instrument that is used to measure the presence, frequency, and severity of symptoms that are characteristic of individuals who develop PTSD. The DTS measures categories of symptoms associated with PTSD, including intrusive reexperiencing of the trauma, the avoidance of people or places that remind individuals of the traumatic experience, and the symptoms of NUMBING and hyper-arousal. The DTS is useful to make a preliminary determination as to whether the symptoms may meet the *Diagnostic and Statistical Manual-IV* criteria for PTSD.

Another structured clinical interview is the Clinician-Administered PTSD Scale (CAPS), a scale designed for the use of trained and experienced clinicians. The CAPS assesses all 17 possible symp-toms of PTSD, along with the social and occupational functioning of the traumatized individual. It has separate ratings for the frequency and intensity of each symptom. There are several different versions of the CAPS.

The Posttraumatic Stress Diagnostic Scale (PSDS) is a 49-item self-report instrument developed by Edna Foa to assist in the diagnosis of posttraumatic stress disorder (PTSD). The PSDS can be used to screen for PTSD in large groups and gauge the symptom severity and functioning of individuals already identified with PTSD features. The PSDS asks respondents to checkmark any traumatic event they have witnessed or experienced, and they are asked to briefly describe the event. The PSDS can be used as a paper and pencil test or can be taken online in 10 to 15 minutes.

The Stroop Test was developed from the results of a doctoral dissertation published in 1935 by John Riley Stroop. In his study, Stroop presented subjects with words printed in different colors. Since words are read more quickly and automatically than naming colors, it was easier to read words than colors printed in words. For example, if the word *blue* is printed in the color green, then the word *blue* is said more readily than the naming of the color in which it is displayed, in this case green. In the test itself, subjects are asked to name the colors of the printed word and not the word itself. This sounds easy, but it is actually a difficult task. This test has been used in batteries of tests with posttraumatic stress disorder syndrome (PTSD) patients and seems to have some predictive and diagnostic value.

Instruments Measuring Issues Associated with Trauma

The Brief Betrayal Trauma Survey (BBTS), developed by Jennifer Freyd in 1996, assesses the subject's exposure to both traumas high in betrayal (for example, abuse by a caregiver, such as a parent) and traumas low in betrayal but high in life-threat (such as a natural disaster). The results are based on self-reported experiences, all retrospective in nature, and it is assumed that the client is truthful in his or her responses.

The Dissociative Experiences Scale is a psychological screening test developed by Eve Bernstein

Carlson and Frank W. Putnam, M.D. It comprises 28 questions given to individuals who may have dissociative identity disorder (formerly known as multiple personality disorder). The individual responds to each question on a continuum of percentages, from 0 percent to 100 percent. For example, one question in the scale is "Some people have the experience of looking in a mirror and not recognizing themselves. Circle a number to show what percentage of time this happens to you." Another item the individual is asked to respond to is "Some people sometimes have the experience of feeling that their body does not belong to them."

Another instrument, the Somatoform Dissociation Questionnaire, is a 20-item screening device for dissociative processes. The theory behind the SDQ assumes that there is a failure of integrative process such that two or more different parts of the individual emerge in the experience. For example, an abused child may appear normal at school and emotional and frightened at home. Pain, inhibitions of movement, lack of body feelings (all of which can be seen in somatoform disorders) may be part of the child's traumatic memories and experiences. The SDQ includes many negative and some positive dissociative symptoms.

Instruments Measuring Impact of Events on Life

Some instruments measure the impact of traumatic events on an individual's life. The Impact of Event Scale (IES) was originally developed by Mardi Horowitz, Nancy Wilner, and William Alvarez in the 1970s in order to assess psychological stress reactions after major life events, such as bereavement, rape, war, and motor vehicle accidents. The Impact of Event Scale is the most widely used self-report questionnaire to assess the frequency of intrusive and avoidant phenomena after a variety of traumatic experiences.

Intrusions include intrusive thoughts, nightmares, intrusive feelings, and visual imagery of the traumatic event. Avoidance behaviors try to block out intrusive images. Examples of avoidance are numbing of responsiveness, loss of interest, and avoidance of situations or locations of the traumatic event. Although maladaptive, these responses are coping strategies.

The IES contains 15 items that are added into two subscales: IES intrusion (seven items) and IES avoidance (eight items). In a self-report format, the subject is asked to report in the past seven days the frequency of symptoms on a four-point measurement scale, with zero indicating not at all, one indicating rarely, three indicating sometimes, and five indicating often. The IES is a short and easily administered questionnaire that is also easily scored. It can be used repeatedly with the subjects to gauge progress. The IES has been translated into several languages, including Arabic, Hebrew, Dutch, German, Swedish, and Croatian.

The Impact of Event Scale, Revised is a self-report scale developed by Daniel S. Weiss and Charles Marmar in 1997 to help evaluate an individual's current distress over a severe life event and address hyperarousal symptoms, the third major symptom cluster of posttraumatic stress disorder (PTSD), with seven additional questions not addressed in IES. The IES-R has been translated into several languages, including Spanish, Japanese, and Chinese, and is one of the most widely used instruments to assess PTSD, partly because of its reliability, construct validity, and ease of administration.

There are 22 items in the Impact of Event Scale, Revised (IES-R). Individuals rate items on the scale based on events in the past seven days from zero (not at all) through four (extremely). An earlier Impact of Event Scale was developed in the 1970s by Horowitz and colleagues to evaluate bereaved individuals, and it was later used to assess the psychological response to many traumas. Two examples of items that individuals respond to and rate on the Impact of Event Scale, Revised, include the following: "My feelings about it were kind of numb" and "Reminders of it caused me to have physical reactions, such as sweating, trouble breathing, nausea, or a pounding heart."

Another test, the Global Assessment of Functioning (GAF), is a 100-point scale that measures psychological, social, and occupational functioning on a hypothetical continuum of mental health/illness. Each 10-point range had two components: symptom severity and functioning ability. For example, a GAF score from 61 to 70 indicates mild symptoms (such as depressed mood and mild INSOMNIA) or some difficulty in social, occupational, or school functioning. But generally, individuals with this score function well and have meaningful interpersonal relationships.

Other Important Instruments

The Rosenberg Self-Esteem Scale was developed by Morris Rosenberg in 1965 and is now in the public domain. It has been translated into French and Norwegian for use as an educational and research tool. The scale is a global unidimensional measure of self-esteem that was originally developed for use with adolescents. It measures overall feelings of self-worth and self-acceptance. Answers are given on a four-point intensity scale that can also be administered through an interview. Scores range from 0 to 30 with higher scores indicating higher self-esteem.

The Social Adjustment Scale is a self-report form used to assess a two-week period on a broad range of social functioning. It is also available in an interview version. There are 42 questions rated on a scale from one to five (a higher number signifies greater impairment). There are six subscales, and each subscale falls into four major categories: the respondent's performance at expected tasks, the amount of friction with other people, interpersonal behavior, and feelings and satisfaction. The six subscales are:

1. Work-impaired performance
2. Social and leisure activities—decreased activities with friends, relationships
3. Relationships with extended family—parents, in-laws, siblings, adult children
4. Marital role as a spouse—sexual problems, impaired communications
5. Role as a parent—lack of involvement with or attention to children
6. Role as a member of the family—economic inadequacies, resentment, guilt

The SAS has been used with a variety of populations of patients with depression to traumatic brain injury.

The COPE Inventory, a 60-item instrument, helps to measure the individual's current style of coping, including effective and ineffective means. It was first developed by Charles S. Carver, Michael F. Scheier, and Jagdish Kumari Weintraub in 1989. A significantly shorter version, the Brief COPE, was later developed by the researchers based on adults who were recovering from Hurricane Andrew.

The COPE Inventory allows an evaluation of 15 factors that reveal a person's active or avoidant coping behavior. These factors include:

- active coping (actively taking steps to remove the stressor or mitigate its effects)
- planning (considering means and strategies to deal with a stressor)
- seeking instrumental social support (seeking advice or information)
- seeking emotional social support (seeking understanding, sympathy, or moral support)
- suppression of competing activities (to enable the individual to concentrate on managing the stressor)
- religion (using spiritual means to cope with stressors)
- positive reinterpretation and growth
- restraint coping (waiting for an opportunity to take action and avoiding acting prematurely)
- resignation/acceptance
- focus on and venting of emotions
- denial (a coping method that may be helpful at some times, such as in the initial stages of a traumatic event, but which is ultimately not helpful)
- mental disengagement (a negative means of coping in which the person is distracted from acting to reduce the stressor, such as by daydreaming, watching many hours of television, and so forth)
- behavioral disengagement (a negative means of coping in which the individual behaves in a helpless manner)
- alcohol/drug use
- humor

The questionnaire asks responders what they generally do and feel when confronted with a stressful event, maintaining that people respond differently to different events and that there are no "right" or "wrong" answers.

The Brief COPE is an abbreviated version of the COPE Inventory to minimize time demands on participants and the redundancy in the original version. The Brief COPE has only two items per scale and eliminates two scales from the original COPE. It also adds a self-blame scale. The Brief COPE scales include:

1. Active coping
2. Planning
3. Positive reframing
4. Acceptance
5. Humor
6. Religion
7. Using emotional support
8. Using instrumental support
9. Self-distraction
10. Denial
11. Venting
12. Substance use
13. Behavioral disengagement
14. Self-blame

Secondary Traumatization

Many individuals who assist traumatized people, such as medical and emergency professionals, as well as mental health professionals, may become traumatized as they empathize with the extreme suffering of the traumatized individuals they assist. There are several instruments that measure secondary traumatization (also known as compassion fatigue).

The Compassion Satisfaction and Fatigue Test is a self-test devised by Beth Hudnall Stamm and Charles R. Figley in the 1990s to help individuals assess their level of compassion satisfaction or compassion fatigue. The Compassion Satisfaction and Fatigue Test has respondents answer questions about themselves by self-rating on a five-point intensity scale.

The items include such statements to respond to with the appropriate number for their situation as "I force myself to avoid certain thoughts or feelings that remind me of a frightening experience," and "While working with the victim, I thought about violence against the perpetrator."

The Professional Quality of Life Scale (ProQol) is a self-test devised by Beth Hudnall Stamm that allows users to measure their own levels of compassion satisfaction, burnout, and trauma/compassion fatigue. It is the most widely used measure of secondary traumatization.

Individuals using this scale respond with numbers ranging from zero (Never) to five (Very Often) to such statements as "I am preoccupied with more than one person I help," and "I am losing sleep over traumatic experiences of a person I help." Responses are based on how the individual has felt over the past 30 days.

Baumert, J., H. Simon, H. Gundel, G. Schmitt, and K. H. Ladwig. "The Impact of Event Scale-Revised: Evaluation of the Subscales and Correlations to Psychophysiological Startle Response Patterns in Survivors of a Life-Threatening Cardiac Event: An Analysis of 129 Patients with an Implanted Cardioverter Defibrillator." *Journal of Affective Disorder* 82, no. 1 (October 1, 2004): 29–41.

Blake, Dudley David, et al. "A Clinician Rating Scale for Assessing Current and Lifetime PTSD: The CAPS-1." *The Behavior Therapist* 13 (September 1990): 187–188.

Briere, J., *Trauma Symptoms Inventory Professional Manual.* Odessa, Fla: Psychological Assessment Resources, 1995.

Briere, J., et al. "The Trauma Symptom Checklist for Young Children (TSCYC): Reliability and Association with Abuse Exposure in a Multi-Site Study." *Child Abuse & Neglect* 25, no 8 (2001): 1,001–1,014.

Elhai, J. D., M. G. Gray, T. B. Dashdan, and C. L. Franklin. "Which Instruments Are Most Commonly Used to Assess Traumatic Event Exposure and Posttraumatic Effects?: A Survey of Traumatic Stress Professionals." *Journal of Traumatic Stress* 18, 5 (October 2005): 541–545.

Kubany, Edward S., et al. "Development and Validation of the Trauma-Related Guilt Inventory (TRGI)." *Psychological Assessment* 84, no. 4 (1996): 428–444.

Newman, E., D. Kaloupek, and T. Keane. "Assessment of Posttraumatic Stress Disorder in Clinical and Research Settings." In *Traumatic Stress,* edited by B. van der Kolk, A. McFarlane and L. Weisaeth. New York: Guilford Press, 1996.

Renner, W. I. Salem and K. Ottomeyer. "Cross-Cultural Validation of Measures of Traumatic Symptoms in Groups of Asylum Seekers from Chechnya, Afghanistan, and West Africa." *Social Behavior and Personality* 34, no. 9 (2006): 1,101–1,114.

Sundin, Eva C. and Mardi J. Horowitz. "Impact of Event Scale: Psychometric Properties." *British Journal of Psychiatry* 180 (2002): 205–209.

Weathers, Frank W., Terence M. Keane, and Jonathan R. T. Davidson, M.D. "Clinician-Administered PTSD Scale: A Review of the First Ten Years of Research." *Depression and Anxiety* 13 (2001): 132–156.

associated disorders Psychological and emotional reactions, problems, and diagnoses that may occur among people who are suffering from TRAUMATIC STRESS disorders and which disorders have developed as a direct result of a TRAUMATIC EVENT. In addition, if the individual previously experienced a problem with a psychiatric disorder such as DEPRESSION or an ANXIETY DISORDER, the disorder may become greatly exacerbated by the traumatic event. Associated disorders may prevent people from seeking treatment for a traumatic stress disorder, especially if the individual feels helpless or hopeless as a result of the associated disorder, combined with the trauma stemming from the event itself.

Disorders that may develop in response to the event include associated disorders such as AFFECTIVE DISORDERS, anxiety disorders (particularly POSTTRAUMATIC STRESS DISORDER), SUBSTANCE ABUSE or ADDICTION, attachment disorders, (see ATTACHMENT STYLES/DISORDERS), DISSOCIATIVE DISORDERS, and AMNESIA. Some examples of traumatic events include a wartime combat experience, a natural disaster (such as a tornado, flood, or extreme blizzard), a severe illness (such as a diagnosis of cancer or early Alzheimer's disease), a physical assault (such as a rape or an extreme beating), or a severe motor vehicle accident.

Hurricanes and other natural disasters are traumatic events, as are the evacuation and relocation efforts they sometimes require. Individuals who experience natural disasters and their subsequent aftermath sometimes develop disorders associated with the trauma. The same is true of individuals who are diagnosed with a severe and/or terminal illness. The person may be consumed by the threat of death as well as by the pain from the illness and its treatments, such as chemotherapy or repeated surgical procedures. Sometimes the effects of the illness or diagnosis can cause changes in relationships with others, even among close family members, such as spouses and children. These relationships can become problematic as some individuals distance themselves from the ill person as if his or her illness were somehow contagious to others, or because they cannot accept the diagnosis of a terminal illness in someone they love.

Many traumatized individuals experience profound GRIEF, which is a state of intense sadness over one or more serious losses that are directly or indirectly related to a traumatic event. This feeling is often normal, such as the grief over losing a family member or friend, or sometimes even the grief suffered over the loss of important property or personal objects, such as when a person's home and belongings (irreplaceable family photos, mementos, etc.) have been destroyed by a hurricane or other natural disaster. However, if the grief is extreme and prolonged beyond about six months, it may lead to the development of posttraumatic stress disorder.

A condition known as POSTTRAUMATIC EMBITTERMENT DISORDER (PTED) can occur following a traumatic event. Sometimes an event that primarily affects only one person, such as a job firing or a demotion, can be extremely traumatic to the individual and may trigger intensely negative emotions. Posttraumatic embitterment disorder can lead to aggression against oneself or other persons, as well as marked feelings of hopelessness.

Emotions are strongly affected by experiencing traumatic events. Some individuals may cope with the traumatic event by displaying an extremely abnormal emotional response, which is also known as AFFECT MODULATION. It may seem to others that they are displaying "too much" or "too little" emotion. This response is seen especially among sufferers of posttraumatic stress disorder (PTSD) and is largely an unconscious process.

Individuals with an abnormal affect modulation may show little or no emotion. They may appear to be cold and unresponsive. This response in a traumatized person often seems strange and unreasonable to others, who may believe that it signifies that the individual lacks feelings about the traumatic event's effects on him or herself or others. For example, a person who has been raped may testify in court in a flat and unemotional voice, leading some jurors to believe that the person was not actually raped despite evidence to the contrary. Others may think that a person who was assaulted would or should show extreme emotion, as they imagine that they would feel in the same circumstances, rather than affective flatness. However, those who make this assumption have not experienced the same trauma.

Conversely, the affect modulation of the traumatized person may be emotionally volatile. The person may scream, yell, and appear hysterical and out of control to others. In this case, others may perceive the individual as behaving irrationally and unreasonably, and they may question the reliability of what the person says.

Sleep disorders such as PARASOMNIAS may occur in individuals who are suffering from traumatic stress disorders. Parasomnias are nocturnal behaviors occurring during sleep, such as sleepwalking, binge eating, moving objects about, or even manipulating weapons and harming others while still in a sleep state. The person often has no MEMORY of these acts on the next day. Individuals with traumatic stress disorders are also prone to suffering from NIGHTMARES.

Affective Disorders

Affective disorders (mood disorders) are also a response to severe trauma. Affective disorders include depression or CLYCLOTHYMIA, a milder form of depression, as well as BIPOLAR DISORDER.

Some symptoms of depression are difficulty thinking or concentrating, a lack of interest in activities that were formerly pleasurable, and feelings of hopelessness and emptiness. Depression is treatable with therapy and medications, particularly antidepressants. It is very important for the clinically depressed person to receive treatment because he or she may be at risk for SUICIDE. The National Institute of Mental Health reports that major depressive disorder affects approximately 19 million adults in the United States and is the leading cause of disability among individuals ages 15 to 44.

Bipolar disorder is another type of affective disorder in which individuals alternate, or cycle, between periods of mania and depression. Trauma may either trigger or exacerbate the symptoms of bipolar disorder. Bipolar disorder is treated with medications and therapy.

PTSD and Other Anxiety Disorders

Anxiety disorders are commonly associated with traumatic stress, particularly posttraumatic stress disorder, PANIC DISORDER, and GENERALIZED ANXIETY DISORDER (GAD), which is sometimes also referred to as global anxiety. Some experts are seeking to have PTSD defined as a separate traumatic stress disorder.

PTSD develops in some individuals after they experience a horrific event, such as wartime combat, rape, or physical abuse. PTSD may develop soon after a terrifying event, or it could occur months or even years later. It is characterized by hypervigilance, FLASHBACKS, and nightmares. Any reminders of the trauma can cause the person to relive the traumatic experience in his or her mind. This is not the same as remembering the event. Instead, the person feels as if he or she is actually reexperiencing the event as it happened. The person with PTSD may also actively seek to avoid people or places that bring reminders of the traumatic event.

Individuals with PTSD may feel distant, cold, and preoccupied toward others.

There is a higher than average incidence of suicide and DIVORCE among PTSD sufferers than among nonsufferers.

Treatment for PTSD includes medications, such as antidepressants, as well as therapy, such as COGNITIVE BEHAVIORAL THERAPIES, EXPOSURE THERAPY, and EYE MOVEMENT DESENSITIZATION AND REPROCESSING (EMDR). The aim of therapy is to help traumatized individuals move away from their reexperiencing of the past to become fully engaged in the present.

Abnormal affect modulation may occur with PTSD, as may hypervigilance; for example, a soldier returning from combat may dive for cover upon hearing a car backfire, reacting to the possible gunfire or bombings that he or she faced in the war zone.

Another anxiety disorder that may develop as a result of a traumatic stress disorder is panic disorder. Panic disorder is a condition in which a person suffers from chronic and debilitating PANIC ATTACKS. Many people who are having a panic attack mistakenly believe that they are experiencing a heart attack or that they are dying. Sometimes individuals with panic disorder become so fearful that they are afraid to leave their homes at all, which is a condition known as agoraphobia.

Generalized anxiety disorder is another form of anxiety disorder that can develop among those with traumatic stress disorders. Individuals with generalized anxiety disorder (GAD) have extreme and unrealistic worries for at least six months, even when the individual fully realizes that the worrying is excessive and unreasonable. They cannot stop the worrying unless the GAD is treated. Individuals suffering from GAD also often have physical symptoms related to their disorder, such as chronic headaches, irritability, sweating, and trembling. They may have difficulty with concentrating, and may also experience trouble getting to sleep or have frequent awakenings and other sleep disorders. GAD is treated with therapy as well as with benzodiazepines and antidepressants.

Substance Abuse or Addiction

Some individuals cope with stress in maladaptive ways, using drugs and/or alcohol to attempt to block out the memory of the trauma by using intoxicants or drugs that temporarily blur and/or distract the mind, preventing them from thinking about the traumatic event. In some cases, they may develop an addiction to the substance, which means that they have both a physical and a psychological need for it. Often these individuals will develop a tolerance for the substance, and need greater amounts of it to achieve the same effect.

Individuals who are addicted or dependent on a substance are obsessed with it as well as with the methods used to obtain it. Their addiction negatively affects their functioning at home and at work. If they do not or cannot use the substance (whether it is illegal drugs, abused prescribed narcotics, or alcohol), they will experience the symptoms of psychological and/or physical withdrawal, which can include vomiting, diarrhea, seizures, hallucinations, craving for the drug, and other effects depending upon the substance. Self-help groups such as Alcoholics Anonymous or Cocaine

Anonymous help many people to overcome their substance dependence. There are also some prescription medications, such as naltrexone, that can control the craving for alcohol or drugs.

Adults who were severely physically or sexually abused as children are more likely to abuse alcohol and/or drugs than nonabused adults, according to *The Encyclopedia of Child Abuse*. In addition, people who are physically or sexually assaulted during adulthood, as in the case of spouse beatings in domestic violence, may sometimes turn to alcohol or drugs for relief from their emotional pain.

Attachment Disorders

Children can become severely traumatized from abuse or neglect that occurs during childhood. They seek their parents' love and attention, and if their parents repeatedly reject them, it can lead to trauma. Even more confusing is the case of parents who are alternately kind and cruel with no discernible pattern. This intermittent reinforcement causes children to seek parental love even more, always hoping that maybe this time they will find the love and validation that they seek.

In addition to the trauma that a child suffers from abuse or neglect, the child may also develop an attachment disorder if normal attachment to a parent or other parental figure does not occur. Bonding refers to the process of connecting with a caregiver (parent, foster parent, or whoever is the primary caregiver) as an infant or small child, while attachment refers to the actual connection. If bonding is a pathological, or destructive, form of bonding , then it will be difficult for the individual to have a normal and healthy life unless treatment helps the child. For example, if the parent or other primary caregiver is intermittently cruel and kind to a child, and there is no discernible pattern to this behavior that the child can predict (for example, it is not related to the child's "bad" or "good" behavior), and if the child receives no treatment, then the child may become very anxious, distressed, insecure, and avoidant of emotional connections. Growing up in this type of environment, the child will not have the experiences to build confidence in himself or herself or to trust others. In adulthood, this individual may have great difficulty attaching to a significant other who is emotionally healthy, and he or she may instead seek someone who exhibits the same pathological behavior patterns of the parent.

Children who are raised in crowded orphanages and who receive little personal attention or affection may develop attachment disorders, even if they are later adopted. This is particularly true if the child remains in the orphanage beyond the age of three or four years according to *The Encyclopedia of Adoption*. Foster children in the United States who have moved from home to home may also have attachment disorders.

The child with an attachment disorder may be very inhibited and resistant to accepting comforting from others. In contrast, children with the disinhibited form of attachment disorder are unusually friendly and sociable to everyone and have no particular attachment to any one person. Although the disinhibited form of attachment disorder may seem more positive, it is not so for the caregiver, who is no more important to the unattached child than any other person who provides care or even mild interest in the child.

Attachment disorders in children are difficult to treat because no clear treatment has emerged and there is considerable disagreement on how such children should be treated. Traditional psychotherapeutic approaches are often not effective because these children have great difficulty trusting and forming alliances necessary for basic therapy. As for the caregiver, the most important intervention is to be emotionally available so as to begin focusing on stable, sensitive, and positive interactions. Caregivers of children with attachment disorders should consult only therapists with specific expertise in this field and with a track record of success that can be confirmed through other experts.

Dissociative Disorders

In the most extreme case, the individual may develop a psychological disorder subsequent to a traumatic event, such as a dissociative disorder in which the individual extremely distances, or dissociates, from the traumatic event. Dissociation is a state within a state in which the person's perception of reality is altered, but the person usually stays in contact with the traumatic experience within this duality.

Dissociation is not abnormal in and of itself. It is a common coping mechanism that many people use in stressful or extremely stressful situations to help them act almost mechanically in order to save their lives or the lives of others. Dissociation becomes abnormal when it is used chronically and prevents the person from processing, remembering, or working through difficult situations in his or her life.

A dissociative disorder is characterized by a sudden sense of being outside one's self, observing from a distance as if watching a movie of ongoing events, with a distortion of body image and time slowing and the world seeming unreal. These symptoms may last a few moments or could come and go for years. Again, the frequency and intensity are the defining factors as to whether dissociation is an abnormal response.

Formerly known as multiple personality disorder, dissociative identity disorder (DID) is a severe disorder in which the individual actually develops separate and distinct personalities, called "alters," usually in response to horrific CHILD ABUSE AND NEGLECT or CHILD SEXUAL ABUSE. The number of alters can be as few as two and as many as 100 or more. According to the National Alliance on Mental Health (NAMI):

> The different identities, referred to as alters, may exhibit differences in speech, mannerisms, attitudes, thoughts, and gender orientation. The alters may even differ in "physical" properties such as allergies, right-or-left handedness, or the need for eyeglass prescriptions. These differences between alters are often quite striking.

A well-known example of a person with DID is the story about a woman who had been severely abused in childhood as told in the book *The Three Faces of Eve* (1957) by Corbett Thigpen. The story of the woman named Eve and her 22 distinct personalities was also the subject of a 1957 movie starring Joanne Woodward.

In the case of severe childhood abuse, a child's psychological coping response to severe abuse is often to distance, or dissociate, himself or herself from the event, as if he or she were watching it from afar in a clinical and unfeeling manner. This is a means of coping with the pain and terror associated with the suffering the child is experiencing. Dissociative identity disorder is difficult to diagnose and treat. Some experts are dubious that dissociative identity disorder is a valid diagnosis, particularly when it is used in defense of a criminal act.

Amnesia

Another severe (albeit usually nonpsychotic) response to a traumatic event is amnesia, which is a serious loss of memory that is unrelated to the normal forgetting of information and which is not due to such brain disorders as Alzheimer's disease or other forms of dementia. Amnesia may result from a severe physical trauma, such as from a TRAUMATIC BRAIN INJURY. In addition, it may also be caused by extreme sustained psychological stress or an unusually stressful situation in which an individual unconsciously blocks the traumatic event from his or her memory.

The individual may experience a loss of memory surrounding and including the time when the traumatic event occurred. In rare cases, the individual forgets his or her own name and details of his or her personal identity, which is itself a traumatic event. This state is known as a DISSOCIATIVE FUGUE. Significant distress and impairment along with the assumption of a new identity may occur, particularly if the identity does not come back to the person. A dissociative fugue state varies in the length of time that it lasts, and it may last for hours, weeks, months, or even years. Often memories come back in fragments and later may flood the individual.

If a traumatic brain injury causes amnesia, it produces a condition usually referred to as POST-TRAUMATIC AMNESIA (PTA). With this disorder, which is a disorder caused by a brain malfunction rather than a psychiatric disorder, the person is unable to store or retrieve new information after the brain is injured.

Secondary Traumatic Stress

Individuals are often distressed when they observe the severe effects of trauma that has been directly experienced by others, such as when they hear an intense and detailed description of the traumatic incident from a person who has been brutally beaten or otherwise physically or emotionally harmed. This reaction is known as SECONDARY TRAUMATIC STRESS. *Primary traumatic stress disorder* results from an individual's direct exposure to a traumatic event. SECONDARY TRAUMATIZATION is also referred to as VICARIOUS TRAUMATIZATION and COMPASSION FATIGUE, and it affects those who care for people who have been directly traumatized. Examples of individuals who may experience secondary traumatic stress are medical responders, therapists, and others who seek to help the person who suffered a primary traumatization. (This secondary traumatization is sometimes called "countertransference" when it is experienced by a therapist as an overidentification with the patient's description of his or her reactions to the traumatic event.) Some symptoms of secondary traumatic stress are fatigue, a hypersensitive startle response, and avoidance of reminders of the traumatic event.

Tertiary traumatization is traumatization that is experienced thirdhand by the individuals who support the supporters, such as the adult family members and children of the first responders (such as emergency medical technicians or police officers), or the individuals who respond to traumatic events and actively seek to help traumatized individuals with primary traumatization.

Symptoms of tertiary traumatization may include anxiety and difficulty sleeping or nightmares, as the individual responds to listening to others describe how they tried to help traumatized individuals (or viewing videos or photographs), and the person with tertiary traumatization deeply empathizes with the distressing stories. Therapy may help individuals who experience either secondary or tertiary traumatization.

Clark, Robin, and Judith Freeman Clark. *The Encyclopedia of Child Abuse,* 3rd ed. New York: Facts On File, 2007.

Doctor, Ronald M., Ada P. Kahn, and Christine Adamec. *The Encyclopedia of Phobias, Fears, and Anxieties,* 3rd ed. New York: Facts On File, 2008.

Miller, M. D., Laurie C. and Christine Adamec. *The Encyclopedia of Adoption,* 3rd ed. New York: Facts On File, 2006.

National Alliance on Mental Health (NAMI), Dissociative Identity Disorder. Available online. URL: http://www.nami.org. Accessed July 21, 2008.

attachment disorders   See ATTACHMENT STYLES/
DISORDERS; TRAUMA AND ATTACHMENT BELIEF SCALES
(TABS); TRAUMA BONDING.

attachment styles/disorders   The term *attachment* refers to the bonding or connection that
one has to the environment. Most children form
bonds to their caregivers as infants, receiving not
only food and shelter but also love and attention.
The process of forming a close relationship with
a caregiver is called "bonding," and the resulting
relationship is called an "attachment." However,
in some cases, because of abuse, neglect, or absent
parents, bonding and attachment does not occur
or is damaged.

Attachment theory was developed by John
Bowlby, an English psychoanalyst. In the 1950s,
Bowlby observed that separation from their parents in very young children followed a pattern of
anger and rage first, then DEPRESSION and withdrawal, and finally detachment from their social
and physical environment. He noted that children
develop an "inner working model" of their environment that guides their perceptions, emotions,
and behavior throughout their lives. Early abuse
breeds a lifelong distrust and social turmoil.

Bowlby based his concept on his observations
of children in orphanages who had lost their parents in World War II. Based on these observations,
Bowlby believed that if children could not form an
attachment to a caregiver by the age of 2.5 years,
then the child could never form a normal attachment to anyone. Other more recent experts, such
as British psychiatrist Michael Rutter, have stated
that there may be a later age at which attachments
can still be formed, such as age four years. He has
also said that attachment may be possible beyond
the age of four years. Rutter based his findings on
his observations of orphaned children who were
later adopted.

Ainsworth studied infant-mother relationships
and concluded that secure and predictable bonding
leads to competent and secure children and adults.
Abused children, on the other hand, were more
resistant to adults, neglected infants became passive, and children from supportive environments
were more cooperative and secure.

Symptoms and Diagnostic Path

The symptoms follow along with the type of
attachment disruption. For example, an "insecure"
attachment leads to ambivalence and distrust as an
adult. Intimacy is very difficult as well as commitment to a relationship. An "anxious" attachment
with the mother may lead to insecurity, doubt, and
excessive worry about oneself or others.

Treatment Options and Outlook

The psychodynamic therapists argue that attachment disorders can be dealt with only by reconstructing the individual's life history through
analysis and allowing unconscious, repressed elements to emerge into consciousness. Behaviorists,
on the other hand, look to the here and now and
develop methods to retrain or relearn old patterns
associated with the bonding disruption. They see
the need to help the client develop new behaviors
for deficits produced by the biasing relationship
with the mother.

Risk Factors and Preventive Measures

Problems with forming a close bond to another
person may occur because of past severe traumas.
The trauma may be related to child abuse or abandonment, or it could stem from another issue or
incident such as CHILD SEXUAL ABUSE that the child
suffered at the hands of relatives, neighbors, or
others. The younger the child is when placed with
a safe and secure parental figure, the more likely
the child will resolve the causes of early trauma.

Research on Attachment and Bonding

Since the 1970s, research and clinical studies have
refined the studying of bonding and have focused
on the "attunement" of baby and mother and the
degree to which the baby feels felt by the mother
and this FELT SENSE is communicated to and experienced by the infant. Attunement centers are
located in particular areas of the BRAIN, namely
the orbitofrontal areas adjacent to the LIMBIC SYSTEM (the emotional center) and the frontal areas
responsible for delay, planning, and higher human
functions. By helping regulate affect (mood), the
caregiver (generally the mother) helps the infant
(and the eventual adult) to experience an inner
self-regulation or attunement and the brain growth

that physiologically supports this experience. This self-regulation process is known as neurohormonal regulation.

The caregiver's own neurohormonal regulation and attunement to the infant helps regulate the developing infant's neurohormonal management. So, under stress when CORTISOL and other neuro-hormones are released in the infant's brain, the mother provides comfort and connection (attun-ement) to help bring down these stress-enhancing hormones. In other words, the mother serves as a calming agent to the infant, and this helps pro-mote the development of internal mechanisms and structures that will provide the infant with stress relief throughout its life span. Abuse and neglect obviously prevent this attunement and the ability to self-regulate, leading to added stress, DYSREGULA-TION, and eventual disease, as well as poor coping and interpersonal skills.

There is support for the role of caregiver inter-action in numerous psychotherapy studies. These studies have shown that when patients recount what was most helpful to them in the therapy, they do not usually recall specific insights or interactions but remember most the quality of the relationship with the therapist.

The Dynamics of Trauma, Attachment, and Stress

Differentiation and the development of the brain occur through social and environmental interac-tion. The brain operates with plasticity, or the ability to mold its structures and functions in response to outside and usually social experiences. It retains its ability to renew and modify its struc-ture based on experience—especially social experi-ence—throughout the lifetime.

Attachment or bonding that occurs early in life sets a lifelong template for thoughts, feelings, behavior, and reactivity. "Good-enough" attach-ment leads to good-enough brain structure and function. But failed attachment, often caused by abuse, neglect, emotional unavailability, or other forms of trauma will have negative effects through-out the developmental cycle. Neural dysregulation and memories of a failed attachment relationship become the basis for adult difficulties with rela-tionships and also put the individual at risk for

developing PTSD, drug abuse, and other psychiatric conditions.

Scientific studies have shown that numerous damaging effects occur to the brain with early abuse and even severe trauma later in life. For example, DeBellis and colleagues found that sexually abused girls showed a much higher incidence of suicidal thoughts and attempts and of depression than did the controls. Many of their critical brain hormones were deviant, and there was clear evidence of "dys-regulatory disorder of the HPA axis." Driessen, et al., found that borderline personality subjects, who are presumed to have experienced early trauma, had 16 percent smaller volumes (sizes) of the HIP-POCAMPUS and 8 percent smaller volumes of the AMYGDALA than the healthy control subjects.

Gaensbauer observed that the body remembered a traumatic experience that was preverbal and that these traumas affected the developmental cycle. Gurvits, et al., has shown that early trauma leads to subtle neurological impairment and puts the person at significant risk for developing PTSD as an adult under conditions of traumatic experience.

Ito and associates showed the presence of abnor-mal left hemisphere frontal, temporal, and anterior region dysfunction in children who had been physically abused, leading to greater use of the right hemisphere and consequent greater negative emotions from the unconscious painful storage of childhood memories in the right side. Schore and Siegel have written about the neurobiology of "secure" and disorganized/disoriented attachment associated with abuse and neglect. They point out that disorganized/disoriented attachment is associ-ated with abuse and neglect. They also note that disorganized/disoriented attachment affects the regulatory capacity in the orbitofrontal cortex, leading to poor stress coping and many of the symptoms of PTSD.

Finally, van der Kolk has examined the psy-chobiology of trauma in relationship to memory processes and points out that "when people are traumatized, the emotional impact of the event may interfere with the capacity to capture the experience in words or symbols."

See also BODY MEMORY; CHILD ABUSE AND NEGLECT; TRAUMA AND ATTACHMENT BELIEF SCALE (TABS); TRAUMA BONDING; TRAUMATIC BRAIN INJURY.

Bowlby, John. *Maternal Care and Mental Health*. Geneva, Switzerland: World Health Organization, 1951.

DeBellis, M.D., et al. "Urinary Catecholamine Excretion in Sexually Abused Girls." *Journal of the American Academy of Child and Adolescent Psychiatry*, 33, no. 3 (1994): 320–327.

Driessen, et al. "Magnetic Resonance Imaging Volumes of the Hippocampus and the Amygdala in Women with Borderline Personality Disorder and Early Traumatization." *Archives of General Psychiatry* 57 (2000): 1,115–1,122.

Gaensbauer, T. J. "Trauma in the Preverbal Period." *Psychoanalytic Study of the Child* 50 (1995): 122–149.

Gurvits, T. V., et al. "Neurologic Soft Signs in Chronic Posttraumatic Stress Disorder." *Archives of General Psychiatry*, 57, no. 2 (2000): 181–186.

Howe, David. *Child Abuse and Neglect: Attachment, Development and Intervention*. New York: Palgrave Macmillan, 2005.

Ito, Y., et al. "Increased Prevalence of Electrophysiological Abnormalities in Children with Psychological, Physical and Sexual Abuse." *Journal of Neuropsychiatry and Clinical Neurosciences*, 5, no. 4 (1993): 401–408.

Schore, A. N. "The Effects of Early Relational Trauma on Right Brain Development, Affect Regulation, and Infant Mental Health." *Infant Journal of Mental Health*, 22 (2001): 201–269.

Siegel, D. "Toward an Interpersonal Neurobiology of the Developing Mind: Attachment Relationships, 'mindsight,' and neural integration." *Infant Journal of Mental Health*, Special Edition on Contributions of the Decade of the Brain to Infant Psychiatry. 22 (2001): 67–94.

van der Kolk, B. A., "The Body, Memory, and the Psychobiology of Trauma." In Judith L. Alpert (Ed.), *Sexual Abuse Recalled: Treating Trauma in the Era of the Recovered Memory Debate*, edited by Judith L. Alpert, 29–60. Northvale, N.J.: Jason Aronson, 1995.

attitudes toward mental illness, public   Societal views toward mental illness, including POSTTRAUMATIC STRESS DISORDER (PTSD). In 1996 a team of researchers published their results of a survey of public attitudes on mental illness. In order to assess attitude changes, the researchers included questions from a 1950 study of attitudes toward mental illness. In 1950 researchers found that the public had a strongly negative view of the mentally ill, particularly regarding their perceived unpredictability and violent behaviors. Mentally ill people were stigmatized and socially ostracized at that time.

The 1996 survey revealed that the public had a more accepting and scientific view of the mentally ill, but the strong stigmatization was still present. The public could differentiate normal worry, DEPRESSION, and anxiety from clinical levels. They attributed mental illness to a variety of causes, mainly biological and psychological stress. On the other hand, public attitudes toward psychosis had intensified in terms of fears of violence. Only 13 percent of those surveyed in 1950 mentioned violence, whereas 30 percent mentioned violence in their description of the mentally ill in 1996. The fact is that there is very little risk of violent behavior toward strangers in the mentally ill and some risk toward family and friends, but this risk mainly occurs among psychotic individuals who are noncompliant with taking their medications.

PTSD was first described in the literature in 1980, and there is no historical data on public attitudes toward this condition. However, because the causes of PTSD are linked to events outside the individual, we can speculate that most people are sympathetic to improved diagnostic understanding. The fear of violence levels, however, may persist since many dramatic cases of PTSD result in acting out socially or in violent actions.

See also MEDIA; STIGMATIZATION.

autonomic nervous system (ANS)   The part of the nervous system involved in regulating individual organ function and homeostasis and generally not under voluntary control.

The autonomic nervous system (ANS) is a regulatory system transmitting impulses from the CENTRAL NERVOUS SYSTEM (CNS) to the peripheral organs. It helps regulate blood pressure, the constriction and dilation of blood vessels, pupil size, the heart's electrical activity, and the contraction and relaxation of smooth muscles. The ANS also regulates the movement of the stomach, intestines, and salivary glands.

The ANS is divided into two parts: the SYMPATHETIC NERVOUS SYSTEM (SNS) and the PARASYMPATHETIC NERVOUS SYSTEM (PNS). There is a third part of the ANS that is less commonly considered a part of the system called the "enteric nervous system," regulating digestive organs and thought to be a very early form of the organization or "brain."

The sympathetic nervous system activates the sympathetic adrenal response, which is commonly known as the FIGHT OR FLIGHT RESPONSE. It prepares the body for fear, fight, and escape during high stress. The sympathetic preganglionic fibers originate in the spinal cord and end in the adrenal medulla. Here ACETYLCHOLINE is secreted, which triggers the release of EPINEPHRINE (adrenaline) and NOREPINEPHRINE. This response acts directly on the cardiovascular system and diverts blood flow from the skin to muscle, brain, and heart. The sympathetic nervous system also raises blood pressure, dilates the pupils of the eyes, stimulates heartbeat, and converts glycogen in the liver to glucose used for energy.

The parasympathetic nervous system works to save energy and is often referred to as the "rest and digest" response. There is a slowdown of the heart rate, lowering of blood pressure, and the facilitation of digestion to a calm resting state. The PNS and SNS work together to bring body functions back to normal. In times of danger, the body prepares itself for fight or flight through the SNS, and when the danger or emergency passes, the PNS reverses these actions.

See also AMYGDALA; BRAIN; PHYSIOLOGY OF TRAUMA.

avoidance/avoidance behavior The symptom triad that comprises POSTTRAUMATIC STRESS DISORDER (PTSD) criteria are intrusive symptoms, hyperarousal, and avoidance behaviors. When the individual becomes excessively distressed with reminders of the trauma, all attempts to avoid memories of the traumatic event become a way of coping. The survivor may isolate himself or herself, become detached from feelings, and experience an emotional NUMBING.

An extreme example of avoidance would be someone who lived in Manhattan through SEPTEMBER 11 and who then moved out of state. A lesser type of avoidance behavior would be someone who worked in Manhattan and who changed jobs in order to avoid the area around Ground Zero. Although it is natural to use avoidance as a coping strategy, avoiding thoughts and feelings about

trauma can interfere with moving on with an individual's life. If avoidance behaviors are too extreme, they may lead to more isolation and DEPRESSION.

Initially nearly all people surviving a TRAUMATIC EVENT will use distraction and avoidance in order to go on with their daily activities. Avoiding the news and going out to a social event can distract the mind from the trauma in the short term. The ability to distract oneself allows individuals to return to their normal lives: go to work, do grocery shopping, and find time to spend with family and friends. But once avoidance becomes the primary way to cope, it becomes more difficult to live a normal life, as the survivor cannot overcome the distress without avoidance behaviors becoming a necessary daily activity and returning to pretrauma lifestyle is severely compromised. Often avoidance is subconscious, and the individual naturally or automatically avoids painful reminders of traumatic experiences.

Some actions are designed to stay away from stimuli that are perceived by the individual as extremely dangerous or threatening. For example, if a person was attacked by a dog in the past, in many cases the person will avoid that particular breed of dog in the future. In addition, some individuals will generalize their fear to all dogs. As a result, if friends or relatives own dogs, they will either not visit those individuals or they will request that the dog be placed behind a closed door or securely leashed outside. If such individuals encounter a dog in the course of their day, they will actively seek to avoid the animal.

Individuals who are distressed by or who are phobic about other stimuli will similarly actively seek to avoid those stimuli. Some individuals become so concerned about the feared stimuli that they develop agoraphobia, and rarely (or never) leave their houses.

Avoidance is a major symptom category of PTSD and can occur at physical, behavioral, or mental levels or at the level of the senses (for example, in the case of numbing). Most often avoidance is subconscious and automatic. Experts know that avoidance, while temporarily reducing anxiety, does not reduce the activated response (anxiety) but actually tends to make it more intense in the long run.

See also ANXIETY DISORDERS.

battered child syndrome A phrase denoting child physical abuse, a condition that was named and first clearly described by C. Henry Kempe and his colleagues in their 1962 landmark article in the *Journal of the American Medical Association.* This article awakened in physicians a new and intense interest in the protection of abused children, a problem that physicians rarely discussed and often ignored before the publication of the study, largely because many doctors had great difficulty believing that parents could harm their own children. Instead, prior to the article by Kempe et al., child abuse was perceived as a problem usually perpetrated by a limited number of psychopathic or psychotic individuals.

Symptoms and Diagnostic Path

Kempe and his colleagues were devoted to the issue of child protection, and they had previously created a hospital-based child protective team at Colorado General Hospital. In their article, they discussed their findings that child abuse occurred far more commonly than was generally accepted by most physicians at the time. Said the authors:

> The syndrome should be considered in any child exhibiting evidence of fracture of any bone, subdural hematoma, failure to thrive, soft tissue swellings or skin bruising, in any child who dies suddenly, or where the degree and type of injury is at variance with the history given regarding the occurrence of the trauma.

In addition, the authors said, "A marked discrepancy between clinical findings and historical data as supplied by the parents is a major diagnostic feature of the battered-child syndrome."

Treatment Options and Outlook

There were no treatments for child abuse when Kempe first described it. Instead, the initial efforts focused on diagnosis, separating the parent(s) or caretakers from the child and putting the child in "protective custody" while the parents underwent psychotherapy. The idea was that treating the parents would solve the problem of child abuse and then the family could be restored.

Unfortunately, the picture quickly appeared to be very complicated, and this simple model gave way to more direct and focused approaches. For example, there was the problem of the stepparent or boyfriend abusing the child, persons who had less investment in the child than the parent. There was the immature mother who saw the child as a caretaker for herself or as a source of approval and who viewed any irritation or independence exhibited by the child as a rejection of her. As a result, courses in identifying the language of crying started to appear.

Alcoholism and drug addiction almost always played a role in abuse patterns. There were also some cases of sadistic psychotic parents (often within a cult) who delighted in torturing and inflicting pain on a child. Treatments had to follow diagnosis and distinguish among different forms of child abuse as diagnosis became more differentiating.

Risk Factors and Preventive Measures

In 2003 John M. Leventhal wrote in *Clinical Child Psychology and Psychiatry* that the article by Kempe and his colleagues was still valuable to experts more than 40 years later. According to Leventhal:

> The authors' discussion of the psychiatric aspects of abuse highlights themes that continue to be rel-

evant today. They noted that the abuse of children is not confined to adults with low intelligence, a psychopathic personality, or low socioeconomic status. They were struck with the histories of poor nurturing in the parents who abused and the intergeneration transmission of patterns of child-rearing.

This observation has been empirically validated in that abuse is usually perpetrated by those who have been abused thus recreating the same pattern with their own children. The risk is also double-faceted in that both the abusive parents and their children require intervention. For example, abused children have been found to elicit abuse in normally nonabusive adults, and the children have required intervention to change their provocative behaviors.

Public school personnel have been trained to identify signs of child abuse, and mental health workers not only are required to have training in the identification of abuse, but most states also require them to take continuing educational course to sharpen their diagnostic and treatment skills.

Abuse comes in many forms with all kinds of people. One reliable predictor is whether the parent or caretaker was abused, but this factor is not foolproof in that most abused children do not become abusive adults. Only a small proportion of abused children will eventually abuse their children.

See also BATTERED WOMAN SYNDROME; BETRAYAL TRAUMA THEORY (BTT); CHILD ABUSE AND NEGLECT (CAN); CHILD PHYSICAL ABUSE (CPA); CHILDREN AND TRAUMA; CHILD SEXUAL ABUSE (CSA); CHILD SEXUAL ABUSE ACCOMMODATION SYNDROME.

Kempe, C. H., et al. "The Battered Child Syndrome." *Journal of the American Medical Association* 181 (1962): 107–112.
Leventhal, John M., "Test of Time: 'The Battered-Child Syndrome' 40 Years Later." *Clinical Child Psychology and Psychiatry* 8, no. 4 (2003): 543–545.

battered woman syndrome (BWS) Repeated physical and psychological violence suffered by a woman that results in her emotional, behavioral, and psychological inability to respond in an appropriate manner, such as by resisting or by leaving the abuser. This syndrome was first defined by Leonore Walker in 1979.

Symptoms and Diagnostic Path
Victims of battered woman syndrome exhibit traumatic symptoms in the form of anxiety, DEPRESSION, fear, low self-esteem, and suspiciousness. They often believe that they cannot change their behavior and that they are trapped in their current situation. They often exhibit a LEARNED HELPLESSNESS (e.g., they have been repeatedly been told by their spouses or partners that they cannot leave and that there is nothing they can do, and they believe this to be true, and act in a passive and helpless fashion). Helplessness combined with low self-esteem, fear, and dependency trap the battered wife in a vicious cycle where living in the outer world alone seems impossible.

Battered woman syndrome has been used as a defense in trials in which a woman has injured or killed an abusive partner, as well as in other cases. The Iowa Supreme Court first allowed expert testimony on battered woman syndrome in 1997 in *State v. Griffin*. In this case, the victim, who was the common-law wife of the defendant, had been repeatedly raped in a hotel room and her clothes were taken away from her so she would not leave. She later went to the hospital and told police about the kidnapping and assault. She then recanted her testimony but later testified for the prosecution. The court found that the expert testimony was relevant because it explained why an abused woman might recant her testimony.

Treatment Options and Outlook
Battered women require a safe place to live, and then healing and deeper therapy can begin. The motivation to change, self-evaluation, and the separation from abusive partners are all essential factors. The outlook for battered women is very good if support, safety, self-exploration, and the means to change are available to them.

Risk Factors and Preventive Measures
Women with poor self-esteem are at risk for battered woman syndrome, as are women who cling to abusive partners and are afraid to be on their own. Alcoholism or drug addiction is most fre-

quently associated with abuse. Often, as seen in most adult disorders, there is a pattern established within childhood of dependency, compliance, and repression that gets acted out at the adult level. Prevention is best when it begins early in life when these patterns are clearly developing.

The battered woman syndrome along with child abuse were two uncontested situations that helped lead to including PTSD in the *DSM* in 1980.

See also BATTERED CHILD SYNDROME.

battle fatigue See COMBAT-RELATED POSTTRAU-MATIC STRESS DISORDER; ELECTROENCEPHALOGRAPH (EEG); THERAPY, TYPES OF.

behavioral reenactment A phenomenon of trauma that occurs with both children and adults involving the repetition or reenactment of a TRAU-MATIC EVENT or events. The reenactment may be in imagery (FLASHBACK), physiologically, emotionally (reexperiencing emotions of trauma in a similar situation) or, in this case, behaviorally. Behavioral reenactment is also a therapeutic process involving play or symbolized reproduction of a trauma in a safe setting. Some of the most focused work on therapeutic reenactment was done by child psychiatrist Lenore Terr in her pioneering study of children kidnapped and buried underground in Chowcilla, California, in 1976.

Kidnappers removed 26 preschool and school-age children, put them into darkened vans, and buried them alive in a tractor trailer underground. The children finally escaped after 28 hours in total darkness when the trailer roof collapsed. Terr noticed that many of these child survivors played games that involved burying vehicles and surmised that they were reenacting elements of the original trauma in an effort to process their experiences. She eventually identified aspects of what she called "traumatic play," including compulsive repetitiveness and its failure to alleviate anxiety. On the other hand, behavioral reenactments, unlike traumatic play, involve patterns of everyday behavior that incorporate aspects of trauma.

At a behavioral level, reenactment may take the form of either victim or perpetrator of traumatic material. This is not necessarily reliving an event but more like unconsciously acting as a victim or perpetrator, usually in an adult mode. For example, a portion of abused children reenact their abuse by abusing their own children, thus keeping the cycle of abuse alive.

See also REPETITION COMPULSION.

Terr, L. *Unchained Memories: True Stories of Traumatic Memories Lost and Found.* Basic Books: New York, 1994.

benzodiazepine A type of CENTRAL NERVOUS SYSTEM depressant that is often used to treat ANXIETY DISORDERS as well as to treat individuals who have suffered traumatic experiences. Some benzodiazepines, such as alprazolam (Xanax) and clonazepam (Klonopin), are approved by the Food and Drug Administration (FDA) for the treatment of PANIC DISORDER, which can be a symptom of PTSD. Other medications in the class of benzodiazepines are prescribed for the general treatment of anxiety and are often used in presurgery preparations. In some cases, benzodiazepines are used for an infrequent need; for example, some people who are claustrophobic but must have a closed magnetic resonance imaging (MRI) test will benefit from taking a one-time dose of diazepam (Valium) or another benzodiazepine, which will enable them to deal with their anxiety over the short period of the test.

Benzodiazepines are sometimes used to ease the symptoms of withdrawal from alcoholism. Benzodiazepines are the main category of what are also known as minor tranquilizers to the general public. Minor tranquilizers are drugs that target fear, anxiety and hyperarousal produced by adrenaline uptake. They are generally nontoxic by themselves but can be fatal if combined with large amounts of alcohol. They can be given orally or by intravenous injection. Some examples of commonly used benzodiazepines are alprazolam (Xanax), diazepam (Valium), clonazepam (Klonopin), lorazepam (Ativan), clorazepate (Tranxene), oxazepam (Serax), and chlordiazepoxide hydrochloride (Librium). Some benzodiazepines are used to treat INSOMNIA, such as estazolam (ProSom), temazepam (Restoril), and triazolam (Halcion).

Individuals taking benzodiazepines should consult with their physicians before stopping the drug because even a legitimate use of the drug could create severe withdrawal symptoms such as seizures if benzodiazepine use ends suddenly. The physician may recommend tapering off the drug, steadily taking a lower and lower dosage of the benzodiazepine until the drug use stops.

Benzodiazepines can significantly reduce an individual's reaction time, and thus those individuals who are taking benzodiazepines should avoid driving or using machinery. At higher doses of benzodiazepines, blackouts and confusion may occur. There is short-term memory loss associated with the use of benzodiazepines, and combined with high doses of alcohol the effect can be fatal.

Some individuals abuse or become addicted to benzodiazepines and require treatment. Some studies have shown that alprazolam is a benzodiazepine with a particular risk for causing addiction among those who are prone to drug dependence.

Benzodiazepines can be sedating, and consequently, they should not be combined with alcohol or other depressants.

See also AMPHETAMINE; ANTIANXIETY MEDICATION; ANXIETY DISORDERS; GENERALIZED ANXIETY DISORDER; TREATMENT: PSYCHOTHERAPY, PSYCHOPHARMACOLOGY, AND ALTERNATIVE MEDICINE.

Doctor, Ronald, and Ada Kahn. *The Encyclopedia of Phobias, Fears and Anxieties*. 3rd ed. New York: Facts On File, 2008.
Gwinnell, Esther, M.D., and Christine Adamec, *The Encyclopedia of Drug Abuse*. New York: Facts On File, 2008.

bereavement The grieving feelings that accompany the death of someone highly valued, such as a spouse, partner, parent, sibling, or close friend. Bereavement often also brings to the forefront the feelings of fear and anguish an individual experiences about his or her mortality, aloneness, separation, and isolation. In addition, in many cases, individuals agonize over their last words spoken to the deceased person, especially if they were said in anger; they may also ruminate over what they could have done or not done that would have somehow prevented the death.

Some individuals are extremely traumatized by the loss of a loved one and lapse into a state of DEPRESSION that extends beyond months after the person has died. In addition, some bereaved individuals develop phobias surrounding their loss that may be related to separation anxiety.

Because many people avoid talking about death in their day-to-day life (and deaths that occur on television and in films do not seem real), when a death does occur, it often appears as a shocking event to many individuals. Even the overall language of death is tailored to avoid any emotional pain, and rather than saying that someone has died, it is often said that he or she "passed on" or went to his or her "reward."

Bereaved individuals are often compelled to make many difficult and rapid choices about the person who has died, such as selecting a funeral home, choosing a coffin or urn, determining how to pay for a funeral or cremation, and so forth. In some cases, they must identify the deceased person, such as when the person was in a car accident. It is extremely trying for those in a highly emotional state to make such choices and take such actions. As a result, some individuals choose to plan and pay for their own funeral before they die in an attempt to save their relatives some of the pain that they know would be associated with their death.

See also GRIEF; GUILT.

betrayal trauma theory (BTT) A theory that was developed by Jennifer J. Freyd and discussed in her article in *Feminism & Psychology* in 1997. In essence, the theory describes the situation of children who trust their caregivers (usually their parents) who subsequently betray the child's trust, often with sexual, physical, or emotional abuse. Because such a betrayal is so psychologically painful, the victimized child can repress the memories of the betrayal abuse and develop AMNESIA of the incident(s), which may reappear in consciousness at a later time.

According to Freyd's betrayal trauma theory (BTT), children abused by their caretakers are more likely to experience amnesia following CHILD SEXUAL ABUSE than when they are abused by noncaretakers. These children face a senseless situation, as the perpetrator is the same person on whom they rely for food and shelter, the ultimate survivor goals. To resolve this conflict, BTT maintains that children continue to bond with the perpetrator and block memories of sexual abuse. The theory explains how a woman who was raped during her child-hood by her stepfather would be totally unaware of being sexually abused until years later when, as an adult, she encountered reminders of the TRAU-MATIC EVENTS. BTT generally refers to this predic-tion of unawareness and amnesia represented by the betrayal of a trusted person.

According to Freyd, "Betrayal trauma theory begins with two assumptions about the current social reality in America: first, that childhood sexual abuse happens; second, that memory of childhood sexual abuse is sometimes impaired, even unavailable for periods of time." Freyd also explained that the purpose to the child of blocking such psychological pain is to seek to get rid of the pain and to avoid the need for making a change in response to the pain.

Freyd says that children abused by a parent or other close caregiver may react with adaptive blindness or PSYCHIC NUMBING. *Adaptive blindness* is a term that usually means repressing certain aversive aspects of an abusive situation in order to survive and feel more normal or happy. It is a common cop-ing mechanism in abuse, ADDICTION, and psychotic-dominated families. Children are attached to the individual who is providing them with care, and if they accused that individual of sexual abuse, then the care would end and the child would feel physi-cally and mentally threatened. Thus, the memory of the abuse is blocked, and the relationship continues. Unfortunately, the abuse often continues as well.

See also CHILD ABUSE AND NEGLECT; CHILD SEXUAL ABUSE; DENY, ATTACK, AND REVERSE VICTIM AND OFFENDER (DARVO); FALSE MEMORY SYNDROME; TREATMENT: PSYCHOTHERAPY, PSYCHOPHARMACOLOGY, AND ALTERNATIVE MEDICINE.

Freyd, Jennifer. *Betrayal: The Logic of Forgetting Childhood Abuse.* Cambridge, Mass.: Harvard University Press, 1996.
Freyd, Jennifer J., "II. Violations of Power, Adaptive Blindness and Betrayal Trauma Theory." *Feminism & Psychology* 7, no. 1 (1997): 22–32.

bimodal/biphasic   Opposing ways of responding to severe trauma; for example, when the individual responds bimodally, he or she is hyperaroused and hyperreactive, while at the same time, the person is also numbed, avoidant, amnesiac and possibly anhedonic, or unable to experience pleasure. Both arousal and NUMBING coexist in the bimodal state within POSTTRAUMATIC STRESS DISORDER (PTSD).

Stated van der Kolk, "These responses to extreme experiences are so consistent across traumatic stimulation that this biphasic reaction appears to be the normative response to any overwhelming and uncontrollable experience."

van der Kolk, B., "The Body Keeps Score: Memory and the Evolving Psychobiology of Posttraumatic Stress." In *Trauma Page*. Available online at URL: http: www.trauma-pages.com/a/vanderk4.php. Downloaded March 20, 2007.

biological factors related to the stress response
Trauma affects people on various levels of biological functioning. The body responds to life-threatening danger by mobilizing the brainstem/HYPOTHALA-MUS, the LIMBIC SYSTEM, and the neocortex for sur-vival. This is known as the alarm reaction, which describes the initial bodily reaction to any stressor or challenge. It involves immediate arousal, orient-ing, tension in muscles, and increased heart beat and respiration, reactions that diminish only when the stressor is removed.

In the initial phases, called the alarm reaction, as described by Hans Selye in 1936, parts of the brain involved in assessing new information and dangerous information are activated, resulting in hypervigilance to the threat. This affective state is anxiety, and the degree of anxiety depends on the degree of threat. The BRAIN, body, and mind are linked so that one of these will affect the other two, as mental processes are products of the brain and body interacting with each other through nerve impulses and through chemicals via the blood-stream during the alarm reaction.

The human brain can store and recall emotional and physiological life events, and the SYMPATHETIC NERVOUS SYSTEM plays a major role in effecting the brain to mobilize the entire body at the time of threat. This activation increases blood pressure, dilates pupils, increases blood flow to muscles, and releases such stress-related hormones as ADRE-NOCORTICOTROPIC HORMONE (ACTH), a hormone secreted by the pituitary gland as well as endorphins. Neural hormones, EPINEPHRINE, NOREPINEPHRINE, and CORTISOL are released rapidly into the bloodstream to prepare the body to fight or flight.

The neurobiological activation responses come in rapid sequences that are reversible at the cost of energy and hormone depletion. If there is sufficient time between threatening situations and the removal of the stressor, the body does return to homeostasis (balance), and all internal chemical processes are replenished. This equilibrium is important to maintain an efficient mechanism of the STRESS-responding cycle for survival.

However, when the body is in a constant state of hyperarousal or activation in preparation for action or defense, the brain changes and the mechanism to homeostasis no longer applies. The brain will readjust and put into MEMORY the environmental demands of the threats by setting higher homeostatic levels for the hormones and NEUROTRANSMITTERS in the brain. These new memories, called "state memories," regulate arousal through the sympathetic nervous system, and they also characterize the symptoms for POSTTRAUMATIC STRESS DISORDER (PTSD). States of an increased startle response, anxiety, and hypervigilance all relate to this higher set point of brain neurotransmitter and hormone functioning.

Trauma response is complex, and not everyone will develop PTSD in response to trauma. It is becoming clearer with research that because of the stimulation of biological systems, a profound alteration in stress hormone secretion is found in people with PTSD. It is in understanding this neurophysiology that future treatment will be most effective.

See also CENTRAL NERVOUS SYSTEM; FIGHT OR FLIGHT RESPONSE; MEDICAL ILLNESS-RELATED PSYCHOLOGICAL DISTRESS; MEDICAL STRESSORS; PHYSIOLOGY OF TRAUMA.

van der Kolk, Bessel A. "The body keeps the score: Memory and the evolving psychobiology of posttraumatic stress." In *Essential Papers on Posttraumatic Stress Disorder,* edited by Mardi J. Horowitz, 301–326. New York: University Press, 1999.
Perry B. D., L. Conroy, and A. Ravitz. "Persisting Psychophysiological Effects of Traumatic Stress: The Memory of States," *Violence Update* 1, no. 8 (1991): 1–11.

bipolar disorder   Also known as manic-depressive illness, bipolar disorder is a BRAIN disorder with extreme shifts of mood (low to high), energy (reckless to listless), and ability to function (serious focus to disabling). About 5.7 million adults or 2.5 percent of the U.S. adult population in any given year will have bipolar disorder.

Symptoms and Diagnostic Path

The wide and deep mood swings of bipolar disorder may last for weeks or months. A recurrent episode of mania and DEPRESSION is referred to as Bipolar I. When the mania episodes are mild (hypomania) with depression, the condition is called Bipolar II. Symptoms of the manic phase of bipolar disorder are: euphoria, unusual energy, rapid speech, racing thoughts, increased activities, reckless need for immediate gratification such as spending sprees, decreased need for sleep, inflated self-esteem, and risky behaviors such as drug use. Symptoms of the depressive state of bipolar disorder are: fatigue, depressed mood, hopelessness, loss of interest or pleasure in activities, loneliness, irritability, sleep problems, and suicidal thoughts. Severe episodes of mania and depression may lead to psychosis, a detachment from reality. Bipolar disorder usually develops in late adolescence or early adulthood, and people usually suffer years before it is properly diagnosed because the person denies that he or she is ill. When a person has milder mood swings where the highs and lows are not severe enough to be called mania or major depression, it is diagnosed as CYCLOTHYMIA. Bipolar disorder is a long-term illness and must be managed for a person to live a productive life.

Treatment Options and Outlook

In order for treatment to begin, a complete patient and family history of mood swings and drug use must be taken, and other disorders, such as attention deficit disorder, school phobia, and schizophrenia, must be ruled out. The best treatment for bipolar disorder is a combination of medications and psychotherapy treatment to achieve stabilization of mood swings. It is recommended that a psychiatrist prescribe mood stabilizers such as lithium, carbamazepine (Tegretol) or valproate (Depakote) to prevent the recurrence of mood swings and reduce the risk of SUICIDE. People with bipolar disorder usually are not treated with antidepressants drugs (e.g. Prozac, Paxil, Zoloft) alone, but rather in combination with mood stabilizers because of the risk of switching into manic phase during treatment. Psychotherapy is helpful to the patient and their families in order to help the patient lead a stable and routine life at work and home with fewer hospitalizations. Currently there is no known cure.

Risk Factors and Preventive Measures

There is no one cause for bipolar disorder, and many factors such as genetics, environment, and brain abnormalities contribute to the onset of this disorder. External risk factors that may trigger a bipolar disorder include severe STRESS or trauma, major life events both good (getting married) and bad (losing a job), and seasonal changes (winter brings on DEPRESSION, summer mania). The research of Leverich and Post finds that from one-third to one-half of adults with bipolar disorder report abusive or traumatic experiences in childhood, and those with POSTTRAUMATIC STRESS DISORDER and childhood onset of bipolar disorder were disproportionately represented by those with a history of physical or sexual abuse. Bipolar disorder cannot be prevented, but two in three people will remain symptom free with proper mood-stabilizing medication for life.

Leverich, G. S., R. M. Post. "Course of bipolar illness after history of childhood trauma," *The Lancet* 367, no. 9,516 (April 2006): 1,040–1,042.

body dysmorphic disorder A condition or disorder in which the individual experiences a misperception and distortion of his or her appearance. It is commonly found among individuals with such eating disorders as anorexia nervosa, bulimia nervosa, depressive disorder, POSTTRAUMATIC STRESS DISORDER (PTSD), and OBSESSIVE-COMPULSIVE DISORDER (OCD), but can also occur on its own as a preoccupation with imagined or minor defects in physical features. The most-targeted body areas of concern are skin, hair, nose, weight, stomach, breasts, eyes, thighs, and teeth. When the preoccupation becomes chronic, persistent, and begins to interfere with the individual's social and occupational functioning, then it would be diagnosed by *DSM* standards as body dysmorphic disorder or BDD. About 1 to 2 percent of the population meet all the diagnostic criteria for BDD. There is an obsessive (and usually compulsive) quality to BDD so it is often linked to OCD, but the exact cause is unknown. It appears to be a complex combination of biological factors, personality, and environmental influences. Symptoms generally appear in adolescence or early adulthood, and BDD is found almost equally among men and women.

Symptoms and Diagnostic Path

Individuals with BDD are usually thought to be quite vain and self-absorbed. In fact, they usually feel very ugly, deformed, and unappealing; just the opposite of vanity. The *Broken Mirror* by Katherine Phillips portrays the personal agony of this condition. The psychiatric criteria, based on the *DSM-IV,* for diagnosis of BDD is as follows (with additional items from clinical lore):

- "preoccupation with an imagined defect in appearance—if a slight physical anomaly is present, the person's concern is markedly excessive"
- "preoccupation causes clinically significant distress or impairment in social, occupational, or other important areas of functioning"
- "preoccupation is not better accounted for by another mental disorder (e.g., dissatisfaction with body shape and size in Anorexia Nervosa)"
- chronic obsessive and delusional thoughts about perceived appearance defect
- major depressive disorder symptoms
- social phobias, emptiness, and social isolation
- suicidal ideation
- anxiety; possible panic attacks

- chronic low self-esteem and shame
- avoidance of social encounters, dependency, and difficulty building relationships
- self-medication

BDD is usually associated with much shame, secrecy, and lack of personal insight, and this leads to underdiagnosing by clinicians. It is also not wide spread and co-occurs with other disorders that are more easily diagnosed. Furthermore, individuals with BDD regard their problems as an appearance problem, and therefore they usually seek surgical cosmetic assistance. The high rate of SUICIDE among cosmetic clients suggests that BDD is present but undiagnosed.

If left untreated, the condition generally worsens over time. Likewise, there is a very high rate of suicidal ideation among BDD individuals (80 percent report having suicidal ideation), and an actual suicide rate almost double that seen in major DEPRESSION. Because there are such strong obsessional and compulsive elements to BDD, it has been linked to OCD.

Treatment Options and Outlook

As mentioned, BDD individuals seldom seek psychological treatment and usually do not confide in physicians or friends. Psychotherapy, medications, and COGNITIVE BEHAVIORAL THERAPY (CBT) can usually slow or reverse the velocity of worsening effects. The SELECTIVE SEROTONIN REUPTAKE INHIBITOR (SSRI) medications have proven helpful in treating BDD, but not as robust as cognitive behavioral therapy.

Research indicates that the psychodynamic "talk therapies," or psychoanalysis, are not effective in treating BDD. On the other hand, cognitive behavioral therapy has proven to be effective. For example, in a 1995 study by J. C. Rosen and colleagues in which 54 patients with BDD were randomly assigned to CBT or no treatment, BDD symptoms decreased significantly in those patients undergoing CBT. In fact, BDD was eliminated in 82 percent of cases at post-treatment and 77 percent at follow-up. BDD is a chronic disorder that if left untreated will generally worsen with time, and without treatment, BDD could last a lifetime.

Risk Factors and Preventative Factors

There are no biological or genetic markers found to be consistently associated with BDD. There are indications that teasing by parents or other children is associated but not causative. It appears that a mixture of factors contributes to the development of BDD. In terms of personality, one finds perfectionism, shyness, low-esteem, introvert, and neurotic are commonly seem in pre-BDD individuals. Also, the experience of a major depressive disorder occurs six to seven times more frequently in BDD individuals than in the general population. Research has shown that one-third of BDD individuals will display symptoms of OCD, and a larger than normal proportion will be diagnosed with avoidant personality disorder.

Early identification of these factors is the only preventative strategy at this time, and with the vast overlap with other disorders, it is difficult to predict the adult outcome.

American Psychiatric Association. *Diagnostic and Statistical Manual of Mental Disorders, Fourth Edition.* Washington, D.C.: American Psychiatric Press, 1994.

Rosen, J. C., J. Reiter, and P. Oroson. "Cognitive-Behavioral Body Image Therapy for body dysmorphic disorder." *Journal of Consulting and Clinical Psychology* 63, no. 2 (1995): 263–269.

body memory The concept that the body can recall and reexperience the sensations that were felt at the time of the original experience of trauma or even positive experience. As a result, a body memory may be transformed into chronic pain by some individuals when the trauma remains unresolved. Body memory is also known as implicit memory, or memories that are considered sensation rather than thoughts or images. Note that the concept of body memory is controversial, and it is not accepted by all experts; however, increasing numbers of experts acknowledge that there is a mind-body interaction that may have a profound effect on health and well-being. The basic premise of body memory is that the body does not actually remember past experiences in the same way that the brain remembers them, and instead, body memory is based on sensory associations. In the case of positive body memories, one might delight in a smell of perfume or food associated with positive past events.

It is also true that some individuals with unresolved trauma may somaticize, or be experienced in bodily sensations; for example, individuals who suffered from childhood abuse are more likely to suffer from such chronic muscle disorders as fibromyalgia than those who were not abused. Body memories that cause problems in an individual's daily life may be diagnosed as SOMATOFORM DISORDER.

Other individuals may have a body memory that causes them to resist physical intimacy in adulthood, such as women who were sexually abused as children or women who were raped as adults and have difficulty with physical intimacy. In addition, such women may experience pelvic pain when they attempt to have intercourse with a partner later in life. Body memories are also associated with grief stemming from the loss of a beloved family member or other person.

Body memories may vary from person to person, according to Patricia Hentz, a health professional, in *Qualitative Health Research* on body memories among women who experienced the loss of a loved one. Hentz analyzed the grief of 10 women and considered their responses at the anniversary of the loss of the loved person. One woman became very ill every February and could not understand why she became sick at that time until she made the connection that her mother had died in February. Another woman despised autumn because it was in the fall that her young son had died.

However accepting grief and also learning that others have had similar experiences can help. Said Hentz:

Acknowledging grief and mourning as personal and expanding a view that explores body memory may help to bring out of silence the experiences of these women and others who suffer alone. Body memory is not a rational process that one can work through by using coping strategies. For these women, it requires an honoring and awareness of these deeper experiences of loss. Ignoring them or trying to push the experiences away not only proved to be ineffective but often made it worse. As one participant commented, "One year, I tried

not to experience the loss but it was as if my body took over and I really didn't have any choice."

See also BATTERED CHILD SYNDROME; CELLULAR MEMORY; CHILD ABUSE AND NEGLECT; FELT SENSE; POSTTRAUMATIC STRESS DISORDER; RAPE TRAUMA SYNDROME (RTS); SOMATIC EXPERIENCING; THERAPY, TYPES OF.

Hentz, Patricia. "The Body Remembers: Grieving and a Circle of Time." *Qualitative Health Research* 12, no. 2 (February 2002): 161–172.

bonding See ATTACHMENT STYLES/DISORDERS; TRAUMA BONDING.

borderline personality disorder (BPD) A personality disorder that is characterized by inner chaos, mood changes, raging, and blaming others for one's stress, instability and disorganization in the self-image, combined with distress or impairment in friendships and intimate relations. Many experts, such as the author and psychologist Marsha Linehan in the book *Cognitive-Behavioral Treatment of Borderline Personality Disorder,* believe that the brain development in individuals with borderline personality disorder has been affected by attachment problems and that this underlies the disorder. Recent research suggests that the individual with borderline personality disorder may suffer from a reduced integration between the right and left hemispheres of the brain and that early trauma is present.

There is evidence that the CORPUS CALLOSUM in the brain of people with borderline personality disorders is smaller than normal, and thus communication and coordination between the right and left hemispheres of the brain is affected. This issue could predispose individuals with this disorder to experience abrupt shifts from left- to right-dominated states (e.g., verbal, rational to sensory, emotional) with very different emotional perceptions and memories in any given situation. Thus, friends and associates could be seen in a positive light in one state and then in a negative light when a shift to the opposite hemisphere occurs. This would explain the tendencies toward aggression, emotional instability, difficulty with relationships, mood variations, and empathic variability experienced by the person with borderline personality disorder.

Symptoms and Diagnostic Path

Impulsive behavior, manipulation, distrust of others, emotional instability, and a frequent sense of empty, lonely depression or irritability and anxiety are all symptoms that are frequently present in the individual with borderline personality disorder.

There are inevitable fears of separation and loss and strong reactions to even the possibility of separation and/or loss. SUBSTANCE ABUSE, manipulative suicidal gestures, cutting and other impulsive behaviors are often present in this patient. Estimates are that 10 to 14 percent of the general population in the United States has borderline symptoms to varying degrees.

The 10 common markers or traits that identify the BPD listed in the DIAGNOSTIC AND STATISTICAL MANUAL (DSM) and published by the American Psychiatric Association represent relatively permanent dysfunctional behavioral and emotional dispositions that are manifested mostly within the interpersonal world of the individual. These traits or markers are:

Emotional Regulation

- shifts in mood lasting only a few minutes to hours.

- angry reactions that are inappropriate, out of proportion, intense or uncontrollable and seem to rule the individual

Typical Behavior Patterns

- self-destructive acts, such as self-mutilation, suicidal threats and suicidal gestures that happen relatively frequently usually under stress.

- potentially self-damaging impulsive behaviors. These could include alcohol and drug abuse, compulsive spending, gambling, eating disorders, shoplifting, reckless driving, compulsive sexual behavior.

Identity Confusion

- Marked, persistent identity disturbance shown by uncertainty in at least two areas. These areas can include self-image, sexual orientation, career choice or other long-term goals, friendships, values. People with BPD may not feel as if they know who they are, or what they think, or what their opinions are, or what religion they should be. Instead, they may try to be what they think other people want them to be. Someone with BPD said, "I have a hard time figuring out my personality. I tend to be whomever I'm with."

- Chronic feelings of emptiness or boredom. Someone with BPD said, "I remember describing the feeling of having a deep hole in my stomach. An emptiness that I didn't know how to fill. My therapist told me that was from almost a 'lack of a life.' The more things you get into your life, the more relationships you get involved in, all of that fills that hole. As a borderline, I had no life. There were times when I couldn't stay in the same room with other people. It almost felt like what I think a panic attack would feel like."

Relationships

- splitting: the sense of self and others are viewed as "all good" or "all bad"; forming unstable, chaotic relationships; Alternating clinging and distancing behaviors (I Hate You, Don't Leave Me)

- sensitivity to criticism or rejection, distrust, neediness, reassurance and affection oriented and a high degree of sensitivity, insight, and empathy with others but not self

- transient, stress-related paranoid ideation or severe dissociative symptoms

Other attributes of individuals with BPD

- They are often viewed as bright, witty, funny, life of the party, and quick.

- They may have problems with object constancy. When a person leaves (even temporarily), they may have a problem recreating or remembering feelings of love that were present between themselves and the other. Often, BPD patients want to keep something belonging to the loved one around during separations.

- They frequently have difficulty tolerating alone-ness, even for short periods of time.
- Their lives may be a chaotic landscape of job losses, interrupted educational pursuits, broken engagements, and hospitalizations. Many have a background of childhood physical, sexual, or emotional abuse, or physical/emotional neglect.

While there are some checklists for diagnosing the borderline, for the most part the clinical interview is the most effective diagnostic instrument. These clinical interviews focus on past behavior, developmental stages, emotional modulation, and the nature of interpersonal relationships.

Treatment Options and Outlook

Individuals with borderline personality disorder are difficult to treat and usually require a great amount of structure and directedness within the therapy. If they also have ANXIETY DISORDERS and/or DEPRESSION, these problems can be treated with therapy and medications. Many therapists argue that only in-patient, structured (phase-oriented or stages or progressions) and intense behavioral therapy (guided learning in relaxation, cognitive and emotional control and interpersonal effectiveness) will be effective because the borderline does not have self-guided or self-insightful behavior. Unfortunately, there is little evidence that medications can treat the borderline condition, although they may be used to stabilize chaotic behaviors.

Risk Factors and Preventive Measures

Borderline personality disorder is probably the most controversial of the personality disorders because there seems to be a high percentage of individuals with some or all of these traits, diagnosis is fairly subjective, and variability is enormous among defining characteristics. Recent research, however, points to early trauma, abuse, and interpersonal victimization as potential contributors to the disorder as an adult, with a high percentage of individuals diagnosed with BPD reporting early sexual and interpersonal abuse. Failures in the relationship between mother and infant, particularly during the separation and identity-forming phases of childhood, have been observed in

many people with borderline personality disorder. Because of the tendency to split people in relationships, a borderline can cause grief and chaos within a family unit, pitting members against one another. Likewise, in social relations, close relationship can be shattered quickly with anger, paranoia, distrust, and portrayal of people as "good" or "bad."

There are no known preventive measures to borderline personality disorder. However, strong motivation, training in interpersonal perception and skills, and calming or relaxation procedures can produce widespread and enduring positive changes.

See also ASSOCIATED DISORDERS; DIAGNOSTIC INTERVIEW FOR BORDERLINES-REVISED (DIB-R); TREATMENT: PSYCHOTHERAPY, PSYCHOPHARMACOLOGY, AND ALTERNATIVE MEDICINE.

Linehan, M. *Cognitive-Behavioral Treatment of Borderline Personality Disorder.* New York: Guilford Press, 1993.

brain The brain is a trillion-cell neurological structure contained in the skull that modulates experience of the outside and inside worlds and, in humans, provides a structure for thinking and higher mental processes. Until the 1990s, the human brain was thought to work much like a computer, receiving, sending out, and processing information, but operating within a fixed and prewired structure. Intelligence and most abilities were believed to be set in specialized areas, and consequently, damage to an area in the brain could not be repaired or restored. "Personality" was believed to be shaped by genetics and one's early experiences, but the brain itself was simply the container for personality and was not itself formed by these developmental experiences.

New technology has allowed for advances and discoveries that have dramatically changed the perception of the development, growth, and workings of the brain. No longer seen as a fixed-for-life structure, the brain is now clearly recognized as an experience-dependent social organ that is intimately affected by the external world and that will evolve throughout the individual's lifespan. Its basic construction is designed for survival in the small hunter-gatherer groups of social organization that humankind formed. Since it is a social organ, early life experience has a profound effect on brain growth and functioning. This entry offers a look at the brain's effects on adult functioning.

Physiological functioning seeks homeostasis, or the optimal levels of functioning and operation. All systems, parts, and even the cells of the body work toward a steady, optimal state. The outside world, however, can cause changes and disruptions in the state of the body and the brain. The study of stress disorders such as POSTTRAUMATIC STRESS DISORDER (PTSD), DEPRESSION, anxiety states, learning disabilities, and health problems has allowed experts to see the difference between normal stress responses (where the body returns to a state of regulation or optimal functioning) and traumatic stress responses that dysregulate the organism. Dysregulation in the body is characteristic of PTSD, but the basic structure of the brain should be considered before examining dysfunction.

The Basic Structure of the Brain

Early social experience helps shape the anatomy, neuro-circuitry, and templates for thoughts, feelings, and behavior. The brain is organized into four interconnected major areas: the brainstem, diencephalon, LIMBIC SYSTEM, and cerebral cortex. Each area provides a specialized function and interconnection with the other areas. The hierarchy of brain function begins at the spinal cord termination and the brain cell differentiation level (and areas that have the fewest cells) called the brainstem, or the lower part of the brain where it connects to the spinal cord. Paul Maclean, M.D., a neuroscientist, defined the brainstem as the lowest level of brain function that mediates primitive life functions and is a distinct tie to the reptilian heritage of humans. Since it is similar in structure and functioning to the brain of reptiles, it is also called the *R-Complex*. The cranial nerves also originate at this level.

The diencephalon is the next level up from the brainstem and consists mainly of the thalamus and hypothalamus. These areas of the brain relay the transmission of information about sensation and movement, and controls the mechanism for maintaining homeostasis. Looking only at functional aspects, it is clear that all sensory and motor

information (except olfaction, or the process of smelling) comes through the thalamus and then to specific sensory and motor areas of the cerebral cortex. Consequently, most neural input to the cerebral cortex comes from the thalamus. During times of STRESS, the thalamus works with the HIPPOCAMPUS and AMYGDALA to filter sensory input and coordinate the relay of this information. It may be that the pace of the thalamus slows after traumatic events, thus causing "numbness" and reduced experience, while other areas of the brain activate the body and produce chronic arousal. There has always been some confusion why both arousal and NUMBING occur at the same time in PTSD. Future research will test this hypothesis.

The hypothalamus is under the thalamus at the base of the brain, and it is the major visceral, or sensory information, control center of the brain. It is said that the hypothalamus is "the door from the brain to the body." It is also involved in limbic system functions as well. The hypothalamus controls the AUTONOMIC NERVOUS SYSTEM and the endocrine system, made up of glands that secretes hormones, and organizes behaviors related to survival of the species: fight, flight, freeze, feeding, and mating. The pituitary gland is attached to the lower base of the hypothalamus, and through this connection the hypothalamus controls much of the endocrine or hormonal system. It is here that neurons interface with neuropeptides that travel to the pituitary gland and stimulate the release of hormones throughout the body. These hormones regulate body temperature, appetite, sexual behavior, fear and aggression, and the sleep cycle. The hypothalamus also serves as a gateway for the brain to stimulate STRESS responses in the body, such as increased heart rate, elevated blood pressure, and the divergence of energy to the muscles and the brain.

The limbic system is next on the hierarchy. Its primary function is to overlay the motivational and emotional aspects of experiences. Learning and memory formation and retrieval are centered in the hippocampus area of the limbic system. Emotional memories primarily originate from the amygdala, which also controls feelings and expression of emotions and recognition of the signs of emotions in other people. It evolved from the human need for social organization and interaction and for emotionally fixing upon dangerous predators.

The cerebral cortex is the most complex part of the brain, and it contains more than 50 percent of all the neurons in the brain. The cerebral cortex mediates all conscious activity, including planning, problem solving, language, and speech. It is also involved in perception and voluntary motor behavior. The cerebral cortex has five main parts: the frontal lobes, temporal lobes, parietal lobes, occipital lobes and the CORPUS CALLOSUM. The lobes have somewhat specialized functions for motor behavior, vision, orientation in space and time, hearing, kinesthetic, and comprehension of language. The corpus callosum consists of a large bundle of nerves that connect the right and left hemispheres (sides) of the brain.

The blood-brain barrier is an efficient system that blocks infections from entering the brain, as bacterial molecules are too large to pass through the blood-brain barrier. Throughout the brain there are hundreds of miles of blood vessels that regulate nutrients and prevent toxic substances from entering the brain through a vascular protective system that forms the blood-brain barrier. STRESS can alter the ability of chemical molecules to pass through the blood-brain barrier and compromise the equilibrium of the brain against toxic substances.

Key Brain Systems Involved in Threat, Fear, Trauma, and Stress

The brainstem is the physical survival system and has projections into all areas of the brain. The reticular activating system (RAS) within the brain stem consists of bundles of ascending nerves that alert individuals to changes in stimulation by activating cortical and limbic processes. The RAS is a part of the brain central for arousal and motivation and works to bring relevant information to one's attention. Consequently, the RAS is the driver for arousal, fear, stress, and threats. The primary nuclei in the RAS for the chemical or hormonal activation of the body and brain is the LOCUS COERULEUS, which functions as a specific activator and also sets the general tone for body arousal.

For example, acute stress results in an increase in locus coeruleus activation, which in turn, activates the body and brain. The person could feel aroused or possibly anxious and fearful if activation is intense. If the stressor is released, the body will usually return to normal. Otherwise, the body will remain activated to some extent, and the general physiological state will result in chronic difficulty sleeping, vigilance, restlessness, affective modulation difficulties, and exaggerated startle responses.

The hippocampus is located between the brainstem and the cortex and plays a major role in MEMORY, particularly episodic or body memory for stress events. Exposure to previously stressful or traumatic events or events that are similar will be "remembered" and trigger a hippocampal response which, in turn, results in an arousal/anxiety reaction in the brain and body. As part of the arousal response, CORTISOL is released from the adrenal glands. If arousal remains chronic, cortisol will atrophy the hippocampal structure over time. Atrophy to parts of the hippocampus creates problems with memory and learning and tend to fire up the arousal system too easily.

The amygdala is the second important trauma and stress structure. The amygdala is adjacent to the hippocampus, and it is key to the processing, interpretation and integration of emotional functioning, and it is the command center of the brain's fear system. It receives input from the thalamus, hypothalamus, and hippocampus and determines the emotional value of these inputs both from the outside and the inside world (including the imagination) and activates a body-wide emergency response. In a landmark series of studies, LeDoux has shown that the amygdala plays a key role in terms of emotional reactions to memory and experience. It activates the autonomic system and the cortex to sensations or perceptions of threat.

Specific Brain Response to Trauma

Some parts of the brain are specific responders to traumatic events. Such parts include the amygdala and the corpus callosum.

In the brain, the cingulate gyrus sits above the corpus callosum, and it is part of the limbic system in the brain. The anterior cingulate cortex plays a role in decision making, empathy, and emotion and is the storehouse of old, lifelong memories. It helps individuals come up with a solution when faced with a number of choices. A number of psychiatric disorders (depression, OBSESSIVE-COMPULSIVE DISORDER (OCD)) have been linked with abnormalities of the anterior cingulated cortex.

The posterior area of the cingulate gyrus is involved in processing information in time and space and may be responsible for decisions in life-threatening situations.

The outer folded layer of the cerebrum is the cerebral cortex, or gray matter. The cerebral cortex is two to 4.5 mm thick and divided into lobes named after the overlaying cranial bones: the frontal, parietal, occipital, and temporal bones. The cerebral cortex is responsible for human intelligence, memory, vision, language, thinking ability, social behavior, and consciousness.

The frontal cortex reflects the difference between humans and all other animals, including human ancestors in evolutionary terms. It allows for planning, thinking, and taking action. The medial prefrontal cortex is the area just above the eyes and is responsible for regulating emotion, including the ability to diminish fear responses. Abnormalities to the frontal cortex are linked to most psychiatric disorders, including posttraumatic stress disorder (PTSD).

See also CENTRAL NERVOUS SYSTEM; CHILD ABUSE AND NEGLECT; PARASYMPATHETIC NERVOUS SYSTEM; SYMPATHETIC NERVOUS SYSTEM; TRAUMATIC BRAIN INJURY.

breathing retraining   Individuals under severe STRESS often take rapid and shallow breaths and may gulp in air. Tension in the chest muscles develops and can become chronic with time. This serves to exacerbate the individual's stress level and produce symptoms of HYPERVENTILATION SYNDROME: difficulty breathing, numbness, tingling in extremities, stomachaches, dizziness, and DISSOCIATION of place and time.

Many of these symptoms can be reversed with breathing retraining, but retraining takes time and practice in order to replace the typical tension-mediated patterns. The vagus nerve from the BRAIN controls parasympathetic or calming activity in the body. Activation of the vagus nerve produces slower more rhythmic breaths and a slower heart beat and lowers blood pressure, activities of calm-ing. In the calmer state, the body moves from an acidic state to an alkaline state that is associated with relaxation. Hyperventilation is a chronic state of activation in which the body chemistry is on the acidic side.

One way to activate the vagus response and produce a more relaxed state is through patterned breathing exercises. These involve the production of slow exhalations that allow carbon dioxide in the body to enter the bloodstream and change the pH levels to a more alkaline level. This effect is immediate in terms of the development of noticeable relaxation. Slow exhalations produce immediate reductions in heart rate and pressure. Typically, breath retraining involves learning diaphragmatic or "stomach" breathing so that exhalations can be lengthened.

See also PROGRESSIVE RELAXATION.

Briquet's syndrome   A form of long-term mental disturbance that is expressed in physical complaints, yet there is no valid identified medical basis for these complaints. Briquet's syndrome is a form of HYSTERIA or SOMATIZATION DISORDER. Briquet's syndrome differs from hypochondriasis in that it is usually more severe and longer-lasting and is less responsive to treatment. To receive this diagnosis, a person must display a range of complaints, including pain, gastrointestinal ailments, sexual symptoms, and a neurological-based symptom.

Briquet's syndrome was named after the French physician Paul Briquet, who wrote an article about hysteria in 1859. Briquet's syndrome is most common among women. Affected females generally live a life of chronic invalidism, constantly seek medical attention and relief, and are frustrated by vague or no diagnoses. They may have had multiple surgeries. The symptoms of this syndrome are first seen in adolescence or before the age of 30.

The syndrome is significantly associated with DISSOCIATION according to a 1993 study reported in the *American Journal of Psychiatry* by Pribor, et al. Individuals with Briquet's syndrome dissociate or detach from parts of their body and mentally impose on those parts some serious medical malady.

Symptoms and Diagnostic Path

Based on the DIAGNOSTIC AND STATISTICAL MANUAL *of Mental Disorders, Fourth Edition, Text Revision, (DSM-IV-TR)*, there are specific types of symptoms that are present with Briquet's syndrome. These include a history of medical complaints and pain in at least four areas of the body or with several functions, such as menstruation, urination, or sexual intercourse. In addition, there must be a history of at least two gastrointestinal complaints other than pain, such as nausea and bloating or irritable bowel syndrome without gastrointestinal studies that identify any medical problem. Further, there must be a sexual or reproductive complaint other than pain, such as menstrual difficulties in women or erectile dysfunction in men. Last, there must be a symptom indicating a possible neurological disorder, such as urinary retention, double vision, impaired coordination, and other symptoms.

Before diagnosing Briquet's syndrome, it is important for physicians to rule out general medical conditions that may mimic this syndrome, such as systemic lupus erythematosus, multiple sclerosis, Lyme disease, and chronic parasitic disease.

In a study of 37 women with Briquet's syndrome and 29 women with primary affective disorder (DEPRESSION) reported in *Psychosomatic Medicine* in 1994, the researchers administered the Minnesota Multiphasic Personality Inventory (MMPI) Study to all subjects. They found that the women with Briquet's syndrome were significantly less logical and consistent in their responses than were the women with depression. They also found that the subjects with Briquet's syndrome had more psychological/interpersonal problems and more somatic symptoms than the depressed women.

An earlier study of 188 psychiatric patients, of whom 16 patients (9 percent) had Briquet's syndrome, appeared in the *American Journal of Psychiatry* in 1989. The patients with Briquet's syndrome had experienced multiple surgeries, menstrual symptoms, and general sickliness. The researchers sought to find an association between Briquet's syndrome and other psychiatric disorders, such as major depression, PANIC DISORDER, or agoraphobia. They found that the patients with Briquet's syndrome were more likely to have depression *and* either panic disorder or agoraphobia, rather than having depression or panic disorder or agoraphobia alone.

Said author Orenstein, "The author proposes that Briquet's syndrome may represent the most extreme expression of a tendency for a number of physical and psychological syndromes to aggregate." He added further:

> The diagnosis of Briquet's syndrome is often overlooked, especially in patients with prominent psychological symptoms. In part, this may reflect the fact that depressive symptoms in Briquet's syndrome are identical to those seen in primary depression in the course of other psychiatric illnesses. One implication of the present study is that a high index of suspicion for Briquet's syndrome is advisable whenever evaluating women with a history of both panic attacks and depression.

Treatment Options and Outlook

Briquet's syndrome can be very difficult to treat because the patient is usually convinced that she or he is truly physically ill and that physicians, for unknown reasons, have not yet found the true cause of the illness. Psychiatric treatment is recommended for this syndrome, but the patient may resist it. Whenever possible, accompanying disorders such as depression should be treated. In some cases, treating secondary disorders such as depression seem to improve the primary disorder of Briquet's syndrome.

Risk Factors and Preventive Measures

Less than 1 percent of the population in the United States suffers from Briquet's syndrome, and most are female. However, according to the *DSM*, somatization disorder has been observed in 10 to 20 percent of the female first-degree biological relatives of women with the disorder. In addition, an adoptive parent or biological parent with either antisocial personality disorder, substance-related disorder, or SOMATIZATION DISORDER increases the risk to the child of developing one of these disorders as well. Individuals with Briquet's syndrome have a higher rate of having experienced CHILD PHYSICAL ABUSE and CHILD SEXUAL ABUSE than those without the disorder.

Women with Briquet's syndrome often have other psychiatric problems, such as depression and ANXIETY DISORDERS. Men with Briquet's syndrome are more likely than women to have antisocial personality disorder and to engage in excessive drinking and the commission of criminal acts.

There are no known preventive measures against Briquet's syndrome.

See also HISTORICAL FACTORS; SOMATIC EXPERIENCING THERAPY; SOMATIZATION; SOMATOFORM DISSOCIATION; SOMATOFORM DISSOCIATION QUESTIONNAIRE.

American Psychiatric Association. *Diagnostic and Statistical Manual of Mental Disorders. Fourth Edition. Text Revision.* (*DSM-IV-TR*). Washington, D.C.: American Psychiatric Press, 2000.

Orenstein, Herbert, M.D., "Briquet's Syndrome in Association with Depression and Panic: A Reconceptualization of Briquet's Syndrome." *American Journal of Psychiatry* 146, no. 3 (March 1989): 334–338.

Pribor, E. F., et al., "Briquet's Syndrome, Dissociation, and Abuse." *American Journal of Psychiatry* 150 (1993): 1,507–1,511.

Wetzel, Richard D., et al., "Briquet's Syndrome (Hysteria) is Both a Somatoform and a 'Psychoform' Illness: A Minnesota Multiphasic Personality Inventory Study." *Psychosomatic Medicine* 56 (1994): 564–569.

"bullycide" and bullying *Bullycide* is a slang term that refers to the murder of a bully, while bullying is the act of intimidating specific others, either to cause them to take some action or sometimes solely for the purpose of humiliation. In most cases, individuals victimized by bullies are considerably physically weaker and smaller than is the bully. Children and adolescents with physical or learning disabilities or with illnesses such as diabetes are more likely bullied, as are those who are obese.

Both children and adults are bullied. Being bullied can cause lifelong trauma to victims, who feel that they must be weak and ineffectual since they were bullied. It is also problematic for the bully, who is at risk for increasing acts of violence into adulthood and eventual incarceration.

Some bullied children have lashed out at their tormentors and have murdered them as well as others whom the victim believed had sympathized with the bully. In contrast, bullies usually do not murder their victims, and instead they enjoy watching the suffering of the victim, particularly when both the bully and the victim are in the presence of others. For this reason, most bullies travel in groups to provide a ready audience to the attacks and the victim's anticipated response.

Often parents and others advise bullied children that they should fight the bully, which is irrational and impractical advice. Bullies are nearly always much larger and with significantly greater strength than the victim, and consequently they could cause severe harm to the victim in any altercation. Instead, parents should seek for the bullying to end by making contact with school officials, the parents of the bully, and others. In some cases, legal threats must be made and carried out. It is a very difficult situation for both the child and the parents. However, if the parents do nothing, the child will feel that the parents do not care or do not understand the torment that he or she is suffering.

Most bullies are males, but some females exhibit bullying behavior. In general, female bullies rely far more on psychological torment, such as name calling or passing around unfounded and cruel rumors about the victim, and females usually do not physically attack the victim. In contrast, male bullies use both the threat of physical force and psychological intimidation, such as name calling. Male bullies may carry out their threats of physical violence, although the intimidation and the fear of threats are often sufficiently effective to terrify the victim, which is the goal of the bully.

Sometimes bullies, particularly male bullies, demand money or other items from the victim, and some victims have stolen from their parents to obtain the money or items that the bully demands—all to avoid a beating from the bully.

Bullies may be subjected to abuse at home, and they may be acting out the abuse that they have learned; however, not all bullies are abused children.

Studies have shown that bullies initially harass many children, often at the beginning of the school year, and then they target the particular children who seem to be the most vulnerable to bullying.

It is unfortunate but true that often children who are bullied are shunned by other children, including children who are not associated with the bully or those who surround him or her. The victim is perceived as a person to avoid, in part because the bully might attack any defenders and also because the victim is seen as an unpopular person.

In a study of 853 undergraduate students (59 percent female), reported by Newman et al. in the *Journal of Adolescence* in 2005, the researchers obtained information from these college students on their past experiences with bullying. One-third of the sample said that before high school they were bullied occasionally, and 26 percent said that they were bullied frequently. While they were in high school, 25 percent said that they were bullied occasionally, and 9 percent said they were frequently bullied.

The researchers also analyzed STRESS symptoms and found that bullied females reported more stress symptoms that did males. They also discovered that how isolated the individual felt was a factor in the degree of stress. Said the researchers, "Those who were bullied frequently in high school, but for whatever reason did not perceive a lack of social support, reported fewer stress symptoms in college." The researchers recommended that schools should consider helping to create social support networks for bullied children and teenagers.

Demographics of Bullied Children

Reports on the percentages of bullied children in the United States vary. According to *Indicators of School Crime and Safety: 2005*, 7.2 percent of children ages 12 to 18 reported being bullied in school in the past six months in 2003. Other studies have shown that about a third of all students have reported being ever bullied, while 5 to 10 percent have said that they were regularly victimized by bullies.

Of the bullied children in the school crime and safety study, most (7.8 percent) were male, while 6.5 percent were female. Most (7.8 percent) were white, followed by the category of "Other" (6.8 percent). From grades 6 through 12, the greatest percentage of bullied children (13.9 percent) was in the sixth grade, followed by seventh grade (12.7 percent). Of bullied children, children in rural areas (9.7 percent) were more likely to be bullied than children in urban areas (6.7 percent) or suburban areas (6.6 percent).

Homicides Involving Bullies

Based on a study reported in the *Journal of the American Medical Association* of school-associated violent deaths in the United States, 1994–99, students who commit homicide are said to have suffered bullying by their peers. Homicides at school are rare, but some patterns have been identified. Said the authors:

> In our study, perpetrators were more likely than victims to have been described as having been bullied by their peers. These bullied youth may represent the "provocative" or "aggressive" victims described in recent studies on bullying behavior, who often retaliate in an aggressive manner in response to being bullied.

The researchers also found that violent deaths at school were most likely to occur at the start of school in the morning, during lunch, or at the end of the school day, but were distributed over the school year

Behaviors of Victims and Bullies

According to *Take Action Against Bullying*, a booklet published by the Substance Abuse and Mental Health Services Administration (SAMHSA), some warning signs that a child may be experiencing bullying are a child who

- frequently complains of illness
- brings home damaged possessions or reports them as "lost"
- has few or no friends
- talks about running away and/or SUICIDE
- displays "victim" body language, such as avoiding eye contact, hanging the head, and hunching the shoulders
- threatens violence to oneself or others
- cries easily and talks about hopelessness
- has changes in sleeping and eating patterns
- has or has attempted to take items of protection to school, such as a gun, knife, stick, or other weapons

Warning signs that a child may be a bully are the child who

- enjoys feeling powerful and in control (whether these feelings are valid or not)
- lacks empathy toward others

- has a history of discipline problems
- seeks to dominate and/or manipulate others
- is a poor winner (arrogant and boastful) and a poor loser
- becomes excited by conflicts between others
- has shown uncontrolled anger
- displays a pattern of impulsive and chronic intimidating, aggressive and hitting behaviors
- is adept at hiding behaviors so that adults do not notice what they are doing

Based on school shootings and violent behavior in schools, schools are more likely to take bullying seriously than in past years, and some states have passed laws banning bullying in schools. Prior bullying experienced by the perpetrators, as in the Columbine school shootings of 1999, link to outbreaks of violence later on.

See also CHILD ABUSE AND NEGLECT; CHILDREN AND TRAUMA.

Anderson, Mark, M.D., et al., "School-Associated Violent Deaths in the United States, 1994–1999." *Journal of the American Medical Association* 286, no. 21 (December 5, 2001): 2,595–2,702.

Clark, Robin, and Judith Clark with Christine Adamec. *The Encyclopedia of Child Abuse. 3rd ed.* New York: Facts On File, 2007.

DeVoe, J. F., et al. *Indicators of School Crime and Safety: 2005.* Washington, D.C.: U.S. Government Printing Office, 2005.

Newman, Matthew L., George W. Holden, and Yvon Delville, "Isolation and the Stress of Being Bullied." *Journal of Adolescence* 28 (2005): 343–357.

Substance Abuse and Mental Health Services Administration. *Take Action Against Bullying.* Washington D.C.: U.S. Department of Health and Human Services, 2003.

CAPS, CAPS-1, CAPS-2 & CAPS-CA Clinician-Administered PTSD Scale. See ASSESSMENT AND DIAGNOSIS.

catecholamine Naturally occurring chemical compounds in the body acting as hormones and NEUROTRANSMITTERS. The most common catecholamines are EPINEPHRINE, NOREPINEPHRINE, and dopamine. They are similar to one another chemically by having a catechol to which an amine or nitrogen group is attached. A catecholamine responds to stress by preparing the body for FIGHT OR FLIGHT RESPONSE. In general, they serve to activate the body in preparation for action.

Epinephrine is both a hormone and a neurotransmitter. It is released by the adrenal medulla and plays an important role in stress reaction, such as when the body perceives danger or a threatening situation. Epinephrine increases the heart rate, dilates the pupils, and constricts the small capillaries in the skin while dilating the arteries in muscles. It also increases blood glucose levels. The term *adrenaline* comes from a name given a synthetic form of epinephrine that has come into common usage.

Norepinephrine is a neurotransmitter located mainly in the brainstem, the area known as the LOCUS COERULEUS, which transports signals within the synaptic brain. It is also a hormone released by the adrenal glands. As a stress hormone, along with epinephrine, it affects the fight or flight response through the SYMPATHETIC NERVOUS SYSTEM by increasing heart rate and releasing energy to the muscles and brain. Panic and anxiety attacks are associated with this neurotransmitter.

See also BRAIN; PHYSIOLOGY OF TRAUMA.

causes/risk factors of traumatic stress disorders There are many different risk factors that increase the likelihood that a person will develop a TRAUMATIC STRESS disorder. In many cases, a problem may be both a cause and a risk factor. Some people have a much greater RESILIENCE to the effects of adverse effects than others, and they can seemingly "bounce back," even from great adversity. This is more likely among individuals who have a positive support group and who are basically self-confident.

For example, CHILD ABUSE AND NEGLECT is one cause of traumatic stress in children, and it is also a risk factor for a plethora of problems experienced by the abused person in adulthood. As adults, individuals who were traumatized at an early age by their parents, caretakers, or significant others often have difficulties bonding closely with others and have high DIVORCE rates. They also often show evidence of serious interpersonal problems that are centered on the issue of trust and the lack of trust. Women who are abused by their spouses or partners are at risk for developing BATTERED WOMAN SYNDROME, a type of traumatic stress disorder. Victims of battered woman syndrome exhibit traumatic symptoms in the form of anxiety, DEPRESSION, fear, low self-esteem, and extreme sense of vulnerability.

A TRAUMATIC BRAIN INJURY, which may be incurred in an accident, is also a risk factor and a possible cause for a traumatic stress disorder because of the effects of both the trauma and the injury.

RETRAUMATIZATION, as with a person who is abused or raped more than once, is another cause as well as a risk factor for the development of a traumatic stress disorder. SEQUENTIAL TRAUMATIZATION, or experiencing different traumas one right after the other, such as a death in the family immediately followed by a natural disaster, can also trigger or increase the likelihood of the development of a traumatic stress disorder.

Experiencing DISASTER SYNDROME, or an individual's severe response to distressing and traumatic natural events and their aftermaths, such as tsunamis, hurricanes, blizzards, or other severe weather phenomena, can trigger a traumatic stress disorder in some people. This is particularly true if individuals have lost loved ones in the disaster and/or have lost their own homes. TERRORISM and the fear of terrorist attacks are also causes and risk factors for the development of traumatic stress disorders.

Individuals who have suffered TORTURE often develop a traumatic stress disorder called POST TORTURE SYNDROME. It is distinguished from POST-TRAUMATIC STRESS DISORDER (PTSD) because both the traumatic events themselves and the effects of the torture together produce posttraumatic stress symptoms. Often the underlying goal of torture is to physically and psychologically immobilize the individual. Both the physical pain and the emotional anxiety caused by torture may generate a traumatic stress reaction in the victim.

SECONDARY TRAUMATIZATION develops when an individual does not experience a trauma directly, but clearly sees its effects on others and empathizes with them to the point of developing a traumatic stress disorder. Secondary traumatization is also known as VICARIOUS TRAUMATIZATION or COMPASSION FATIGUE. Individuals affected by secondary traumatization include fire and police officials, as well as emergency and health professionals and mental health professionals.

Sometimes the internal mental process of KINDLING can trigger the development of a traumatic stress disorder. This refers to an external stimulus, such as something that induces extreme fear or dread, that triggers the FIGHT OR FLIGHT RESPONSE in the brain. For example, a major accident may be perceived as life threatening by the victim. Memories of past severe traumas may then be triggered, causing a repetition of the sensations that were experienced at the time of the original trauma. This repetitive cycle of sensation and brain reactions, most often associated with dissociation and

avoidance, is the kindling effect that perpetuates the trauma.

Some people who suffer from stress experience SUBTHRESHHOLD POSTTRAUMATIC STRESS DISORDER, which is a reaction to a traumatic experience that does not reach the definition of posttraumatic stress disorder (PTSD) as defined by the *DIAGNOSTIC AND STATISTICAL MANUAL (DSM)* produced by the American Psychiatric Association. Although not clinically defined as PTSD, subthreshold PTSD can increase the likelihood of the development of depression and SUBSTANCE ABUSE.

Child Abuse and Neglect

The effects of childhood trauma usually show up directly in the child's experience; for example, traumatized children may have an ALTERED PAIN PERCEPTION and consequently, they must learn to perceive tactile stimuli accurately. In addition, traumatized children must also learn to be able to talk about their past traumatic experiences in a safe environment.

Some severely abused children develop DISSOCIATIVE DISORDERS, such as dissociative identity disorder, once known as multiple personality disorder, or the development of separate identities within the same person. This disorder develops as a means to cope with otherwise unbearable trauma, such as the physical or sexual attack of a child by a family member or other trusted person.

Some traumatized children abuse alcohol and drugs, while others may exhibit cutting and self-mutilation behaviors, but the most common forms of coping among children are withdrawal and isolation. Some traumatized children develop paranoid ideas, seeing personal attacks where they are not made, while others seem numb to the activities that other children find stimulating and interesting.

Adults who experienced childhood abuse have an increased risk for the following problems:

- abuse of their children
- substance abuse
- depression and other psychiatric disorders
- chronic pain and chronic diseases
- SUICIDE

In considering psychiatric disorders, according to *The Encyclopedia of Child Abuse,* childhood abuse almost triples the risk of a person suffering from an ANXIETY DISORDER or mood disorder in adulthood, and it also doubles the risk of phobias. In addition, adults who were abused as children have about 10 times the risk of suffering from a PANIC DISORDER in adulthood compared to nonabused adults. The earlier the abuse occurs in a child's life, the more profound the ultimate effects in adulthood.

Emotional abuse in childhood also increases the risk for adult suicide. In a study reported in the *Journal of the American Medical Association* in 2001, the researchers found that of those subjects who experienced no emotional abuse as a child, 2.5 percent attempted suicide; however, among subjects who *had* experienced emotional abuse as children, 14 percent had attempted suicide.

Battered Women

Often women who are repeatedly abused by their spouse or partner believe that they are hopelessly entrapped in their current situation. Domestic violence is a serious problem in the United States, and according to the National Center for Post-traumatic Stress Disorder, an estimated 1.3 million women are physically assaulted by an intimate partner each year. In addition, 20 to 30 percent of women in the United States are physically abused by a partner at least once in their lives, and nearly a third (30 percent) of women who are murdered are killed by their male partners. An estimated 30 to 40 percent of emergency room visits are caused by injuries incurred during incidents of domestic violence.

PTSD is also common among battered women; in one study of 91 battered women, published in the *Journal of Interpersonal Violence* in 2002, the majority (51.6 percent) had PTSD. The National Center for Posttraumatic Stress Disorder says that predictive indicators of abuse include a history of battering in the past, verbal threats of violence by the abuser as well as the abuser breaking objects and using force when arguing. In addition, some warning signs of future battering are

- cruelty to children and animals
- rapid mood changes

- unreasonable jealousy
- verbal abuse and blaming others for problems
- controlling behavior

Battered women may exhibit a LEARNED HELP-LESSNESS, believing that there is nothing they can do to improve their current situation despite the urgings of family members and others to leave the abuser. The reason for this may be *traumatic bonding,* the link between the abused woman and the abuser that develops in part because the abuser is intermittently cruel and kind. Battered women can break away for many reasons; for example, if the batterer begins to attack their or her child or if the abuse is so severe that victim is hospitalized. If the victim is treated for the depression that occurs in an estimated 60 percent of battered women, her improved mood may enable her to break away from the abuser. Therapy can also help battered women realize that the abuser cannot or will not change and that their lives are in danger and they must leave. As with child abuse and neglect, battered women syndrome involves human-against-human violations, and this is one of the greatest risk factors for development of PTSD and trauma-related disorders.

Traumatic Brain Injury

A traumatic brain injury (TBI) is a severe injury of the BRAIN caused by a jolt or blow to the head or by a penetrating injury that impedes the normal functioning of the brain. Psychiatric problems are common among patients with TBIs, and families may find it extremely difficult to deal with the personality and behavioral changes that occur. Patients may exhibit aggression and violence, as well as emotional outbursts. Some patients' personality changes so much that they show many characteristics associated with BORDERLINE PERSONALITY DISORDER although they do not have the life-long pattern seen in this disorder.

Children injured with a TBI may fail to mature emotionally after the injury occurs.

Individuals with TBIs may suffer from severe headaches, as well as sensitivity to light and noise and sleep disturbances. They may also have difficulties with MEMORY, attention, and language.

Often, people with TBIs have serious psychiatric symptoms, such as depression, anxiety, impulsivity, and inappropriate laughter. Some of the symptoms that may be seen with individuals with TBIs may resemble those that are seen among patients with posttraumatic stress disorder (PTSD).

Some patients with TBI suffer from antero-grade or retrograde POSTTRAUMATIC AMNESIA (PTA). Retrograde PTA is an impaired memory of events that occurred *before* the TBI happened, while anterograde PTA is an impaired memory of the events that occurred *after* the TBI. Some TBI patients may also suffer from severe language and communication problems, such as aphasia, which is the difficulty in understanding language and speaking.

Retraumatization and Sequential Traumatization

Retraumatization occurs when the victim experiences the same type of abuse as was suffered in the past, such as when she or he is raped or assaulted again. Retraumatization may also occur in therapy if patients are led to describe a traumatic event in detail. As a result, good therapists are very cautious before asking a patient to relive an event by relating what happened to them.

With regard to sequential traumatization, multiple or "pile-on" tragic events are not only difficult for an individual to cope with, but it also takes a long time to process and resolve these events. Events that are the most likely to have lasting effects on individuals are the early separation from or loss of parents and early traumatization from experiences such as surgeries, isolation, or accidents. Sequential or multiple traumas that occur early in the individual's life have the most profound effect on adult behavior and the risk for the development of some or all PTSD symptoms. Furthermore, normal developmental (physical and psychological) stages are often blunted or disrupted, and these have life effects unless addressed in some form of therapy.

Disaster Syndrome

Disaster syndrome results from experiencing a frightening natural disaster and its aftermath. Common indicators include the following:

- a feeling of disorientation, being in a daze, apathy, passivity, and feeling stunned
- concern for loved ones and the community, altruism, appreciation for help that is received
- a strong identification with the community and a desire to restore it to normalcy again
- the presence of ambivalent feelings and the search for meaning from the traumatic event itself

Treatment focuses on the experience itself. Almost any verified trauma treatment will have a positive effect on single incident trauma such as disaster syndrome.

Terrorism and Post Torture Syndrome

Fear of terrorism can trigger a traumatic stress disorder, even when the individual has not directly experienced torture or a terrorist attack. The psychological impact of terrorism on the public has intensified in recent years due to extended media coverage and Internet Web site postings by many terrorist groups predicting future attacks. Research shows that deliberate violence has more lasting mental health effects than do natural disasters and accidents. Survivors of terrorism and the affected community often feel a sense of injustice, anger, and a helplessness to protect themselves. People may also suffer from a pervasive feeling of being unsafe and vulnerable. A consistent finding is that most people, over time, are resilient to violent terrorist acts, but the people directly exposed to the violence have a higher risk of developing posttraumatic stress disorder (PTSD).

Complex bereavement can result from terrorism, due to the sudden, unexpected, and violent nature of deaths caused by terrorist attacks. An individual's recovery may be long and arduous, as it was for many people after the terrorist attacks of SEPTEMBER 11, 2001, leading families and survivors to experience uncertainty and fear. Even with a great deal of support available to the bereaved through public rituals and the recognition of their needs, exposure to these attacks predicts current PTSD and depression. Traumatized victims of torture may develop a wide range of emotions, including anxiety, depression, feelings of resignation, guilt, apathy, fear, suspiciousness, aggressiveness, sudden weeping, intensive rage, irritability, suicide attempts, introversion, drowsiness, exhaustion, memory difficulties, lack of concentration, disorientation, sleeping difficulties, paresthesia, and sexual and psychosomatic disturbances.

Torture effects are particularly acute and severe because torture is usually administered by another individual who is directly acting against the victim. Human-against-human trauma is typically much more traumatic than an impersonal trauma, such as an accident or a natural event. Typically, torture is used to render the victim ineffectual socially and politically. Death is seldom the goal.

Resilience and Posttraumatic Stress Disorder (PTSD)

Some individuals are far more resilient to stress than others, and researchers have studied this issue to find differences between those who develop traumatic stress disorders in reaction to severe stress and those who do not. The National Vietnam Veterans Readjustment Study tracked 1,632 female and male war veterans and found that 26 percent of the 830,000 men and women who served in Vietnam developed PTSD impairment. However, the researchers also found some protective factors *against* the development of PTSD, including the specific following traits:

- Japanese-American ethnicity
- a high school degree or higher
- an older age at entry to the war
- a higher socioeconomic status
- a more positive paternal relationship

Social support while away from home as well as after the war were also critical elements that supported an increased likelihood of resilience against developing PTSD.

Among abused children, the key factor that seems to enhance their personal resilience is having a person in their lives on whom they feel that they can truly depend. In general, females are more resilient than males. A child's temperament is also a factor, and generally easygoing children are more resilient than others. Another important factor is the ability to *not* blame themselves for the abuse that they suffered as well as the ability to avoid their abusive parents.

Some key characteristics of child resilience were discussed in *Promoting Resilience: A Review of Effective Strategies for Child Care Services,* a publication in the United Kingdom. The following traits were found to be key characteristics among children who were resilient:

- a sense of humor
- positive peer relationships
- personal attractiveness to others
- feelings of empathy
- problem-solving abilities
- academic success
- membership in a faith group
- involvement in extracurricular activities
- possession of good social skills

Subthreshold Posttraumatic Stress Disorder

The creation of the subthreshold posttraumatic stress disorder designation is an effort to identify people who have some (but not all) PTSD symptoms and to study and treat the effects these symptoms have on their lives.

Someone with subthreshold PTSD may never seek traditional trauma-based therapies because they often adapt to the "symptoms," and consequently, they do not perceive themselves as in need of therapy. On the other hand, many individuals with undiagnosed PTSD seek therapy for complaints other than PTSD, such as anxiety, depression, or somatic complaints. A good therapist will help to uncover the traumatic roots of their complaints and will treat that aspect of the problem.

In a study of subthreshold PTSD among Canadian peacekeepers with varying levels of traumatic stress, described in *Stress, Trauma, and Substance Use,* the participants include 1,101 male veterans from the regular and reserve forces of the Canadian military. Most of the soldiers (85 percent) were married, although marriage was not found to be significantly related to PTSD status. The researchers found that the veterans with either full or sub-threshold PTSD had greater levels of depression and health problems when they were compared to the veterans with no PTSD. They also found that those peacekeepers with full PTSD had a significantly greater level of impairment from alcohol use disorders than did those with subthreshold PTSD or no PTSD; however, peacekeepers with subthreshold PTSD had higher levels of impairment than did those with no PTSD. The full PTSD group was found to have clinical levels of depression, while the subthreshold PTSD group *approached* clinical levels of depression.

The researchers stated: "Finally, although the overall findings lend support to the validity of the current diagnostic thresholds for full PTSD, they also indicate that subthreshold PTSD is a meaningful diagnosis, as subthreshold PTSD significantly impacts the affect and mental health of the peacekeeping veterans. For example, a substantial proportion (30.3 percent) of veterans with subthreshold PTSD reported clinical levels of depression. This later finding supports the notion that clinical problems are indeed associated with subthreshold PTSD and suggests that clinical attention to and intervention for subthreshold PTSD would be beneficial for veterans."

Dube, Shanta R., et al. "Childhood Abuse, Household Dysfunction, and the Risk of Attempted Suicide Throughout the Life Span: Findings from the Adverse Childhood Experiences Study." *Journal of the American Medical Association* 286, no. 24 (2001): 3,089–3,096.

Kirkpatrick, D. G., and Resnick, H. S. "Posttraumatic stress disorder associated with exposure to criminal victimization in clinical and community populations." In *Posttraumatic Stress Disorder: DSM IV and Beyond,* 1st ed., edited by J. Davidson and E. Foa, 113–143. Washington, D.C.: American Psychiatric Press, 1993.

Sharhabani, Arzy, Ronit, et al. "The Toll of Domestic Violence." *Journal of Interpersonal Violence* 18, no. 11 (2003): 1,335–1,346.

Shaw, K., and MacFarlane, A. C. "The aetiology of posttraumatic stress disorder following a psychotic episode." *Journal of Traumatic Stress* 15, no. 1 (2002): 39–47.

Yarvis, Jeffrey S., Patrick S. Bordnick, and Christina A. Spivey, "Subthreshold PTSD: A Comparison of Alcohol, Depression, and Health Problems in Canadian Peacekeepers with Different Levels of Traumatic Stress." In *Stress, Trauma, and Substance Use,* edited by Brian E. Briade and Samuel A. MacMaster, 117–135. New York: Routledge, 2008.

cellular memory　Human behavior patterns are learned from information stored at the cellular level as cellular memory. They may be stored in the CENTRAL NERVOUS SYSTEM or the peripheral nervous system. For example, the very complicated skill of riding a bicycle involves both central and peripheral nervous enervation, and the skill is available anytime because the experience, balance, and skill is inherent in the cells of our body. Likewise, when an individual goes into an aversive situation, such as a restaurant where he or she had food poisoning, the body "remembers" by reproducing some of the same reaction previously experienced. This ability of the body to remember situations comes from the storage at the cellular level. If the individual has been traumatized, some of the PTSD reaction will occur in situations that "remind" the body of the traumatic event.

For example, when an individual perceives a TRAUMATIC EVENT as a threat to his or her well-being, complex hormonal messenger molecules are released and encode all the sensory impressions of the perceived threat as cellular memory. This initial memory of the threat can later act as the catalyst to trigger the same reflex response as if it were the original threat and become conditioned to produce the same reactions as those of the original threat, regardless of the environmental stimulus. It is possible for an individual who returns from war to react to a car that backfires in the same way as if he were in combat and immediately ducks down. This process is stimulus generalization.

Survivors of trauma must deal with the conditioned reflex that is encoded as cellular memory. Unless the cellular memory is decoded, trauma survivors must live with the psychological and psychosomatic illnesses through the conditioned reflex. The more times that the memories are activated via stimulus generalization, the greater the likelihood of the individual expressing symptoms of POSTTRAUMATIC STRESS DISORDER.

Over the last decade, a number of therapeutic tools have effectively neutralized, or perceptually reframed, cellular memories. Such methods as meditation, guided imagery, and other mind-body techniques show great promise in helping individuals cope with the traumatic memory and decode the conditioned reflex mechanism at the cellular level.

See also BODY MEMORY; FELT SENSE.

McClaskey, Thomas R. "Decoding Traumatic Memory Patterns at the Cellular Level." *American Academy of Experts in Traumatic Stress*, 1998. Available online. URL: http://www.aaets.org/article30htm. Downloaded March 7, 2008.

central nervous system (CNS)   The BRAIN and spinal cord (all nerves that are encased in bone) make up the central nervous system to control behavior. The spinal cord connects to the brain at the base of the skull, and it is composed of nerve fibers that transmit electrical impulses to and from the brain. Nearly every voluntary muscle below the head depends on the spinal cord for control.

The human brain, on average, weighs three pounds and comprises 100 billion neurons nourished through the blood-brain barrier. It is an extremely complex organ and is the control center of the central nervous system. The largest structure, the *cerebrum*, is the seat of intelligence and memory. It resembles a walnut and has two large hemispheres that are connected by the CORPUS CALLOSUM, a fibrous network of neurons bridging the two sides. The hemispheres' outer layer, the cerebral cortex (gray matter) consists of the cell bodies of the neurons. The inner layer (white matter) is made up of long fibers (axons) emanating from the cell bodies connecting neurons to one another. The fibers are coated with fatty white sheaths called myelin, which act as insulators, allowing signals to travel more efficiently.

In the center of the brain lie two important structures, the HIPPOCAMPUS and AMYGDALA, each playing critical roles in MEMORY and emotional response when exposed to stressful situations. Two other structures in the center of the brain are the hypothalamus and thalamus, regulating information from the brain to the body. The hypothalamus is crucial in signaling the pituitary glands to release stress hormones in threatening situations. The thalamus is the relay center of all incoming sensory information to the cortex. In the back of the brain lies the cerebellum, coordinating fine motor movements, and the brainstem, a highway of nerve fibers connecting to the spinal cord.

The neurons in the brain communicate with one another by converting message signals to electrical current. This electrical signal travels from the cell body of the neuron down the myelin-coated axon to the very end of the neuron where the signal is transformed into a chemical signal through NEUROTRANSMITTERS. Under the microscope, each neuron is separated from the next neuron by a gap called the synapse, through which the neurotransmitter flows to the next neuron and is converted back to an electrical signal. All communication between neurons operates uniquely through a system of electricity and chemicals called the electrochemical system.

The Central Nervous System in Times of Stress

The body is sensitive to any environmental change and communicates this information to virtually every organ of the body as a survival mechanism. As soon as an individual perceives danger or a life-threatening situation, the body immediately releases hormones and chemicals into the bloodstream and brain. These hormones allow the individual to form critical thoughts for survival and shut down normal body processes, such as digestion. During times of STRESS, hormones such as CORTISOL and NOREPINEPHRINE bathe the brain to focus attention on impending danger and recall similar situations of danger enabling the body to either fight, flee, or freeze.

Stress and TRAUMATIC STRESS can have a lasting effect on the brain as well as on other physical areas of the body, leading to physiological and psychiatric disorders, such as POSTTRAUMATIC STRESS DISORDER (PTSD) and DEPRESSION.

See also AUTONOMIC NERVOUS SYSTEM; PHYSIOLOGY OF TRAUMA; SYMPATHETIC NERVOUS SYSTEM.

Bremner, J. Douglas. *Does Stress Damage the Brain?* New York: W.W. Norton, 2005.
Al-Chalabi, Ammar, Martin R. Turner, and R. Shane Delamont. *The Brain.* Oxford: One World Publications, 2006.

cerebral cortex   See BRAIN.

characteristics of survivors (Lifton)   See LIFTON'S CHARACTERISTICS OF A SURVIVOR.

child abuse and neglect (CAN)   The commission of harmful acts to children (child abuse) or the omission of necessary care (neglect), such as the provision of food and shelter. Child abuse and neglect are together often known as *child maltreatment*. In 2004 there were 1,490 deaths in the United States due to abuse and neglect. Most of the children who died (81 percent) were infants to toddlers ages three years old, and 12 percent were ages four to seven years old.

Child abuse and neglect often has lifelong repercussions, directly affecting how the child perceives him or herself as an adult, and sometimes affecting how their own children are reared. An estimated 40 percent of individuals who were abused as children will grow up to abuse their own children.

Childhood abuse and neglect can also affect BRAIN development; for example, a study in a 2004 issue of *Biological Psychiatry* of 26 abused or neglected children admitted for psychiatric evaluation and compared to nonabused healthy subjects, found that the CORPUS CALLOSUM of the brain was 17 percent smaller in the abused sample than the control subjects. It was also 11 percent smaller than the psychiatric patients who had not been neglected or abused. The researchers found that in most cases, neglect was a stronger predictive factor for smaller brain size than abuse, and neglect was associated with a 15 to 18 percent reduction in the corpus callosum regions. However, sexual abuse was the strongest factor for the reduced size of the corpus callosum in girls.

Categories of Abuse and Neglect

Most state laws recognize four types of child maltreatment: physical abuse, neglect, sexual abuse, and emotional abuse. However, many child victims suffer from more than one form of abuse or neglect, although neglect is the most commonly occurring form of maltreatment.

Physical abuse is physical injury that results from beating, shaking, stabbing, burning, throwing, biting, or otherwise harming a child. It is irrelevant whether the perpetrator actually meant to harm the child, and the lack of intent still signifies physical abuse when the child is harmed. States exclude corporal punishment (as with spanking) as physical abuse; however, there are provisions for cases when the spanking exceeds limits considered acceptable by state law.

Sexual abuse includes activities of a parent or caretaker that involve fondling the child's genitals, sexual penetration, oral sex, rape, indecent exposure, incest, and the exploitation of child through the production of child pornography or prostitution. The specific definition of sexual abuse under the Federal Child Abuse Prevention and Treatment Act (CAPTA) is as follows:

> The employment, use, persuasion, inducement, enticement, or coercion of any child to engage in, or assist any other person to engage in, any sexually explicit conduct or simulation of such conduct for the purpose of producing a visual depiction of such conduct; or the rape, and in cases of caretaker or inter-familial relationships, statutory rape, molestation, prostitution, or other form of sexual exploitation of children, or incest with children.

Neglect is the omission of necessary acts, rather than the commission of undesirable acts, as with physical abuse and sexual abuse. Examples of child neglect are failing to provide adequate food or shelter, failing to obtain needed medical care for the child, failing to provide for the child's education, and failure to provide a safe environment for the child. The abandonment of a child is a form of neglect, as when a parent leaves a child in the care of others and does not return or when a parent leaves an infant or small child unattended for hours in an apartment or car.

Federal Guidelines and Demographics of Abused Children

Each U.S. state has its own particular definitions of what specific behaviors constitute child abuse and child neglect, but federal legislation provides a minimum standard for the states to follow. The Keeping Children and Families Safe Act of 2003, an amendment of CAPTA, defines child abuse and neglect as a minimum of the following:

- any recent act of failure to act on the part of a parent or caretaker which results in death, serious physical or emotional harm, sexual abuse or exploitation; or
- an act or failure to act which presents an imminent risk of serious harm

According to the Administration on Children Youth and Families in its 2006 report on child maltreatment, 872,000 children were maltreated in substantiated cases of abuse or neglect in 2004. Most of these children (60 percent) were victims of abuse: 18 percent were physically abused; 10 percent were sexually abused; and 7 percent were emotionally maltreated. Other children fell under other state categories of abuse. See Table 1 for the numbers of children victimized and the rates of victimization. It is important to note that many children are victims of more than one form of maltreatment.

The child population in the United States was more than 73 million children nationwide in 2004. As seen in "Victimization Rates by Maltreatment Type, 2004," table below, there were 152,250 child-age victims of physical abuse, or 2.1 percent of all children in the United States. There was a greater rate of neglect than abuse, or 7.4 percent. In some cases, not all states reported statistical data to the federal government; for example, 38 states reported on medical neglect. Of the reported cases compared to the number of children, less than 1 percent of children experienced medical neglect.

Children with the greatest risk of victimization were those between birth and age three years. Children at the next greatest risk for victimization were those who were ages four to seven years old. In considering children in terms of the type of abuse and the child's age, there are significant differences. (SEE TABLE ON PAGE 60.) For example, the table clearly shows that among those children who were abused and neglected, infants and toddlers up to age three had the greatest risk from neglect (72.9 percent) and medical neglect (2.6 percent). They also had the *lowest* risk of sexual abuse (2.2 percent). In considering the category of physical abuse, abused children who were ages 12 to 15 (22.8 percent of this group) and age 16 and older (24.9 percent) had the greatest risks for both physical and sexual abuse.

According to the report, children of certain races and ethnicities had higher rates of abuse than others in 2004; for example, African-American children, Pacific Islander children, and American Indian or Alaska Native children (grouped together in one category) had the highest rate of abuse, or respectively, 19.9 per 1,000, 17.6, and 15.5. The abuse rate for Caucasian children was 10.7, and it was 10.4 for Hispanic children.

Perpetrators of Abuse

Most victimizers of children (79 percent) in 2004 were parents; other relatives represented 7 percent of victimizers; unmarried partners of parents represented 4 percent; and the category of "other" represented 5 percent. The remaining categories of perpetrators represented less than 1 percent each.

VICTIMIZATION RATES BY MALTREATMENT TYPE, 2004			
Maltreatment Type	Victims	Rate	Number of States
Physical Abuse	152,250	2.1	50
Neglect	544,050	7.4	50
Medical Neglect	17,968	0.3	38
Sexual Abuse	84,398	1.2	50
Psychological Maltreatment	61,272	0.9	47
Other Abuse	126,856	3.2	26
Unknown	2,080	0.1	8

Source: Adapted from Administration for Children and Families, *Child Maltreatment 2004*, Children's Bureau, U.S. Department of Health and Human Services, Washington, D.C., 2006, page 39.

VICTIMS BY AGE GROUP AND MALTREATMENT TYPE, 2004

Age Group	Total Victims	Physical Abuse		Neglect		Medical Neglect		Sexual Abuse		Psychological Abuse	
		Number	Percent	Number	Percent	Number	Percent	Number	Percent	Number	Percent
Age <1–3	232,409	29,733	12.8	169,311	72.9	5,981	2.6	5,145	2.2	11,067	4.8
Age 4–7	187,275	31,389	16.8	119,794	64.0	2,870	1.5	17,018	9.1	11,954	6.4
Age 8–11	160,940	30,973	19.2	96,205	59.8	2,584	1.6	18,294	11.4	11,881	7.4
Age 12–15	158,104	36,089	22.8	85,362	54.0	2,617	1.7	26,133	16.5	10,716	6.8
Age 16 and Older	45,946	11,460	24.9	24,098	52.4	713	1.6	7,480	16.3	2,871	6.2
Unknown or Missing	2,397	532	22.2	1,462	61.0	26	1.1	278	11.6	207	8.6
Total	787,071	139,996		496,232		14,791		74,348		48,696	
Percent			17.8		63.0		1.9		9.4		6.2

Source: Adapted from Administration for Children, and Families, *Child Maltreatment 2004,* Children's Bureau, U.S. Department of Health and Human Services, Washington, D.C., 2006, page 48.

Other perpetrators were in such categories as foster parents, residential facility staff, child daycare providers, legal guardians, other professionals, and friends and neighbors.

Women represented the majority of perpetrators (58 percent). However, of maltreating parents, less than 3 percent sexually abused their children, although 63 percent committed neglectful acts. In contrast, of perpetrators who were friends or neighbors of the family, almost 75 percent committed sexual abuse and 10 percent committed acts of neglect.

In a study published in 2005 by the Office of the Assistant Secretary for Planning and Evaluation of the U.S. Department of Health and Human Services, researchers looked at male perpetrators of child maltreatment. They studied data from 18 states and found that of male perpetrators, 51 percent were biological fathers (in contrast to 86 percent of the perpetrators who were biological mothers), while 25 percent were men in nonparental relationships (relatives, foster parents, day care providers, or friends).

About 20 percent were men in a parental role, such as stepfathers or mothers' boyfriends. In nearly two-thirds of the cases, a male perpetrator acted alone, while in about one-third of the cases, the perpetrator acted with the child's mother. In the remaining cases, the male perpetrator acted with someone other than the child's mother. Biological fathers and father surrogates who abused the child with the mother were about twice as likely to reabuse the child within 12 months as were fathers who acted alone.

Lifelong Trauma from Child Abuse

Adults who experienced childhood abuse have an increased risk for the following problems:

- abuse of their own children
- SUBSTANCE ABUSE
- DEPRESSION and other psychiatric disorders
- chronic pain and chronic diseases
- SUICIDE
- relationship difficulties
- difficulties bonding with children and others
- low self-esteem
- learning problems

In considering substance abuse, adults who were abused as children have a greater risk for alcoholism and/or drug dependence (ADDICTION) compared to nonabused adults; for example, women sexually abused during childhood have nearly three times the risk for drug dependence in adulthood as women not abused as children.

Women who were abused in childhood also have a greater risk for suffering from chronic pain in adulthood. In a study reported in 2004 in the *Journal of Clinical Psychiatry,* the researchers found that childhood sexual abuse was linked to adults with chronic pain that was associated with depression. In addition, according to Kathleen A. Kendall-Tackett in *Childhood Maltreatment*, women abused as children are more likely to experience chronic headaches in adulthood. Chronic pain syndromes occur more commonly among women abused as children, such as irritable bowel syndrome and pelvic pain.

In considering psychiatric disorders, childhood abuse almost triples the risk of an adult suffering from an ANXIETY DISORDER or mood disorder in adulthood, and doubles the risk of phobias. In addition, adults abused as children have about 10 times the risk of suffering from a PANIC DISORDER in adulthood.

Childhood abuse also increases the risk for adult suicide. In a study reported in the *Journal of the American Medical Association* in 2001, researchers found that of subjects with no emotional abuse as a child, 2.5 percent attempted suicide; however, among subjects who had experienced emotional abuse, about 14 percent had attempted suicide.

See also BATTERED CHILD SYNDROME; BODY MEMORY; CHILDREN AND TRAUMA; RAPE TRAUMA SYNDROME; THERAPY, TYPES OF; TORTURE.

Administration for Children and Families. *Child Maltreatment 2004.* Children's Bureau, U.S. Department of Health and Human Services, Washington, D.C., 2006.

Arnow, B. A. "Relationship between Childhood Maltreatment, Adult Health and Psychiatric Outcomes, and Medical Utilization." *Journal Clinical Psychiatry* 6, Supplement 12 (2004): 10–15.

Child Welfare Information Gateway. "Recognizing Child Abuse and Neglect: Signs and Symptoms," Washington, D.C.: Children's Bureau, Administration for Children and Families, April 2006. Available online. URL: http://www.childwelfare.gov/pubs/factsheets/signs.cfm. Downloaded July 15, 2006.

Clark, Robin E., and Judith Freeman Clark with Christine Adamec, *The Encyclopedia of Child Abuse.* 3rd ed. New York: Facts On File, 2007.

Dube, Shanta R., et al. "Childhood Abuse, Household Dysfunction, and the Risk of Attempted Suicide Throughout the Life Span: Findings from the Adverse Childhood Experiences Study." *Journal of the American Medical Association* 286, 24 (December 26, 2001): 3,089–3,096.

Federal Child Abuse Prevention & Treatment Act, Public Law 93–427, 1974, most recently amended 2003, Public Law 108–36. U.S. Code Title 42, Chapter 67.

Kendall-Tackett, Kathleen A. "Chronic Pain Syndromes as Sequelae of Childhood Abuse." *Child Maltreatment.* Kingston, N.J.: Civic Research Institute, 2005.

National Institute on Drug Abuse. "Childhood Sexual Abuse Increases Risk for Drug Dependence in Adult Women." Available online. URL: http://www.nida.nih.gov/NIDA_Notes/NNVol17N1/childhood.html. Downloaded August 2, 2006.

Office of the Assistant Secretary for Planning and Evaluation. *Male Perpetrators of Child Maltreatment: Findings from NCANDS.* Washington, D.C.: U.S. Department of Health and Human Services, January 2005.

Teicher, Martin H., et al. "Childhood Neglect Is Associated with Reduced Corpus Callosum Area." *Biological Psychiatry* 56, no. 1 (July 2004): 80–85.

child physical abuse (CPA)   Actions that cause physical harm to a child, including beating, stabbing, shooting, or any other acts that harm the child temporarily or permanently. The child may receive harm that ranges from minor and treatable injuries to severe harm that causes death. Childhood physical abuse can have lifelong effects. Note that corporal punishment (spanking) is not considered physical abuse in any state; however, if the spanking exceeds the limits of what is allowed under state law, such acts may be considered physically abusive.

According to the Administration for Children and Families, in 2004 139,996 children were substantiated victims of physical abuse in the United States, and in 28.3 percent of all fatality cases, children died as a result of physical abuse only. (More children died from neglect only, or 35.5 percent.)

Of all maltreated children in 2004, 17.8 percent were physically abused compared to 63 percent who were neglected. When considering the total population of victims by age and those who were physically abused in that age group, infants and toddlers up to age three years were the least likely to be physically abused, and older children ages 12 and older have nearly twice the risk for physical abuse as babies and toddlers. (SEE TABLE ON PAGE 62.)

Symptoms and Diagnostic Path
According to the Child Welfare Information Gateway of the Children's Bureau of the U.S. Department of

PHYSICALLY ABUSED VICTIMS BY AGE, 2004

Age Group	Total Victims	Number Physically Abused	Percent
Age <1–3	232,409	29,733	12.8
Age 4–7	187,275	31,389	16.8
Age 8–11	160,940	30,793	19.1
Age 12–15	158,104	36,089	22.8
Age 16 and Older	45,946	11,460	24.9
Unknown or Missing	2,397	532	22.2
Total	787,071	139,996	
Percent			17.8

Source: Adapted from Administration for Children and Families, *Child Maltreatment 2004,* Children's Bureau, U.S. Department of Health and Human Services, Washington, D.C., 2006, page 48.

Children and Families, some signs of physical abuse of a child include:

- The child has unexplained bites, burns, bruises, broken bones, or black eyes.
- The child has fading bruises or other marks that are noticeable after an absence from school.
- The child seems afraid of parents or other caregivers and cries when it is time to go home.
- The child shrinks away from adults.
- The child reports an injury caused by a parent or other caregiver.

In addition, caregiver behavior that may indicate signs of physical abuse include the following behaviors on the part of the caregiver:

- offers conflicting, unconvincing or no explanation for a child's injury
- describes the child as "evil" or in another very negative manner
- uses harsh physical discipline on the child
- has a history of abuse him or herself, in childhood

Treatment Options and Outlook

Physically abused children may be removed from their families and placed into foster care. They and their parents may receive therapy to overcome their problems that led to the abuse, so that the family can be reunited, if possible. The outlook depends on the severity of the abuse and the cause; for example, if the parents were abusive because of alcohol or drug dependence and are unwilling to receive treatment, the likelihood of family reunification is low.

Risk Factors and Preventive Measures

Children are more likely to be physically abused if their parents are substance abusers or dependent on substances. In addition, if their parents were themselves physically abused as children, the risk is increased.

See also BATTERED CHILD SYNDROME; BODY MEMORY; CHILD ABUSE AND NEGLECT; CHILDREN AND TRAUMA; CHILD SEXUAL ABUSE; RESILIENCE TO STRESS; THERAPY, TYPES OF; VULNERABILITY.

Administration for Children and Families. *Child Maltreatment 2004.* Children's Bureau, U.S. Department of Health and Human Services, Washington, D.C., 2006.
Child Welfare Information Gateway. "Recognizing Child Abuse and Neglect: Signs and Symptoms," Washington, D.C.: Children's Bureau, Administration for Children and Families, April 2006. Available online. URL: http://www.childwelfare.gov/pubs/factsheets/signs.cfm. Downloaded July 15, 2006.
Clark, Robin E., and Judith Freeman Clark with Christine Adamec, *The Encyclopedia of Child Abuse.* 3rd ed. New York: Facts On File, 2007.

children and trauma   Extremely distressing and abnormal experiences that may occur to a child, such as CHILD ABUSE AND NEGLECT, CHILD PHYSICAL

ABUSE, and CHILD SEXUAL ABUSE. Childhood trauma may also occur as a result of PEDIATRIC MEDICAL TRAUMATIC STRESS, such as when a child suffers from a very serious medical problem that is either an acute problem such as cancer or a chronic serious problem, such as juvenile arthritis or juvenile diabetes. Another cause of childhood trauma is bullying (see "BULLYCIDE" AND BULLYING), which is usually perpetrated by a child's peers in school and/or in the neighborhood. Bullying can be very distressing to a child, causing him or her to feel powerless and weak. These feelings may transcend into adulthood. The death of a parent or loved one is another form of trauma that may occur in childhood.

A child who has experienced trauma may develop COMPLEX POSTTRAUMATIC STRESS DISORDER (CPTSD), a disorder of those individuals who are exposed to chronic traumas for months or years at a time, such as when children are repeatedly abused or neglected for years in their development. Prolonged and extreme psychological harm can develop through repeated exposure to traumatic situations. One such situation occurs when the victim is under the control of the perpetrator such as a trusted individual. One widespread case of such abuse are young boys who were traumatized by some Catholic priests who abused them in the 1980s and 1990s, when the church turned a blind eye to the abuse. For example, Father John Goeghan, a serial pedophile in the Boston archdiocese, was transferred from parish to parish, although the first complaint about him as a sexual predator was received in 1979 and complaints continued until the 1990s. Geoghan was arrested for molesting a boy in a pool in 2002. He was convicted and later murdered in prison.

BATTERED CHILD SYNDROME is an older term given to a condition of chronic abuse of a child. This is also a medical term that physicians and other medical professionals use to denote the frequent and chronic abuse of children, to the point of causing physical harm. This condition was first identified and named by C. Henry Kempe and his colleagues in their 1962 landmark article in the *Journal of the American Medical Association,* where they discussed symptoms of chronic child abuse, such as the failure to thrive, and soft tissue swellings or skin bruising or other injuries where the degree and type of injury did not match the explanation given to doctors about what had caused the injury. They used the term *battered child syndrome* to describe this condition.

It is now hard to believe, but in the early 1960s many people, including doctors, did not recognize child abuse as a serious problem. However, as a result of the pioneering work of Kempe, teachers and other school officials as well as day-care centers are now trained to recognize the signs of child abuse and to report it to officials.

Unfortunately, in some cases, efforts to identify abuse went too far, and some innocent people were wrongfully accused of child abuse in the 1980s. This was largely driven by therapists who used procedures later proven harmful such as MEMORY RECOVERY THERAPIES. This form of therapy urged children and adults to remember past sexual abuse, even if the individual actively denied that any such abuse had occurred. Eventually, some patients came to believe they had been abused and talked about abuse, with the strong encouragement of the therapist even though later research revealed that they had never actually been sexually abused. In the meantime, serious family damage had occurred, and parents, adult children, and siblings were permanently estranged. The false implanted memories of child abuse eventually became known as FALSE MEMORY SYNDROME. It was itself a form of trauma because it alienated children from their families for years or permanently.

Probably the most famous case of a false accusation was that of Margaret Kelly Michaels in New Jersey. Michaels was a day-care worker who was charged with extreme abuse and convicted of 155 counts of child sexual abuse. This abuse allegedly occurred during the day and no one else noticed, nor did the abuse leave any marks on the children's bodies. Michaels went to jail in 1987, but her conviction was overturned in 1993 by the New Jersey Superior Court Appellate Division. However, others in the same situation as Michaels died in prison before exoneration came.

Symptoms of Child Traumatization

The symptoms of child trauma are often very similar to those found in traumatized adults, such as arousal and anxiety, behavior problems, sleep difficulties, sudden anxiety, FLASHBACKS, insecurity, and a general feeling of being unsafe. Without psychotherapeutic intervention, these symptoms tend to persist or become worse. Traumatized children must become able to talk about their past traumatic experiences and find safe ways to process the psychic and somatic experiences. In addition, they need to feel safe and be given rules, boundaries, and a sense of predictability. Children who have been traumatized may have an ALTERED PAIN PERCEPTION, and they often need to learn to accurately perceive tactile stimuli. In addition, they must relearn how to relax, which the therapist can often help the child achieve through play therapy.

Experts such as van der Kolk say that the most common feature of traumatized children is a lack of self-regulation, leading to problems with poor impulse control and the child's uncertainty about the predictability and reliability of others. The child may be poor at reading social cues accurately and may also be more likely to engage in bullying behaviors than are other children. Some traumatized children also develop paranoid ideas, seeing personal attacks where they are not made, while others are numbed to activities other children find stimulating and interesting.

Severely abused children may develop problems with attachment disorders (see ATTACHMENT STYLES/DISORDERS), where the normal bonding with a parent or other parental figure does not occur. Likewise, attachment difficulties early in life often set children up for later traumatic reactions. They may also develop a problem with dissociative identity disorder, formerly called multiple personality disorder. To cope with extremely severe abuse, the child dissociates him or herself from his or her own body, separates into an observer and another (or more) identity, and may develop "alters," or other personalities that help to cope with the ongoing traumatic environment. Even years after the abuse has ended, the dissociative disorder remains unless or until it is treated.

Nightmares and Sleepwalking NIGHTMARES are extremely unpleasant dreams that often cause the dreamer to wake up. In children, nightmares may be frequent when the child is suffering from trauma. Sleepwalking (somnambulism) is a sleep disorder that occurs in some children. This disorder may stem from a traumatic event. Somnambulism frequently occurs when the individual is under STRESS. It is common in the teenage years and usually declines in frequency with age.

Cutting and Self-Mutilation Some children who have been traumatized resort to CUTTING themselves, particularly girls. Females have about four times the rate of cutting behavior as males. As painful as it is, cutting proves to the child that he or she is the one in control. Early emotional abuse is commonly associated with self-harm. Cutters are usually not suicidal; however, a child could accidentally hit a vein or artery and cause serious bleeding, necessitating treatment in the emergency room of a hospital. Adult females who are cutters often have a history of child sexual abuse or complex trauma.

Self-harm seems to arise as a coping mechanism involving DISSOCIATION, or mentally removing oneself from the unbearable situation, and also from unresolved emotional discomfort. There is no category in the *DIAGNOSTIC AND STATISTICAL MANUAL* published by the American Psychiatric Association for cutting and self-mutilation behavior. Those with DEPRESSION, phobias and BORDERLINE PERSONALITY DISORDER are the most at risk for this behavior.

Child Abuse and Neglect

Child abuse and neglect is together known as *child maltreatment* and represents the worst form of childhood abuse and one of the most difficult to treat. In general, abuse is the commission of harmful acts to children, while neglect refers to the *omission* of necessary care (neglect), such as the failure of the parent or guardian to provide food, shelter, and medical care or if the parent abandoned the child. In 2004 there were 1,490 deaths due to abuse and neglect, according to a 2006 report on child maltreatment by the Administration for Children and Families (ACF). Most of the children who died were very young: infants to toddlers ages three years old.

The Administration for Children and Families also reported that most abused or neglected children (60 percent) were victims of neglect, while 18 percent were physically abused, 10 percent were sexually abused, and 7 percent were emotionally maltreated. Other children fell under other state-defined categories of abuse. Note that many children are victimized by more than one form of maltreatment.

As with all the other years in which data has been captured by the federal government, most perpetrators of child abuse in 2004 were parents (79 percent), and women were also the majority of perpetrators (58 percent), except in the case of sexual abuse. Of perpetrators who were friends or neighbors of the family, almost 75 percent committed acts of sexual abuse, and 10 percent committed acts of neglect.

Physical Abuse   Physical abuse of a child is any act that causes physical harm, including beating, stabbing, shooting, or other acts that may harm the child temporarily or permanently. The child may receive treatable injuries or broken bones, or the harm could cause scars, or may be even more severe, up to and including causing death. It should be noted that corporal punishment (spanking) is not considered physical abuse in any state; however, if the spanking exceeds the limits of what is allowed under state law, such as a spanking that leaves severe welts or scars, then it is generally considered physically abusive.

According to the Administration for Children and Families, in 2004, 139,996 children were substantiated victims of physical abuse in the United States, and in 28.3 percent of all fatality cases, children died as a result of physical abuse only. More children died from neglect only, or 35.5 percent.

Sexual Abuse   The sexual abuse of a child includes behaviors ranging from sexual touching to assault and up to and including intercourse. Less than 1 percent of sexually abused children die from sexual abuse. However, child sexual abuse causes severely negative lifelong consequences to the child and to the adult that the child becomes. Most victims of sexual abuse are females. Small children diagnosed with sexually transmitted diseases (STDs) are usually victims of sexual abuse. In the case of adolescents, however, teenagers may have had consensual sex and contracted the disease from each other. As adults, sexually abused children will tend toward extremes of sexual behavior. For example, studies have shown that 100 percent of identified prostitutes were sexually abused as children. Other sexually abused children will become inhibited and anxious with sexual activities and tend to refrain from them.

Child Neglect   Child neglect is the failure of a parent or caregiver to provide needed food, shelter, or medical care, and it is often more dangerous than child abuse, particularly in the case of infants and toddlers. The abandonment of a child is a form of neglect, as when a parent leaves an infant or small child in an apartment or car, unattended for hours, days, or longer. An infant or toddler can die in a hot locked car within a relatively short period.

Neglect is emotionally traumatic for the child who is a toddler or older and wonders where his or her mother or father is and who is often fearful of being with strangers, even when they are kind and compassionate relatives or foster parents. The child may think that a parent left because of something that he or she did or failed to do, or it was because the child was not "good" or at least not good enough. In fact, the neglectful or abusive parent may have told the child that the maltreatment was the child's fault, and the child may internalize this view.

Some children are removed from their families by the state because of abuse or neglect and placed in foster care with strangers for their own protection. This is a very traumatic experience for most children. It often causes them to act out. Sometimes the acting out is extreme as the child tests the foster parents. The foster parents may become frustrated and tell social services authorities that they cannot handle the child, so the child is placed with another foster family. According to sources such as *The Encyclopedia of Child Abuse,* with each successive move, the child's behavior usually becomes worse. Eventually, the child may be placed in a group home or a psychiatric facility until the child "ages out" of the system at age 18.

Bullying and "Bullycide"

Bullying is the act of one child or a group of children intimidating other children, either to cause them to take some action or sometimes solely for the purpose of humiliation. Bullying is very common among children. *Bullycide* is a slang term that refers to the murder of a bully by the victim, which is very rare. Children and adolescents with physical or learning disabilities or with illnesses such as diabetes are more likely to be bullied by other children, as are those who are obese.

Often parents mishandle the bullying of their child, telling the child to either "ignore" it or to "fight back." Yet, often the bullies will not allow the child to ignore them, and instead they will get "in their face." In addition, they are usually physically much bigger and stronger than the bullied child; thus, if the bullied child were to fight back, he or she would receive a beating. A better course is to discuss the problem with the child's teachers and possibly with other parents whose children may also be experiencing victimization from the bully. Often it is *not* a good idea to contact the bullying child's parents, who may be very unreceptive and even hostile or aggressive. Another course of action is to contact school authorities to seek help.

Being bullied can cause lifelong trauma to victims, who may believe that they must be weak and ineffectual, since they were bullied. They internalize the negative comments that the bully makes about them, as weak, stupid, babyish, and so forth. They may believe that nobody likes them, particularly since many times other children do not provide any help because they fear and/or admire the bully. If unchecked, bullies may escalate their violence, and the behavior may continue into adulthood until they commit worse crimes.

Most physically abusive bullies are males, but some females also exhibit violent bullying behavior. In one case in 2008, female bullies beat a classmate and videotaped the beating, later showing it to others on the Internet. This evidence caused the bullies to be arrested. However, in general, female bullies rely far more on psychological torment, such as name calling or passing around unfounded and cruel rumors about the victim.

Some bullies, particularly male bullies, extort money or other items from the victim, and some victims have stolen from their parents to obtain the money or items that the bully demands, in order to avoid a beating from the bully.

According to *Indicators of School Crime and Safety: 2005,* early adolescence is when bullying often reaches a peak. From grades 6 to 12 the greatest percentage of bullied children (13.9 percent) was in the sixth grade, followed by seventh grade (12.7 percent).

Pediatric Medical Traumatic Stress

The key symptoms of pediatric medical traumatic stress are the core ACUTE STRESS DISORDER (ASD) symptoms of arousal, fear, shock, denial, and avoidance. In families of a child diagnosed with cancer, the rates of ASD are often actually higher in the parents than they are in the child with cancer. In pediatric injury cases, an estimated one in five injured children and their parents will develop POSTTRAUMATIC STRESS DISORDER (PTSD) symptoms lasting more than four months.

A 2003 issue of the *Journal of the American Medical Association* reported on a study of seriously injured children and their parents and the risk for persistent stress. The researchers found that 22 percent of the children and 33 percent of their parents had ASD symptoms. Of course it is very distressing for the child to be injured or ill, but parents can become even more distressed because as caregivers they feel that it is their job to protect the child. Yet at the same time, they may feel helpless or even terrified as they struggle to obtain information and answers from medical personnel about the child's prognosis.

General Response to Childhood Trauma

Children may respond to childhood trauma in a variety of mostly predictable ways, including feeling guilty for being abused, neglected, or bullied or even for having a medical disorder that causes distress to their families. Guilt is a feeling that the individual has somehow caused the problem or at least contributed to the cause, although in the case of childhood trauma, the child may often not know *how* he or she caused it. Unresolved guilt may lead to self-condemnation, depression, suicidal feelings, and SUBSTANCE ABUSE. It can also keep a person "stuck" in their suffering and can prevent recovery. Adults who were abused or neglected as children may still carry guilt from the past and believe that they are somehow defective, since they were rejected by their parent or parents.

Therapies for Child Trauma

Traumatized children urgently need therapy, as often do adults who were traumatized as children and who never received therapy. Treatments that employ COGNITIVE BEHAVIORAL THERAPIES combined with some form of play therapy for younger children, or therapies that help the individual challenge his or her own thinking about the trauma, are often useful. For example, if the child blames him or herself for past abuse, as is common, the child can be taught that it was *not* his or her fault that the abuse occurred.

With cognitive behavioral therapy that focuses on the trauma, children can describe their feelings in a safe environment and learn to tolerate feelings related to the trauma. The therapist teaches traumatized children how to identify, evaluate, and change their thoughts and behaviors to feel better.

Other techniques, such as NARRATIVE MEMORY are used to help the child. With narrative memory, as people become more aware of different aspects of their traumatic experience in childhood, they construct a story, or a narrative memory, to help them explain what happened to them.

Some therapies employ SOMATIC EXPERIENCING, in which the child imagines how he or she felt when the trauma occurred and learns how to work with the body sensations associated with the event. EYE MOVEMENT DESENSITIZATION AND REPROCESSING (EMDR) is a therapy that is also effective with sexual trauma. It is described as an information-processing form of therapy. EMDR is an eight-phase treatment approach that identifies the past events that traumatized the child, current situations that trigger disturbance, and types of experiences needed to help the child recover. In the adult who was traumatized as a child, he or she might need to develop social skills that are missing because the client was traumatized in childhood. EMDR processes both the negative experiences that cause dysfunction and positive experiences that need to be incorporated. Client preparation is the second part of treatment to assure that the client can stay present with the therapist no matter what is coming to consciousness internally. The client is taught a variety of self-control techniques to help him or her return to equilibrium at any time.

Younger children may benefit from ART THERAPY, expressing feelings, which they cannot say aloud, through their drawings and paintings. Older children and adults can benefit through writing about their feelings in a journal.

PROLONGED EXPOSURE THERAPY may be used with adolescents or adults who experienced childhood sexual abuse and who suffer from posttraumatic stress disorder (PTSD) as a result. Individual therapy sessions cause clients to think about anxiety-provoking traumatic events or feared objects over eight to 12 sessions in order to reduce or extinguish intrusive thoughts, fear, anxiety, and the startle response. Often relaxation techniques are practiced with patients prior to the therapy because the therapy itself can be quite intense. Prolonged exposure therapy is used to reduce PTSD symptoms that are associated with child sexual abuse, and criminal assaults.

Another form of therapy is TRAUMATIC INCIDENT REDUCTION, in which the patient is taught to "see" the traumatic event as if it were a videotape. Repeated viewings enable the patient to reduce the level of trauma. The purpose of this form of therapy is to help the client integrate unresolved aspects of the trauma through repeated viewings.

Lifelong Effects of Traumatic Experiences

Numerous studies have documented that childhood trauma often leaves emotional scars on the adult, and traumatized children are more likely than others to grow up to have problems with substance abuse and dependence, according to *The Encyclopedia of Child Abuse* and many other sources. In addition, experiencing childhood abuse nearly triples the risk of an adult suffering from depression or an anxiety disorder. Adults who were sexually abused in childhood have a 40 percent greater risk of marrying a person with alcoholism compared to adults who were not sexually abused in childhood.

SUICIDE is another increased risk for adults who were abused in childhood; for example, according to researcher Shanta Dube, et al., in the *Journal of the American Medical Association,* among adults who were not emotionally abused in childhood, 2.5 percent attempted suicide as adults. Among those who were emotionally abused in childhood, 14.3

percent attempted suicide in adulthood. Among those not physically abused in childhood, 2.2 percent attempted suicide in adulthood; among those who were physically abused as children, 7.8 percent attempted suicide as adults. Yet there is hope, and adults who were traumatized as children can still benefit from therapy and learn to overcome the trauma that they faced as children.

Clark, Robin E., Judith Freeman Clark, with Christine Adamec. *The Encyclopedia of Child Abuse.* 3rd ed. New York: Facts On File, 2006.
DeVoe, J. F., et al. *Indicators of School Crime and Safety: 2005.* Washington, D.C.: U.S. Government Printing Office, 2005.
Dube, Shanta, et al. "Childhood Abuse, Household Dysfunction, and the Risk of Attempted Suicide throughout the Life Span: Findings from the Adverse Childhood Experiences Study." *Journal of the American Medical Association* 286, no. 24 (December 26, 2001): 3,089–3,096.
van der Kolk, Bessel A., M.D., "The Neurobiology of Childhood Trauma and Abuse." *Child and Adolescent Psychiatric Clinics* 12 (2003): 293–317.

child sexual abuse (CSA) Touching, fondling, or the sexual assault of a child, up to and including intercourse. Less than 1 percent of sexually abused children die from the abuse. However, child sexual abuse causes severely negative lifelong consequences to the child and the later adult. Most victims of sexual abuse are females.

In 2004, according to the Administration for Children and Families, 74,348 children were victims of sexual abuse in the United States. Most perpetrators of child sexual abuse are males under age 30, and they are often known to the child, such as a friend or a neighbor.

Children who appear to have sexually transmitted diseases or who are diagnosed with STDs are usually victims of sexual abuse. In the case of adolescents, however, teenagers may have had consensual sex with each other.

According to the Child Welfare Information Gateway, some signs of sexual abuse are as follows:

- difficulty walking or sitting
- NIGHTMARES or bedwetting
- a change in appetite
- sophisticated or advanced sexual knowledge or behavior
- sudden refusal to change in gym class or participate in physical activities
- a pregnancy or the appearance of an STD in a child under age 14
- running away

In addition, the possibility of child sexual abuse may exist when the parent or other adult caregiver exhibits any of the following behaviors:

- is unusually protective of the child or severely limits the child's contact with other children, particularly children of the opposite sex
- is isolated and secretive
- is controlling and jealous with family members

Sexual abuse is traumatic for children who suffer it, whether they are females or males; for example, many boys who were victimized by Catholic priests report lifelong problems and DEPRESSION. In addition, teenage boys who are seduced by older women often have confusion about their sexuality, despite the popular view that such boys are "lucky" to have had such experiences.

Treatment for Sexually Abused Children
Therapy is usually indicated for sexually abused children as well as for adults who were sexually abused as children. As with most abuse victims, therapy will take a long time to deal with the abuse and with the skills and behaviors that did not develop because of the abuse. An understanding, compassionate but detached therapist is needed to help build developmental skills that did not develop because of abuse.

Relationship and talk therapy are usually the first step. Dealing with the abuse is both an "in-the-present" and "in-the-past" seesaw: Work may begin with a present experience and quickly move to past roots of the individual's reaction. COGNITIVE BEHAVIORAL THERAPIES are helpful, and SOMATIC EXPERIENCING THERAPY and EYE MOVEMENT DESENSITIZATION AND REPROCESSING (EMDR) are also effective with sexual trauma. In general, sexually abused individuals will either act out sexually as an adult or become repressed and inhibited sexually, both patterns being maladaptive and aversive to the individual.

According to the Administration for Children and Families, among children who were sexually abused in the United States in 2004 compared to all child abuse victims, the largest percentage were ages 12 to 15 years and older (16.5 percent), and the fewest percentage were infants and toddlers up to age three (2.2 percent). In considering race only, the largest percentage of sexually abused children (8.4 percent) were white, compared to 8.3 percentage who were unknown or missing. (SEE TABLE BELOW.)

Perpetrators of Sexual Abuse

As can be seen in the table above right, among those who abuse children, friends or neighbors are the most likely to commit sexual abuse (73.8 percent), followed by the category of "Other" (30.9 percent). Of other relatives who are abusive, 29.7 percent were sexual abusers. Abusive parents were the least likely to commit sexual abuse (2.6 percent).

Problems into Adulthood

Childhood sexual abuse is associated with many problems in adulthood, such as depression, prostitution, SUBSTANCE ABUSE, and SUICIDE. In a 2005 study published in the *American Journal of Public*

PERPETRATORS OF SEXUALLY ABUSED CHILDREN AND THEIR RELATIONSHIP TO THE VICTIM, 2004

	Number	Percent
Parents	13,957	2.6
Other Relatives	13,271	29.7
Foster Parents	191	6.2
Residential Facility Staff	131	12.1
Child Day-care Provider	1,115	22.5
Unmarried Partner of Parent	3,150	11.0
Legal Guardian	34	2.7
Other Professionals	264	21.4
Friends or Neighbors	1,302	73.8
Other	11,022	30.9
Unknown or Missing	3,459	12.8
Total Number	47,896	6.9

Source: Adapted from Administration for Children, and Families, *Child Maltreatment 2004*, Children's Bureau, U.S. Department of Health and Human Services, Washington, D.C., 2006, page 79.

Health, researchers studied the age at the time of the first injection among adult injection drug users and found that childhood sexual abuse was associated with an earlier initiation of injection drug use. (Most subjects were male.) In this study, 5.4 percent of the drug users had been forced to have sex before age 13, and 7.2 percent were compelled to have sex between the ages of 13 and 17 years.

Some studies have shown that survivors of childhood sexual abuse have abnormally suppressed levels of CORTISOL years after the abuse had occurred.

See also BATTERED CHILD SYNDROME; BODY MEMORY; CHILD ABUSE AND NEGLECT (CAN); CHILD PHYSICAL ABUSE; CHILDREN AND TRAUMA; CHILD SEXUAL ABUSE ACCOMMODATION SYNDROME; POSTTRAUMATIC STRESS DISORDER (PTSD); RAPE TRAUMA SYNDROME; RESILIENCE TO STRESS; THERAPY, TYPES OF; VULNERABILITY.

Administration for Children and Families. *Child Maltreatment 2004*, Washington, D.C.: Children's Bureau, U.S. Department of Health and Human Services, 2006.
Child Welfare Information Gateway. "Recognizing Child Abuse and Neglect: Signs and Symptoms." Washington, D.C.: Children's Bureau, Administration for Children and Families, April 2006. Available online. URL: http://www.childwelfare.gov/pubs/factsheets/signs.cfm. Downloaded July 15, 2006.

RACE OF SEXUALLY ABUSED VICTIMS, 2004

Race	Number	Percent
African American	9,350	5.7
American Indian or Alaska Native	307	3.9
Asian	322	4.8
Pacific Islander	99	5.6
White	29,716	8.4
Multiple Race	465	4.0
Hispanic	8,905	7.1
Unknown or Missing	3,183	8.3
Total	52,347	
Percent		7.4

Source: Adapted from Administration for Children and Families, *Child Maltreatment 2004*, Children's Bureau, U.S. Department of Health and Human Services, Washington, D.C., 2006, page 53.

Clark, Robin E., and Judith Freeman Clark, with Christine Adamec. *The Encyclopedia of Child Abuse*. 3rd ed. New York: Facts On File, 2007.

Dube, Shanta R., et al. "Long-Term Consequences of Childhood Sexual Abuse by Gender of Victim." *American Journal of Preventive Medicine* 28, no. 5 (2005): 430–438.

Lewis, Angela, ed. *Child Sexual Abuse*. New York: Thomson Gale, 2005.

child sexual abuse accommodation syndrome (CSAAS)   Childhood behavior that was regarded as directly associated with the child being subjected to CHILD SEXUAL ABUSE, based on the description of the syndrome by psychiatrist Roland C. Summit, M.D., in his article for *Child Abuse & Neglect* in 1983. Summit's theories in his article were used in many subsequent court cases of alleged child sexual abuse, with some convictions that were directly tied to his theories. However, Summit later stated in the *Journal of Child Sexual Abuse* in 1992 that his theory was *not* meant to be used for diagnosis and that it had instead been exploited.

In his earlier 1983 article, Summit stated that there were five categories within the syndrome of child sexual abuse accommodation syndrome, including secrecy, helplessness, entrapment and accommodation, a delayed and an unconvincing disclosure, and a retraction of an abuse allegation. Stated Summit, "The accommodation syndrome is proposed as a simple and logical model for use by clinicians to improve understanding and acceptance of the child's position in the complex and controversial dynamics of sexual victimization."

In this model, secrecy of the sexual abuse was present in most cases, and the average child never asked what was happening and never told anyone else about the abuse. Helplessness referred to the child's subordinate role to adults, such as to adult relatives. The concept of entrapment and accommodation referred to the child's feeling that since he or she could not reveal the abuse to others and it was likely to continue, then the child would have to accept it and somehow accommodate it. One way to accept it was to assume that it was his or her fault. In some cases, sexually abused children developed DISSOCIATIVE DISORDERS.

With regard to a delayed and unconvincing disclosure, Summit said that most ongoing sexual abuse was never disclosed or was only disclosed years later. Last was the concept of retraction. According to this model, if a child said that he or she had been sexually abused, the child was highly likely to retract the allegation later on in order to regain the love and positive attention of family members. Likewise, a similar pattern of denial, secrecy, and retraction is seen in cases of child sexual abuse (molestation) by priests or valued authority figures.

As Summit later wrote in his 1992 article, his concept of child sexual abuse accommodation syndrome was never meant to be used as it was by the legal community and others. Summit wrote in the *Journal of Child Sexual Abuse* in 1992:

> The Child Sexual Abuse Accommodation Syndrome (CSAAS) is a clinical observation that has become both elevated as gospel and denounced as dangerous pseudoscience. The polarization which inflames every issue of sexual abuse had been kindled further here by the exploitation of a clinical concept as ammunition for battles in court. The excess that has been generated by false claims advanced by prosecutors as well as a primary effort of defense interest to strip the paper of any worth or relevance.

Summit said that if he had known that lawyers and courtrooms would consider the word *syndrome* to be somehow synonymous with *diagnosis*, he would have instead used the term *pattern* to Child Sexual Abuse Accommodation Pattern to describe his model.

Studies of Abused Individuals

Kamala London, et al., compared their findings to Summit's CSAAS in their analysis of a retrospective look at studies of adults who were abused as children as well as concurrent or chart review studies of children who were receiving an evaluation or treatment for child sexual abuse. They described their findings in a 2005 issue of *Psychology, Public Policy, and Law*.

As with Summit, they also found that the majority of children did not reveal sexual abuse during childhood. Stated the authors, "However, the evidence fails to support the notion that denials, tentative disclosures, and recantations characterize the disclosure patterns of children with validated histories of sexual abuse."

However, the authors said that CSAAS had been greatly misused in the courtroom, and they cited the case of *State v. Michaels* in 1993 as the best example of CSAAS being used as a diagnosis and proof of child sexual abuse. In this case, Margaret Kelly Michaels was found guilty of 115 counts of sexual abuse with 20 children at the Wee Care Day Nursery in Maplewood, New Jersey. Stated the authors:

> Expert testimony was presented at trial by Eileen Treacy, who stated that children in the case showed behavior consistent with CSAAS and thus their testimony and conduct was consistent with CSS [child sexual abuse]. After 5 years in prison, Michaels' conviction was overturned for reasons including the inadmissibility of testimony that uses CSAAS as a tool to diagnose abuse.

With regard to the concept of inevitable recantations, the authors took issue with Summit, based on their analysis and stated, "The research on denial and recantation shows that when directly questioned in a formal setting, only a small percentage of abused children demonstrate these behaviors."

However, child sexual abuse has lasting traumatic effects throughout the developmental cycle into adulthood where negative interpersonal and sexual consequences are invariably evident.

See also BATTERED CHILD SYNDROME; BODY MEMORY; CHILD ABUSE AND NEGLECT; CHILDREN AND TRAUMA; FALSE MEMORY SYNDROME; RAPE TRAUMA SYNDROME.

London, Kamala, et al. "Disclosure of Child Sexual Abuse: What Does the Research Tell Us About the Ways That Children Tell?" *Psychology, Public Policy, and Law* 11, no. 1 (2005): 194–226.
Summit, Roland C., M.D. "Abuse of the Child Sexual Abuse Accommodation Syndrome." *Journal of Child Sexual Abuse* 1, no. 4 (1992): 153–163.
Summit, Roland C., M.D. "The Child Abuse Accommodation Syndrome." *Child Abuse & Neglect* 7 (1983): 177–193.

circumscribed posttraumatic stress disorder (PTSD)
A term that is synonymous with what today is called "single incident" trauma, whereas COMPLEX POSTTRAUMATIC STRESS DISORDER (CPTSD) refers to multiple or chronic abuse or trauma that leads to PTSD. The idea of "circumscribed" does not mean that an event was a minor event. On the contrary, the TRAUMATIC EVENT could range from a relatively minor or distant event to one that is very intense and intimate, such as a rape, kidnapping, sniper attack, and so on.

Symptoms and Diagnostic Path
Circumscribed PTSD shows the same symptoms as the A–E criteria (life or injury threatening event, intrusive recollection, avoidance and numbing, increased arousal, and impairment) in the *DIAGNOSTIC AND STATISTICAL MANUAL* for PTSD. With time, the particular incident (single incident trauma) often becomes vague, distorted, or even forgotten. The body, however, remembers and any exposure to a similar incident will produce a strong fear reaction, sensations associated with the trauma, and sometimes, FLASHBACKS.

Treatment Options and Outlook
In the cognitive behavioral literature, circumscribed traumas are best treated with EXPOSURE THERAPY in which the evocative stimulus (the trauma event) is gradually presented in small doses without the aversive (traumatic) event occurring. In this way, "extinction" or the termination of the traumatic response (symptom) can occur.

During the initial traumatic exposure, avoidance was not possible, but during exposure trials, each approach step is taken only when some reduction has occurred in that exposure step. Avoidance can occur if arousal to a particular step is too great. The cognitive behaviorists point out that extinction for many traumatic events naturally occurs when people cannot avoid the safe reexposure to the situation (i.e., where the aversive or traumatic event no longer occurs). For example, it is known that the events of SEPTEMBER 11 produced considerable symptoms of POSTTRAUMATIC STRESS DISORDER (PTSD) in New Yorkers and many travelers and people throughout the country. However, since they continued to go to work and to be exposed to elements of the trauma without reexperiencing the full trauma itself, it was assumed that some extinction occurred.

In 2002 David Vlahov, Ph.D., director of the Center for Urban Epidemiological Studies, presented an update on New York Academy of Medicine's (NYAM) research on the incidence of PTSD, DEPRESSION, and substance use in the New York metropolitan area following 9/11.

Vlahov reported longitudinal data expanding the initial NYAM study from four to eight weeks after 9/11 to six to nine months after 9/11, and a follow-up at one year was under way at the time of the conference. "Approximately one-third of the residents of New York City were directly affected by the events of September 11," Vlahov said, summarizing results from the NYAM studies. "Since 9/11, more than 1 million people in New York City have had symptoms consistent with at least subthreshold PTSD. Symptom prevalence has declined over time, but by six to nine months there remained an estimated 90,000 persons with probable PTSD in New York City."

The estimates of new cases of PTSD and/or depression reported by the NYAM researchers are not significantly different from those given in other published studies, but methodological differences prevailed and criteria for diagnoses varied, calling into question the true values. However, each of the studies reported significant percentages of the population of New York having PTSD, probable PTSD, or subthreshold PTSD so even after six to nine months, significant effects were still present.

Circumscribed PTSD usually involves a single incident usually confined to a particular period of time (such as 9/11). On the other hand, complex PTSD is a traumatic disorder in which the individual has a history that is characterized by repeated trauma, the effects of which are much more pervasive and profound on the individual and his or her functioning. An example might be a woman whose husband abused her for many years. Or, more typically, an adult who was abused as a child during many years of development. Here neglect, chronic physical or sexual abuse, and other forms of impersonal trauma that extended over a number of years often produce lasting effects into adulthood and throughout life unless treatment is attempted.

Risk Factors and Preventive Measures

Circumscribed PTSD can rarely be anticipated or avoided. Trauma is a part of life. One would have to live in a totally controlled environment with absolute control to prevent trauma and, even then, the experience of isolation and feeling unsafe could be traumatic.

See also THERAPY, TYPES OF.

Rosack, J. "Psychiatric symptoms tied to 9/11 resolving, but long-term impact still unclear." *Psychiatric News* 37, no. 17 (September 6, 2002): 1.

civilian trauma   See TRAUMA, COMBAT VERSUS CIVILIAN.

Clinician-Administered PTSD Scale (CAPS)   See ASSESSMENT AND DIAGNOSIS.

cognitive behavioral therapy/interventions (CBT)/ (CBI)   A form of therapy in which the therapist helps clients identify their primary irrational thoughts that produce distress, DEPRESSION, anxiety, and so on, and then teaches them to challenge these irrational (and almost invariably negative) ideas that are impeding their lives.

Examples of such irrational thoughts are that it is unfair and terrible that the individual is suffering or that others should be more understanding of an individual's hardships, and it is extremely bad when they are not. It often *is* unfair and terrible that individuals suffer from traumatic reactions; however, ruminating on this unfairness usually prevents the individual from taking actions to improve his or her situation. If the situation cannot be improved, then the individual needs to learn to accept the situation and make it as palatable as possible.

When CBT is trauma-focused, as when children ages three to 18 years old are treated for traumas ranging from past or existing abuse, war trauma, community violence, or other forms of trauma, the traumatized children may develop an extreme fear of anything that reminds them of the traumatic event. Using CBT that focuses on the trauma, the children can talk about their feelings in a safe environment and learn to become less fearful and avoidant and better able to tolerate feelings that are related to the trauma. Using CBT, the therapist teaches children how to identify, evaluate, and change their thoughts and behaviors so that they can feel better. Many studies have found that CBT is an effective form of therapy for traumatized children and adults.

CBT is different from many other forms of therapy; for example, with psychoanalysis the therapist must spend many sessions over years to seek out the root causes for problems that may have occurred in the individual's childhood. CBT is a more rapid and more practical form of therapy that is useful for many patients.

The two most popular forms of CBTs are Rational Emotive Behavior Therapy (developed by the late Albert Ellis) and Cognitive Therapy (developed by Aaron Beck). Rational Emotive Behavior Therapy works to identify irrational, demanding, and excessive belief patterns, such as "I must be loved by everyone" or "I have to be perfect," and so on, that produce disturbing behavior and affect (mood). The therapist works to help the individual substitute more rational and less demanding thoughts, eliminating "musts" or "shoulds." Cognitive Therapy attacks illogical thinking processes and helps clients recognize their negative thoughts, biased interpretations, and errors in logic. "Overgeneralization," for example, is the illogical idea that because one thing goes wrong (such as a dent in a car fender in the morning as you leave for work) that everything else will go wrong that day as well.

See also ANXIETY DISORDERS; COGNITIVE PROCESSING THERAPY; THERAPY, TYPES OF.

cognitive processing therapy (CPT)   A form of therapy specifically designed to work with POST-TRAUMATIC STRESS DISORDER (PTSD) in sexual assault survivors. Cognitive processing therapy (CPT) combines an information-processing approach with observational and self-report information obtained from exposure treatments.

The theory is that information about the traumatic event is stored in the nervous system in the form of memories and bodily responses and meanings to the individual. The entire network stimulates avoidance behavior as a survival mechanism supported by internal and external AVOIDANCE BEHAVIORS. These networks also create beliefs and expectations that direct attention and support and trigger avoidance behaviors and establish personal or self-attitudes and beliefs.

For example, studies have found that rape survivors who experience conflict between their prior beliefs and the rape experience usually have great difficulty recovering, and they maintain severe reactions. An example is a woman who believes that "Rape does not happen to nice women." If she was raped, this woman would no doubt experience shame, humiliation, self-doubt, and feelings of angry betrayal, and these characteristics are often seen in PTSD rape victims.

Information-processing therapy can help the victim assimilate this new experience with the old beliefs in order to change the meaning of the traumatic experience. These schemata "stuck points" or conflicts must be modified and assimilated so that the personalized, victim, and self-condemnation aspects of the experience are changed into more realistic, rational, and less personal beliefs. The process also requires using exposure-based therapies to treat the PTSD.

See also EXPOSURE THERAPY; RAPE TRAUMA SYNDROME; THERAPY, TYPES OF.

collective trauma   In the aftermath of a tragedy, collective trauma is the psychological effect shared by individuals in a community, and its broader scope, an entire society. It is the pain the individual radiates onto the community due to the TRAUMATIC EVENT that can influence cultural norms and mass action. Community healing begins with the development of a secure community group and family connections that help to address losses and severe post-trauma symptoms. Normalization of trauma reactions and acknowledgment of multiple losses enhances the long-term healing process.

Some examples of collective traumas include President John F. Kennedy's assassination, SEPTEMBER 11, the Indian Ocean Earthquake Tsunami, and Hurricane Katrina. Likewise, smaller scale collective traumas such as kidnapping and murder of a child also can be viewed as collective traumas.

combat fatigue   See COMBAT STRESS REACTION.

combat-related posttraumatic stress disorder (C-PTSD) Posttraumatic stress disorder arising from combat or combat-related situations is common among military personnel. Because neither the Department of Defense nor the Veterans Administration adequately track PTSD in returning veterans, precise statistics are not available. However, empirical self-report studies that have been carried out indicate the between 15 and 50 percent of returning combat veterans will eventually develop PTSD. Furthermore, from a clinical standpoint, subsequent traumas, even rather minor events such as an auto accident, can trigger a large-scale reaction in a surviving veteran previously exposed to TRAUMATIC EVENTS.

Symptoms and Diagnostic Path

Many combat veterans do not want to talk with others about their experiences. Friends and family do not understand, nor do they have the experiences to relate to the horrors of combat. As a result, their symptoms tend to be greater and have a general effect on their lives.

Symptoms of combat-related PTSD tend to occur in three areas (FLASHBACKS, NIGHTMARES, and fear and anxiety) of the lives of combat veterans. (Note that the DIAGNOSTIC AND STATISTICAL MANUAL (DSM) criteria for PTSD were developed mainly from combat veteran's experiences.) Intrusiveness (re-creation of traumatic events) shows up as flashbacks of horrific events during periods of wakefulness, as nightmares of combat images, and as anxiety or fearfulness they experienced in the war zones. Another, complicating factor, is that a fairly high proportion of combat veterans also have BRAIN injury caused by concussions from explosions and rockets. Government assessments find 15 to 20 percent of combat veterans with brain concussions. Brain injury complicates and amplifies the effects of traumatic stress.

Because combat survivors experience these incidents, they feel unsafe wherever they are and feel particularly vulnerable at home. Consequently, they frequently have dogs, guns, alarm systems, and many locks on their doors. Avoidance is another category of symptoms. By definition, thoughts, feelings, memories, and so on, are actively avoided in the combat-related PTSD group through suppression, distraction, and self-medica-

tion with drugs and alcohol. The body remembers, however, and the combat-related PTSD veteran may be plagued with emotional numbness, aggressiveness, easy startle responses, panic and anxiety attacks and irritability, loss of interest in normal activities and detachment from others, difficulty with MEMORY and strange body sensations, or some combination of these reactions.

Stimulus triggers are a third category of symptoms and may include any external event that is similar to the war experiences. Movies, sounds, movement, smells, situational events, and even reading magazines and newspapers can set off a distorted conditioned reaction in the combat veterans with PTSD.

Treatment Options and Outlook

Currently, TRAUMA MANAGEMENT THERAPY is proving to be the most effective treatment for chronic combat-related PTSD. This form of therapy is a multicomponent approach, and it recognizes the complex nature of the often chronic nature of combat-related disorders.

For several reasons, simple drug therapies and exposure are not sufficient to treat combat-related PTSD. First, there are almost always comorbid conditions, such as addiction, depression, anxiety, and so on, present, in addition to the PTSD symptoms. Second, combat-related disorders are often associated with social maladjustments that were present prior to the combat experiences. These "negative symptoms" must be addressed along with the PTSD and can actually slow or interfere with treatment approaches.

EXPOSURE THERAPY, desensitization, and EYE MOVEMENT DESENSITIZATION AND REPROCESSING (EMDR) are helpful with treating PTSD reactions, but social skills training and anger management are also required. To address these negative symptoms, Trauma Management Therapy uses education about trauma and exposure work, homework, social skills training within small group settings and exposure therapies combined with cognitive modification as its basic tools.

Risk Factors and Preventive Measures

As with most PTSD, the intensity of the combat experience will affect the severity. Past psychiatric problems such as DEPRESSION or anxiety are predictors and risk factors for developing PTSD. Past trauma and isolation are also risk factors. But just the intensity of war and the suddenness of attack make the war experience itself a high risk factor for PTSD.

See also COMBAT STRESS REACTION; POSTTRAUMATIC STRESS DISORDER; THERAPY, TYPES OF; TRAUMA, COMBAT VERSUS CIVILIAN.

Sherman, Michelle D., Dona K. Zanotti, and Dan E. Jones. "Key Elements in Couples Therapy with Veterans with Combat-Related Posttraumatic Stress Disorder." *Professional Psychology Research and Practice* 36, no. 6 (2005): 626–633.

combat stress reaction (CSR)   A psychological response to the stress of combat that makes a soldier unfit for combat. *Battle fatigue* is the term for combat stress reaction that occurs while on the battlefield; however, a combat stress reaction can occur before a battle or just after a battle. (A reaction that occurs months or years later is a form of POSTTRAUMATIC STRESS DISORDER [PTSD].) Note that some experts use the terms *combat stress reaction* and *battle fatigue* interchangeably. *Soldier's heart* is a term that was used in the Civil War to describe symptoms that stemmed from what was later called battle fatigue and was also called SHELL SHOCK in World War I. Soldier's heart has also been called Da Costa's syndrome or irritable heart. Da Costa's syndrome represents a syndrome with a set of symptoms that are similar to those of heart disease, though a physical examination does not reveal any physiological abnormalities. The condition was named for Jacob Mendes Da Costa, who investigated and described the disorder during the American Civil War. *Combat stress reaction* is the term that is used today.

Symptoms and Diagnostic Path

The chief symptoms of combat stress reaction are fatigue and an increased heart rate, but there are no medical problems. Some symptoms of a combat stress reaction include:

- severe anxiety
- DEPRESSION
- PANIC ATTACK
- insomnia
- headache
- pounding heart
- nausea and vomiting
- diarrhea
- difficulty speaking and communicating
- inability to concentrate
- easily startled by movement, light, or noise
- crying
- anger

If the combat stress reaction is severe, the following symptoms may be exhibited:

- shaking
- paralysis
- inability to hear, see, or feel
- staggering
- speech that is inappropriate or too rapid
- MEMORY loss
- severe NIGHTMARES
- visual or auditory hallucinations
- hysterical outbursts

Treatment Options and Outlook

Sometimes the soldier with a combat stress reaction can recover with such simple measures as an opportunity for sufficient sleep, nutritious food, and water. Sleep alone is vitally important, and experts report that every 24 hours of lost sleep impedes the mental performance of the individual by 25 percent. Stimulants such as caffeine in soft drinks, chewing gum, and candy bars can temporarily improve the situation, but sleep deficits build up quickly even with such short-term aids.

According to information from the U.S. Army on combat operational stress reaction (COSR) in Technical Guide 241, friends and leaders of the soldier should take the following actions, with the understanding that even serious combat stress reactions can often improve within minutes if they are handled well immediately:

- If the soldier's behavior endangers the mission, control the situation.

- If the soldier is upset, talk calmly and try to enlist the soldier's cooperation; assign a simple task.

- Make a quick check for physical injuries.

- Reassure the soldier that recovery can occur quickly.

- If the soldier is no longer reliable:
  - unload the soldier's weapon;
  - take the weapon only if you are seriously concerned;
  - physically restrain only if necessary for safety.

- Get the soldier to a safer place.

- Do not leave the soldier alone.

- Get the soldier to drink water, eat, and sleep if tired.

- Warm, cool, and/or dry the soldier if needed.

- Assign the soldier to appropriate, realistic tasks, and eventually, to a return to duty.

- Get a medic's advice if signs could be from injury, drugs, or disease.

- Get the soldier to talk about what happened.

- Evacuate the soldier to an aid station if the soldier does not improve, but reassure the soldier of recovery and return to duty.

- If unable to evacuate, ensure the soldier's safety while continuing to give reassurance and support.

According to the authors of a 2005 Rand report on combat stress reactions, the key principles for the treatment of battle fatigue can be simplified into four "R's." According to the authors, these R's include:

> *Reassurance* of a quick recovery from a confident and authoritative source; *respite* from intense stressors; *replenishment* in the form of water, a hot meal, sleep, regulation of body temperature, and hygiene; *restoration* of perspective and confidence through conversation and working.

Another acronym for treatment is PIES, or *proximity* (treating the soldier close to the battlefront), *immediacy* (treating right away or as soon as possible), *expectancy* (telling the soldier that he or she is expected to recover) and *simplicity* (using a simple approach to treatment). The "new" army employs these techniques to help reduce posttraumatic stress disorder and restore personnel to the battlefield. This was termed *forward psychiatry* during World War I. Talking about a traumatic event shortly after it occurs has a long military tradition that is set in the PIES crisis intervention principles. During World War II, U.S. and British forces reintroduced PIES as an effective method to return soldiers to active duty. The role of the military psychiatrist in these situations was to tell the soldier that he or she is neither sick nor a coward, but rather one that just experienced an extremely stressful event and is in need of some rest, and with time will get better. Returning soldiers to their unit and to perform their duties is the primary goal of forward psychiatry.

Risk Factors and Preventive Measures

According to the authors of a 2005 Rand report on combat stress reaction, the best predictor of the development of combat stress reactions is the intensity of the combat. In addition, as the number of physical casualties of military men and women escalate, so will the number of combat stress reactions.

It is interesting to note, however, that elite units usually report extremely *low* rates of combat stress reactions and other psychiatric problems. According to the Rand report, elite groups rarely have more than 5 percent psychiatric casualties. Stated the authors, "Factors that may protect these units include increased cohesion due to high retention of members, intense training and the self-respect that comes from being viewed as elite, as well as briefer combat engagement periods than conventional divisions."

There are some variables that are linked to a higher risk for the development of a combat stress reaction, according to the authors of the Rand report. Stress at home and low educational levels are both linked to an increased risk for combat stress reaction among soldiers. Poor morale and low self-confidence increase the risk as well. Combat that occurs in an urban situation is more stressful than combat in the field, partly because of the risk of civilian casualties.

Stressors from home may include concern over a sick parent or child. In addition, positive stress is also a factor, such as with a recent marriage or the birth of a child before or after being sent to combat. The receipt of a "Dear John/Jane" letter severing a personal relationship is also extremely stressful and may exacerbate the risk of a combat stress reaction.

Extrapolating from data obtained from World War II, inexperienced troops have their highest risk of combat stress reactions in the initial five to 21 days of combat. Veteran troops last longer but are also at risk. The risk of breakdowns among veteran troops is greatest between 30 to 250 days of combat. Some experts estimate a soldier's "emotional lifespan" in combat at about 80 to 90 days.

In general, soldiers who are moving are less likely to have a combat stress reaction than are soldiers who are located in a stationary situation on a static battlefield, such as in an urban warfare situation.

Note that one factor that has *not* been shown to predict combat stress is personality, and thus individuals at risk for combat stress reaction cannot be screened out with personality tests.

If the combat stress reaction is severe and it cannot be mitigated by the actions of the soldier's fellow combatants or leaders, the individual may need to be evacuated and treated by psychiatrists in a hospital location. Some soldiers are able to return to duty after treatment.

With regard to preventive measures to combat stress reaction, some experts, such as the Rand authors, believe that combat stress reactions can be significantly reduced by military leaders and training in specific actions. For example, they recommend that before sending troops to combat, some tasks be overlearned through repetition so that they become automatic to the soldier. As a result of this overlearning, soldiers are less likely to freeze up in the confusion of combat.

Experts also recommend that after soldiers have completed their initial training in firing their weapons (and their confidence has been built up), the training should then include distractions, since there are many distractions on the battlefield.

It is also important to prepare troops beforehand with regard to how they may react in a combat situation; for example, anxiety and confusion are normal reactions in the face of combat, as are heart palpitations. If troops are not given this information, they may become overly anxious and think their reactions are abnormal and consequently may be less effective in the battlefield.

Teamwork is extremely important in the battlefield, and team skills should be an integral part of training for combat missions. Unit cohesion is especially important, and research has revealed that soldiers who are serving with strangers are more likely to suffer from combat stress reactions than are those who are working with others whom they know and trust.

Historical Background

Da Costa's syndrome was a posttraumatic stress syndrome-like disorder that was first identified among soldiers by internist Jacob Mendez Da Costa during the Civil War. In an article published in the *American Journal of Military Sciences* in 1871, Da Costa wrote that he found a soldier who was anxious before a Civil War battle and had sharp pains, palpitations, and difficulty moving following the battle. Repeated occurrences of these symptoms were noted until the soldier was wounded at Gettysburg and was bedridden. In the absence of any structural deficiencies of the heart, Da Costa concluded that this syndrome was caused by nerve irritability or damage to the sympathetic nerves to heart, hence the alternate name, irritable heart syndrome.

In later years, the terms *anxiety neuroses, combat fatigue* or *neuroses,* and *shell shock* became the more commonly accepted terms to describe these symptoms. However, undaunted by the vagueness of the symptom pattern and the specific and quite traumatic nature of its onset in war, medical researchers later identified civilian cases in which individuals hyperventilated in reaction to stress and named the condition "neurocirculatory asthenia."

The fact that 45 percent of the soldiers in World War I who were diagnosed with Da Costa's syndrome reported a family history of "nervousness" strengthened the prevailing theory of constitutional weakness or DEGENERACY.

Convoy fatigue was a term for combat stress reaction that was used prior to and during World War

II. At the time, the United States used some 6,000 ships manned by Merchant Marines for trade. This fleet was commissioned by President Franklin D. Roosevelt as part of the country's economic recovery program. However, these ships were defenseless against predators and enemies and were often sunk or boarded. In 1940 the *Jean Mecolinty* was sunk, and its surviving crew suffered great personal shock and trauma. Mental health centers responded and formed group therapy programs for the Merchant Marines to treat emotional injuries from attacks and convoy fatigue. These sailors were not covered by the GI Bill and had no other benefits, even though they experienced one of the highest causality rates in World War II. Finally, in 1988 the Defense Department granted them full veteran status and benefits.

See also COMBAT RELATED POSTTRAUMATIC STRESS DISORDER; ELECTROENCEPHALOGRAPH; POST-VIETNAM SYNDROME (PVS); THERAPY, TYPES OF; TRAUMA, COMBAT VERSUS CIVILIAN.

Helmus, Todd C., and Russell W. Glenn. *Steeling the Mind: Combat Stress Reactions and Their Implications for Urban Welfare.* Santa Monica, Calif.: Rand Corporation, 2005. Available online. URL: http://www.rand.org/pubs/monographs/2005/RAND_MG191.pdf. Downloaded August 15, 2006.

Jones, Edgar, and Simon Wessely. "War Syndromes: The Impact of Culture on Medically Unexplained Symptoms." *Medical History* 49 (2005): 55–78.

Noy, Shabtai. "Gradations of Stress as Determinants of the Clinical Picture Immediately After Traumatic Events." *Traumatology* 6, no. 3 (2001): 1–9.

Oppenheimer, B. S., and M. A. Rothchild. "The Psychoneurotic Factor in the Irritable Heart of Soldiers." *Journal of the American Medical Association* 70 (1918): 1,919–1,922.

U.S. Army, Combat Operational Stress Reaction (COSR) ("Battle Fatigue"), undated. Available online. URL: http://chppm-www.apgea.army.mil/documents/TG/TECHGUID/TG241.pdf#search=%22batt ele%20fatigue%20normal%20common%20signs%20self%20buddy%20army%22. Downloaded August 17, 2006.

compassion fatigue Emotional exhaustion and numbness that may occur after consistently providing empathy and assistance to one or more needful individuals with TRAUMATIC STRESS symptoms.

Compassion fatigue is seen in mental health professionals, health-care professionals, child protection workers, and members of the clergy. In addition, nonprofessionals also experience compassion fatigue, such as the constant caregivers of ill parents or other relatives. The term *compassion fatigue* was first coined by C. Figley in 1995 in his book *Compassion Fatigue: Coping with Secondary Traumatic Stress Disorder in Those Who Treat the Traumatized.* Some individuals use the term *compassion fatigue* interchangeably with the phrases SECONDARY TRAUMATIZATION or VICARIOUS TRAUMATIZATION.

A variety of studies have been made on compassion fatigue, particularly among helping professionals. In one study, the results of a survey of 236 social workers living in New York City, 80 percent of whom were involved in disaster counseling after the SEPTEMBER 11 attacks, was reported in a 2004 issue of the *International Journal of Emergency Mental Health.* The researchers considered compassion fatigue a construct that comprised both secondary traumatization and job burnout. The researchers also defined compassion fatigue as "the reduced capacity or interest in being empathic."

They found that social workers who had worked with traumatized victims experienced a greater risk for compassion fatigue, and World Trade Center recovery involvement was the factor with the greatest risk for secondary trauma: 52 percent of those with high recovery involvement were determined as potential secondary trauma cases, versus 25 percent of the social workers with low involvement in recovery. Recovery included such actions as supporting rescue or recovery efforts, helping to lower rescue workers' stress, and providing shelter to displaced people. Note that if the social workers had been directly involved when the World Trade Center disaster occurred, they would have experienced a primary trauma, and working with victims would then have exacerbated this trauma further.

In contrast, high counseling involvement yielded lower but significant rates: 35 percent of those determined to have high counseling involvement with September 11 victims were considered to be at risk for secondary trauma versus 25 percent of those with low involvement in counseling. However, it is not known if this study can be generalized to other social workers working with trauma victims because of the uniqueness of the September 11 tragedy and the high rate of involvement of the social workers; for example, more than 90 percent of the studied social workers said that they were directly involved with recovery, rescue, or counseling in the World Trade Center disaster.

In another study on compassion fatigue and burnout, the researchers analyzed rabbis who worked as chaplains to determine which factors increased their risk for compassion fatigue. This study was reported in the *Journal of Pastoral Care & Counseling* in 2006. The researchers found that compassion fatigue was low among the 66 male and female respondents; however, rates were higher for chaplains who were divorced and increased for those who spent many hours each week working with trauma victims and their families. In addition, compassion fatigue rates were high among those who were divorced women.

It appears that, as with traumatic experiences, compassion fatigue is more likely to develop in people with previous traumatic and psychiatric conditions.

See also COMPASSION SATISFACTION AND FATIGUE TEST; PRIMARY/SECONDARY/TERTIARY TRAUMATIC STRESS DISORDER; SECONDARY TRAUMATIC STRESS (STS)/SECONDARY TRAUMATIC STRESS DISORDER (STSD).

Boscarino, Joseph A., Charles R. Figley, and Richard E. Adams. "Compassion Fatigue following the September 11 Terrorist Attacks: A Study of Secondary Trauma among New York City Social Workers." *International Journal of Emergency Mental Health* 6 no. 2 (2004): 1–9.

Rothschild, Babette, with Marjorie Rand. *Help for the Helper: The Psychophysiology of Compassion Fatigue and Vicarious Trauma.* New York: W.W. Norton, 2006.

Taylor, Bonita E., et al. "Compassion Fatigue and Burnout among Rabbis Working as Chaplains." *Journal of Pastoral Care & Counseling* 60, nos. 1–2 (Spring–Summer 2006): 35–42.

Compassion Satisfaction and Fatigue Test   A self-test that was devised by Beth Hudnall Stamm and Charles R. Figley in the 1990s to help individuals assess their level of compassion satisfaction or COMPASSION FATIGUE. Individuals respond to questions about themselves by self-rating on a five-point intensity scale.

The items include such statements as, "I force myself to avoid certain thoughts or feelings that remind me of a frightening experience," and "While working with the victim, I thought about violence against the perpetrator."

The Compassion Satisfaction and Fatigue Test has been largely replaced by the more comprehensive PROFESSIONAL QUALITY OF LIFE SCALE (Pro Qol), a measure created by Hudnall Stamm that looks at more "quality of life" factors. Quality of life is a general measure of overall functioning in one's life and has been used to assess changes in trauma-related disorders as well as other forms of mental illness.

See also PRIMARY/SECONDARY/TERTIARY TRAUMATIC STRESS DISORDER; VICARIOUS TRAUMATIZATION.

complex posttraumatic stress disorder (CPTSD)   Complex posttraumatic stress disorder, also known as disorders of extreme stress not otherwise specified (DESNOS), describes individuals exposed to chronic traumas that last for months to years at a time. This prolonged, extreme psychological harm develops through repeated trauma, as when the victim is under the direct control of the perpetrator, such as with the sexual abuse of children, adult abusive relationships, or prisoner of war captivity. This diagnosis is currently not included in the *DIAGNOSTIC AND STATISTICAL MANUAL OF MENTAL DISORDERS (DSM-IV)*, but it is under consideration for inclusion in *DSM-V* (to be published in 2011) as a formal diagnosis.

Symptoms and Diagnostic Path

Individuals with complex PTSD have impaired affect regulation and difficulty regulating their internal emotional states. The National Center for PTSD of the Department of Veterans Affairs, describes the symptoms for complex PTSD as:

- alternations in emotional regulation, which may include symptoms such as persistent sadness, suicidal thoughts, explosive anger, or inhibited anger
- alterations in self-perception, which may include a sense of helplessness, shame, guilt, stigma, and

a sense of being completely different from other humans

• alterations in the perception of the perpetrator, such as attributing total power to the perpetrator or becoming preoccupied with the relationship to the perpetrator, including a preoccupation with revenge

• alterations in relations with others, including isolation, distrust, or a repeated search for a rescuer

• alterations in the individual's system of meanings, which include a loss of sustaining faith or a sense of hopelessness and despair

Treatment Options and Outlook

Complex PTSD will take longer to treat and will require greater therapist skills and focus than will single incident trauma. Generally, a phase-oriented approach is needed in which interventions are introduced sequentially. The therapist must establish a solid and trusting relationship before any trauma or historic work. Affect modulation or containment must be established, and any current disorder must be addressed. Trauma work requires patience and attention to details.

COGNITIVE BEHAVIORAL THERAPIES have proven effective as well as EYE MOVEMENT DESENSITIZATION AND REPROCESSING (EMDR). Additionally, new patterns of behavior to replace old maladaptive ones are needed for better adjustment and interpersonal success. Sometimes traditional therapy can be combined with EMDR administered by another therapist.

Risk Factors and Preventive Measures

B. A. van der Kolk and colleagues reviewed the *DSM-IV* research database and found that people who were traumatized early in life tended to have all of the trauma symptoms listed in the *DSM-IV.* The longer the trauma lasted, and the less protection that was received from the perpetrator, the more pervasive was the damage to the self. The field trials confirmed that trauma had its most profound effect during the first 10 years of life. People who were exposed to early and prolonged interpersonal trauma developed the psychological problems in the DESNOS syndrome. The older the

people were, with the shorter duration of trauma, the more likely were the development of core PTSD symptoms.

In his book, Scaer refers to individuals with complex PTSD as primed to dissociate and experience many perceptual states associated with DISSOCIATION, such as depersonalization, AMNESIA, an altered sense of time, and feelings of unreality.

See also BATTERED CHILD SYNDROME; CHILD ABUSE AND NEGLECT; THERAPY, TYPES OF.

Scaer, Robert. *Trauma Spectrum.* New York: W.W. Norton, 2005.
van der Kolk, B. A., S. Roth D. Pelcovitz, and F. Mandel. *Complex PTSD: Results of the PTSD Field Trials for DSM-IV.* Washington, D.C.: American Psychiatric Press, 1993.

concentration camp syndrome   See KZ SYNDROME.

conditioned emotional reactions   Refers to emotional responses that are elicited by particular stimuli after some trials in which the two are paired. The result is comparable to having both an image and a positive feeling when someone smells the perfume that an old girlfriend used to wear. Another example might be of a person thinking about a favored restaurant (stimulus) and then starting to feel hungry (conditioned emotional reaction).

On the aversive side, when negative emotions are conditioned, an individual might find fear (conditioned) reactions arising whenever the brake lights (conditioned stimuli) of another car appear in front of him or her after a rear end collision. Another example of an aversive conditioned emotional reaction occurs when a person has a nauseated (conditioned) reaction when seeing or thinking about some food (conditioned stimulus) that he or she ate before getting sick.

The study of these reactions has been a central focus in psychology and physiology because they represent important aspects of life and can also create quite restrictive effects on functioning. For example, almost all the ANXIETY DISORDERS involve aversive emotional conditioning (anxiety) to internal or external stimuli. Phobias are a good example of situations in which anxiety toward to a particular object or event develops after conditioning has occurred. This usually leads to escaping or running away from that stimulus or avoiding it altogether. In both cases, functioning is restricted.

How Conditioned Emotional Reactions Arise

Some of the earliest scientific work on this question comes from studies in 1889 by Pierre Janet, who argued that overwhelming emotions are split off from the consciousness and are stored separately in the body. Thus, they never get "processed" or worked through on a verbal or symbolic level and any reexperiencing of the event (stimulus) can trigger some of the original traumatic reaction.

Freud in 1919 adopted Janet's views, and he also linked them to psychopathological reactions, arguing that "the patient has undergone a physical fixation to the trauma." However, it was Ivan Pavlov (1926) who demonstrated empirically the process by which common, neutral stimuli (e.g., a bell) could condition (elicit) a particular response that was associated with the neutral stimulus (such as salivation). In his initial experiments with dogs, a bell would ring followed immediately by food (meat paste, in this case) being served to the animals. After a few pairings, the ringing of the bell alone elicited salivation (conditioned response) in the dogs.

Pavlov coined the term *defensive reaction* in situations where innate aversive reactions (such as fear) were conditioned to environmental threats or events. Reexperiencing some aspect of the aversive (traumatic) environmental event (such as a person seeing a stranger following behind on the street, long after he or she had been robbed) would trigger or elicit the defensive reaction of fear. In this way, a protective reaction or response was developed to prevent future harm or traumatization. Watson and Rayner, two experimental behavioral psychologists working in the 1920s, actually demonstrated the acquisition of defensive fear reactions with a toddler. They paired a loud noise with the presence of a rabbit and quickly conditioned the baby to fear both rabbits and furry animals in general. (Such an experiment would be frowned upon today.)

Physiological Mechanisms

Today scientists are beginning to understand some of the physiological mechanisms involved in trau-matization and conditioned emotional reactions. In particular, the lower or subcortical brain centers seem to play a central role in the development of PTSD and aversive emotional reactions. The AMYGDALA and HIPPOCAMPUS areas of the brain, in particular, seem to be crucial for the storage of trauma-related stimuli or memories that seem to drive the hormonal and autonomic responses.

In the 1990s, Joseph LeDoux, an experimental physiologist, showed that animals retain the memory of traumatic events when the amygdala and hippocampus are intact, even when the cortical areas associated with MEMORY are damaged or nonfunctional. Furthermore, subcortical areas of the BRAIN are intimately connected to bodily sensations that are associated with TRAUMATIC EVENTS (Peter Levine) that serve as triggers for defensive behavior. As researchers discover more about the physiological and hormonal (and possibly cellular) aspects of POSTTRAUMATIC STRESS DISORDER (PTSD), interventions will improve and victims will begin to find consistent relief from the barriers to human functioning that are imposed by PTSD.

See also BODY MEMORY.

convoy fatigue   See COMBAT STRESS REACTION.

COPE Inventory/Brief COPE   An instrument that helps measure the individual's current style of coping, including effective and ineffective means. The COPE Inventory, a 60-item test, was first developed by Charles S. Carver, Michael F. Scheier, and Jagdish Kumari Weintraub in 1989. A significantly shorter version, developed in 1997, the Brief COPE, was developed based on the coping skills of adults who were recovering from Hurricane Andrew.

The COPE Inventory evaluates 15 factors or scales that reveal a person's active or avoidant coping behavior. These scales include:

1. Active coping (actively taking steps to remove the stressor or to mitigate its effects)
2. Planning (considering means and strategies to deal with a stressor)
3. Seeking instrumental social support (seeking advice or information)

4. Seeking emotional social support (seeking understanding, sympathy, or moral support)
5. Suppression of competing activities (to enable the individual to concentrate on managing the stressor)
6. Religion (using spiritual means to cope with stressors)
7. Positive reinterpretation and growth
8. Restraint coping (waiting for an opportunity to take action and avoiding acting prematurely)
9. Resignation/acceptance
10. Focus on and venting of emotions
11. Denial (a coping method that may be helpful at some times, such as in the initial stages of a traumatic event, but which is ultimately not helpful)
12. Mental disengagement (a negative means of coping in which the person is distracted from acting to reduce the stressor, such as by daydreaming, watching many hours of television, and so forth)
13. Behavioral disengagement (a negative means of coping in which the individual behaves in a helpless manner
14. Alcohol/drug use
15. Humor

The questionnaire asks responders what they generally do and feel when confronted with a stressful event, maintaining that people respond differently to different events and that there are no "right" or "wrong" answers. The COPE has been used in many health-related studies assessing the importance of the coping process, and it is predictive of prospective physiological effects, such as human immunodeficiency virus (HIV) and breast cancer.

The Brief COPE, an abbreviated version of the COPE Inventory, is designed to minimize time demands on participants and eliminate the redundancy in the original version. The Brief COPE has only two items per scale and eliminates the Restraint Coping and Suppression of Competing Activities scales from the original COPE and adds a Self-Blame scale.

The Brief COPE scales include:

1. Active coping
2. Planning
3. Positive reframing
4. Acceptance
5. Humor
6. Religion
7. Using emotional support
8. Using instrumental support
9. Self-distraction
10. Denial
11. Venting
12. Substance use
13. Behavioral disengagement
14. Self-blame

See also ASSESSMENT AND DIAGNOSIS.

Carver, Charles S., Michael F. Scheier, and Jagdish Kumari Weintraub. "Assessing Coping Strategies: A Theoretically Based Approach." *Journal of Personality and Social Psychology* 56, no. 2 (1989): 267–283.
Carver, C. S. "You Want to Measure Coping But Your Protocol's Too Large: Consider the Brief COPE." *International Journal of Behavioral Medicine* 4, no. 1 (1997): 92–99.

coping mechanism Coping is the ability to manage the demands placed upon the individual without exceeding the resources available. Coping with a traumatic event is quite different from dealing with everyday stress, and most individuals do not practice or have in their repertoire the behaviors needed to deal with such tragedy.

As a result, emotional NUMBING, FLASHBACKS, INSOMNIA, and cognitive impairment are the initial reactions to such events. Active coping strategies are the cognitive and behavioral responses designed to terminate the exposure to stressors and help the individual resume "normal living," actively challenging oneself to engage in "doing something" to change how one thinks about the traumatic experience. Conversely, passive coping strategies lead the individual to disengage from the situation, even to the point of freezing in his or her life, becoming avoidant, withdrawn, and in denial.

Coping mechanisms or coping strategies are survival strategies. Two dimensions of coping styles have received attention in research, and they are used to categorize other strategies. These coping styles are (1) problem-focused coping, which is aimed at altering person-environment relationships, and (2) emotion-focused coping, which is aimed at regulating emotional distress. According to Higgin and Endler (1995), problem-focused coping predicts a better recovery from stressors, while emotion-focused coping, such as avoidance and self-blame, can lead to more psychological distress following stressful events.

In 1993 Lahad studied coping mechanisms under stress and identified six coping styles: cognitive, affective/emotional, social, imagination, belief and values, and physical. The individual with the cognitive style prefers information gathering, problem solving, self-navigation, and internal conversations. The person with the affective or emotional coping style uses emotional expression through crying, laughter, talking, or through nonverbal methods, such as writing or drawing. The individual with the social coping style receives support from belonging to a group, such as family. The fourth type of coping style uses imagination to deal with the horrific facts by daydreaming or diverting attention through pleasant thoughts, or by finding solutions in imaginative ways, improvising as necessary. The belief and values coping style relies on the individual's belief system to guide him or her through times of crisis. It is not only religious belief but also encompasses the person's political expressions or need for self-expression that is meaningful. Last, the individual with the physical coping style reacts to stress by using physical expressions in body movements, such as exercise or relaxation activities.

Higgins, J. E., and N. S. Endler. "Coping, Life Stress, and Psychological and Somatic Distress." *European Journal of Personality* 9 (1995): 253–270.

Lahad, S., "Tracing Coping Resources through a Story in Six Parts—The "BASIC PH" model." In *Psychology at School and the Community During Peaceful and Emergency Times*. Tel Aviv, Israel: Levinson-Hadar (in Hebrew), 1993.

corpus callosum   An area of the BRAIN consisting of thick bundles of nerves connecting the right and left hemispheres of the brain. In the 18th century, the corpus callosum was thought to be the site of the human soul. It was not until the 1950s that researchers realized that the corpus callosum was the mechanism for the transfer of information between the two hemispheres of the brain.

Studies of intractable epilepsy (in which even drugs had little or no effect on seizures) found that severing portions of the corpus callosum (and leaving a small section intact) relieved the epilepsy but still allowed some communication between hemispheres. This work has been called split-brain research. Splitting the two hemispheres into separate structures allowed for the study of each hemisphere separately and the means of communication between the two sides.

In an intact brain, information is received in the right hemisphere and then quickly passed from the right hemisphere to the left via the corpus callosum. This path from right (sensory) to left (verbal and language-mediated) has important implications for the study of trauma and its effects on the individual, as well as for the forms of effective treatment. Surprisingly, in the split-brain person, cognitive functions appear to the observer to be within normal limits. It is only when specific neurological tests are administered that symptoms of disconnection become apparent.

As mentioned, the left hemisphere is primarily responsible for language, logical thought based on language, and motor activity on the right side of the body. The right hemisphere is responsible for motor activity on the left side of the body, but more important, it also deals with context and holistic perception. The sensory receptors or terminals in the brain primarily feed the right side. The left side has access to this sensory stimulation only through transmission across the corpus callosum.

Another important area of the brain is the orbitofrontal cortex (which lies directly behind the eyes and is adjacent to the LIMBIC SYSTEM). This area is responsible for integrating emotional responses generated in the limbic system with the higher cognitive or executive functions, such as planning, delay of action, use of logical, language-based understanding and strategies that reside in the functions of the cerebral cortex's prefrontal lobes. The left orbito-frontal cortex handles MEMORY creation or encoding, while the right orbital-frontal cortex is responsible for memory retrieval. Healthy functioning requires the integration of both the right and left hemispheres.

The corpus callosum is not yet developed at birth; consequently, most of the experience of the infant is in the right or sensory side, and it is not accessible to declarative or EXPLICIT MEMORY (long-term memory that can be communicated verbally). Explicit memory relies on encoding, decoding, and processing functions that reside on the left side.

In cases of substantiated abuse and neglect, children have been shown to have smaller and more poorly integrated corpus callosum bundles. This would appear to result in deficient integration and coordination of the hemispheres and a general underdevelopment in the orbito-frontal cortices or executive functions. Poor development or communication with the orbitofrontal cortices would account for trauma-related symptoms, such as difficulty regulating emotions, lack of cause-effect thinking, an inability to accurately recognize emotions in others, an inability to articulate emotional states, an incoherent sense of self and one's history, poor inhibition, and deficits in social skills and in attunement with others.

Early attachments to parental figures and individual interpersonal experiences have a profound effect on brain development. The brain circuits that are responsible for social perception are also those that integrate functions, such as the creation of meaning, the regulation of body states, emotional regulation, the organization of memory, and the capacity for interpersonal understanding and empathy. Neuroendocrine impairment also occurs, which further enhances brain structure deficits.

Secure early attachment seems to be critical to the physical and hormonal sculpting of the brain and its eventual functioning. For example, it is known that an infant uses the parents' state to regulate his or her own mental and emotional processes. The child's developing capacity to regulate emotions and develop a coherent sense of self requires sensitive and responsive parenting. Failures in bonding or attachment are called attachment disorders (see ATTACHMENT STYLES/DISORDERS).

The corpus callosum seems to be essential to the synchronization of neural activity within a particular frequency band. Split-brain research and fragmented consciousness studies suggest that the corpus callosum helps synchronize the brain patterns that organize conscious experience. The rhythmic eye movements that are associated with EYE MOVEMENT DESENSITIZATION AND REPROCESSING (EMDR) may establish a background of synchronic rhythm across cerebral hemispheres that allow the processing of traumatic material toward some form of resolution.

See also AMYGDALA; AUTONOMIC NERVOUS SYSTEM; CENTRAL NERVOUS SYSTEM; CHILD ABUSE AND NEGLECT; SYMPATHETIC NERVOUS SYSTEM.

corticosteroid A class of steroids that is produced in the cortex of the adrenal gland. Two main groups of corticosteroids include GLUCOCORTICOIDS, which are essential in carbohydrate, fat, and protein metabolism and are involved in the body's stress response system, and mineralocorticoids, which regulate electrolytes and saltwater balance within the body. The main hormone produced by the adrenal cortex that seems to be indicative of POSTTRAUMATIC STRESS DISORDER (PTSD) is CORTISOL. This substance is associated with chronic stress reactions and seems to be involved in sustained autonomic arousal.

Corticosteroids are secreted as part of the hypothalamus-pituitary-adrenal gland (HPA) pathway when ADRENOCORTICOTROPIC HORMONE (ACTH) triggers the adrenal cortex. Eventually, the corticosteroids signal the HIPPOCAMPUS, the part of the brain that seems to control emotional memories, and the hippocampus helps to inhibit or abate the stress arousal.

cortisol A GLUCOCORTICOID steroid hormone that is produced by the adrenal glands. It is also referred to as hydrocortisone when it is in synthetic form. Cortisol plays a significant role in the body when safety is threatened, and it is referred to as the stress hormone because its output is increased during FIGHT OR FLIGHT RESPONSE. This hormone is critical to survival.

Cortisol acts to increase blood sugar levels for greater energy, heightens memory functioning, increases the pain threshold, and increases immune function. Cortisol also brings the body back to homeostasis once the STRESS reaction passes. Immune dysfunction results from chronic, long-term stress upon the body as frequent higher levels of cortisol in the bloodstream have negative effects on health. Excessive cortisol can also interfere with how NEUROTRANSMITTERS function for MEMORY retrieval, resulting in confusion or the mind going "blank" during a crisis situation.

Corticotrophin-releasing factor (CRF) is a protein in the BRAIN that drives the release of cortisol. Normally, CRF is released from the hypothalamus, then CRF stimulates the pituitary gland to release ADRENOCORTICOTROPIC HORMONE (ACTH), which in turn stimulates the release of cortisol to the adrenal gland.

Stress hormones can have detrimental long-term effects. Excessive cortisol levels result in the thinning of the stomach lining, which increases the risk for gastric ulcers. It also can result in a thinning of the bones of older people and an impairment of the reproductive system in younger people. Interestingly, people with POSTTRAUMATIC STRESS DISORDER (PTSD) usually show lower than normal levels of cortisol.

counterphobic   An attempt by a phobic person to avoid the appearance of anxiety in the presence of phobic stimuli. *The International Dictionary of Psychoanalysis* defines a counterphobic person as "The person who seeks out one or more external objects or phenomena, whether consciously or unconsciously, to escape from the manifestations of anxiety linked to his or her phobias." At the extreme, many people who are known as "daredevils" have this quality, and they may appear fearless in spite of the enormous risks that they are taking.

Traumatized people may also try to look normal even though they experience intense anxiety and discomfort. The true counterphobic, however, may actually gain control of the anxiety experience and not consciously feel its effects.

Interestingly, students of the Enneagram (a 9-category personality typing system), attribute counterphobia to the person who is a "loyalist." Loyalists are believed to make good law enforcement, armed services, and uniformed personnel because they know and adhere to a standard set of rules set down for them by authority figures. Since adherence occurs in spite of any personal fears or anxieties, they are often seen as counterphobic prototypes. They are dedicated to a cause or set of principles that they choose to adhere to, and hence, are loyalists. In psychoanalytic terms, counterphobia is a way to bind anxiety so that it does not intrude into consciousness and disrupt the psychic mechanism.

See also ANXIETY DISORDERS.

coupling   A term from SOMATIC EXPERIENCING THERAPY that refers to a close association between or among the elements of sensation, image, behavior, affect (mood), and MEMORY, such that the arousal in one element can trigger the arousal in other elements (overcoupling) or it can restrict arousal in other elements (undercoupling).

Traumatic coupling can produce either over- or undercoupling, and these responses become the template for discharging and/or binding any arousal that is strong or overwhelming to the individual. Obviously, a great deal of energy is expended in both forms of trauma response. The individual then organizes behavior around these templates, which are triggered when almost any arousal takes place.

Overcoupling is evident in body constriction within the same elements, such as sensation (for example, warmth in one part leads to a headache), image (a FLASHBACK triggers a flood of images), behavior (the hand starts to tremble, the shoulder gets stiff, the neck gets stiff, and so on), affect (anger turns to sadness), and meaning (one thought after another). On the other hand, constriction in one element may cross over to another element. Within somatic experiencing therapy, the therapist often has to work to uncouple responses (if responses are overcoupled) or to find ways to couple them (if the responses are undercoupled) in order for therapy to progress and to help the individual to restore balance in his or her emotional life.

See also ELABORATED POSTTRAUMATIC STRESS DISORDER (EPTSD); THERAPY, TYPES OF.

crime   See NATIONAL CRIME VICTIMIZATION SURVEY.

crisis management briefings (CMB)   A key component of the CRITICAL INCIDENT STRESS MANAGEMENT system (CISM) developed by Everly and Mitchell, which is generally used with schools, businesses, and community populations that are affected by a crisis event. It is a four-phase crisis intervention system designed for use with small or large groups of people (10 to 300) and takes 45 to 75 minutes to conduct. Not designed as a stand-alone crisis intervention tool, it is intended to be followed up with CRITICAL INCIDENT STRESS DEBRIEFINGS (CISD) and one-on-one individual interventions.

Phase 1 consists of gathering the groups of people who have experienced a common crisis event in a safe environment, such as an auditorium, hotel conference room, business meeting room, or any large gathering facility. Phase 2 is to have authoritative sources present the facts of the crisis or traumatic event. The purpose of reporting the facts is to control rumors and reduce anxieties by providing what is known and what is still unknown.

Phase 3 involves having a mental health professional provide information on stress-related symptoms and address common reactions to TRAUMATIC EVENTS, such as grief, anger, and SURVIVOR GUILT. Phase 4 includes providing educational information on how one can mitigate distressing symptoms that may occur following such a crisis event. Each individual receives a helpful fact sheet describing stress management techniques and contact information for local professionals.

See also DEBRIEFING; MULTIPLE STRESSOR DEBRIEFING MODEL.

Mitchell, J. T., and G. S. Everly, Jr. *Critical Incident Stress Debriefing (CISD): An Operations Manual for the Prevention of Traumatic Stress Among Emergency Service and Disaster Workers.* 2nd ed. Elliott City, Md.: Chevron, 1997.

critical incident stress debriefing (CISD) One component of the model that uses Jeffrey T. Mitchell's CRITICAL INCIDENT STRESS MANAGEMENT (CISM), and which is used with homogeneous groups of individuals, usually 24 to 72 hours following a critical incident or three to four weeks after a major disaster, such as an earthquake or a hurricane. A critical incident is any negative situation that exceeds the normal experiences of an

individual and that can potentially overwhelm the individual's ability to cope and function effectively. The situation can be devastating, catastrophic, or traumatic, and may bring on unusually strong emotional feelings and thoughts.

The formal CISD is a seven-phase process that is led by a mental health professional and a peer facilitator.

The phases are as follows:

1. Introduction: The facilitators introduce themselves and describe the rules of confidentiality, the discussion process, and expectations. (Critical incident stress debriefing is not psychotherapy, nor is it an operational debriefing.)
2. Fact: The group participants are asked to describe the critical incident event from their own perspective and discuss what activity they performed during the event.
3. Thought: The participants are asked to describe their first thoughts of the event and to facilitate cognitive reactions.
4. Reaction: The facilitators ask participants such questions as, "What was the worst part of the incident for you?" to identify their emotional reactions.
5. Symptom: Personal symptoms of stress are identified and participants describe how their lives have changed since the event.
6. Teaching: Participants are educated on stress management, coping techniques, and normalizing crisis reactions to extraordinary events.
7. Re-entry: To provide closure, the facilitators summarize the debriefing process by answering any questions, re-emphasizing normalization of reactions and providing follow-up referrals for those who may need further intervention.

CISD has been used by emergency service workers, rescue workers, police and fire personnel, as well as trauma/disaster survivors.

CISD Process with Children

There are several modifications of the CISD process when working with children. With children below the age of six, the children might best be brought together in their natural group with a familiar person, such as their teacher, to reassure them of safety and provide emotional support. This type of group is also called CRISIS MANAGEMENT BRIEFING. There is little structure to the group, and the information given to the children should offer a sense of reassurance and hope. Children should not feel terrified by new information in this debriefing. For children ages six to 12, a modified five- phase CISD model is advised, including Introduction, Fact, Reaction, Teaching, and Re-entry.

The group leader must always use age-appropriate language, and children must not be forced to speak. A more active role of the group leader is required when talking of emotions. Asking the children, "How many of you were frightened today? Show me your hands" allows participation. For children age 13 and older, the full seven-phase CISD process can be used. Teens may need supportive encouragement to participate in a group, whereas adults participate as they see fit. Practical advice and information can be immediately useful for teens as they try to recover from a traumatic event.

In recent years there has been confusion and controversy over crisis-intervention practices called debriefings, specifically CISD. There has been an erroneous assumption that a single session of CISD intervention can prevent PTSD from developing in traumatized individuals. CISD was never intended to be a substitute for psychological treatment nor a stand-alone intervention. Rather, it is a form of crisis-intervention and a component of the larger crisis-intervention program referred to by Mitchell and Everly as CRITICAL INCIDENT STRESS MANAGE-MENT. Addressing criticism that debriefings are not effective, Mitchell and Everly have acknowledged as one of the difficulties "the confusion over terms and the failure of methodologies to evaluate their specific model of debriefing in the situation for which it was developed [i.e., emergency services]." Specifically, these studies applied the CISD format to individuals when the CISD model was developed and used extensively for group intervention. When addressing the efficacy of debriefings, in the future, outcome research needs to focus on the type of crisis intervention, who provides this intervention and to whom, and in what specific situation.

See also DEBRIEFING; MULTIPLE STRESSOR DEBRIEF-ING; MODEL NATURAL DEBRIEFINGS.

Everly, G. and J. Mitchell. "The Debriefing Controversy and Crisis Intervention: A Review of Lexical and Substantive Issues." *Journal of Emergency Mental Health* 2, no. 4 (2000): 211–225.
Mitchell, J. T., and G. S. Everly, Jr. *Critical Incident Stress Debriefing (CISD): An Operations Manual for the Prevention of Traumatic Stress among Emergency Service and Disaster Workers.* 2nd ed. Ellicott City, Md.: Chevron, 1997.

critical incident stress management (CISM)   A comprehensive integrated multicomponent crisis intervention system. The origins of critical incident stress management (CISM) can be traced back to the early 1970s. It was formalized by Jeffrey T. Mitchell and George S. Everly in their writings and training in the last several decades to describe a stress management strategy for individuals who were affected by a critical incident, a stressor event. CISM was originally developed for use with emergency response personnel (first responders), but it is now applicable to all persons exposed to trauma in settings such as schools, businesses, hospitals, and the military. A cultural traumatic event, such as the SEPTEMBER 11 terrorist attack on New York City, was as complex a disaster as the world had ever seen and required more than one type of crisis intervention technology.

CISM utilizes seven core crisis-intervention components to stabilize and mitigate crisis symptoms in individuals. CISM is summarized as follows:

1. Precrisis preparation. This component includes stress management education, stress resistance, and crisis mitigation training for individuals and organizations.
2. Disaster, terrorist, or other large-scale incident interventions, including but not limited to
   a) demobilizations for emergency response personnel, a shift-change decompression;
   b) CRISIS MANAGEMENT BRIEFINGS (CMB) for school, corporate, and general civilian populations;
   c) town meetings; and
   d) incident command staff advisement.
3. Defusing. This is a three-phase, structured small group discussion provided within hours of a crisis for purposes of assessment, triaging, and acute symptom mitigation.

4. CRITICAL INCIDENT STRESS DEBRIEFING (CISD) refers to the International Critical Incident Stress Foundation seven-phase structured group discussion, usually provided one to 10 days post crisis (two to four weeks post disaster) designed to mitigate acute symptoms, assess the need for follow-up, and provide a sense of postcrisis psychological closure.

5. One-on-one crisis intervention/counseling or psychological support throughout the full range of the crisis spectrum.

6. Family crisis intervention as well as organizational consultation and pastoral crisis intervention.

7. Follow-up and referral mechanism for assessment and treatment if necessary.

CISM interventions cover the entire temporal span of a crisis from precrisis to acute crisis, and into postcrisis phases. It is considered comprehensive since it applies to individuals, families, small and large groups, as well as to communities. CISM distinguishes itself from psychotherapy and is recognized more as a form of PSYCHOLOGICAL FIRST AID (PFA). CISM programs exist in many federal government agencies, such as the U.S. Coast Guard, the Federal Bureau of Investigation, the U.S. Secret Service, and the Bureau of Alcohol, Tobacco, and Firearms.

See also DEBRIEFING; MULTIPLE STRESSOR DEBRIEFING; NATURAL DEBRIEFINGS.

Mitchell, J. T., and G. S. Everly, Jr. *Critical Incident Stress Debriefing (CISD): An Operations Manual for the Prevention of Traumatic Stress among Emergency Service and Disaster Workers.* 2nd ed. Ellicott City, Md.: Chevron, 1997.

cultural trauma   The trauma experienced by a large percentage of the population or culture following a large-scale TRAUMATIC EVENT. Some cultural traumatic events include the atom bomb blasts in Japan during World War II, the Armenian genocide carried out by the Ottoman Turkish government from 1895 to 1915, the tsunami in the Indian Ocean in the 21st century, the Holocaust in World War II, the Vietnam War, and the SEPTEMBER 11, 2001, terrorist attack on the United States.

A large proportion of the survivors of these events develop POSTTRAUMATIC STRESS DISORDER (PTSD) as do people related to or close to them. Furthermore, there is considerable evidence that the effects of these cultural traumas may even be passed on to subsequent generations in the form of TRANSGENERATIONAL TRAUMA. For example, the Jewish Holocaust was an attempt to extinguish a whole race of people. Survivors displayed PTSD symptoms, but the children of the survivors have also displayed PTSD symptoms and had PTSD levels of CORTISOL in their bodies, as demonstrated by Yehuda, et al., in 2002.

Similarly, in the case of the Armenian genocide, more than 1.5 million Armenian civilians were slaughtered. Transgenerational effects were also noted in terms of abnormal DEPRESSION and PTSD scores, according to Topdijian in 2007. The transgenerational effects of trauma include abnormal hormone levels, a biological vulnerability to develop trauma symptoms, character deficiencies, a greater life stress than with nontraumatized populations, relationship problems, and difficulty with commitment to others.

See also LIFTON'S CHARACTERISTICS OF A SURVIVOR.

Topdjian, V. "Post-generational Trauma in First, Second and Third Generational Children of Armenian Genocide Survivors." Master thesis, California State University at Northridge, 2007.

Yehuda, R., S. L. Halligan, and L. M. Bierer. "Cortisol Levels in Adult Offspring of Holocaust Survivors: Relation to PTSD Symptoms Severity in the Parent and Child." *Psychoneuroendocrinolgy* 27 (2001): 171–180.

cutting and self-mutilation/self-harm   Deliberate self-inflicted injuries often associated with early emotional abuse.

Some individuals, often those experiencing severe anxiety based on past traumas, feel compelled to make tiny cuts on their skin with a razor, knife, or other sharp object to the point of causing minor bleeding and sometimes scarring. These acts seem to release the cutter's intense anxiety. Some cutters report a feeling of depersonalization when they self-injure. However, the tension eventually builds up again, and without treatment the individual returns to cutting. Individuals who engage in cutting behavior are usually not psychotic, and they realize that their behavior is irrational. Cutters are more likely to be females than males. Cutters are often ashamed of and embarrassed by their behavior, yet without treatment they feel compelled to continue the cutting.

The injuries made by cutters are evident to those who see them; however, cutters may hide some of the cuts by wearing pants or long-sleeved shirts or cutting in parts of the body that are not normally exposed. Cutters are usually not suicidal; however, they may accidentally hit a vein or artery and cause serious bleeding, necessitating treatment in the emergency room of a hospital.

Studies have shown that females who are cutters are about three times more likely to engage in risky sexual behavior than are women who are not cutters. Often there is a history of CHILD SEXUAL ABUSE or COMPLEX POSTTRAUMATIC STRESS DISORDER (CPTSD).

Some experts consider cutting and self-mutilation to be a subset of OBSESSIVE-COMPULSIVE DISORDER, a type of ANXIETY DISORDER, and treat such patients with antidepressants such as SELECTIVE SEROTONIN REUPTAKE INHIBITORS (SSRIs). Therapy is often useful, although patients may be more likely to cut themselves after a stressful session that causes them to recall past traumas, such as incidents of abuse. In such cases, BENZODIAZEPINES can be useful to limit the acceleration of anxiety subsequent to therapy.

Reviews of the literature on cutting and self-mutilation indicate that there are three distinct categories of self-harm. The first category involves major but infrequent acts that produce clear tissue damage. This category is associated with severe conditions such as psychosis and acute intoxication in which contact with the body and with reality is impaired. The second form of self-harm is associated with mental retardation and rhythmic, recurrent, and fixed behavior without any particular symbolism. The third category, the most common form of self-harm, involves superficial skin cutting, burning, scratching, punching, self-biting, insertion damage, and ingestion of damaging substances or objects.

Self-harm is not considered a form of suicidal behavior but seems to arise as a coping mechanism involving DISSOCIATION and emotional discomfort. There is no category for this behavior in the *DIAGNOSTIC AND STATISTICAL MANUAL* published by the American Psychiatric Association, nor is there an ICD-10 diagnostic category for such self-harm since it is seen as a symptom of an underlying disorder.

It is difficult to describe who engages in self-harm because most individuals with this behavior do not report it, and only the most extreme cases, which usually result in hospitalization, are recorded. However, European studies estimate that among 15- and 16-year-olds one in 10 have attempted deliberate harm to themselves, and one in 12 do so between the ages of 11 and 25 years. Females engage in self-harm at four times the rate of males. Those with DEPRESSION, phobias, and BORDERLINE PERSONALITY DISORDER are the most at risk for this behavior.

Attention does not seem to be reinforcement for the behavior since most sufferers cover their self-inflicted wounds so as not to draw attention to themselves. Dissociation is often present, and most clinicians believe that the physical pain of self-harm distracts the individual from emotional discomfort and pain. As a COPING MECHANISM, self-harm can become quite addicting and may occur as an act of self-punishment.

Several Web sites offer self-harm information and referrals, including http://www.lifesigns.org.uk; http://www.recoveryourlife.com; http://www.self-injury.org; and http://www.helpguide.org.

In general, however, it is difficult to generalize about self-harm, and it is best to look at each individual who exhibits this behavior on a case-by-case basis.

See also SUICIDE; THERAPY, TYPES OF.

cyclothymia (cyclothymic depression) Cyclothymia is a milder form of BIPOLAR DISORDER, also known as manic depressive disorder. It has less exaggerated mood swings than does bipolar disorder and less effect on the individual's ability to function intelligently and socially. When the cyclothymic mood is up (hypomania), the person may experience not only good feelings, but also enhanced productivity and social functioning. Depressive symptoms, when they occur, are not as severe as in MAJOR DEPRESSION. Alternations in mood, however, must be persistent for at least two years for the person to be diagnosed with cyclothymic disorder.

Symptoms and Diagnostic Path

People may go undiagnosed for years, unaware that their mood swings can be treatable. With cyclothymic disorder, people may experience low-level depression, dysthymia, and periods of high energy, irritability, and creativity, known as hypomania. Cyclothymia is a chronic illness with symptoms occurring daily, weekly, or months at a time. People with cyclothymia have been described as having a personality disorder of alternating mood swings from mania to mild depression. Those who frequently feel good and energized may never seek treatment, while those who live in a mild depressive state for months usually find treatment helpful through medications and psychotherapy. There is no laboratory test or BRAIN imaging study to detect a cyclothymic disorder.

The signs and symptoms of the cyclothymia are:

- increased energy and restlessness
- euphoric moods
- irritability
- racing thoughts
- distractibility
- unrealistic beliefs
- impulsivity in action and judgment
- increased sexual drive
- aggression
- blaming of others

The symptoms of the depressive swing are similar to those with major depression, but they are less severe.

Treatment Options and Outlook

The same treatments used with bipolar disorder are also used with cyclothymic disorder, with the exception that lithium is seldom used. COGNITIVE BEHAVIORAL THERAPIES are most helpful with cyclothymic disorders and have proven to be the first choice of treatment. Often, the cyclothymic person does not see the shifts in mood (and often behavioral energy) until too late. Identifying triggers can often prevent shift or reduce their effects. Likewise, learning to shift one's thinking is essential to moderating mood and behavioral shifts. The bipolar disorders will require medications and a strong willingness to stick with the medications because compliance is a serious problem.

Major depression, as mentioned, usually gets better within one year. Medications, such as antidepressants or SSRIs, will speed recovery. In chronic cases, individuals may need such medication for the rest of their lives. However, most people recover from major depression and return to normal functioning within the year span. Psychotherapy, particularly cognitive behavioral therapy (CBT), has proven to be the most effective intervention, even superior to medications. With CBT, depressive or irrational thoughts are targeted and changed through work with the therapist to more realistic, nondepressive, and more normal ways of thinking.

Risk Factors and Preventive Measures

There is no known cause of cyclothymic disorder, but frequently these individuals come from homes in which standards and expectations are high and often unrealistic for parents and their children. Early intervention might prevent later development of cyclothymic disorder. In contrast, bipolar disorder is associated with strong genetic factors. There are no preventive measures for bipolar disorder, and the disorder can only be treated once it has been identified. Early identification and intervention (with medications and therapy) are essential to help the individual cope with the progressive increase in the intensity of this disorder.

Da Costa's syndrome/disease   See COMBAT STRESS REACTION.

Davidson Trauma Scale   See ASSESSMENT AND DIAGNOSIS.

death guilt   Feelings of guilt about surviving a catastrophic event that the individual did not cause, and in which circumstance others have died. This is sometimes called SURVIVOR GUILT for that reason. The survivor may be plagued by irrational thoughts, believing, for example, that the catastrophic event could have been prevented if he or she had taken certain actions. For example, one might think, "If I had left home earlier . . . ," or "If I had only taken my lucky rabbit's foot, this might not have happened."

Death guilt or survivor guilt is very common in war situations in which friends can die suddenly and the survivor feels that "It might have been me" or "Why wasn't it me?" Survivor guilt is often very subtle and unconscious, but it can affect the mood and behavior of the individual.

See also LIFTON'S CHARACTERISTICS OF A SURVIVOR; SURVIVOR SYNDROME; THERAPY, TYPES OF.

death imprint   See LIFTON'S CHARACTERISTICS OF A SURVIVOR.

debriefing   A therapeutic group intervention process for individuals to talk about their TRAUMATIC EXPERIENCE soon after a catastrophe or life-threatening situation. Debriefing is the main therapeutic intervention with survivors of catastrophic events.

It was developed as a part of CRITICAL INCIDENT STRESS DEBRIEFING (CISD), referred to as a psychological debriefing. The purpose of debriefing is to mitigate acute stress symptoms and educate individuals about normal reactions following exposure to stressful events and not put psychological labels to those reactions; that is, to "normalize" the reaction. Debriefings are generally conducted by mental health professionals and peer facilitators who have not been involved in the crisis event. Confidentiality is highly valued and recommended. There are many formal group debriefings, such as the critical incident stress debriefing (CISD) and MULTIPLE STRESSOR DEBRIEFING MODEL (MSDM).

According to Joseph Ruzek and Patricia Watson in their article for *PTSD Research Quarterly,* a psychological debriefing is:

> A single-session intervention delivered to groups or individuals with the aims of promoting disclosure [detailed description of events experienced] of traumatic experiences, normalizing reactions to trauma [traumatic reactions are normal under these circumstances], educating participants about stress reactions [that they are not crazy, weird, or over reactive], enhancing coping [what you can do next to stabilize your reaction and return to a more normal life], and identifying those who may benefit from more intensive services [further therapeutic interventions].

The victims may have been traumatized by a MOTOR VEHICLE ACCIDENT, a crime, a natural disaster, or other traumatic events. The psychological briefing is taken to alleviate or ameliorate the subsequent development of POSTTRAUMATIC STRESS DISORDER (PTSD). According to Choe in a 2005 article in *The New School Psychology Bulletin,* such an intervention was used after battle by commanders in World War I to boost morale, and it was at that time that techniques were developed to enable traumatized soldiers to return to battle.

The concept was later expanded to encompass traumatized emergency responders as well as others dealing with traumatized victims, such as police officers, firefighters, and many other professionals.

According to Choe, results are mixed on the effects of psychological debriefings, and some evidence indicates that such debriefings are least effective among victims of criminal acts, car crashes, and in some other cases. It is difficult, however, to conduct a study on the effects of psychological debriefings because to do so would mean creating a control group that was denied the debriefing. The ethics of such a study are questionable. Although lacking evidence on their effectiveness, debriefings have a cultural value in bringing compassionate people to the aid of distressed others.

See also CRISIS MANAGEMENT BRIEFINGS (CMB); CRITICAL INCIDENT STRESS MANAGEMENT; GROUP STRESS DEBRIEFING; NATURAL DEBRIEFINGS; PSYCHOLOGICAL FIRST AID.

Choe, Injae. "The Debate over Psychological Debriefing for PTSD." *The New School Psychology Bulletin* 3, no. 2 (2005): 71–82.

Everly, G. S., and J. T. Mitchell. *The Basic Critical Incident Stress Management Course*. 3rd ed. Ellicott City, Md., 2001.

Ruzek, Josef, and Patricia Watson, "Early Intervention to Prevent PTSD and Other Trauma-Related Problems." *PTSD Research Quarterly* 12, no. 4 (Fall 2001): 1–3.

defusing   A shortened version of the DEBRIEFING, defined as a group meeting or discussion about the TRAUMATIC EVENT within eight hours of exposure. The concept of defusing was originally developed by Jeffrey T. Mitchell, Ph.D., and was designed for targeting small groups (six to eight people) comprising emergency workers, such as police officers, fire fighters, hospital emergency room staff, ambulance crew, and paramedics who might have emotional reactions to the scene and the emergency work they are asked to do.

The goal of a defusing is to mitigate the impact of the incident by reducing cognitive, emotional, and physiological symptoms and to accelerate the recovery process and the return to more normal ways of life. It is also an opportunity to identify individuals who will require mental health follow-ups. A defusing is a group process that is conducted in a nonthreatening environment, allowing people to speak freely or be silent, facilitated by a trained critical incident stress debriefer.

Components of Defusing

There are three main components or phases of a defusing: introduction, exploration, and information. The facilitator meets the group in the introduction phase and explains the purpose of the meeting, stresses confidentiality, defines goals, and sets the tone for the group so that they will feel comfortable and motivated to participate. The group is reassured that this is not an investigatory process.

The second phase is the exploration of facts: What happened? Where were you when the traumatic event occurred? What did you see? What did you think? This phase opens up discussion about how individuals experienced the event and how they reacted to it.

The third phase, information, is used to summarize participants' exploration of the traumatic event and normalize their experiences and reactions. This phase emphasizes the need for individuals to take care of themselves and teaches them STRESS survival skills, including exercise and relaxation techniques and the importance of maintaining balanced nutrition and avoiding alcohol and sugar.

See also CRISIS MANAGEMENT BRIEFINGS (CMB); CRITICAL INCIDENT STRESS DEBRIEFING (CISD); DEBRIEFING; MULTIPLE STRESSOR DEBRIEFING MODEL (MSDM); NATURAL DEBRIEFINGS.

degeneracy   The view in psychiatry and medicine that humans are analogous to machines or clocks and that mental disorders are the result of a breakdown in one aspect of the mechanism. Some experts continue to believe in some form of this view. Degeneracy refers to this breakdown, whether it is constitutional, hereditary, or biological. Constitutional inadequacies in the past were treated as unforeseen causes of most mental disorders. For example, a common phrase used during the turn of the 20th century was, "Poor protoplasm poorly put together" as a descriptor of a sociopath or a person with antisocial personality disorder. This phrase reflected the constitutional deficiency or degenerative nature of pathology.

A hereditary view would be that children inherit the deficient behaviors of their parents, and children who are born to sociopaths or criminals are more likely to exhibit the same or similar behavior when they grow into adulthood. A biological view of degeneracy would be that there is some problem in the brain or elsewhere that leads to sociopathic behavior, such as a "chemical imbalance" (although it is not known which, if any, chemicals are out of balance).

On the other hand, because of the belief in constitutional factors in mental illness and retardation, a "eugenetics" movement emerged in the late 1800s that promoted the idea of planned parents in order to "improve the human stock." This movement was campaigned by Sir Francis Galton (1822–1911), a prominent geneticist, psychologist, and statistician who was interested in the area of "individual differences" among people. Galton was a half cousin of Charles Darwin.

delayed posttraumatic stress disorder Refers to the situation where symptoms of POSTTRAUMATIC STRESS DISORDER (PTSD) show up six months or more after the trauma experience. Many people who experienced severe traumatic childhood abuse may have no recollection until well into adulthood. Often, their own abuse is activated emotionally and through images when their children reach the age in which the parent was abused. Unlocking these memories can be the result of virtually any stressor or major life event that reactivates feelings of helplessness followed by delayed PTSD symptoms. Very little is known about how the brain can turn the key to unlock these traumatic MEMORIES.

Delayed onset is seen in Holocaust survivors and World War II and Vietnam veterans. The rate of acute COMBAT STRESS REACTIONS (CSR) seen in World War II veterans, however, was much lower than the rate seen in Vietnam veterans, who developed PTSD symptoms more than a year after returning from combat duties when civilian life became more difficult to handle.

In his book *Combat Stress Reaction: The Enduring Toll of War,* Solomon states that clinicians who treated Vietnam veterans had "raised questions as to the validity of the diagnosis of delayed PTSD when instances of malingering in pursuit of disability compensation, factitious symptoms, drug abuse and precombat psychopathology were mistakenly diagnosed as delayed PTSD." Another argument as to the validity of delayed PTSD is that time lapse is not a true latency period because usually there are untreated symptoms that may never have been acknowledged or accepted due to the fear of stigmatization for having a chronic mental health disorder.

Delayed PTSD is not well understood even today. There is little empirical research in the area of why individuals who coped effectively at the time of their trauma should experience full-blown PTSD years or decades later.

The argument may not be in questioning the validity of delayed PTSD, but why a certain population exposed to TRAUMATIC EVENTS such as sexual abuse or combat initially have no apparent psychiatric disturbances and are asymptomatic months to years after the event. While clinically the phenomenon of delayed PTSD has been documented, much research is still needed to determine the conditions that produce delay and the individual characters associated with these reactions.

Solomon, Z. *Combat Stress Reaction: The Enduring Toll of War.* New York: Plenum Publishing, 1993.

dementia praecox The name for individuals with a variety of deteriorating "early in life" praecox (dementia) and psychotic and psychological symptoms, first described in an 1896 textbook by Emil Kraepelin, a German physician. Many of the symptoms that were included in dementia praecox by Kraepelin were later redefined by Bleuler as schizophrenia. *Dementia praecox* as a term is no longer used by psychiatrists in making a diagnosis. However, the term emphasizes the view of that time that "constitutional" factors were the cause of these disorders and also that they would become progressively worse with time. Today, however, schizophrenia is divided into the "rule of thirds" in which one-third of individuals with schizophrenia get better within a brief period of time (usually six months), another third are in and out of schizophrenia, but usually can maintain themselves on the outside, and the last third need structure and supervision throughout their lives.

According to Glenn Shean in *Understanding and Treating Schizophrenia: Contemporary Research, Theory, and Practice,* Kraepelin based his argument that dementia praecox was a single disorder on the following three key points:

First, he emphasized that the subtypes of dementia praecox have many symptoms in common, such as hallucinations, impaired judgment, delusions, withdrawal, impulsiveness, shifting attention and interest, disturbances of emotion and volition, and loss of inner unity of activities of intellect, emotion, and volition. Second, he provided a rationale for grouping these subtypes beyond their symptomatic similarities by emphasizing that they begin early in life and lead to progressive decline to a similar "demented" end state. Third, Kraepelin argued that all forms of dementia praecox must be the result of a single underlying cerebral disease process.

Kraepelin also believed that the complete deterioration of the individual was the only possible outcome of dementia praecox. His work was consistent with the thinking of the time that "constitutional" or genetic factors caused mental illness and were incurable, lifelong, and gradually got worse.

Shean, Glenn D., *Understanding and Treating Schizophrenia: Contemporary Research, Theory, and Practice.* New York: Haworth Clinical Practice Press, 2004.

deny, attack, and reverse victim and offender (DARVO) A concept introduced by Jennifer Freyd in her 1997 article on BETRAYAL TRAUMA THEORY (BTT) in *Feminism & Psychology.* The concept is based on clinical/observational evidence and not on empirical research. In essence, the concept is that perpetrators, especially those who are guilty of sexual offenses, often deny the behavior and then attack the person who has accused them. Then the perpetrator attempts a role reversal such that he or she is perceived as the person being victimized.

Freyd explained in her article that denial itself is not evidence of guilt. Stated Freyd:

I hypothesize that if an accusation is true, and the accused person is abusive, the denial is more indignant, self-righteous and manipulative, as compared with denial in other cases. Similarly, I have observed that actual abusers threaten, bully and make a nightmare for anyone who holds them accountable or asks them to change their abusive behavior. This attack, intended to chill and terrify, typically includes threats of lawsuits, overt and covert attacks on the whistle-blower's credibility, and so on. The attack will often take the form of focusing on ridiculing the person who attempts to hold the offender accountable.

Denial and attack have become clinical red flags for identifying perpetrators of abuse.

Freyd, Jennifer J. "II. Violations of Power, Adaptive Blindness and Betrayal Trauma Theory." *Feminism & Psychology* 7, no. 1 (1997): 22–32.

depression Forms of severe sadness and also forms of mental illness. Depression is an emotional state that is marked by great sadness and apprehension, feelings of worthlessness and guilt, withdrawal from others, changes in patterns of sleep, appetite, and sexual desire, and either lethargy or agitation. It is present frequently in POSTTRAUMATIC STRESS DISORDER (PTSD) as part of the syndrome or as a condition that is reactivated by the traumatic experience and was present in the individual's life in the past. Depression affects an individual both at work and at home. Depression usually occurs without psychosis (loss of reality), but it can also occur in conjunction with psychosis. A less intense but chronic form of depression is called CYCLOTHYMIA, in which the individual cycles between a slight to moderate depressed state and a mild to moderate manic or activated state. Cycles may occur within a day or months apart.

Double depression is a situation in which dysthymic disorder leads to a major depressive disorder. *Dysthymia* is a long-lasting, but not disabling, moderate form of depression in which the individual is functional but has many mild to moderate symptoms of depression (see below). The intensity of the depression usually fluctuates over time but never truly goes away. It is also possible for someone with chronic or long-lasting dysthymia to develop a more intense or MAJOR DEPRESSION that is disabling and pervasive. Often these major depressive episodes are triggered by traumatic stress.

Major Depression

One of the most serious and frequently occurring forms of mental illness is major depression, which is often the result of a traumatic experience. In a given year, about 5 percent of the population in the United States may experience a major depression, which is persistent and insidious and invades all aspects of the person's functioning. Major depression is also called unipolar depression and dysthymia, which refers to moderate cases. While no one cause of depression is known, brain chemicals, heredity, and life experience all play a role.

Depression symptoms include sadness, crying, drug use, sleep difficulties, concentration problems, lack of motivation, suicidal ideation, loneliness, self-condemnation, and low self-esteem. Depressed persons may also experience physical pain, digestive disorders, diminished energy, and headaches. Treatment for major depression usually includes a combination of COGNITIVE BEHAVIORAL THERAPY and antidepressant medications. With effective treatment, most patients recover within a year. Anyone can suffer from depression, but more women than men usually experience major depression. Soldiers returning from combat are at increased risk for depression. Evaluation by a mental health professional is the best preventive measure against major depression.

Cyclothymia

A mild form of BIPOLAR DISORDER is cyclothymia. With less extreme mood swings than in bipolar disorder, those suffering from cyclothymia may experience good feelings, enhanced productivity, and better social functioning when their mood is up. When their mood swings are low, their depressive symptoms are less severe.

Cyclothymia symptoms occur daily, weekly, or for months at a time. The main signs and symptoms of the disorder are increased energy and restlessness, euphoric moods, irritability, racing thoughts, distractibility, unrealistic beliefs, impulsivity in action and judgment, increased sexual drive, aggression, and blaming others for things that are not their fault.

Treatments for cyclothymia are similar to those for bipolar disorder or major depression. Cognitive behavioral therapies are the first choice. Treatment may also involve medication. The cause of cyclothymic disorder is unknown, but there appears to be a link to growing up in a family with very high or unrealistic standards and expectations.

See also ANXIETY DISORDERS; BENZODIAZEPINES; SELECTIVE SEROTONIN REUPTAKE INHIBITOR; SEROTONIN NOREPINEPHRINE REUPTAKE INHIBITOR; THERAPY, TYPES OF.

developmental history relating to posttraumatic stress disorder (PTSD) in children There are three factors that increase the likelihood of children developing POSTTRAUMATIC STRESS DISORDER (PTSD). These are: (1) the TRAUMATIC EVENT; (2) the parental reaction to the threat; and (3) the physical proximity to the traumatic event. The way the symptoms of PTSD appear in children and adolescents may not be the same as they present in adults.

Young children may have very few PTSD symptoms because the *DIAGNOSTIC AND STATISTICAL MANUAL* (*DSM-IV-TR*) list includes eight of the PTSD symptoms that describe verbally one's feeling and experience. Very young children will not possess the verbal skills to accurately report their true feelings. Instead, they will report fears of strangers or separation anxiety, avoidance of situations that remind them of the trauma, sleep disruption, and a preoccupation with words or symbols that are unrelated to the traumatic event. It is not uncommon for traumatized children to regress and to lose some acquired developmental skills, such as toilet training.

Elementary-age schoolchildren may not experience visual FLASHBACKS or AMNESIA of the trauma. Instead, children experience time skew and "omen" formation, which are typically not reported in adults with trauma. Time skew refers to the rearranging or missequencing of trauma events when recalling the traumatic MEMORY.

Children may also believe that there were warning signs (omens) that predicted the trauma. School-age children often believe that if they pay attention to their surroundings, they will recognize warning signs and avoid future trauma. These children tend to reenact the trauma in play, by drawings or through verbalization. After a school shooting, for example, children may be seen recreating the trauma by playing shooting games. This reenactment is a literal representation of the trauma, and it does not reduce anxiety.

Adolescents who are exposed to traumatic events tend to experience symptoms that resemble adult PTSD. As children reenact the trauma through play, adolescents also may engage traumatic reenactment by incorporating aspects of the trauma into their daily lives. They can exhibit aggressive and impulsive behaviors.

The salient developmental impact to the child or adolescent is often overlooked in an effort to immediately address PTSD reactions. The traumatic experience involves the failure in evolving developmentally how one assesses and confronts dangerous situations. These may include the failure of alarm reactions, protective shielding, the inability to resist forced violation, failure of heightened emotions to protect against harm, and the sense of resignation in having to surrender to an unavoidable moment of danger.

Hamblen, Jessica. *PTSD in Children and Adolescent, A National Center for PTSD Fact Sheet.* Washington, D.C.: U.S. Department of Veterans Affairs, 2005.

Pynoos, R. S., A. M. Steinberg, and A. Goenjian. "Traumatic Stress in Childhood and Adolescence, Recent Developments and Current Controversies." In *Traumatic Stress,* edited by B. A. van der Kolk, A. C. McFarlane, and L. Weisaeth. New York: Guilford Press, 1996.

dexamethasone suppression test A diagnostic test that is given to measure feedback regulation in the HYPOTHALAMIC-PITUITARY-ADRENAL (HPA) AXIS, using a measurement of the level of CORTISOL hormone in the blood and urine after the ingestion of dexamethasone (a synthetic steroid similar to cortisol), a glucocorticoid drug. In a person who is in normal health, the dexamethasone should suppress both the corticotrophin releasing factor (CRF) and the ADRENOCORTICOTROPIC HORMONE (ACTH) production, which in turn will cause decreased levels of cortisol in both the blood and the urine of the individual. However, if the person has Cushing's syndrome, a rare endocrine disorder of the pituitary gland, the cortisol levels will stay at high levels despite the ingestion of dexamethasone.

The abnormal secretion of cortisol can have several root causes, including Cushing's syndrome, an adrenal tumor, a pituitary tumor, or a tumor in the body that inappropriately produces ACTH.

The dexamethasone suppression test is sometimes used in psychiatric studies, and some studies have found abnormal cortisol levels with this test in individuals who have POSTTRAUMATIC STRESS DISORDER (PTSD) or DEPRESSION or in individuals who have suffered from domestic violence. Cortisol levels may remain at abnormal levels even years after the TRAUMATIC EVENT occurred.

A study in 1993 by Rachel Yehuda and her colleagues and reported in the *American Journal of Psychiatry* used a low dose of dexamethasone to determine if patients with PTSD had a greater suppression of cortisol than did normal subjects. If so, this would indicate possible abnormalities in the HPA axis. The researchers found that patients with PTSD did show a greater suppression of dexamethasone.

See also ASSESSMENT AND DIAGNOSIS; BRAIN.

Yehuda, Rachel, et al. "Enhanced Suppression of Cortisol Following Dexamethasone in Posttraumatic Stress Disorder," *American Journal of Psychiatry* 150 (1993): 83–86.

Diagnostic and Statistical Manual (DSM) A manual that categorizes psychiatric disorders for both adults and children that is published by the American Psychiatric Association. It is the handbook most used by psychiatrists, psychologists, social workers, counselors, nurses, rehabilitation therapists, and other mental health professionals who make psychiatric diagnoses in the United States and other countries. The *DSM* has gone through five revisions since its introduction in 1952 as a brief 130-page pamphlet with 106 categories. In 1968 the *DSM II* was issued with 134 pages and 182 categories. In 1980 the *DSM III* had 494 pages and 265 categories, including POSTTRAUMATIC STRESS DISORDER (PTSD). By 1987 and the *DSM IIIR*, there were 567 pages and 292 categories. The current edition as of this writing is *DSM-IV-TR*, which was published in 2000 and has 886 pages and 297 categories. Page size increased because the *DSM* has slowly moved from defined categories (listing symptoms) to a more dimension formulation of disorders and sampling of symptoms in order to improve reliability of diagnosis. The *DSM-IV-TR* represents a text revision of the *Diagnostic and Statistical Manual-IV (DSM-IV)* and is the manual used by mental health professionals as of this writing. More than a thousand professionals and numerous professional organizations conducted a comprehensive review of the literature to establish a firm empirical basis for making changes to the previous edition, *DSM-III-R*. Major changes were made to add, delete, and reorganize classification to the diagnostic criteria sets and to the descriptive text of the various mental disorders. The *DSM-IV-TR* was introduced in May 2000.

The goal of the *DSM-IV-TR* was to maintain currency of the *DSM-IV* text that was based on literature up until 1992. Changes were made to the descriptive text and to correct errors in the diagnostic criteria. Some diagnostic codes were changed to reflect updates to the *International Classification of Diseases, Ninth Revision, Clinical Modification (ICD-9)* coding system adopted by the U.S. government. The next revision is due approximately in 2012 and will be the *DSM-V.*

Mental health professionals use this manual to diagnose their patients based on an understanding of their illness, as the *DSM* lists known causes of the disorder, the prognosis, and optimal treatment approaches. Before *DSM*, communication among mental health professionals was not uniform, and thus it was difficult to facilitate objective psychiatric research.

The criteria for inclusion of a mental disorder are decided on a process of consultations by a committee of mental health clinicians, mainly psychiatrists. What is considered a mental disorder may change with time; for example, homosexuality was once considered a psychiatric disorder, but today it is seen as a normal sexual orientation by most psychiatrists and mental health clinicians. Posttraumatic stress disorder was first included in *DSM-III* in 1980, which was then a new diagnosis for an age-old psychological disorder.

The *DSM* is divided into the diagnostic classification, diagnostic criteria, and the descriptive text. The diagnostic classification is a list of mental disorders that are labeled with a diagnostic code, which is used by institutions for data collection and billing purposes. The diagnostic criteria indicates the symptoms that must be present, as well as the symptoms that must be excluded, in order for the individual to be given a diagnosis. The descriptive test describes each disorder in subsections under "Diagnostic Features," "Subtypes and/or Specifiers," "Recording Procedures," "Associated Features and Disorders," "Specific Culture, Age, and Gender Features," "Prevalence," "Course," "Familial Pattern," and "Differential Diagnosis."

The Five DSM Axes

The *DSM* uses a multidimensional approach to diagnosing patients by assessing the following five axis, each of which refers to a set of information to help the clinician plan treatment and predict outcome.

Axis I: Clinical disorders. This axis is for reporting the major disorders, such as mood, schizophrenia, substance-related disorders, anxiety, somatoform, factitious, dissociative, eating, sexual and gender identity, bipolar, impulse control, adjustment, and other conditions that may be a focus of clinical attention.

Axis II: This axis records mental retardation and personality disorders, such as obsessive-compulsive personality, paranoid, schizoid, antisocial, borderline, narcissistic, avoidant, dependent, and histrionic personality disorders. Pervasive developmental disorders, such as Asperger's disorder and autistic disorders, which are first evident in childhood and which are often associated with some degree of mental retardation are coded on Axis II.

Axis III: General medical conditions such as brain injury that can result in mental illness are recorded in this axis to promote communication among health-care professionals and provide a thorough evaluation of the individual.

Axis IV: Psychological and environmental problems are reported here. Events such as unemployment, the death of a loved one, or marriage may have an impact on the disorders indicated in Axis I and II.

Axis V: This axis indicates the clinician's assessment of the person's highest level of functioning in the present and in the past year with regard to the GLOBAL ASSESSMENT OF FUNCTIONING (GAF) scale from 0 to 100.

The *DSM* states its "diagnostic criteria for each mental disorder is offered as a guideline" to help the clinician make a diagnosis. It is intended for use only by professionals and should not be used by laypersons to make diagnostic conclusions.

American Psychiatric Association. *Diagnostic and Statistical Manual of Mental Disorders-IV-TR.* Washington, D.C.: American Psychiatric Publishing, Inc., 2000.

Diagnostic Interview for Borderlines-Revised (DIB-R)

A structured clinical interview to evaluate the presence of BORDERLINE PERSONALITY DISORDER in an individual by evaluating the occurrence of specific symptoms or behaviors that are grouped into four areas of functioning, including affected (helplessness, hopelessness, loneliness, anger); impulsivity (suicidal gestures, sexual deviance, SUBSTANCE ABUSE); cognition (distorted perceptions, odd thinking, nondelusional paranoia); and interpersonal relations (stormy relationships, abandonment, dependency, entitlement). The DIB-R assesses 22 symptoms in these four areas of functioning and provides five measures of borderline pathology, the four section scores, and a total DIB-R score. The DIB-R is considered the best means for diagnosing bipolar personality disorder.

The original Diagnostic Interview for Borderlines was developed by Gunderson and Kolb in 1980, and it was revised in 1989 to better differentiate between borderline personality disorder from other personality disorders as well as from disorders such as schizophrenia and neurotic depression.

Many researchers see a connection between psychological trauma and borderline personality disorder in the form of COMPLEX POSTTRAUMATIC STRESS DISORDER (CPTSD). For example, the permanent result of early childhood traumatic experiences can place the sufferers in alternating states of hyperarousal and numbness in response to their stressful environments. Researcher Judith Herman believes that bipolar personality disorder is a name that is given to a particular manifestation of PTSD when the elements are identity and relationship disturbances. In 2003 Golier, et al., compared subjects without BPD to subjects with BPD and found significantly higher rates of childhood/adolescent physical abuse in those with BPD (52.8 percent versus 34.3 percent), and these subjects were twice as likely to develop PTSD in the group with BPD.

Golier, J., et al. "The Relationship of Borderline Personality Disorder to Posttraumatic Stress Disorder and Traumatic Events." *American Journal of Psychiatry* 160 (November 2003): 2,018–2,024.

Herman, J. *Trauma and Recovery.* New York: Basic Books, 1997.

Kolb, J. E., and J. G. Gunderson. "Diagnosing Borderline Patients with a Semistructured Interview." *Archives of General Psychiatry* 37, no. 1 (1980): 37–41.

See also ASSESSMENT AND DIAGNOSIS.

Diagnostic Interview Schedule (DIS)

The development of the National Institute of Mental Health Diagnostic Interview Schedule (DIS) for use in a large-scale, multicenter epidemiology study that began in 1978. This instrument was administered by laypersons or clinicians. The DIS was originally a one-hour, highly structured psychiatric interview. The major goals of the DIS program were to survey adults across the United States and provide prevalence data of specific psychiatric disorders in large samples, as many psychiatric disorders were rare and a large sample was required to provide accurate numbers.

The *DIAGNOSTIC AND STATISTICAL MANUAL*, third edition (*DSM-III*) was the standard diagnostic system in the country in 1980, and the DIS used *DSM-III* criteria to cover many of the major diagnosis. In order to make selected *DSM-III* diagnosis, a diagnostic interview had to capture the lifetime history and clinical significance of all symptoms in the *DSM-III* criteria. No survey had previously performed this task. The closest was the Renard Diagnostic Instrument (RDI), and the first version of the DIS adapted and modified the RDI, while the second revision, DIS-II, was coproduced by the authors of the Research Diagnostic Criteria from Columbia University, who were leading the development of *DSM-III.*

The uniqueness of the DIS was the ability to make a diagnosis without requiring a clinical mental health professional for interviewing or scoring. There are clear rules as to how a question is asked and coded. The coded responses are input directly into the computer where the diagnosis is made.

Version III-A of the Diagnostic Interview Schedule added these new diagnostic categories: generalized anxiety, POSTTRAUMATIC STRESS DISORDER, and bulimia.

The DIS-IV version has updated questions in terms of how they served the *DSM-IV* criteria. Unnecessary questions were dropped, and questions that did not match *DSM-IV* criteria were rewritten. Due to these revisions, the DIS takes approximately 90 to 120 minutes to administer.

There is another version of DIS, the Diagnostic Interview Schedule for Children. It is also a highly structured interview given by lay interviewers. It has a parent and child's version with questions about the child's psychiatric symptoms.

See also ASSESSMENT AND DIAGNOSIS.

direct therapeutic exposure (DTE)   A class of exposure treatments used with individuals who are experiencing severe distress due to TRAUMATIC EVENTS. The primary focus of treatment is the exposure of the individual to the stimuli that evoke high levels of anxiety. Exposure continues until the individual's anxiety peaks and eventually diminishes. Lyons and Scotti found that DTE is effective in reducing anxiety and DEPRESSION through reexperiencing the trauma, physiological arousal, and avoidance of trauma-related cues. Long-term follow-ups are needed to show the durability of this approach.

Patrick A. Boudewyn's research with Vietnam veterans and with patients suffering from POSTTRAUMATIC STRESS DISORDER (PTSD) first called this technique *direct therapeutic exposure,* which is the use of FLOODING and IMPLOSIVE THERAPY techniques, described in his book *Flooding and Implosive Therapy: Direct Therapeutic Exposure in Clinical Practice.*

See also EXPOSURE THERAPY; THERAPY, TYPES OF.

Boudewyns, Patrick A., and Robert H. Shipley. *Flooding and Implosive Therapy: Direct Therapeutic Exposure in Clinical Practice.* New York: Plenum Press, 1983.
Lyons, Judith A., and Joseph R. Scotti. "Behavioral Treatment of a Motor Vehicle Accident Survivor: An Illustrative Case of Direct Therapeutic Exposure." *Cognitive and Behavioral Practice* 2, no. 2 (Winter 1995): 343–364.

disaster syndrome   An individual's severe response to traumatic events. First coined by Andrew Wallace in 1956 to discuss the response to a tornado, the term has subsequently been used to allude to reactions to other natural or manmade disasters. Natural disasters are a source or event that leads to POSTTRAUMATIC STRESS DISORDER in many victims.

According to Wallace, disaster syndrome includes the following phases:

- disorientation, daze, apathy, passivity, feeling stunned
- concern for loved ones and the community, altruism, appreciation for help that is received
- strong identification with the community and a desire to restore it
- ambivalent feelings and the search for meaning from the event

As with other "single incident" traumas, treatment focuses on the experience itself. In particular, both the body and cognitive reactions to the trauma must be addressed. Almost any verified trauma treatment will have a positive effect on single incident trauma. The treatment outlook is excellent.

No one can predict or anticipate most traumatic events. By nature they surprise the survivor and create great terror and fears of death. Risk factors include previous history of mental illness, including anxiety and DEPRESSION, multiple exposures to traumatic events, social support, and the degree of emotional adjustment.

disorders of trauma   One or more severe traumatic events can lead to a physical disease or psychological disorder resulting from a trauma, including such traumatic disorders as ACUTE STRESS DISORDER and POSTTRAUMATIC STRESS DISORDER (PTSD). There are also special types of PTSD such as CIRCUMSCRIBED POSTTRAUMATIC STRESS DISORDER, COMPLEX PTSD, and DELAYED PTSD. In addition, other special forms of trauma include RAPE TRAUMA SYNDROME, TYPES I, II AND III TRAUMA, and VICARIOUS TRAUMATIZATION.

These disorders have been increasingly recognized by acknowledged experts as valid issues of individuals who have suffered from one or more severe traumas, such as the trauma of experiencing wartime combat, the trauma of rape/sexual assault or of CHILD ABUSE AND NEGLECT, the trauma of living through a major natural disaster such as Hurricane Katrina and then dealing with its aftermath, and many other major traumas.

Whether a traumatic disorder develops depends on many different factors, such as whether the trauma is a prolonged event, whether it has been experienced more than once, whether the individual was a child or an adult when it occurred, whether others have suffered the same or similar trauma, and many other factors, such as the individual's mental health and RESILIENCE at the time of the traumatic event. (In general, *resilience* refers to the individual's ability to cope with, adapt to, and overcome serious threats to safety without developing a traumatic stress disorder.) It will also depend on the degree of social support for the individual, their prior psychiatric history, whether the event is intentionally produced by humans or a natural catastrophe, and other variables.

In addition, trauma can lead to other serious disorders, such as BORDERLINE PERSONALITY DISORDER, which is a serious personality disorder that impedes the individual's happiness and success. POSTTRAUMATIC PSYCHOSIS is another possible outcome of a traumatic event. Trauma may also trigger some physical diseases, particularly autoimmune disorders or fibromyalgia, according to some experts.

Acute Stress Disorder

With an acute stress disorder (also known as *acute traumatic stress disorder*), the individual suffers a reaction immediately or soon after an event, which may lead subsequently to the development of posttraumatic stress disorder.

According to the *DIAGNOSTIC AND STATISTICAL MANUAL of Mental Disorders IV-TR (DSM-IV-TR)*, published by the American Psychiatric Association, acute stress disorder is a trauma-based anxiety disorder in which the individual experiences at least three of five different dissociative symptoms in anticipation (peritraumatic), during, or after experiencing a traumatic event, including:

1. a subjective sense of numbing, detachment, or absence of emotional responsiveness
2. a reduction in an awareness of the individual's surroundings (e.g., feeling like the person is in a "daze")
3. derealization or a feeling of unreality surrounding the traumatic event
4. depersonalization or the feeling that the individual is not personally affected by the traumatic event, even though he or she is both deeply and profoundly affected
5. dissociative AMNESIA (the inability to recall important aspects of the trauma)

The disturbance in an acute stress disorder can start immediately or after two or more days and it can persist for up to four weeks. Beyond that time it would be classified as PTSD. Individuals with acute stress disorder may relive the event in their minds over and over again, and they may also suffer from increased states of arousal and anxiety, as well as suffering from significant distress in social and/or occupational functioning.

Individuals suffering from acute stress disorders are generally best helped with somatic therapy to work to process the experience and EYE MOVEMENT DESENSITIZATION AND REPROCESSING (EMDR) or one of the exposure-based therapies. Simply talking about the incident is not a good way to resolve the trauma because talking alone usually stimulates emotional reactions and delays and prolongs emotional healing. COGNITIVE BEHAVIORAL THERAPIES have proven helpful with acute traumas, as have some medications such as antidepressants or antianxiety drugs.

Posttraumatic Stress Disorder

PTSD is an anxiety disorder that may be triggered by life-threatening events such as natural disasters (earthquakes, hurricanes, and floods), violent personal attacks (physical and sexual abuse, kidnapping, rape, or violent crime), military combat, or serious accidents. Victims of PTSD can be any age, gender, or race, but some predisposing conditions make some people vulnerable to developing PTSD. These include individuals who have had early psychiatric problems, as well as those who have DEPRESSION, who have had previous traumatic reactions, and who have not received emotional support from others.

People with PTSD may reexperience the traumatic event as FLASHBACK episodes, memories, somatic sensations, and nightmares. Reminders of the trauma, including anniversary dates, can trigger symptoms of reliving the tragedy all over again. Many sufferers of PTSD say that they can no longer feel any emotions toward their loved ones, and they begin to feel distant and cold as they become increasingly preoccupied with the traumatic event. This behavior often leads to poor relationships at work and a decline in work performance. Avoiding places and people that remind them of the traumatic event(s) can create isolation from others, as well as depression and an overall lack of personal initiative. The individual with PTSD may also suffer from NIGHTMARES and other sleep disturbances, as well as from severe anxiety.

Hypervigilance is another common symptom of PTSD. Military war veterans, such as those newly returned from Iraq or Afghanistan, may have an exaggerated startle response. Hearing a low-flying helicopter or fireworks, they may feel that they are back again in a battlefield and find themselves diving for cover. This is sometimes referred to as a COMBAT STRESS REACTION.

PTSD can interfere greatly with normal social and family functioning, and there is a higher than average incidence of SUICIDE and DIVORCE among PTSD sufferers than is found among nonsufferers.

A common side effect of PTSD that is often neglected is the experience of not feeling safe. Victims invariably report that they do not feel safe or that they feel safe only in well-circumscribed areas or with certain people.

PTSD is also often linked to the presence of serious physical illness. According to researcher Joseph Boscarino in his article for the *Annals of the New York Academy of Science* in 2004, a study of chronic PTSD in 2,490 Vietnam veterans several decades after the war ended revealed that those with chronic PTSD were more likely than others to have developed serious autoimmune diseases, such as rheumatoid arthritis, insulin-dependent diabetes, and thyroid disease. Other studies have also correlated the presence of PTSD to an increased risk for fibromyalgia, chronic fatigue syndrome, cardiovascular disease, gastrointestinal disorders, and musculoskeletal disorders.

PTSD is usually treated with cognitive behavioral psychotherapy and pharmacological agents such as antidepressants and antianxiety medications (BENZODIAZEPINES). Cognitive behavioral therapies include cognitive restructuring and exposure experiences. Another effective treatment for PTSD is eye movement desensitization and reprocessing. The primary aim of any therapy is to help traumatized individuals move on from constantly reexperiencing the past to becoming fully engaged in the present.

Circumscribed PTSD

In the case of a circumscribed posttraumatic stress disorder, the individual experiences a "single incident" trauma. This does not mean that the event was minor; for example, anyone involved in New Orleans when Hurricane Katrina hit is likely to be affected for life by what he or she experienced there. However, the traumatic event of circumscribed PTSD could range from a relatively minor event such as a public humiliation (e.g., in school) to one that is very intense and intimate, such as when the individual suffers from a rape, kidnapping, sniper attack, or a variety of other assaults and attacks.

With time, the single incident trauma may be forgotten or distorted in the minds of those who experienced it. However, the body itself remembers the experience, and any other exposure to a similar incident will often induce a strong fear reaction, as well as the sensations associated with the initial trauma. For example, if the single incident that traumatized the individual was a severe car crash in which some people important to the traumatized person were severely harmed or killed, then if the traumatized person is hit in the future in a minor fender-bender accident, he or she may have a flashback to the experience of the first severe car crash, and may overreact. Or, someone sexually abused as a child may find that situations in which he or she is dominated result in overreactions as an adult.

Circumscribed traumas are usually treated with EXPOSURE THERAPY, in which the traumatic event is gradually presented in imagination or, if possible, in the real situation (but with the therapist). In this way, the "extinction," or the termination, of the traumatic response can occur.

Complex PTSD

In contrast to circumscribed PTSD, another form of PTSD is complex posttraumatic stress disorder, also known more simply as complex trauma and sometimes also by the older term ELABORATED PTSD. This type of PTSD develops as a result of long-term situations of repeated abuse and includes the experience of individuals who are exposed to chronic traumas that lasted for months to years at a time, such as with torture victims in prisoner of war camps or concentration camps, children who are repeatedly beaten and/or raped by their tormentors, and individuals who have been severely bullied. This disorder is also sometimes referred to as disorders of extreme stress not otherwise specified or DESNOS.

The symptoms for complex PTSD may include alternations in the normal emotional regulation, such as persistent sadness, suicidal thoughts, explosive anger, or inhibited anger. The individual may also experience major alterations in self-perception, which may include feelings of hopelessness, helplessness, shame, guilt, and feeling stigmatized. The person with complex PTSD may feel completely different from and separate from all other humans, and he or she may feel that others cannot ever possibly understand what he or she has gone through.

There may also be significant alterations in the individual's perception of the perpetrator of the abuse. The victim may attribute total power to the perpetrator or become preoccupied with his or her relationship to the perpetrator to the exclusion of other people and events in life. Sometimes the individual develops an overwhelming fixation with obtaining revenge against the perpetrator, as with

the bullied victim who plots to murder the bully in a "BULLYCIDE." (Rarely does such a murder actually occur.) The individual may also have intense feelings of isolation or distrust.

Because of the repeated nature of the trauma, complex PTSD is difficult to treat; generally, a phase-oriented approach is taken in which interventions are introduced sequentially. A solid and trusting relationship must be established between the therapist and the client before even minimal progress may be made. Usually, the client must be "resourced" or prepared to tolerate the emotional arousal and regulation needed before addressing the traumatic experience itself. Cognitive behavioral therapies have proven effective, as well as EMDR. Additionally, the patient must learn new patterns of behavior to replace old maladaptive ones for better adjustment and interpersonal success.

Delayed PTSD

Not all traumatic stress disorders are immediately evident when the traumatic event ends. Some individuals, such as combat veterans or abused children, may react months or even years later to the distressing experiences they suffered. Delayed PTSD is defined as PTSD that occurs at least six months after the traumatic event. Many people who experienced severe traumatic childhood abuse may have no recollection of it, having blocked out their memories completely until well into adulthood. Unlocking these memories may result from virtually any stressor or major life event that reactivates the individual's extreme feelings of helplessness.

Rape Trauma Syndrome

Rape trauma syndrome (RTS) results from a specific form of traumatization experienced by an individual who has suffered from the inhumanity of rape. Generally, it alludes to a disorder of females, although it is also possible for men to be raped, particularly men who are incarcerated in prison. Some experts consider RTS to be a subset of posttraumatic stress disorder.

Rape trauma syndrome was named by Ann Wolbert Burgess and Lynda Lytle Holmstrom in their article for the *American Journal of Psychiatry* in

1974, which was based on their interviews of rape victims in Boston, Massachusetts. According to the researchers, in the acute phase of rape trauma syndrome, the individual suffers from fear, anxiety, and anger. Sleep disturbances are common, and women who were awakened from sleep by their assailant and subsequently raped found themselves later waking up at the same time as when the rape had occurred. Many women experience stomach pains and appetite loss, as well as gynecological symptoms and general pain throughout the body. Emotional reactions may include fear, humiliation, embarrassment, anger, and a desire for revenge.

Over the long-term, women with RTS may experience severe nightmares. Many rape victims become phobic, and they fear being inside, although women who were attacked outside their homes may fear being outside. Many victims fear being alone, and many are afraid of crowds. Some victims fear people being present behind them, who they unconsciously (or consciously) worry will attack them. Sexual difficulties are common among the rape victims.

Rape counselors and therapists need to be understanding, patient, and supportive. Some studies have shown that the majority of rape victims experience acute stress disorder, and many of them develop PTSD after one month. Medical treatment is also imperative, including an examination and blood tests for sexually transmitted diseases, as well as pregnancy tests and counseling if the pregnancy test is positive.

Victims of RTS suffer long-term health problems, even years after assaults. Clinicians use insight therapy and cognitive behavioral therapy as the primary treatment modalities. Somatic experiencing therapy and EMDR are exceptionally useful in treating the traumatic psychological and somatic reactions to rape.

Types I, II, and III Trauma

Type I and Type II Trauma were initially described in 1991 by Lenore Terr, a psychiatrist who specialized in childhood trauma. According to Dr. Terr, Type I Trauma is characterized by an acute reaction to a single, unexpected, highly traumatic experience that was difficult to forget because of persistent flashbacks, avoidance behavior, and high levels of arousal. Dr. Terr believes that if the child was older than three years when the event occurred, he or she retained memories of the event even if only in a distorted form.

While a Type I Trauma is caused by one major event in one's life, the Type II Trauma involves chronic or repeated exposure to traumatic events over a period of time. Because of the chronic nature of the Type II Trauma, the victim often relies on coping skills such as massive denial, NUMBING, dissociation, or rage. If the victim was less than three years old at the time of the trauma, the reaction is stored as a sensory or body memory, which could result later in the victim's experiencing physical sensations.

In 1999, Eldra Solomon and Kathleen Heide proposed a Type III Trauma which divided the Type II Trauma created by Dr. Terr into two separate categories based on the severity of the intrusion or traumatic experiences. The first category was the Type II as described earlier, but the second category was based on multiple and pervasive violent events beginning at an early age and continuing for years. There were severe boundary violations such as those seen in the case of rituals conducted in cult cultures, involving multiple perpetrators, use of force, and sadistic intrusions. Usually both physical and sexual abuse occurred along with torture and severe violent physical and sexual acts. Likewise, children beaten or forced into sexual acts with caretakers on a regular basis would be classified here.

Type III Trauma victims may feel suicidal and hopeless for no obvious reason to others. Their initial evaluation of their childhood is usually positive, but taking a careful and extensive history will uncover patterns of prolonged severe abuse. The PTSD symptoms are usually intense, but the individual's memory, emotions, and body sensations are difficult to identify due to their automatic dissociative behaviors. The past life history of clients with Type III Trauma is usually littered with disappointing and abusive relationships, an avoidance of intimacy, and major trust issues. There is often a clear pattern of somatization and frequent headaches, and often a history of substance abuse or dependence as well.

The treatment of Type III Trauma clients is complex, long-term, and multiphasic. It requires a longer period of treatment than with Type I or Type II clients. Since trauma, particularly in its early forms, often adversely affects the development of many age-appropriate behaviors, the teaching and development of new adult-level behaviors, particularly social behaviors, is necessary. Self-esteem, containment, and learning to modulate feelings, as well as the integration of client identity and disempowering past events, are just some of the therapeutic goals.

Vicarious Traumatization/Secondary Stress Traumatization

Some individuals are not directly traumatized by an event they experience, but instead they are traumatized upon hearing about the details of traumatic events directly experienced and reported on by others. This form of traumatization may be referred to as either vicarious traumatization or secondary stress traumatization. Vicarious traumatization is also known as COMPASSION FATIGUE. For example, individuals who assist others who have been traumatized by combat, a natural disaster, violent abuse, or another dire event can themselves become traumatized by the accounts, emotions, and reliving of the event by the victims they are assisting. When helping individuals are themselves traumatized, they also need assistance from others.

In their article on vicarious traumatization in disaster and trauma workers (such as disaster professionals, healthcare workers, emergency service personnel, mental health professionals, and journalists) for *Prehospital and Disaster Medicine,* Kathleen M. Palm, Melissa A. Polusny, and Victoria M. Follette described the key symptoms of vicarious traumatization. Said the authors, "Vicarious trauma reactions may include intrusive imagery and thoughts, avoidance and emotional numbing, hyperarousal symptoms, somatization, and physical and alcohol use problems similar to those experienced by direct trauma survivors. Further, working with trauma survivors may lead to changes in self-identity, world-view, spirituality, and general psychological functioning."

They recommended that the professional actively work to maintain a balance between the professional and emotional aspects of living, and say, "For example, therapists working with disaster survivors should consider ways to provide more balance at work by developing a caseload of clients with different types of problems; working with populations other than trauma survivors; limiting caseloads, avoiding the scheduling of difficult clients one after another; scheduling breaks during the day and finding opportunities to work with colleagues." They also recommended limiting television exposure to traumatic material, especially before going to sleep.

Trauma Triggering Serious Disorders

A major trauma may lead to the development of borderline personality disorder (BPS). BPS is a personality disorder thought to be characterized by inner chaos, mood changes, raging and blaming others for one's internal stress, and by instability and disorganization in one's self-image. It is a disorder also characterized by distress or impairment in both friendships and intimate relations.

A traumatic event may also trigger a posttraumatic psychosis, or a psychotic state in which the individual can no longer distinguish reality from unreality. In the histories of many people who are suffering from psychosis, there is a high incidence of past physical and sexual abuse, and there is also a high incidence of PTSD in people who have a primary diagnosis of psychosis. In some cases, the psychosis may be trauma-induced. Both PTSD and psychosis are characterized by intrusion and avoidance. Negative beliefs and dissociation are several factors that may implicate both the development of PTSD and psychosis after the occurrence of traumatic life experiences.

Boscarino, Joseph. "Posttraumatic Stress Disorder and Physical Illness: Results from Clinical and Epidemiologic Studies." *Annals of the New York Academy of Sciences* 1032 (2004): 141–153.

Palm, Kathleen M., Melissa A. Polusny, and Victoria M. Follette. "Vicarious Traumatization: Potential Hazards and Interventions for Disaster and Trauma Workers." *Prehospital and Disaster Medicine* 19, no. 1 (2004):73–78.

dissociation/dissociative disorders　A disruption in memory, identity, or consciousness. Dissociation is a state within a state in which reality is altered, but the person usually stays in contact with the traumatic experience within this duality. Dissociation is not abnormal in and of itself. In fact, it is a common coping mechanism that many people use in stressful or extremely stressful situations. It becomes abnormal when dissociation is chronic and prevents people from processing, remembering, or working through difficult situations in their lives. Dissociation is inherent in some people, but for most individuals, it is a coping device to deal with traumatic events and situations that would otherwise overwhelm the individual and make functioning difficult.

Symptoms and Diagnostic Path

The experience of dissociation may take various forms. Following are some of the more common experiences taken from Steinberg (2001), with examples of how people characterize them:

1. detachment from one's self or one's sense of his or her body. People might characterize the experience as "floating" out of their body, or looking down on themselves in the room, or watching themselves in a traumatic situation as if "in a movie."
2. feelings of unreality; being there but feeling detached and observing the traumatic event like it is unreal
3. numbing of emotions. A feeling of being numb, of not reacting to what is going on, of being there but not emotionally, like a "robot" or acting automatically without thought
4. sharpening of one's senses and slowing of time such that time seems to stand still, every detail is clear and vivid, and one's thoughts might be racing and speeded up
5. changes in one's perception of the environment and quickening of thoughts where everything is unreal, distorted, and sometimes "in a fog." Often only parts of the environment that signal escape or safety are present.
6. reliving memories, such as "my life flashed before me" or forgotten memories suddenly appear in the situation

There are several distinctions between normal dissociation and abnormal or dysfunctional dissociation. One major difference is in the duration and frequency of dissociation in one's life. At the abnormal end is dissociative identity disorder (DID), in which the person may "switch" among different distinct personalities without a conscious awareness of doing so. Normal dissociation would be infrequent and somewhat conscious, such as "tuning out" when driving to work or on a trip, so that an individual thinks about different things other than the ongoing experience.

Normal memory retrieval usually produces pleasant memories, but people with dissociative disorders usually experience frightening or alarming fragments or FLASHBACKS in their memories. Similarly, normal people often find speeding up of thoughts in stressful or traumatic situations, whereas those with dissociative disorders will usually "blank out" or suffer confusion or clouding of their experience. Normal people also tend to dull or numb their emotions under stress whereas those with dissociative disorders will usually experience heightened anxiety and emotional distress under stressful conditions.

Treatment Options and Outlook

Treatment, as with all the dissociative disorders, takes a long time and involves various phases. First, the disorder must be accurately identified or diagnosed. These patients often feel isolated from themselves and others, as if something is missing in them. Patients must bond with the therapist and trust that he or she will do no harm. The therapist, in turn, will generally start to introduce the sub-personalities to each other through methods such as hypnosis and drug therapy.

The abusive and traumatic roots of each personality must be processed. Here EYE MOVEMENT DESENSITIZATION AND REPROCESSING is helpful in speeding healing. As trauma is processed, efforts are made to integrate the sub-personalities or fuse them into a comprehensive identity. Once a high degree of fusion occurs, efforts are made to maintain the complete personality and to teach social and coping skills that may help prevent setbacks and further dissociation. This process not only takes years to complete but also requires high levels of motivation on the patient's part and on the part of the sub-personalities.

The physiological or psychological mechanisms that control the dissociative reactions are unknown.

However, two things are apparent. The first is that psychology and biological studies must work together to unravel these disorders. Second, the disorders themselves affect the very foundation of perception, memory, and identity that are so vital to human functioning and growth. The fragility of human life certainly comes into focus here.

Risk Factors and Preventive Measures

Severe childhood abuse is a risk factor for dissociative disorders. There are no preventive measures.

Forms of Dissociative Disorders

The forms of dissociative disorders are listed below. It is important to remember that these disorders usually have a traumatic history that has led to patients' excessive use of dissociation in managing their lives.

Dissociative amnesia (DA) is a disorder that is characterized by the loss of memory for traumatic events or by periods of one's life, especially from childhood, that are absent from memory. People with DA ordinarily do not complain of memory losses. The lost period of time usually has a distinct onset (such as a year or season of the year) and an end point where memories continue from then. The extent of trauma during these periods of time usually correlates with the development of AMNESIA.

Dissociative amnesia can be localized, selective, generalized, or continuous. Localized amnesia is the loss of memory for all events that took place within a particular limited period of time, almost always beginning with a traumatic event. This is the most common form of amnesia.

The second most common form is selective amnesia, in which only certain events within a limited period of time are not remembered. For example, a conversation may be recalled but not the particular situation in which it occurred (such as a funeral). Generalized amnesia occurs when events that long preceded a trauma are forgotten, along with the upsetting event itself. With continuous amnesia, new events and ongoing events in the present, along with past events, are forgotten. Continuous amnesia is rare. In all cases of amnesia with dissociation, episodic material (i.e., relating to experiential memories of events) is forgotten, but semantic or more verbal factual material tends to be unaffected by amnesia.

DISSOCIATIVE FUGUE is a condition that separates one from one's sense of identity. People with dissociative fugue retain their capabilities and their faculties but they lose the sense of who they are. They also usually leave their environment to live elsewhere with a new identity and name and no memory of their background or previous identity. A fugue state can last for hours, months, or even years. Usually there is great disorientation, DEPRESSION, and anger when the fugue lifts and they return, and there is a general forgetting of their fugue behavior and identify. Fugues tend to end abruptly. Most people with fugue recover their memories and never have a recurrence. Often repressive environments in which the person feels stifled or excessively controlled by others or by their community restrictions are breeding grounds for fugue states.

Depersonalization disorder is a new diagnosis in the *DIAGNOSTIC AND STATISTICAL MANUAL-IV-TR*. It is characterized by a sudden sense of being outside one's self, observing from a distance as if watching a movie of ongoing events, with a distortion of body image, time slowing, and the world seeming unreal. These symptoms may last a few moments or could come and go for years. Again, the frequency and intensity are the defining factors as to whether it is abnormal.

Occasionally, parts of the body seem foreign to individuals with depersonalization disorder, and they may seem unusual in size. The mind can feel as though it is floating above them—a condition known as doubling. The emotional state is also disproportionate or distorted, and individuals experiencing depersonalization may report feeling "mechanical" or "dreamlike" states or feeling disoriented. They are aware of these distortions, which are disturbing and frightening.

Depersonalization can also be accompanied by derealization, the feeling that the external world itself appears unreal and strange. Objects and people may change shape, smell and touch may seem strange, and people and objects may lose their sense of life. This disorder is usually confined to adolescents and young adults and rarely occurs to those older than 40 years. Its onset is sudden but is typically triggered by extreme fatigue, pain, intense stress, anxiety, depression, or recovery from substance abuse. Symptoms will come and go over time but the condition tends to be long-lasting. Feelings of depersonalization and derealization are also common in other disorders such as panic disorders and, certainly, in the psychoses. Little systematic research has been conducted on depersonalization and derealization, so treatments tend to be eclectic in nature.

Dissociative identity disorders, formally known as multiple personality disorder, involves "switching" to various alternate identities when under stress. Each identity is separate with its own name, personal history, and personality, including marked differences in manner, voice, gender, and even physical characteristics. Researchers have also discovered that the sub-personalities differ in physiological and autonomic reactivity.

Brain electroencephalogram (EEG) patterns differ among sub-personalities as will other objective measures, such as blood pressure, allergic reactions, and systemic diseases. The different identities ("alters") usually are unaware of each other. DID is thought to begin in childhood in response to repeated traumatic or overwhelming life experiences, most of which are physical or sexual in nature. It is usually diagnosed in adulthood and often after numerous instances of misdiagnosis or unsuccessful medical and psychological workups. Women receive this diagnosis at least three times more often than men do.

The nature of the relationship of the various sub-personalities or alters has been studied clinically with the following summary: in general, two types of relationship are present, mutual amnesic and mutual cognizant. In mutual amnesic relationships, the various sub-personalities are unaware of each other and operate independently. On the other hand, mutually cognizant patterns involve full or partial awareness of each different sub-personality by every other. They may interact by talking with each other and the host may hear their voices or they may talk among themselves without host involvement.

Conflicts and harmony may exist among the sub-personalities. There are also coconscious sub-personalities or quiet observers who watch the actions of the other sub-personalities but do not interact with them. These sub-personalities might express themselves through internal voicing or automatic writing behavior to communicate with the host. The average number of sub-personalities for women with this disorder is 15 and for men it is eight. Theories attempting to explain or identify critical elements of DID emphasize "state dependent learning" (behavior learned in a particular state of mind or situation that returns when the conditions are reproduced) as a phenomenon and self-hypnosis (where people essentially hypnotize themselves to forget unpleasant events).

See also DISSOCIATIVE EXPERIENCES SCALE; THERAPY, TYPES OF.

Dissociative Experiences Scale A psychological screening test developed by Eve Bernstein Carlson and Frank W. Putnam, M.D., for identifying dissociative processes in individuals. It is comprised of 28 questions given to individuals who may have dissociative behavior or even dissociative identity disorder (formerly known as multiple personality disorder). The individual responds to each question on a continuum of percentages, from zero to 100 percent. For example, one question in the scale is "Some people have the experience of looking in a mirror and not recognizing themselves. Circle a number to show what percentage of time this happens to you." Another question is "Some people sometimes have the experience of feeling that their body does not belong to them." The individual is instructed to circle the percentage that best represents how often this circumstance has occurred to him or her.

In 1993, E. B. Carlson et al. analyzed 1,051 individuals with and without dissociative identity disorder to determine the validity of the scale. They found that the scale was valid (measuring what it purported to measure) as well as reliable (different individuals administering the test would receive the same result).

See also ASSESSMENT AND DIAGNOSIS; DISSOCIATION; DISSOCIATIVE FUGUE.

Carlson, E. B., et al. "Validity of the Dissociative Experiences Scale in Screening for Multiple Personality Disorder: A Multicenter Study." *American Journal of Psychiatry* 150 (1993): 1,030–1,036.

dissociative flashback episodes (flashback)   See DISSOCIATION; DISSOCIATIVE EXPERIENCES SCALE.

dissociative fugue   A disorder in which episodes of AMNESIA cause the individual to suddenly travel away from home with the inability to recall his or her past. Significant distress and impairment along with the assumption of a new identity may occur. It is estimated that fewer than 1 percent (or 0.2 percent) of the population experience dissociative fugue, although research shows the prevalence increases following traumatic or stressful life events, such as war, accidents, or natural disasters.

Symptoms and Diagnostic Path

Often dissociative fugue states occur spontaneously, and they may last for several hours to weeks, months, or even years. It is not a faked state, although it is often thought that the person is seeking to avoid his or her circumstances. During the fugue state, the person may not attract much attention, may assume a new identity, move to a new residence, and act appropriately in complex social encounters. However, at some point the person may find confusion in his identity, such as when memories of the life before the fugue state are triggered. Once the fugue state ends, symptoms of grief, shame, and DEPRESSION and suicidal or aggressive impulses may appear.

Diagnosis of dissociative fugue for a person confused about his or her identity or past must be carefully approached by a complete physical and psychological examination corresponding to the recent memory loss, or amnesia. It may also be diagnosed after the fugue state, when the person finds himself or herself in strange and unfamiliar circumstances. Dissociative fugue is treated with hypnosis or drug-induced interviews. The person may regain all past memories but lose memories of what occurred during the fugue state.

Treatment Options and Outlook

Dissociative fugue usually responds well to psychotherapy. Since this state represents a stress reaction within a life space such as a family, often significant others are asked to participate in the therapy. Gradually, memory returns with therapy, and with the therapist's guidance, restructuring of the family or living unit can occur. In some cases, if the living unit is not amenable to change, the individual may be supported and encouraged in leaving. Since dissociative fugue states tend to occur in isolated communities where there is a great deal of repression and lack of awareness of inner feelings, the community itself may be resistant, and the individual may have to move to a more normal community and develop relationships there.

Risk Factors and Preventive Measures

Little is known about dissociative fugue disorder because it is relatively rare in incidence and usually shows up in isolated rural communities that have little contact with the outside world. One of the risk factors would be that of living in such a community. Appalachia and some Mormon isolated groups might produce a higher incidence of dissociative disorders. Also, fundamentalist communities are at risk. There are, however, no known preventive measures for these rarely occurring disorders.

See also DISSOCIATION/DISSOCIATIVE DISORDERS; DISSOCIATIVE EXPERIENCES SCALE.

dissociative identity disorder (DID)   See DISSOCIATION/DISSOCIATIVE DISORDERS; DISSOCIATIVE EXPERIENCES SCALE.

dissociative response   See DISSOCIATION; PSYCHIC NUMBING.

divorce   The permanent legal dissolution of marriage. In contrast, an annulment is a declaration from the court that the marriage was never valid. Divorce can be an extremely traumatic experience for both men and women, as well as for their children. A significant part of an individual's identity is usually linked to the role of being a spouse, and when that role is severed, the person must redefine himself or herself in many different ways. It is particularly painful if one of the individuals opposes the divorce. Divorce is usually traumatic for everyone involved, but POSTTRAUMATIC STRESS DISORDER is not a predictable outcome.

According to the Centers for Disease Control and Prevention in a 2006 issue of the *National Vital Statistics Report,* the divorce rate in 2005 was 3.6 per 1,000 people, slightly down from 3.8 in 2003 and 3.7 in 2004. There are many reasons for divorce, such as infidelity, financial problems, sexual incompatibility, and poor communication. Unfortunately, if the divorced person remarries, the same or similar problems may arise again if they have not yet been resolved.

In considering the number of divorces for 2005, the greatest number of reported divorces occurred in Florida (81,346), followed by Texas (74,023) and New York (53,507). SEE TABLE BELOW for the reported divorce rate in most other states.

Effects of Divorce on the Adults Involved

In addition to the psychological trauma that is involved with divorce, there are also health risks, including an increased risk of death. For example, according to a study on work stress and marital dissolution published in the *Archives of Internal Medicine* in 2002, thousands of men without evidence of coronary heart disease but with above average risk for heart disease were recruited for the Multiple Risk Factor Intervention Trial and were followed for nine years. The researchers found that both work stress and marital stress increased the risk of death in the subjects. Marital stress was associated with a significantly increased risk for death from coronary heart disease, and an increasing degree

NUMBER OF DIVORCES IN SELECTED STATES IN THE UNITED STATES, 2005

State	Number	State	Number
Alabama	22,076	Montana	3,537
Alaska	3,861	Nebraska	5,975
Arizona	24,535	Nevada	18,618
Arkansas	16,578	New Hampshire	4,335
California	Not available	New Jersey	25,343
Colorado	20,504	New Mexico	8,837
Connecticut	9,354	New York	53,507
Delaware	3,260	North Carolina	32,711
District of Columbia	1,145	North Dakota	1,495
Florida	81,346	Ohio	41,720
Georgia	Not available	Oklahoma	19,966
Hawaii	Not available	Oregon	15,527
Idaho	7,020	Pennsylvania	29,143
Illinois	32,408	Rhode Island	3,138
Indiana	Not available	South Carolina	12,423
Iowa	8,108	South Dakota	2,359
Kansas	8,638	Tennessee	27,575
Kentucky	18,898	Texas	74,023
Louisiana	Not available	Utah	9,992
Maine	4,656	Vermont	2,078
Maryland	17,111	Virginia	29,129
Massachusetts	14,308	Washington	25,264
Michigan	34,747	West Virginia	9,185
Minnesota	Not available	Wisconsin	16,504
Mississippi	12,968	Wyoming	2,686
Missouri	20,952		

Source: Adapted from Centers for Disease Control and Prevention. "Births, Marriages, Divorces, and Deaths: Provisional Data for 2005," *National Vital Statistics Reports* 54, no. 20 (July 21, 2006): 6.

of stress was also associated with a significantly increased risk of death from all causes.

In addition, work stress and marital stress appeared to be related, and the number of subjects who reported a separation or divorce increased with the number of work domain stressors. However, both work stress and marital separation and divorce were independently linked to an increased risk of death. Said the authors,

> In particular, stress may increase levels of circulating catecholamines, ambulatory blood pressure, and cortisol, may reduce heart rate variability and impair vagal tone, and may enhance platelet reactivity and release of platelet products. Stress also increases susceptibility to infectious disease and contributes to rapid progress in [those with] human immunodeficiency virus. Work stress and marital dissolution may result in poor decision making, causing risky behaviors.

Similar effects can be seen in DEPRESSION and loss situations.

Other studies have shown that divorce in midlife also significantly affects the cardiovascular health of women, even more so than among men.

In another study on the psychological adjustment patterns of divorced custodial parents published in a 2004 issue of the *Journal of Divorce & Remarriage,* the researchers analyzed divorced custodial mothers and fathers in terms of depression, alcohol use, hostility, and overall well-being. They found that custodial mothers were less likely to cohabit with lovers than custodial fathers (17 percent of the mothers versus 31 percent of the fathers) and that the mothers also experienced more economic strain and less income. The average total household income for custodial mothers was $25,077 compared to $34,565 for the fathers.

Most of the custodial mothers were younger than the custodial fathers, with an average age of 36.8 years for the mothers, compared to an average age of 39.1 years for the fathers. Custodial mothers also had significantly higher rates of hostility and depression than fathers, but they were less likely than fathers to drink alcohol to excess. The well-being of custodial mothers and fathers was about the same.

The researchers said, "We concluded that custodial parents differ in their negative adjustment, but not their positive adjustment, and that custodial fathers have fewer problems with adjustment than custodial mothers."

Effects of Divorce on Children

Children are often at least initially traumatized when their parents divorce. The trauma is compounded when parents continue to disagree and especially if court and custody battles continue. Parents may try to win children over to "their" side, causing children to suffer from torn loyalties. Parents may also seek information from their children about the other parent, causing the child to feel like a spy or a traitor.

Most courts award joint custody of children to the parents, unless there is a compelling reason against this arrangement, such as one parent who is violent, alcoholic or drug-addicted, or has other serious issues that could pose a danger to the child.

In a study reported in the *Journal of the American Medical Association* in 2002, the researchers studied 218 families that included adolescents between the ages of 15 and 19 years old to determine the effects of divorce in children. The control group was adolescents in preventive programs designed to alleviate the impact of divorce. The researchers found that adolescents not in preventive programs were more likely to drop out of school, to have mental health problems, to have more sexual partners, and to become pregnant. In addition, they were more likely to abuse marijuana, alcohol, and other substances and to exhibit externalizing or blaming behaviors.

For example, 23.5 percent of the adolescents not in preventive programs had mental health problems, compared to 11 percent of the children in such programs. Said the authors,

> Program benefits were found in the context of a rigorous efficacy trial, which included numerous eligibility criteria, extensive evaluation, and exception fidelity of program implementation. Given the promising findings, large-scale trials in ethnically and economically diverse samples that test whether these programs can be delivered with fidelity and effectiveness in natural service delivery systems is a critical next step.

Divorce is a major social problem with potentially harmful effects on children, parents, and extended families. Social programs have had little impact. The churches have had little impact. Future programs and thinking that will diminish this problem in society are needed.

Centers for Disease Control and Prevention. "Births, Marriages, Divorces, and Deaths: Provisional Data for 2005." *National Vital Statistics Reports* 54, no. 20 (July 21, 2006): 1–7.

Hilton, Jeanne M., and Karen Kopera-Frye. "Patterns of Psychological Adjustment Among Divorced Custodial Parents." *Journal of Divorce & Remarriage* 41, no. 3–4 (2004): 1–30.

Matthews, Karen A., and Brooks B. Gump. "Chronic Work Stress and Marital Dissolution Increase Risk of Posttrial Mortality in Men from the Multiple Risk Factor Intervention Trial." *Archives of Internal Medicine* 162 (February 11, 2002): 309–315.

Wolchik, Sharlena A., et al. "Six-Year Follow-up of Preventive Interventions for Children of Divorce: A Randomized Controlled Trial." *Journal of the American Medical Association* 288, no. 15 (October 16, 2002): 1,874–1,881.

dopamine   See CATECHOLAMINE.

double dissociation   A term that refers to a loss or separation of one or several functions as a way of studying brain localization and interaction. The term was developed in neuropsychology to describe a method of studying independent brain functions or perceptions. The analogy that is often used is one of the television picture. If the color is lost, the person perceives the picture, but has lost the color. Picture and color are independent. On the other hand, if the picture was lost, nothing would be perceived, and this would be a case of single dissociation. If one set had sound, but no picture, while another television set had a picture, but no sound, it could be concluded that sound and picture are independent or separate functions, and this would be a case of double dissociation.

Likewise, if a patient has lost language perception but not primitive speech, while another patient had lost speech but not language perception, then this would represent double dissociation and it could be concluded that speech and language perception are separate and independent functions of the brain. Further research would then help to identify the particular areas responsible for each function.

DSM-IV/DSM-IV-TR   See DIAGNOSTIC AND STATISTICAL MANUAL.

dual representation theory of posttraumatic stress disorder   A theory that trauma experiences may need two levels of representation to understand the complex phenomenon of trauma. The multiple memory systems of verbally accessible memory (VAM) and situationally accessible memory (SAM) provide a cognitive architecture to explain the unique characteristics POSTTRAUMATIC STRESS DISORDER, including the experience of reliving the traumatic event.

Verbally accessible memories are higher forms of memory that can be deliberately retrieved from the memory bank of autobiographical experience, and thus the individual can provide verbal accounts of the event. These memories can be edited as time passes so that new meanings can be assigned to the trauma, and there is an opportunity to change or embellish these memories.

Situationally accessible memories represent stored sensory information, especially visuo-spatial images, or images within a context, accessed automatically when people are exposed to relevant cues to cause spontaneous experiences of intrusive emotionally laden FLASHBACKS while in the context of the traumatic situation. The context can be internal, as with thinking about the trauma, or may be external, as in viewing the news on television about a similar traumatic event.

Holmes et al. compared SAM to raw film footage with incoherent images that trigger flashbacks and VAM to a news broadcast with narration to explain each event and put meaning to them.

Brewin, C., T. Dalgleish and S. Joseph. "A Dual Representation Theory of Posttraumatic Stress Disorder." *Psychological Review* 103, no. 4 (1996): 670–686.

Holmes, E., C. Brewin, and R. Hennessy. "Trauma Films, Information Processing and Intrusive Memory Development." *Journal of Experimental Psychology* 133, no. 1 (2004): 3–22.

dysregulation Both psychological and physiological systems require a regulatory mechanism to maintain constancy or proper regulation. The concept of a negative feedback loop is used to conceptualize the necessary aspects of a regulation system.

There are four essential elements to any regulation or negative feedback loop mechanism including:

1. a system variable—a characteristic to be regulated, such as an emotion, arousal or temperature in the body; something that is measured. As an example, take temperature in a room as a system variable.
2. a set point—a value that the system uses as a standard to return to. Using our example, we might set the temperature at 72 degrees. With emotions, we might have a set point of no arousal or activation or emotion as a set point.
3. a detector—a device that monitors the value of the system variable. In our example, we might use a thermostat to monitor or detect the temperature in the room and determine its deviation from the set point. So, if the temperature is 74 degrees the "detector" would note that temperature is too high (or too low, if the temperature is below 72 degrees). We could do the same with emotions but would have outside detectors (such as physiological measuring equipment) to detect increases and degree of increase.
4. a correctional mechanism—a mechanism that restores the system variable to the set point. With room temperature, we might have a heater/air conditioner that is turned on when the detector indicates too high (above set point) or too low (below set point). The negative feedback referring to deviations from the set point or standard are fed back to the correctional device. With emotions, we might give a tranquilizer or teach the individual relaxation procedures in order to reset the emotional level.

The same process occurs in the body to provide homeostasis for all essential systems and responses, such as hunger and thirst, temperature, blood pressure, hormonal values, arousal, and so on. Likewise, the emotional-psychological system requires the same four elements in order to return to a set point or to emotional homeostasis where the person can effectively function.

Dysregulation occurs when the feedback loop malfunctions and responses are not well modulated or it maintains too high or too low a set point on a chronic basis. Affective or emotional dysregulation is characterized by too great or too little an emotional response for both positive and negative emotions; for example, a minor comment might trigger a blowup or an excessive withdrawal and nonresponsiveness when dysregulation is present.

Emotional dysregulation is the hallmark of POSTTRAUMATIC STRESS DISORDER (PTSD), and it is particularly noticeable in complex trauma conditions and with BORDERLINE PERSONALITY DISORDER (both of which seem to have roots in traumatic experiences). It is also evident in mood disorders. Other terms used to describe emotional dysregulation are problems in affect tolerance and AFFECT MODULATION.

Causes of Dysregulation

It is generally thought that hyperarousal as a result of trauma makes it difficult for the person to correct or modulate his or her responses back to a functional set point. In time the set point actually moves up, and this creates even further difficulty with the detector system as well as with the correctional mechanisms. The central memory storage, neurological pathways, and hormonal responses all are compromised.

For example, when traumatic symptoms occur (in posttraumatic stress disorder or complex trauma) the person is usually in a hyperaroused state on a chronic basis. In terms of the AUTONOMIC NERVOUS SYSTEM alone, this means that the sympathetic arousal side is constantly "on" (causing sleep difficulties, concentration problems, and affect modulation dysregulation). It also means that the parasympathetic system cannot bring the system back to a resting set point (because it is either weakened or it too is locked into a frozen high-level state).

Along with sympathetic and parasympathetic dysregulation are also changes in hormone levels (e.g., chronically high or low levels of CORTISOL, NOREPINEPHRINE, and so on), changes in brain functions and anatomy (e.g., shrinkage of AMYGDALA and hippocampal sizes) and behavioral changes. Physiologists call this rise in set point tuning or ergotropic tuning, or sympathetic arousal dominated responses. In contrast, trophotropic tuning is parasympathetic dominated behavior.

Both PTSD and complex trauma disorders are marked by dysregulation. The borderline personality disorder, thought to be a complex trauma disorder, in particular is characterized by extremes of mood and affect, and recent evidence suggests that it is also related to early traumatic abuse. The earlier that abuse or trauma occurs in the development cycle, then the more likely that the individual will have emotional dysregulation problems. For this reason, and because the caretaker is critical for helping develop adequate modulation, this early damage seems to be also related to attachment issues. In fact, there is an effort within the mental health community to rename borderline personality disorder to emotional dysregulation disorder. Correcting attachment problems in adulthood is a long and complex therapeutic problem.

See also BRAIN; CENTRAL NERVOUS SYSTEM.

Girdano, D. A., G. S. Everly Jr., and D. E. Dusek. *Controlling Stress and Tension,* 7th ed. New York: Pearson Books, 2005.
Pert, C. *Molecules of Emotion.* New York: Simon and Schuster, 1999.

echoic memory   Memory is the retention of infor-mation over time. It has three general processes: encoding, storage, and retrieval. Storage refers to how information is retained and in what form it is retained. Echoic memory is information that is stored in an auditory-sensory form. Consequently, echoic memory is information that has been received by audition or through the ear-hearing mechanism. Other sensory modalities have their own storage facilities. In some cases, traumatic experiences can impede memory, over a short or a long term.

The eyes (iconic memory), olfactory, tactile, and taste senses each retain their unique impressions. Obviously, these storage facilities interact so that individuals can retrieve memories and, for example, bring a picture of a restaurant to mind and even imagine tasting the food that was enjoyed in the past. Likewise in their minds, people can hear a musical composition (echoic memory) and picture being in the auditorium and seeing the production. Musicians have well-developed echoic memory systems. Blind individuals have to develop other sense modalities and forms of memory in order to function in the world.

See also AMNESIA.

elaborated posttraumatic stress disorder (EPTSD)
A situation in which the individual is exposed to repeated interpersonal trauma over an extended period of time. Examples of elaborated posttrau-matic stress disorder (EPTSD) include the repeated physical, sexual, or emotional abuse of children over a period of time. EPTSD is also known as com-plex trauma or relational trauma.

Symptoms and Diagnostic Path

While the symptoms of CIRCUMSCRIBED POSTTRAU-MATIC STRESS DISORDER closely follow the A–E criteria in the DIAGNOSTIC AND STATISTICAL MANUAL-IV (DSM), EPTSD often shows many individual differences in expression. The DSM A–E criteria are: life- or injury-threatening event, flashbacks, avoidance and numbing, arousal, and interfer-ence with work or social life. In particular, EPTSD has many negative effects on social and personal relationships.

Complex or relational trauma can arise from pro-longed periods of aversive stress usually involving entrapment (psychological or physical), repeated violations of boundaries, betrayal, and rejection and confusion that is marked by a lack of control and helplessness. Common situations include bul-lying, harassment, physical, sexual and emotional/verbal abuse, domestic violence and substance abuse, stalking, threats, separation and loss, unre-solved grief, and neglect. The following eight areas of functioning, taken from an unpublished paper by Ronald Doctor in 2002, are affected by relational trauma in some way:

1. alterations in relations with others. Symptoms include:
   a. a general feeling of distrust and use of isola-tion as a defense against hurt, rejection and disapproval
   b. problems keeping personal boundaries and recognizing the boundaries of others; dif-ficulty attuning to emotional states and per-spectives of others
   c. difficulty asking for help and often a relent-less search for a rescuer or savior from the outside
   d. revictimization and/or victimizing others
   e. preoccupations with revenge
   f. attachment problems—ambivalent, avoidant, or disorganized relationships

2. biological and bodily effects. Symptoms include:
   a. hypersensitiveness and aversion to physical contact, analgesia or under-responsiveness and need to seek sensations
   b. autonomic nervous system "set-point" is chronically too high or too low, leading to over-coupling (excessive sudden arousal) or under-coupling (excessive inhibition and dissociation) of traumatic experience
   c. sensorimotor and coordination problems—developmental lags
   d. somatization and systemic medical problems such as chronic fatigue, digestive problems, spastic colon/irritable bowels, allergies, endocrine problems, and other auto-immune disorders
   e. predisposition to develop POSTTRAUMATIC STRESS DISORDER (PTSD) to subsequent traumatic stressors
   f. poor response to prolonged exposure therapy
3. alterations in affect regulation. Symptoms include:
   a. persistent moods of sadness, suicidal thoughts and feelings, explosiveness or greatly inhibited anger, unmodulated sexual behavior, excessive risk taking
   b. difficulty self-regulating emotions
   c. difficulty describing feelings, sensations, and internal experience
   d. difficulties communicating wishes and desires
4. alterations in attention and consciousness. Symptoms include:
   a. exaggerated amnesia for or reliving traumatic events
   b. episodes of dissociation involving derealization and/or depersonalization, or under-coupling of traumatic experience
   c. impaired memory for state-based events
5. difficulties with behavioral control. Symptoms include:
   a. cutting, self-mutilation, and self-destructive behaviors
   b. excessive self-soothing—binge eating, substance abuse, interpersonal dependencies
   c. poor impulse modulation with anger and aggression
   d. extremes of compliance or oppositional behavior
   e. difficulty understanding and complying with rules
   f. arousal problems manifest in sleep disturbance, eating disorders, and learning problems
   g. inability to inhibit behavior when aroused
6. cognition. Symptoms include:
   a. difficulties with sustained attention, attention regulation, and executive functioning
   b. problems focusing, planning, anticipating, and completing tasks
   c. difficulties seeing own role in events
   d. learning, language, and orientation in time and space problems
   e. object constancy problems and visual-spatial pattern difficulties
   f. high levels of competence and interpersonal sensitivity coexisting with self-hate, lack of self-care, and interpersonal cruelty
   g. poor response to cognitive restructuring behavioral therapy
7. alterations in self-perception and self-concept. Symptoms include:
   a. sense of helplessness, shame, guilt, and self-blame
   b. feeling stigmatized and perceived as difficult by others
   c. low self-esteem and poor sense of individuation from others
   d. conviction of being unlovable and permanently damaged
8. alterations in systems of meaning. Symptoms include:
   a. despair and hopelessness
   b. loss of previously sustained beliefs
   c. belief in a foreshortened future

Treatment Options and Outlook

Treating EPTSD or relational trauma requires using a phase-oriented approach. Following the diagnosis and assessment the therapist must establish a solid, trusting, working relationship with the client.

The first phase of actual treatment involves stabilizing symptom management and containment. The client often must learn effective ways to manage and contain his or her symptoms. This may take quite a long time to develop but is an essential part of providing effective therapy. Next, psychological and emotional resources must be strengthened in order to improve affect (mood) control and modulation and to help build a sense of safety in the individual. The next phase is to identify his or her internal states and their effect on the individual's behavior.

Traumatic memories are brought into the treatment process only after these phases are in place (which may take years). The client is now ready to work on and resolve these experiences. Usually the client also needs to learn and practice new and effective interpersonal and boundary skills.

Risk Factors and Preventive Measures

EPTSD has a lasting effect on development and adult personality and emotional stability. In particular, as an adult, the traumatized individual with EPTSD will have difficulty with trust and interpersonal intimacy. EPTSD usually has more profound effects than circumscribed PTSD (CPTSD) or circumscribed trauma, in which there is one or a few traumatic experiences that are specific in nature. With CPTSD, specific events can be identified and worked on in therapy, but EPTSD has a more pervasive effect on social interactions and the development of the self and of private events, thus making therapy more difficult and prolonged. The therapeutic relationship itself becomes a vehicle for developing trust and intimacy with another person without aversive consequences.

See also BATTERED CHILD SYNDROME; CHILD ABUSE AND NEGLECT; CHILD PHYSICAL ABUSE; CHILD SEXUAL ABUSE; THERAPY, TYPES OF.

Doctor, Ronald. *The Complex/Relational Trauma Syndrome in Children and Adults.* Unpublished paper, 2002.

electroencephalograph (EEG)   The instrument that measures brain waves and pathological responses, producing a record known as an encephalogram (EEG). The quantitative electroencephalogram (qEEG) is a more complex type of electroencelphalogram. Abnormal brain wave patterns on the EEG or the qEEG may indicate a seizure disorder or another neurological problem. It may also indicate the presence of POSTTRAUMATIC STRESS DISORDER (PTSD). In addition, individuals who have been traumatized may have abnormal sleep patterns, as measured by electroencephalography.

In a study of 18 combat veterans with PTSD and 20 healthy nonveterans, reported in 2001, the researchers compared the qEEG of the two groups of subjects. They found that the subjects with PTSD had increased theta (daydream, fantasy) and beta (arousal, active brain engagement) activity but there were no differences in the two groups with regard to delta (sleep but not dreaming) and alpha (nonarousal states) activity. According to the researchers, the results indicated a neurobiological basis for PTSD, meaning the disorder is connected to changes in the state of the nervous system.

Said the researchers, "Various explanations (cortical hyperexcitability, prolonged wakefulness, or attention disturbances) have been offered for the beta activity increase in PTSD subjects." They also speculated that the increased theta activity might be part of the explanation for changes in the hippocampal volume of the brain.

See also BRAIN.

Begić, Drazen, Ljubomir Hotujac, and Nataša Jokić-Begić. "Electroencephalographic Comparison of Veterans with Combat-Related Post-Traumatic Stress Disorder and Healthy Subjects." *International Journal of Psychophysiology* 40 (2001): 167–172.

EMDR   See EYE MOVEMENT DESENSITIZATION AND REPROCESSING; THERAPY, TYPES OF.

emotional detachment   See EMOTIONAL NUMBING.

emotional numbing   One of the primary symptoms of POSTTRAUMATIC STRESS DISORDER (PTSD) or complex trauma is emotional numbing or emotional anesthesia. It is also sometimes referred to as PSYCHIC NUMBING. This often appears as a pervasive feeling of being detached from other people, from the outside world, and from activities that used to be enjoyable. Sufferers experience a greatly diminished ability to experience emotion, especially tenderness and the feelings associated with intimacy and sex. Other symptoms reflect an overaroused AUTONOMIC NERVOUS SYSTEM.

Sufferers have difficulty falling asleep or staying asleep; they are keyed up and their startle response is heightened. Anxiety and DEPRESSION are common in those with PTSD. Irritability is a further problem. GUILT about surviving when others did not and about the behavior that was necessary for survival may be constant and painful. Some of those with this disorder turn to alcohol or drugs for escape; others may become self-defeating or suicidal. In times of war, psychic numbing helps the soldier face the threat of death and the horrors of the war, including seeing civilian deaths as well as fallen comrades. Soldiers report acting like robots to get the job done on the battlefield. This numbing effect protects the soldiers against the most unbearable sights of horror, guilt, and inescapable fear, but psychic numbing can soon become dysfunctional.

During the course of deployment to a war zone, psychic numbing can prevent soldiers from fully absorbing vital information and responding to it, and if prolonged, it can lead to a breakdown of functioning by continually stifling their feelings. This opens the door for returning soldiers to have difficulty integrating well with their loved ones and sustaining close relationships and to suffer from intense feelings of isolation. If treatment is not sought, PTSD symptoms can lead to severe dysfunctions in everyday life.

emotional personality (EP)   A broad term used to describe people who like other people and who communicate and socialize. It is the emotional or feeling part of relationships. If there is damage to the personality from traumatic experiences, then the emotional personality would suffer the most. These people tend to be optimistic and expect good things from situations and people. Like the Tin Man in the *Wizard of Oz*, emotional personalities have a "heart" and are compassionate and outgoing.

There are many tests for emotionality or the emotional personality. Historically the search for emotional personalities was accomplished by body assessments and fluids. For example, Hippocrates ("The Father of Modern Medicine," 460 B.C.–370 B.C.) identified four types of disorders from sampling bodily fluids or humors. An excess of yellow bile was believed to cause mania, while an excess of black bile was believed to cause melancholia (DEPRESSION). Hippocrates was instrumental in pointing toward internal causes of personality and derangement.

Modern knowledge of physiology has led to some interesting approaches to personality assessment. For example, using highly sophisticated temperature devices, researchers have noted differences between the temperatures of the right and left ears of children. Although these differences are slight and must be accumulated over many measurements, asymmetry in temperature is associated with negative emotionality. Specifically, people who exhibit higher right side temperature relative to the left side tend to have more negative and less positive emotional dispositions as determined by parental ratings. Recorded temperatures are external ways of measuring the blood flow to the right and left frontal cortexes.

See also BRAIN.

endogenous stress hormones   Refers to stress hormones such as CORTISOL, EPINEPHRINE, and NOREPINEPHRINE. The body responds to STRESS as "danger," and it activates the nervous system, releasing specific endogenous stress hormones. The adrenal glands are signaled by the hypothalamus to release cortisol, epinephrine and norepinephrine into the bloodstream. The immediate reaction to this release is the speeding up of the heart rate, breathing rate, metabolism, and blood pressure. The muscles are put on alert for a FIGHT OR FLIGHT RESPONSE by opening up blood vessels to the major muscle groups. The liver responds by releasing glucose for energy and producing sweat to cool down the body.

Many other endogenous stress hormones are also released, such as ADRENOCORTICOTROPIC HORMONE, which stimulates the release of GLUCOCORTICOIDS, glucagons to mobilize energy, ENDORPHINS to block pain, and vasopressin, which also plays a role in cardiovascular stress response.

See also PHYSIOLOGY OF TRAUMA.

endorphins   Opioid-like peptides (chains of amino acids) that are produced in the nervous system and pituitary gland and which result in natural morphine-like numbing effects to relieve pain. The name *endorphin* is derived from the phrase "endogenous morphine-like substance." The first neuropeptides were discovered in 1975 by John Hughes and Hans Kosterlitz of Scotland and were named *enkephalins,* a short chain of five amino acids. Since then, two other peptide groups of endorphins have been identified as beta-endorphin (shortened to endorphin) and dynorphin.

In addition to their analgesic properties, endorphins also appear to produce a feeling of euphoria or a "runner's high." This euphoria occurs when endorphins are released after vigorous exercise such as running, swimming, bicycling, and aerobics. In trauma research, van der Kolk wrote in 1989 that "endorphinergic influences might also contribute to the phenomenon of compulsive trauma reenactment," that is, the tendency to repeat elements of the trauma in one's life.

People with POSTTRAUMATIC STRESS DISORDER (PTSD) who are reexposed to a stimulus resembling the original trauma will secrete endorphins that serve to help protect against or modulate extreme emotional reactions.

See also BRAIN; CENTRAL NERVOUS SYSTEM; NEUROPEPTIDE Y; PHYSIOLOGY OF TRAUMA.

van der Kolk, B. A., M. S. Greenberg, S. P. Orr, and R. K. Pitman. "Endogenous Opioids and Stress Induced Analgesia in Post Traumatic Stress Disorder." *Psychopharmacology Bulletin* 25 (1989): 108–112.

energetic field of trauma   The AUTONOMIC NERVOUS SYSTEM controls 90 percent of bodily functions. Feeling good brings this system into balance or resets the set point of this system to a balanced or regulated level. In contrast, trauma distorts this balance toward the sympathetic end, causing chronic arousal. Regulation is a balance between the sympathetic (arousal) and parasympathetic (relaxation) sides of the autonomic nervous system.

The heart's electrical field has 400–600 times more amplitude than the electrical field of the BRAIN. Furthermore, the electromagnetic field of the heart is more than 5,000 times stronger than that of the brain (pulsing electromagnetic energy). The heart's electromagnetic energy is strong enough to broadcast to others. In addition, research has shown that brain wave patterns of another person can be transmitted at least 10 feet to a receiving person. Psychic lore indicates that this transmission distance may be much greater.

Individuals are trained to use their minds to guide their behavior and affect (mood). If the heart is regarded as the resonating center of the body, then the question becomes how individuals can bring the heart into participation with perception and life to provide coherence, harmony, and fulfillment. This involves making room for heart energy in thinking, attitudes, and self-concept. Traumatic experience tends to distort and skew energy and to create a state of DYSREGULATION.

epinephrine/adrenaline   A CATECHOLAMINE, epinephrine is both a hormone and a NEUROTRANSMITTER. It is released by the adrenal glands and plays an important role in stress reaction, such as when the body perceives danger or a threatening situation. It is also released in response to anxiety and exercise. Epinephrine is carried in the bloodstream and increases the heart rate, dilates the pupils, and constricts the small capillaries in the skin while dilating the arteries in muscles. It also increases blood glucose levels. The term *adrenaline* comes from a name given a synthetic form of epinephrine that has come into common usage.

Epinephrine is a FIGHT OR FLIGHT RESPONSE hormone and is rapidly released during emergency situations that may be life-threatening as well as exciting, as when a hurricane nears. Because a perceived threat can be both a physical threat and a psychological threat (Can I overcome my fears?), the human body can become overstimulated and maladaptive due to an overabundance of epinephrine in the bloodstream. Too much epinephrine can lower the immune system, resulting in health problems, such as colds and flu, and more serious problems, such as heart disease, if the body's stress response is repeatedly triggered.

See also NOREPINEPHRINE.

eustress   Nonharmful arousal or stress responses in the body. Hans Selye, M.D., is credited with developing the concept of *stress*. His classic publication, *The Stress of Life,* described the stress response as "wear and tear" on the body that eventually leads to death or chronic disease if is it not dealt with. To Selye, stress was arousal in the body in preparation for action, to either fight or flee. The arousal pattern would diminish or return to normal once the stressor was removed.

To account for arousal that was not fearful or protective, such as sexual arousal, laughing, games and action, and so on and which do not seem to be destructive or harmful to the person, Selye distinguished between "distress" (harmful stress) and "eustress" (from the Greek *eu* meaning good, as in euphoria). Said Selye,

> During both eustress and distress the body undergoes virtually the same nonspecific responses to the various positive or negative stimuli acting upon it. However, the fact that eustress causes much less damage than distress graphically demonstrates that it is "how you take it" that determines, ultimately, whether one can adapt successfully to change.

In other words, what makes something distressful or not is the individual's interpretation of the event and not the event itself. It is how an individual perceives a situation that can create destructive effects. Cognitive behavior therapists understand Selye's theory and have developed approaches to help modify interpretations that are destructive and unproductive.

See also STRESS.

Selye, Hans. *The Stress of Life.* New York: McGraw-Hill Books, 1956.

explicit memory   There are two forms of memory related to traumatic experiences. The first is explicit memory (sometimes called declarative memory). The second is implicit (sometimes called procedural). Implicit memory is subconscious but can influence behavior through implicit cues like body sensations. Explicit memory, however, involves the recall of events into awareness or consciousness. This requires focused attention, and this is often difficult for children to accomplish at young ages. Traumatic experience is thought to be stored mostly as implicit memory. We use consciousness to recall and verbalize memories about a specific time and place or events or facts that an individual chooses to remember, such as a person's birthday celebration.

Explicit memories tend to be holistic in that they not only represent the different aspects of a situation but also the context in which the event occurred, such as the time of day, place, and people who were present at the event. Recall of explicit memories involves an image and the details of the situation. It is what is asked of witnesses in a trial. Van der Kolk points out that explicit memories are seriously affected by lesions of the frontal lobe and HIPPOCAMPUS, which have been linked to the neurobiology of POSTTRAUMATIC STRESS DISORDER (PTSD).

See also MEMORY; MEMORY CONSOLIDATION.

van der Kolk, B. "The Body Keeps the Score: Memory and the Evolving Psychobiology of Post Traumatic Stress." *Harvard Review of Psychiatry* 1, no. 5 (1994): 253–265.

exposure therapy   A form of behavior therapy in which an individual who is phobic (extremely fearful) or traumatized confronts the person, animal, event or place associated with their reaction or trauma. Whenever possible, this is done in the real situation; otherwise imaginal, pictorial, or video material is used for the exposure experience.

Exposure is always done in a controlled manner where escape or termination of the stimulus event is possible. The goal of exposure treatment is to reduce the distress, both physical and emotional, felt in these traumatic or scary situations. Exposure therapy is generally used to treat anxiety disorders, phobias, and POSTTRAUMATIC STRESS DISORDERS. The goal is that eventually the individual can face the feared or threatening item and not react with fear. The treatment includes a mild exposure at first that is gradually increased to a direct exposure to the feared thing.

In exposure treatment, a therapist accompanies the client into the feared or traumatic situation in a gradual manner and helps the client become aware of and release emotions or physical reactions that arise from the situation. In the exposure process, thoughts that cause stress, distress, or fear and anxiety are examined and confronted. It is important to confront and begin to modify these fear-associated thoughts because they trigger fear reactions on their own. Reducing or changing these thoughts helps relieve symptoms and reactions in the fear situation.

Exposure can be used with hypnosis or virtual reality methods. Often relaxation skills are developed before attempting exposure so the client has coping skills for arousal (fear) and can modulate his or her reactions. Generally, exposure treatments gradually lead to a more intimate presence with the stimulus situation. Sometimes flooding is used, and this involves exposure directly with the feared situation without gradual exposure. For example, with fear of riding in elevators, there is a point where the door closes, and the elevator proceeds to its destination. Graduated exposure is not possible here. Exposure combined with relaxation training and cognitive behavior therapy is usually called exposure therapy. If the exposure period is extensive, it is called PROLONGED EXPOSURE THERAPY. VIRTUAL REALITY EXPOSURE therapy involves wearing a helmet that projects images in 180-degree format; the client is exposed to animated or video images, usually in graded stages. This procedure is called virtual reality graded exposure therapy.

See also IMAGE HABITUATION THERAPY (IHT); THERAPY, TYPES OF.

extreme events   Usually refers to unusual events that are outside the range of usual human experience, such as a sexual assault, a hurricane, a tsunami, or an individual's being victimized in a crime, especially a crime of violence. The term *extreme event* is preferred by some experts to *traumatic event*, because the phrase *traumatic event* implies that the event is inevitably traumatic to everyone who experiences it; yet some individuals who experience an extreme event are traumatized, while others are not.

Only about 3–5 percent of people exposed to extreme events actually become traumatized. This difference in terminology highlights the fact that the event itself is not traumatizing, because obviously most people exposed to the extreme event do not develop trauma disorders. It is the impact it has on a given individual that produces a traumatic reaction. This is an important distinction, between an event causing a traumatic reaction versus a traumatic reaction developing in an individual exposed to the extreme event. The acquisition of a traumatic response is within the individual rather than the event. With this in mind, it is important to find the risk factors associated with the development of traumatic reactions within individuals in order to find preventive strategies against developing trauma disorders.

eye movement desensitization and reprocessing (EMDR)   An information processing therapy that uses bilateral stimulation of the brain to process traumatic reactions and that has proven effective in treating trauma-based conditions. Eye movement desensitization and reprocessing (EMDR) was developed in 1987 by Francine Shapiro. It has been refined over the years into a comprehensive therapy for trauma, although the procedures can also be used to treat clients with other problems and disorders. Since its inception, hundreds of case studies and controlled empirical studies have validated the effectiveness of EMDR for clients with trauma and other clients.

EMDR therapy assumes that trauma causes an overload of an information processing system that exists in all people. This processing system takes perceptions of the present and links them into already existing networks of memories in order to make sense of them. An event may be initially disturbing, but if the processing system is functioning well, the person learns from the experience, and it is then stored in memory with the appropriate feelings, thoughts, and sensations. However, if a trauma disrupts the system, then the event is stored in the brain in the form that it was experienced.

Memories of an event contain the image, thoughts, physical sensations, and emotions that occurred at the time. External or internal reminders can trigger that memory, and these images, thoughts, sounds, emotions, and sensations arise and can cause the symptoms of POSTTRAUMATIC STRESS DISORDER (PTSD). Even if all the symptoms of PTSD do not exist, recent research has indicated that general life events, even those which are not officially designated as trauma, can cause many of these symptoms and debilitate the person. The symptoms can stem from one event or a series of events that are stored in the memory networks.

EMDR is a form of therapy that integrates aspects of other orientations, such as psychodynamic, cognitive-behavioral, and experiential. It differs from the other therapies in that it focuses on the physically stored memories in the brain, with specific procedures and protocols to process the memories to an adaptive resolution. What is useful is learned and stored with useful associations in the brain, and the negative aspects are discarded. Unlike with hypnosis, the client is always aware of what is occurring and does not take the suggestions of the therapists. Rather, the client's own processing mechanism activates the insights and associations that arise.

EMDR is an eight-phase treatment approach. The first phase is a history-taking session, during which the therapist assesses the client's readiness for EMDR and develops a treatment plan. Client and therapist identify possible targets for EMDR processing. These include recent distressing events, current situations that elicit emotional disturbance, related historical incidents, and the development of specific skills and behaviors that will be needed by the client in future situations.

During the second phase of treatment, the therapist ensures that the client has adequate methods of handling emotional distress and good coping skills and that the client is in a relatively stable state. If further stabilization is required, or if additional skills are needed, therapy focuses on providing these. The client is then able to use stress-reducing techniques whenever necessary, during or between sessions. However, one of the goals is not to need these techniques once therapy is complete.

In phases three through six, a target is identified and processed using EMDR procedures. These involve the client identifying the most vivid visual image related to the memory (if available), a negative belief about self, and related emotions and body sensations. The client also identifies a preferred positive belief. The validity of the positive belief is rated, as is the intensity of the negative emotions.

After this, the client is instructed to focus on the image, negative thought, and body sensations while simultaneously moving his or her eyes back and forth following the therapist's fingers as they move across his or her field of vision for 20 to 30 seconds or more, depending upon the need of the client. Although eye movements are the most commonly used external stimulus, therapists often use auditory tones, tapping, or other types of tactile stimulation. The kind of dual attention and the length of each set is customized to the need of the client. The client is instructed to just notice whatever happens. After this, the clinician instructs the client to let his or her mind go blank and to notice whatever thought, feeling, image, memory, or sensation comes to mind.

Depending upon the client's report, the clinician will facilitate the next focus of attention. In most cases a client-directed association process is encouraged. This is repeated numerous times throughout the session. If the client becomes distressed or has difficulty with the process, the therapist follows established procedures to help the client resume processing. Occasionally processing will become blocked, and the client "loops" around that same material and cannot move on. When LOOPING occurs, the therapist will first change the direction or speed of bilateral stimulation. If looping persists, the therapist might offer an "interweaver" or rational statement to move the process along. For example, a client might be stuck on being beaten in the home and feel he or she should have defended himself or herself. The therapist might say, "You were only a child and your parents were much bigger than you" as a way to move out of the loop. When the client reports no distress related to the targeted memory, the clinician asks him or her to think of the preferred positive belief that was identified at the beginning of the session, or a better one if it has emerged, and to focus on the incident, while simultaneously engaging in the eye movements. After several sets, clients generally report increased confidence in this positive belief. The therapist checks with the client regarding body sensations. If there are negative sensations, these are processed as above. If there are positive sensations, they are further enhanced.

In phase seven, closure, the therapist asks the client to keep a journal during the week to document any related material that may arise and reminds the client of the self-calming activities that were mastered in phase two.

The next session begins with phase eight, reevaluation of the previous work, and of progress since the previous session. EMDR treatment ensures processing of all related historical events, current incidents that elicit distress, and future scenarios that will require different responses. The overall goal is to produce the most comprehensive and profound treatment effects in the shortest period of time, while simultaneously maintaining a stable client within a balanced system.

After EMDR processing, clients generally report that the emotional distress related to the memory has been eliminated or greatly decreased and that they have gained important cognitive insights. Importantly, these emotional and cognitive changes usually result in spontaneous behavioral and personal changes, which are further enhanced with standard EMDR procedures.

These phases also include a form of bilateral stimulation (eye movements, taps, or tones) that many researchers believe stimulate an "orienting response" causing new positive associations to arise, as the negative ones are discarded. Some researchers have compared the progressions to those that occur in Rapid Eye Movement (REM) sleep, which is believed to be the body's own mechanism for processing survival information.

During the reprocessing phases, the trauma memory is transformed with new insights, emotions, sensations, and beliefs that automatically arise. The rape victim can move from a sense of shame and guilt to the feeling of being a strong and resilient woman. Research has indicated that these changes can occur very rapidly, often within three sessions.

EMDR sessions end with a closure phase that resolves any distress from incomplete treatment and prepares the client for any continued processing between sessions. As homework, the client keeps a log of any new thoughts, feelings, or images that may arise. The next session begins with a reevaluation to check on the previous work and guide the clinician to choosing the next target.

In addition to treating PTSD, EMDR can also address any clinical complaint that is based upon, or made worse by, disturbing life experiences. These more general disturbances are called small "t" trauma. That is, while humiliations in grade school may be commonplace, they can also have long-lasting negative effects (small "t" trauma) and they felt "traumatic" when they occurred. They also appear to be stored in the BRAIN in a way that holds the original negative emotions, thoughts, and body sensations. Processing these types of memories can help resolve a wide range of pathologies.

Empirical support has been established for the efficiency and effectiveness of EMDR. Furthermore, physiological studies find positive structural changes occur in the brain following successful EMDR therapy. In 1995, a professional organization was independently formed to establish ethical and training standards for therapists practicing EMDR. This organization is called the Eye Movement Desensitization and Reprocessing International Association or EMDRIA. Both the EMDR Institute and EMDRIA have Web sites available for more information and help finding a trained therapist.

See also DISSOCIATION/DISSOCIATIVE DISORDERS; THERAPY, TYPES OF.

Shapiro, F. *Eye Movement Desensitization and Reprocessing: Basic Principles, Protocols, and Procedures.* 2nd ed. New York: Guilford Press, 2001.

false memory/false memory syndrome A memory can be a false memory because the event never happened or because the event in recall is too distorted to remember it correctly. When people recall events, this recall is vulnerable to omissions of details and the natural tendency to "fill in the gaps." This reconstruction of the event is very important to the false memory controversy. The controversy centers around the question as to whether these "memories" are real or fabrication from outside subtle suggestion. The memories of individuals may be permanently stored in the brain, but they are not retrieved with 100 percent accuracy, as individuals mix up facts or combine unrelated experiences and wrongly conclude it as an authentic, single memory. The more individuals rehearse a memory incorrectly, the more that they come to believe that it is a valid memory.

The false memory syndrome is the term used to describe a condition in which the person's identity and relationships are centered on vivid but false memories of abuse during their childhood. The controversy and debate over false memory syndrome is centered on child abuse, as adult children have claimed repression of the trauma until later in life when the memory resurfaced on its own or during the psychotherapeutic process. The controversy is not whether children are abused. The controversy is about the claims of how accurate these recovered memories are of the abuse. Henkel et al. found that the most compelling false memories may occur when fragments of real experiences (as with viewing photographs or hearing other eyewitnesses recount events) play a role in how memories can get muddled and confused. The false memory syndrome does not have diagnostic criteria in the *DIAGNOSTIC AND STATISTICAL MANUAL of mental disorders* (DSM).

See also IMPLICIT MEMORY.

Henkel, Linda, Nancy Franklin, and Marcia K. Johnson. "Cross-Modal Source Monitoring Cofusions Between Perceived and Imagined Events." *Journal of Experimental Psychology: Learning, Memory and Cognition* 26, no. 2 (March 2000): 321–335.

felt sense A bodily sensation that guides human perceptions, thoughts, and emotions, which was first described by Eugene Gendlin in his book, *Focusing*. Felt sense is formed from past experiences, and it guides an individual's responses, particularly to traumatic events. According to Gendlin, the felt sense is not an emotion: "Think of it as a taste . . . or a great musical chord that makes you feel a powerful impact, a big round unclear feeling." Focusing on the felt sense is said to help to change and shift or neutralize negative experience to a more neutral state.

Gendlin says there six movements, or steps, to focusing on the felt sense, including:

1. The individual clears a space in the mind to identify problems while not concentrating on any problem. All problems, large and small, are to be "stacked" until they are all present.
2. The individual then identifies which problem feels or seems the worst. Then he or she is instructed to think not about the problem itself but rather how it makes the body feel. Gendlin says the individual should not evaluate or judge the sense of the problem, but should merely experience it.
3. The next step is to find a quality about the felt sense, such as "sticky," "heavy," "helpless," or "tight" or a phrase, such as feeling like the

person is "in a box." At this point, the problem begins to change to the individual. Gendlin says that when the person notices a shift in the bodily experience of the problem, this is a "handle."

4. The fourth movement is "Resonating Handle and Felt Sense." In this stage, the individual is instructed to use the word or image that was derived from the third movement and then compare it to the felt sense (second step) and make sure that there is a perfect fit. Said Gendlin, "When you get a perfect match, the words being just right for the feeling, let yourself feel that for a minute . . . allow it to be."

5. In the next movement, or the asking stage, if a shift has not yet occurred, the individual is to ask the felt sense itself what it is, using the handle to allow the felt sense to be more vivid.

6. In the last movement, or "Receiving," the individual is instructed to take whatever comes into focus and to welcome it. Said Gendlin, "Take the attitude that you are glad your body spoke to you, whatever it said."

Experiencing the felt sense is the basis for SOMATIC EXPERIENCING THERAPY developed by Peter Levine and used to treat traumatic reactions.

See also BODY MEMORY; THERAPY, TYPES OF.

Gendlin, Eugene. *Focusing.* New York: Bantam, 1982.

fight, flight, and freeze phenomenon   Methods of dealing with threat. Orienting is the first behavior, and it is guided by the lower brain centers that are organized for survival. When a stimulus is identified as a threat, individuals orient toward it as they mobilize for fight or flight. Freezing is usually engaged if fight or flight will not work or is not possible.

FIGHT OR FLIGHT RESPONSES involve high levels of AUTONOMIC NERVOUS SYSTEM activation, as these reactions involve whole body reactions. If fight/flight fails in some way, the individual goes into freeze, which is an autonomic nervous system disorganization involving inhibition, primarily of the muscular system. In freeze there are high levels of sympathetic activation combined with high levels of parasympathetic activation as a counterbalance. The freeze response in humans is often described as

being in shock, a state of arousal but disconnected and dissociated from ongoing events. Much of the knowledge of the fight, flight, and freeze phenomenon comes from research and observation of animals, since human culture imposes restrictions on performance of these responses.

fight or flight response   The adaptive response of the SYMPATHETIC NERVOUS SYSTEM that prepares the body to "fight" or "flee" the perceived threat to human survival. It is also known as acute stress response. The fight or flight response was first described by physiologist Walter Cannon in the 1920s as one that was hardwired into the brain and was genetically embedded from the earliest humans who had to fight off threats from predators and other outside threats to life. It was later recognized as the first stage of a general adaptive syndrome that regulates STRESS responses.

When a person experiences stress and the fight or flight response is activated, the sympathetic nervous system releases adrenaline and NOREPINEPHRINE from the adrenal glands into the bloodstream. The body changes dramatically, and the heart rate and breathing increase. Blood is diverted from the digestive tract to the muscles, where the body prepares to fight or run. ENDORPHINS are released to reduce the perception of pain. The pupils of the eyes dilate and the individual is acutely aware of his or her surroundings. Mental focus shifts to immediate danger and bypasses the rational mind. All is prepared for survival.

Once the danger or threat passes, the PARASYMPATHETIC NERVOUS SYSTEM restores the body to normal, using the NEUROTRANSMITTER known as ACETYLCHOLINE.

See also BRAIN; CENTRAL NERVOUS SYSTEM.

flashback   An experience wherein a person has a sudden image and feeling of experiencing a past experience, often a distressing one. Flashbacks can take the form of visual images, sounds, smells, feelings, or body sensations as the person believes that the traumatic event is happening all over again. The person does not lose consciousness, but may have difficulty distinguishing what is real from the flashback experience. This may last for a few seconds, minutes, or hours, and rarely, days. The emotions are reexperienced almost in the same manner as they were felt during the original experience, such as feeling trapped or powerless, causing the heart to beat faster and adrenalin to flow. A flashback may occur among individuals suffering from POSTTRAUMATIC STRESS DISORDER (PTSD).

Flashbacks are often triggered by something the survivor may see, smell, or hear that reminds them of a past trauma, and the emotions are charged just as they were during the actual trauma. It is evident that the "body keeps the score," as stated by van der Kolk, in that it stores experiences that are retriggered by memories or by coming into contact with environmental triggers.

Flashback was a term originally used in the film industry. Psychiatrists first used the term in the 1960s to refer to visual and perceptual disturbances with individuals who used hallucinogenic drugs (LSD) and later used the term to refer to trauma recollections of Vietnam veterans.

See also BODY MEMORY; FELT SENSE.

van der Kolk, B. A. "The Body Keeps the Score: Memory and the Evolving Psychobiology of Posttraumatic Stress." In *Essential Papers on Posttraumatic Stress Disorder,* edited by M. J. Horowitz, 301–326. New York: New York University Press, 1999.

flooding A therapeutic procedure involving the exposure of the individual to distressing stimuli for a prolonged period without the individual's experiencing anxiety-avoidance behaviors. Flooding is sometimes called implosive therapy. If EXPOSURE THERAPY is analogous to first dipping your toe into the water and gradually moving your body further in as comfort permits, flooding is equivalent to being tossed into the water fully. With flooding, however, the individual is immersed fully in the scary situation until the anxiety begins to subside. Obviously, this requires great dedication and trust by the client and a high degree of confidence by the therapist, who must have extensive training in the procedures. Flooding can be conducted in vivo (in real life) or imaginal (in the imagination). In vivo flooding is used primarily to treat phobias and obsessive compulsive disorder.

Imaginal exposure to one's traumatic memory is a core treatment for posttraumatic stress and ACUTE STRESS DISORDER. According to Moulds and Nixon (2006), in vivo flooding to fear-eliciting situations is also a common treatment procedure for POSTTRAUMATIC STRESS DISORDER (PTSD), targeting phobic avoidance reminders of the trauma. The major criticisms of flooding are the discomfort it produces for the individual receiving the treatment and the prolonged distress that it causes. Both these factors make the method aversive to many clients, who avoid such techniques. There is also some question as to the long-term success of flooding, in that many studies show regression of effects at six-month and one-year follow-ups.

See also EXPOSURE THERAPY; IN VIVO THERAPY; THERAPY, TYPES OF.

Moulds, M. L., and R. D. Nixon. "In Vivo Flooding for Anxiety Disorders: Proposing its Utility for the Treatment of Post Traumatic Stress Disorder." *Journal of Anxiety Disorder* 20 (2006): 498–509.

forward psychiatry See COMBAT STRESS REACTION.

fright neuroses Fright neurosis is an old term that was used to describe POSTTRAUMATIC STRESS DISORDER when very little was known about it. In Freudian terms, it was a form of *neurosis* or a disorder that arises from repressed, unconscious conflictual experiences, much as the "anxiety neurosis." Fright neurosis was included in Emil Kraepelin's 1909 early diagnostic system in which he said that fright neurosis was a condition arising from a response to overwhelming stress. Over time the term was lost in a deluge of psychological labels used to describe the shock, FIGHT, FLIGHT, AND FREEZE PHENOMENON that is currently called posttraumatic stress disorder (PTSD). Other terms were also used to describe the disorder, such as SHELL SHOCK, combat/war neurosis, traumatic neurosis, compensation neurosis, and SURVIVOR SYNDROME. According to Freud,

"Anxiety" describes a particular state of expecting the danger or preparing for it, even though it may be an unknown one. "Fear" requires a definite object of which to be afraid. "Fright" is the name given to the state a person gets into when he has run into danger without being prepared for it; it emphasizes the factor of surprise.

Freud also is said to have pointed out that it is this element of surprise that distinguishes anxiety from fear as well as fear from fright.

See also COMBAT STRESS REACTION.

fugue state   Fugue states are dissociative events in which the individual loses his or her sense of personal identity, memories of the past and, to some extent, his or her unique personality before the fugue. So, these are people who generally leave their environment and their identity behind and unconsciously move to a new place and identity that is more satisfying and free from any stressors from their old life. The process is unconscious and involves dissociative amnesia that is not drug- or injury-produced. There is no medical or physical precipitant. The fugue state seems to occur in individuals who are highly repressed and live in a very repressed environment in which feelings and personal reactions are not discussed or supported. Multiple episodes are possible, but generally there is just one dramatic break from the old life to a new life and new identity. Fugue states are a very rare occurrence and usually start with a reminder of a traumatic event or a traumatic and dissatisfying way of life.

See also AMNESIA.

gamma-aminobutyric acid (GABA) An inhibitory NEUROTRANSMITTER in the brain that is associated with anxiety, DEPRESSION, PANIC DISORDER, and POSTTRAUMATIC STRESS DISORDER (PTSD). It is hypothesized that excitability or anxiety states involve a state of generalized arousal or excitability throughout the BRAIN, and that GABA release is part of a feedback system to reduce the level of excitability. Some researchers believe that malfunctions of this feedback system can cause increased anxiety, generalized anxiety, or the chronic arousal states seen in PTSD.

Increased GABA levels in the brain can bind with GABA receptors to produce sedation. Likewise, drugs that also bind with these receptors, such as anesthetics, BENZODIAZEPINES, sedatives, or alcohol, typically have relaxing and antianxiety effects. GABA, discovered in 1950, and glycine (the smallest of the 20 amino acids, an inhibitory neurotransmitter with high concentrations in collagen), seem to be the most important inhibitory neurotransmitters in the brain. Unfortunately, research on GABA's effects has been conducted mainly on animal subjects and, consequently, its generalization to humans seems rather simplistic to date.

In 2006, French investigators G. Vaiva et al. evaluated 78 survivors of traffic accidents at one year posttrauma and found that the GABA levels were significantly lower among the survivors who met all or nearly all the criteria for PTSD. The authors concluded that a return to normal levels of GABA may be a marker of recovery from PTSD.

Vaiva, G., et al. "Relationship between Posttraumatic GABA Plasma Levels & PTSD at 1 Year Follow-Up." *American Journal of Psychiatry* 163 (August 2006): 1,446–1,448.

Ganser syndrome A controversial disorder in which a patient's behavior mimics symptoms of psychosis; however, the individual is not psychotic. It is a form of pseudodementia that is often associated with prison or torture environments. Many experts consider it to be a form of malingering (faking illness). However, some experts believe that a TRAUMATIC BRAIN INJURY could lead to the symptoms of Ganser syndrome, while others believe that organic dementia may cause these symptoms.

Ganser syndrome was first recognized in 1898 by German psychiatrist Sigbert J. Ganser, who described prisoners who sought to avoid prosecution. The DIAGNOSTIC AND STATISTICAL MANUAL (DSM) categorizes Ganser syndrome as a dissociative disorder, not otherwise specified or diagnosed, although it has its own ICD-10 medical code. The ICD-10 is a mental illness coding system used in other parts of the world.

The syndrome may occur subsequent to a stressful or traumatic event, such as problems in the sexual, domestic, or financial areas of life. It is believed to occur as a result of an event that is intolerable to the individual.

Symptoms and Diagnostic Path

Symptoms of Ganser syndrome are varied and may include hysterical seizures, paralysis, visual and olfactory hallucinations, a disorientation of time and place, and AMNESIA. One unique symptom is that when questioned, individuals with Ganser syndrome give approximate answers to questions with clear right and wrong answers; for example, if the person is shown a glove and asked what the item is, he or she may state that it is a hand. The answer is wrong, but it approximates the correct answer.

A case of a man with both acquired immune deficiency syndrome (AIDS) and Ganser syndrome was described in *Psychosomatics* in 2003. The man was traumatized by his AIDS diagnosis, became depressed, and reported several SUICIDE attempts. During the Mini-Mental State Examination, when asked what year it was, he responded with the prior year. He was asked what city he lived in, and he named a city in another state. He did not answer one question correctly. This patient also reported visual and auditory hallucinations. One week later, the patient's performance improved. Said the doctors,

> In Ganser's syndrome, symptoms are unconsciously produced, although they may appear to have secondary gain. In this case, the patient was confronted regarding his knowledge of giving approximate answers, and he responded with indifference, demonstrating no awareness of the occurrence. Moreover, he showed no anxiety or fear of being discovered. He did not appear to be particularly guarded or bothered by the inconsistencies in his reporting of symptoms. Further, when the clinician exited the room and the patient was left without supervision, his presentation did not appear to change significantly as observed from another room through a one-way mirror.

Treatment Options and Outlook

Ganser syndrome is very difficult to treat; generally, only accompanying psychiatric disorders such as DEPRESSION can be treated. The syndrome often resolves on its own. There is little research or clinical data on this syndrome and certainly no specific treatment for this condition.

Risk Factors and Preventive Measures

Prisoners seem to have a higher risk than others for this syndrome. There are no known preventive measures. Otherwise, there is not enough known about this condition to make statements about incidence or risk factors.

Cosgray, R. E., and R. W. Fawley. "Could it Be Ganser's Syndrome." *Archives of Psychiatric Nursing* 3, no. 4 (August 1989): 241–245.

Deibler, Marla Wax, et al. "Ganser's Syndrome in a Man with AIDS." *Psychosomatics* 44, no. 4 (July–August 2003): 342–345.

generalized anxiety disorder (GAD)   A common form of anxiety disorder that is experienced by 2.1 percent of the United States population in a given year and 4.1 percent within a lifetime. It is also sometimes called global anxiety, but this term is seldom used professionally. The onset of generalized anxiety disorder (GAD) can occur at any age, but the median age of onset is 31 years. Many people with GAD also have other psychiatric disorders, such as DEPRESSION, other forms of ANXIETY DISORDERS, and SUBSTANCE ABUSE/DEPENDENCE. Individuals who have suffered from traumatic experiences have an elevated risk for developing GAD.

According to author and psychiatrist Aaron Beck, there are three types of precipitating psychological factors that can lead to the development of GAD. Often GAD develops because the individual feels overloaded. For example, when demands increase such that he or she feels in danger of failure, this is a potentially precipitating factor for GAD. A job promotion with many new expectations of the employee is another example of such a situation.

Another example of a precipitating factor is an increased amount of threat in a life situation, such as a new mother with a very sick infant, who becomes fearful that she cannot properly care for her child.

A third precipitating factor may be a stressful event that severely undermines the confidence of the individual, such as in the case of an attorney who knows that he or she must pass the bar examination to be accepted by his or her company, but who then fails the examination.

Beck and Emery said in *Anxiety Disorders and Phobias: A Cognitive Perspective:*

> In cases of GAD, we often see that the problems reported by the patient did not start with the precipitating events but actually extended far back into the developmental period. The precipitating stressors are potent only insofar as they strike at a person's specific vulnerabilities. The mother who was chronically anxious after the birth of her child had experienced long-standing "feelings" of inadequacy. However, the problem now was: Her inadequacy could risk the baby's life and thus become a source of danger. A person faced with the threat of failure in his career now thinks seriously for the first time, "I may not be successful in my career and thus I can never be happy."

Symptoms and Diagnostic Path

The primary symptom of GAD is an unrealistic worry and overconcern about several issues and problems that has lasted for six months or longer. This worrying continues even when the individual realizes that his or her worrying is excessive and unreasonable. The person may feel a sense of impending doom at most times and be unable to relax. Some individuals worry about financial issues, while others may worry about a partner's fidelity or even world problems that the individual has no control over. Although the types of worries vary considerably from person to person, the intensity of the worrying is extreme and debilitating in all who have GAD.

The worrying is also accompanied by such physical symptoms as fatigue, INSOMNIA, and irritability. Muscle tension is a somatic symptom that often appears in individuals with GAD. Other symptoms that may occur with GAD include:

- headaches
- difficulty swallowing
- lightheadedness
- irritability
- excessive sweating
- nausea
- a frequent need to urinate
- feeling out of breath
- difficulty concentrating

The anxiety and the physical symptoms negatively affect the person both at work and at home.

Diagnosis is often made by a mental health professional, usually from extensive interviews on developmental history, who notes the severe concerns of the patient as well as the physical symptoms that accompany this anxiety. Medical problems such as hyperthyroidism should be ruled out (from blood work) before the diagnosis of GAD is made, because individuals with hyperthyroidism may exhibit many of the same symptoms that are found with GAD.

Treatment Options and Outlook

GAD is treated with antianxiety medications, particularly drugs in the BENZODIAZEPINE class. Antide-pressants are also sometimes used to treat anxiety disorders, such as SELECTIVE SEROTONIN REUPTAKE INHIBITORS (SSRIs). In addition, bupropion (Wellbutrin), a dopamine reuptake inhibitor, is used to treat GAD. COGNITIVE BEHAVIORAL THERAPY is often helpful to teach the patient to adopt more realistic and favorable ideas about life and its risks and challenges. The cognitive behavioral therapies are usually combined with medications. Here the client is encouraged to identify irrational cognitions that produce anxiety and worry. Working with the therapist, the client is encouraged and coached in bringing in new, more realistic and rational self-statements that do not lead to worry and anxiety and help him or her function better with minimal arousal.

Risk Factors and Preventive Measures

Women have about twice the risk of developing GAD as do men, according to the National Institute of Mental Health. Individuals with a family history of anxiety disorders, particularly GAD, have an increased risk for this disorder. Early shyness and perfectionism are risk factors for developing GAD. Also, excessive worry and feelings of guilt and responsibility contribute greatly.

See also ANTIANXIETY MEDICATION; THERAPY, TYPES OF.

Beck, Aaron T., M.D., and Gary Emery. *Anxiety Disorders and Phobias: A Cognitive Perspective*. New York: Basic Books, 2005.

Grant, B. F., et al. "Prevalence, Correlates, Co-morbidity and Comparative Disability of DSM-IV Generalized Anxiety Disorder in the USA: Results from the National Epidemiologic Survey on Alcohol and Related Conditions." *Psychological Medicine* 35, no. 12 (2005): 1,747–1,759.

genetic influences on trauma   Issues that impinge on the response of individuals to traumatic events. Following exposure to traumatic stressors, POST-TRAUMATIC STRESS DISORDER (PTSD) develops in only a small subset of people. The question then becomes, "Are there people who are predisposed genetically to develop PTSD from traumatic experiences?" Heredity and environment cannot be separated and studied separately; both factors are always interacting and working together, and therefore, the heredity-environment issue is unsolvable. However, it is possible to determine whether hereditary factors provide a potential risk for developing PTSD.

The study of twins exposed to trauma helps researchers to estimate hereditary risks. For example, the Vietnam War provided an unfortunate laboratory for studying trauma in all its aspects. In one study, 4,029 male-male pairs of twins who had both served in Vietnam were examined, and the results were reported in the *American Journal of Medical Genetics* in 1993. Monozygotic (MZ) twins, also known as identical twins, were compared with dizygotic (DZ), or fraternal twins, for the incidence of PTSD.

However, a cautionary note is required. These twin pairs were established based on verbal reports from the subjects. Monozygotic twins are very rare and are usually classified by appearance alone and not DNA studies. Thus, the MZ group may have been more heterogeneous, making comparisons with DZ twins less meaningful. There is no way to know this from this type of study.

The MZ group in this study showed higher concordance rates (agreement with both twins engaged in the same activity) in terms of volunteering for military service, volunteering to go to Vietnam, and volunteering for combat. The conclusion was that heredity played a moderate role in these experiences and accounted for about 30 percent of these effects.

A second study reported by Stein et al. in 2002 examined trauma exposure and PTSD in 184 male and female pairs of DZ twins and 222 pairs of MZ twins in nonveteran and noncombat volunteers. Unlike the first study, which concentrated on uniform trauma, this study looked at many different kinds of civilian traumas and separated them into person-assaultive traumas (such as rape, robbery, etc.) and nonassaultive traumas (such as auto accidents, natural disasters, etc.) for both male and female twin sets. Assaultive trauma (person against person) showed a moderate genetic influence, whereas nonassaultive trauma was mainly a function of environmental factors.

Although it is difficult to determine the proportional role of heredity and environment because the two coexist, it can be assumed from these studies that when there is a person-against-person traumatic experience, genetics plays a moderate role in the development of PTSD, whereas in nonassaultive trauma, the experience of environment plays the major role in the development of PTSD.

Lyons, M. J., et al. "Do Genes Influence Exposure to Trauma?" *American Journal of Medical Genetics* 48 (1993): 22–27.
Stein, M. G. "Genetic and Environmental Influences on Trauma Exposure and Posttraumatic Disorder Symptoms." *American Journal of Psychiatry* 159 (2002): 1,675–1,681.

global anxiety See GENERALIZED ANXIETY DISORDER (GAD).

Global Assessment of Functioning (GAF) A clinician's report of an individual's overall level of functioning, as described in the *DIAGNOSTIC AND STATISTICAL MANUAL of Mental Disorder*, Volume 4. The GAF is a 100-point scale that measures psychological, social, and occupational functioning on a hypothetical continuum of mental health/illness. Each 10-point range has two components: symptom severity and functioning ability. For example, a GAF score from 61–70 indicates mild symptoms (such as depressed mood and mild INSOMNIA) or some difficulty in social, occupational, or school functioning. Generally, individuals with this score function well and have meaningful interpersonal relationships.

In a 1998 study, Steven Weine et al. worked with 20 Bosnian survivors of ethnic cleansing who resettled in Chicago. After each survivor provided TESTIMONY THERAPY as a way of telling his or her survival story, describing life in war and as a refugee, Weine found that the rate of POSTTRAUMATIC STRESS DISORDER (PTSD) diagnosis decreased from 100 percent to 74 percent immediately after testimony and then to 53 percent at six months. There was also substantial improvement in their functioning as measured by GAF scores.

See also ASSESSMENT AND DIAGNOSIS; INSTRUMENTS/SCALES/SURVEYS THAT EVALUATE POSTTRAUMATIC STRESS DISORDER (PTSD).

Weine, S., et al. "Testimony Psychotherapy in Bosnian Refuges: A Pilot Study." *American Journal of Psychiatry* 155, no. 12 (December 1998): 1,720–1,726.

glucocorticoids   A class of steroids and hormones of which CORTISOL is the most abundant in the body. Its name is derived from the early observation that these hormones played a critical role in glucose metabolism and body activation. In response to physical or mental STRESS, corticotrophin-releasing hormone (CRH) is released from the hypothalamus, which in turn triggers the production of ADRENOCORTICOTROPIC HORMONE (ACTH). It is ACTH that stimulates the release of cortisol and other glucocorticoids.

The maleficent effects of glucocorticoids seem to be a recurring theme in nearly every discussion of these hormones and in just about every context; however, experts report that despite their bad reputation, stress hormones have protective as well as damaging effects on the body such as inhibition of bone formation, suppression of calcium absorption, and delayed wound healing. The side that predominates is dependent on the time-course of the hormonal stress response, as well as the body's exposure to the stress hormones. To this end, glucocorticoids promote the conversion of proteins and lipids into usable carbohydrates. In the short term, this conversion is useful in replenishing an individual's energy reserves after a period of activity. On the other hand, chronic high levels of these hormones can damage body organs and are associated with weight gain and possibly serious diseases.

Glucocorticoids also act on the BRAIN to increase the appetite for food and to increase locomotor, or behavioral, activity and food-seeking behavior. This is beneficial after a period of physical activity, but it can also be damaging when, for example, a person is eating junk food while cramming for an examination.

Inactivity and a lack of energy expenditure lead to the chronic elevation of glucocorticoids, which impede the action of insulin to promote glucose uptake. This interaction results in an elevated insulin level coupled with elevated glucocorticoids, which promote the deposition of body fat. Additionally, this combination of hormones also contributes to the formation of atherosclerotic plaques in the coronary arteries.

See also CORTICOSTEROIDS.

grief   Intense sadness over a loss. Coping with the loss of a loved one is one of life's shared experiences, but if it is prolonged, unresolved, and intense, grief can lead to POSTTRAUMATIC STRESS DISORDER (PTSD). According to experts who study the grief cycle, it can be broken down into overlapping but discrete stages. In her study of the grief process, Elizabeth Kubler-Ross described the stages of grief as denial, anger, bargaining, DEPRESSION, and, finally, acceptance.

There are, of course, individual differences in dealing with grief, and sometimes not all of these stages are present. For example, men tend to resolve a significant loss by thinking and taking action, while women typically talk it out, cry, and express their emotions.

No matter what method is used to cope and resolve one's grief, grieving individuals usually suffer from impaired immune system effects as well as difficulty sleeping. DEPRESSION and anxiety may also be present and sometimes lead to chronic states. Researchers have found that people who have strong spiritual or philosophical beliefs seem to resolve their grief more rapidly and completely than those who have no such belief systems.

It is important to note that grief is different from depression. With grief, there is a longing in some way for the lost person, as well as memories and experiences that come to mind and frequent thinking about that person. Grief is a normal response. Depression, on the other hand, involves prolonged lethargy, fatigue, and emotional distress for reasons other than the death. Depression is usually related to oneself.

The traumatic aspects of grief often arise from the sudden shock of a loss and feelings of personal responsibility as well as blaming others. There is also often grief for the loss of safety and security that the deceased person had provided. There may also be issues of attachment and dependency. Psychological interventions are necessary for long-term difficulties that are related to traumatic or complicated grief. These interventions include COG-NITIVE BEHAVIORAL THERAPIES that help the person think about and understand the impact of the loss on their lives and help him or her make behavior changes, while gradually rebuilding self-confidence. Therapeutic interventions are long lasting.

See also BEREAVEMENT; THERAPY, TYPES OF; TRAUMATIC GRIEF.

Gross Human Rights Violation (GHRV) See TORTURE.

gross stress reaction The historical term to describe POSTTRAUMATIC STRESS DISORDER (PTSD) and ACUTE STRESS DISORDER following World War I, when young men returned home from trench warfare suffering deep trauma from their experiences in combat. The descriptive syndrome at the time was called SHELL SHOCK or combat fatigue. By World War II, a formal diagnostic category called gross stress reaction was created. It was a time that brought together psychiatrists and medical professionals to talk about the common vocabulary and to discuss the diagnoses observed in soldiers at war's end.

The American Psychiatric Association created its first manual, *DIAGNOSTIC AND STATISTICAL MANUAL of Mental Disorder-I (DSM-I)*, in 1952; it covered victims of stress by the diagnosis of gross stress reaction. When *DSM-II* was published in 1968, at a time when the United States was not engaged in a major war, gross stress reaction was not included as a diagnosis. It was not until 1980, when *DSM-III* was published following the Vietnam War, that PTSD was introduced as the new term for gross stress reaction. By the time *DSM-IV-TR* was published in 2000, acute PTSD was categorized as acute stress disorder.

group stress debriefing Interventions with groups of people following major traumatic events, such as natural disasters, wars, terrorist attacks, MOTOR VEHICLE ACCIDENTS, fires, assaults, or witnessing tragic deaths. Stress debriefings are also known as psychological debriefings. The purpose of the stress debriefing is to reduce ongoing stress reactions by promoting emotional processing through ventilation or expression of emotions and the normalization of reactions within one to 10 days after the event.

One of the most widely used group stress debriefing models is Jeffrey Mitchell's CRITICAL INCIDENT STRESS DEBRIEFING (CISD), a seven-step group discussion model in which survivors share their experiences with others for the purpose of minimizing the adverse psychological effects after a traumatic event.

The seven steps or phases of a group stress debriefing are:

1. introduction: The facilitator and participant group members introduce themselves, define expectations (this is not psychotherapy) and address confidentiality.
2. fact phase: Participants describe what happened and what role they may have played in the incident.
3. thought phase: exploring cognitive processing by asking, "What were your first thoughts?"
4. reaction phase: The facilitator may ask, "What was the worst part for you?" to allow emotions to be expressed by all.
5. symptom phase: Participants are asked to identify symptoms or distressing emotions as a result of their experience. Questions the facilitator may ask include "How are you different now because of the traumatic event?" or "What has life been like since the incident?"
6. teaching phase: normalizing the reactions and giving the participants helpful tips (stress management tools) to their recovery
7. reentry phase: summarizing the group process and finding closure for the group by answering questions and facilitating follow-up needs for participants who may need it (further mental health services)

Mitchell's CRITICAL INCIDENT STRESS MANAGEMENT (CISM) model is a comprehensive integrative multi-component crisis intervention system that includes the need for follow-up and psychological service to ensure the health of an organization's personnel. CISM consists of the following seven core components:

1. pre-crisis preparation. Just as police and fire departments prepare for dangerous situations, psychological preparedness education should occur, according to Jeffrey Mitchell, to help workers prepare for traumatic events and recognize the symptoms and distress that accompany such crises. Stress management education and crisis-mitigation training should be provided to businesses and community organizations.
2. large scale incident or disaster: demobilization for first responders to a disaster by providing food and rest as well as information on stress management when their shift is over. Community support programs and crisis management briefings or town meetings should be provided to the civilian population.
3. DEFUSING. This is a small group discussion provided within hours of the incident or disaster designed to reduce psychological distress, mitigate acute symptoms, assess, and triage for later CISD groups.
4. Critical Incident Stress Debriefing.
5. individual crisis intervention. This is the most frequently used CISM intervention, consisting of the individual's receiving one to three contacts lasting from 15 minutes to several hours. The individual is allowed to express emotions and be reassured that his or her reactions are normal in an abnormal situation.
6. family/organizational crisis intervention. This is a debriefing given to families, community organizations, or business units that follows the CISD model.
7. follow-up and referral. Individuals are assessed for further treatment that is psychological, medical, or spiritual in nature.

There are other well-known group stress debriefing models, including MULTIPLE STRESSOR DEBRIEFING MODEL (MSDM) and National Organization of Victim Assistance (NOVA).

MSDM addressed the needs of the American Red Cross when engaging in relief operations that extended over a great period of time during the 1989 San Francisco earthquake. First-responder rescue workers faced long hours, multiple contacts with victims, the fear of continuing aftershocks, living away from home, and dealing with the dif-

ficult political climate and negative publicity of the Red Cross. MSD model was developed to help the rescue personnel transition to the home environment after their lengthy deployment in the disaster zone. The four-phase multiple stressor debriefing model was developed by Armstrong, O'Callahan, and Marmar in 1991. It includes:

1. disclosure of events. The initial contact allows participants to talk about distressing events during their work and allows the workers a break from their jobs to reflect on positive and negative aspects of their work.
2. feelings and reaction phase. The group participants are encouraged to talk about their feelings and thoughts about the distressing events. The facilitator helps normalize these stressful experiences, and time is set aside to talk about feelings associated with positive events.
3. coping strategy phase. The facilitator educates the participants about the stress response syndrome, identifying stress-coping strategies used by the group such as self-care through good nutrition, staying in touch with family and friends, and being supportive and connected to their coworkers.
4. Termination phase. The participants talk of their transition to home life, saying good-bye to those they have gotten close to and talking about their accomplishments and positive aspects of their recovery work. They are also referred for further mental health services as needed.

NOVA's crisis intervention model evolved from helping victims of crime immediately after the assault and through the criminal justice system. NOVA's crisis intervention team also helps survivors of natural and man-made disasters. NOVA emphasizes the following three phases:

1. safety and security: providing victims with as much information as possible to allow them to feel safe again and shielding them from media questioning
2. ventilation and validation. Advocates help victims and survivors to tell their story, which helps them ventilate emotions and understand their experience. Validation comes to survivors by advocates listening and reassuring them that

their reactions are "not uncommon." They do not use the phrase "normal reactions to abnormal situations."

3. prediction and preparation. Victims and survivors take back control of their lives when they understand what has happened and what will happen. They are provided with information of what to expect physically, emotionally, financially, and legally if dealing with insurance companies when rebuilding their homes.

It is important to point out that group stress debriefings are only the first steps to help victims and survivors recover from such great public tragedies such as the SEPTEMBER 11 terrorist attack.

See also NATURAL DEBRIEFINGS.

Armstrong, K., W. O'Callahan, and C. Marmar. "Debriefing Red Cross Disaster Personnel: The Multiple Stressor Debriefing Model." *The Journal of Traumatic Stress* 4, no. 4 (1991): 581–593.

Gamino, L. A. "Critical Incident Stress Management and Other Crisis Counseling Approaches." In *Living with Grief Coping with Public Tragedy,* edited by M. Lattanzi-Light and K. J. Doka. New York: Brunner-Routledge, 2003.

Mitchell, J. T., and G. S. Everly Jr. *Critical Incident Stress Debriefing (CSID): An operations manual for CISD, defusing and other group crisis intervention services.* 3rd ed. Elliot City, Md.: Chevron Publishing Corporation, 2001.

guilt   An unpleasant feeling associated with feelings of wrongdoing from the past. Conscious and unconscious guilt may undermine relationships and control behaviors. Following a traumatic event or loss, thoughts of the experience may be faulty as individuals assess the outcome, as if their action or lack of action had somehow resulted in the pain and suffering of others. Unresolved guilt may lead to self-condemnation, DEPRESSION, suicidal feelings, and substance abuse. It can also keep a person "stuck" in his or her suffering and can prevent recovery.

On the other hand, guilt is also a motivation for change: a person can make adjustments to allay "feeling guilty" and make changes in his or her life that put the guilt to rest. For those who are responsible for others, it may be difficult to put the guilt to rest, as in the case of a parent, a leader, or persons of authority, such as police officers. These groups are vulnerable to feeling a sense of failure to protect those around them.

SURVIVOR GUILT occurs when the person survived the traumatic event while others were injured or killed. This form of guilt may come from a feeling that the individual who survived was unable to rescue someone or had to leave someone behind in a disaster. One way in which survivors have dealt with their guilt is by visiting the relatives of the deceased to offer information about their lost or missing loved ones. Any positive approaches to helping others, including rescue work, have helped individuals to process their guilt toward healing the self.

See also THERAPY, TYPES OF.

Hamilton Anxiety Scale (HAS) Developed in 1959 by Max Hamilton, the Hamilton Anxiety Scale (HAS) is a 14-item clinical interview test that measures the severity of anxiety symptoms in adults and children who were previously diagnosed with anxiety. The HAS was not designed to discriminate between anxiety and DEPRESSION or to diagnose anxiety but rather was designed to measure the clinical status of patients diagnosed with neurotic anxiety states. HAS is also used in assessing the impact of ANTIANXIETY MEDICATIONS so that the dosage of the medication can be adjusted based on the patient's test results.

During the test, an interviewer rates the responses to the 14 semi-structured questions on a five-point scale. The interviewer has little subjective value when interpreting and scoring the test. The 14 items address areas of psychic anxiety (psychological distress) and somatic anxiety (physical complaints). The 14 items are:

1. anxious moods
2. tension and nervousness
3. fear
4. insomnia
5. difficulty in concentration and memory
6. depressed mood
7. somatic complaints—muscular
8. somatic complaints—sensory
9. cardiovascular symptoms
10. respiratory symptoms
11. gastrointestinal symptoms
12. genitourinary symptoms
13. autonomic symptoms
14. behavior at time of interview

There is a concern that the HAS confounds symptoms of anxiety and depression, and its value as a severity-measuring instrument is often debated. Originally, the Hamilton Anxiety Scale included depression items, its proponents arguing that anxiety produces depressive symptoms and that a measure of the severity of anxiety would be helpful in making a diagnosis.

One reason for the popularity of the Hamilton Anxiety Scale is its reliability in measuring anxiety symptoms in a consistent way. The high measure of validity for HAS is supported in research by Shear et al. (2001), who made the finding as they developed a structured interview guide for the HAS (SIGH-A). They employed specific instructions for administration and scoring, since the original HAS had no reliability aids. The study provided confirmation of the convergent validity of the two forms of the instruments.

See also ANXIETY DISORDERS; ASSESSMENT AND DIAGNOSIS.

Shear, K., et al. "Reliability and Validity of a Structured Interview Guide for the Hamilton Anxiety Rating Scale (SIGH-A)." *Depression and Anxiety* 13 (2001): 166–178.

Harvard Trauma Questionnaire (HTQ) See ASSESSMENT AND DIAGNOSIS.

heart rate/response (HR)/(HRR) See HEART RATE VARIABILITY.

heart rate variability (HRV) A measure that is derived from the beat-to-beat variations or changes of the heart rate. Parasympathetic (e.g., calming) activity or activation produces a slowing of the heart rate or a wider beat-to-beat interval. On the other hand, sympathetic activation (e.g., activation or arousal) produces an increase in heart rate and a narrowing or decrease in the beat-to-beat interval.

The AUTONOMIC NERVOUS SYSTEM (ANS) controls many of the body's functions, including heart rate, movement, activation, the immune and hormonal systems, and gastrointestinal activities, and it also interacts with mental and emotional states. The autonomic nervous system is comprised of two separate and relatively independent systems, including the SYMPATHETIC NERVOUS SYSTEM (SNS), which regulates arousal activities, and the parasympathetic nervous system (PNS), which regulates calming and digestion. Until recently, it has been difficult to study the parasympathetic system because there were no direct physiological indices such as there are in the sympathetic system (heart rate, galvanic skin response, etc). Heart rate variability now provides a means to study the PNS and the relationship between PNS and SNS activity.

Heart rhythms change with thoughts, emotional changes, and physical activities. These changes also affect the brain's decision-making ability, problem solving, and creativity. This makes the study of HRV a powerful tool for understanding the dynamics of a person's mental, emotional, and physical functioning. Essentially, it can be a biofeedback tool for (1) measuring arousal activity or (2) a feedback tool for assisting relaxation training.

See also POWER SPECTRAL DENSITY.

hierarchy of fears   A method to resolve anxiety symptoms that is also known as the anxiety hierarchy. Psychiatrist Joseph Wolpe developed SYSTEMATIC DESENSITIZATION (SD) in the late 1950s to inhibit anxiety symptoms. He found that anxiety symptoms were reduced when stimuli to the anxiety were presented in a hierarchical order and systematically paired with a relaxation response. Research has shown that systematic desensitization can be effective with any phobia when a client and therapist use the three steps to SD: (1) learning a relaxation skill, (2) constructing a hierarchy of fears, and (3) pairing the relaxation response with the situations in the hierarchy of fears.

An example of constructing a hierarchy of fears uses the situation "fear of flying." The hierarchy contains scenes relating to making a plane flight,

both in real and imagined situations. An imagined situation might be a flight that is ready for departure, doors closed, when the captain delays the flight because the FBI is coming aboard to remove suspected terrorists from the plane. The validity of this scene is that it would produce varying degrees of anxiety. Once the scenes are described it is important to provide sufficient details of each situation to fully imagine the scene during recall.

An individual may begin the hierarchy by writing down 15 to 20 steps involved in preparing for his or her trip. These steps would include making the flight reservations, the trip to the airport, going through the security checkpoints, checking in, boarding the flight, interactions with flight attendants, takeoff, turbulence, landing, and exiting the aircraft. Since it is important to get a graded fear hierarchy, a progression is necessary, and the best way to grade each step is to assign a number from 1 to 100 to each situation (where 100 represents the highest anxiety and 0 represents no anxiety). Because the list must be graded from low anxiety to high anxiety, there must be at least two situations each from 1–20, 21–40, 41–60, 61–80, and 81–100 to have a progressive hierarchy for the fear of flying.

The following is an example of the Fear of Flying hierarchy and the level of anxiety (parentheses):

1. calling the airlines for tickets (5)
2. packing for the trip (10)
3. the night before the flight, praying for a safe trip (65)
4. taking the trip to the airport by shuttle van (25)
5. making the decision to make a flight (35)
6. walking into the airport and trying to locate the airline counter (45)
7. standing in a long line and waiting for a long time until a counter opens up (50)
8. going through the security checkpoints and seeing the alarms go off with other passengers (55)
9. boarding the plane, finding a seat near the window, and adjusting the air vents (60)
10. listening to the flight attendants go through the safety checklist (67)
11. The plane is ready to depart the gate when the captain comes over the speakers to let the passengers know that a security breach is in

progress in the airport, and the FBI will be boarding the plane to investigate before clearing it for takeoff. (This is the imagined scene that almost never actually occurs, but which is still feared.) (75)

12. lifting off and the feeling of gravity holding you back in your seat (85)

13. The captain comes on the intercom and says that there will be a brief period of turbulence soon. (95)

14. encountering turbulence, with everyone in their seats (100)

Once the hierarchy of fears list is complete, the systematic desensitization process begins with the individual confronting each situation and pairing it with a state of deep relaxation, which is learned through progressive relaxation training.

See also PROGRESSIVE RELAXATION; THERAPY, TYPES OF.

hippocampus   A sausage-like structure of the BRAIN that lies beneath the cortex in the area known as the LIMBIC region, and which is important in MEMORY, learning, and navigation. The role that the hippocampus plays in long-term memory and learning formation is complex.

The role of the hippocampus is more complex than simple storage of new facts and lists. It is described as placing an individual in the context of both space and time. It tells individuals where they are and what is happening in relation to both the future and the past, relating present information to other memories and experiences already collected. Thus, the hippocampus plays an integrative role. This may be the reason that damage to the hippocampus, or conversely, the electrical stimulation from the hippocampus, is associated with increases in symptoms of DISSOCIATION.

A breakdown in the function of the hippocampus leads to disintegration of the sense of self and a loss of the context of memories, with associated gaps. In the most extreme case of dissociation, which is dissociative identity disorder, there is a breakdown of the individual's sense of identity in the sense that patients will attribute different identities or personality states to their selves, memories, and experiences. Each personality may experience a distinct history, self-image, and identity. Consistent with the idea that hippocampal damage as a result of STRESS contributes to these disabling systems is the finding that, in traumatized patients, the greatest decrease in the volume of the hippocampus is associated with the most profound symptoms of dissociation.

Some imaging studies of individuals with POST-TRAUMATIC STRESS DISORDER (PTSD) have found atrophy in the hippocampus and a 25 percent decrease in the volume on one side of the hippocampus. Although there is extensive debate as to the cause of this atrophy, one possibility might involve a class of steroid hormones called GLUCO-CORTICOIDS. During physical or psychological stress, the adrenal glands secrete large amounts of glucocorticoids. The hippocampus has many receptors for glucocorticoids, thus, it is the part of the brain that is the most sensitive to hormones.

Laboratory experiments have demonstrated that elevated glucocorticoid levels over a few days can endanger a hippocampal neuron, making it less likely to survive a seizure. Elevated levels over weeks or months can cause glucocorticoids to shrivel the branch-like connections between hippocampus neurons. Once stress or glucocorticoid exposure ends, the branches slowly grow back. When glucocorticoid levels are high enough for months or years, they can destroy hippocampal neurons.

Experts believe that only 15 to 30 percent of soldiers returning from combat develop PTSD, and it may be true that these individuals had a smaller hippocampal size before their exposure to trauma. Also, as a result of this smaller hippocampal size, they may be more susceptible to PTSD. Soldiers with PTSD have a higher than average rate of soft neurological signs or red flags, such as delayed developmental landmarks or a higher than average rate of learning disorders.

While memories are formed continuously, there is a process called consolidation that allows memories to be strengthened over a period of weeks and months, and then stored permanently in the cerebral cortex. This window of consolidation presents a limited time span during which TRAUMATIC MEMORIES can be altered before they become permanently engraved in the mind. If they are not consolidated, then isolated images, bodily sensations, and sounds can be stored separately from other life experiences and the individual will feel alienated. Hippocampal dysfunction may also play a role in dissociative symptoms when an individual is exposed to traumatic stress.

See also AUTONOMIC NERVOUS SYSTEM; CENTRAL NERVOUS SYSTEM; SYMPATHETIC NERVOUS SYSTEM.

van der Kolk, Bessel A., Alexander McFarlane, and Lars Weisaeth, eds. *Traumatic Stress.* New York: Guilford Press, 1996.

historical factors The phrase POSTTRAUMATIC STRESS DISORDER (PTSD) is relatively new in the understanding of traumatic stress disorders, but many physicians and mental health professionals have known about key underlying concepts of PTSD since at least the Civil War era. Some of these conditions or syndromes are identified with the experiences of soldiers in wartime, such as Da Costa Syndrome/Disease, or combat stress syndrome, while other concepts, such as STOCKHOLM SYNDROME or BETRAYAL TRAUMA THEORY are tied to particular and unique types of civilian trauma. The names and phrases describing traumatic stress disorders have changed over time and as knowledge has been updated and improved, but the history behind these conditions is instructive for a better overall understanding of trauma disorders.

Military Trauma Syndromes throughout History

Doctors in the Civil War were aware of the effects of combat stress, although they perceived the problem through the lens of their knowledge at the time. For example, internist Jacob Mendez Da Costa wrote in an 1871 issue of *American Journal of Military Sciences* about a soldier who was extremely anxious before a Civil War battle. Da Costa described the soldier's symptoms of sharp pains, palpitations, and difficulty moving about following the battle.

Dr. Da Costa concluded that this syndrome was caused by a nerve irritability or by damage to the sympathetic nerves to the heart, hence his name for the problem, *irritable heart syndrome*. It was also referred to as *soldier's heart*. SEE TABLE BELOW for

SOMATIC SYMPTOMS COMMONLY ASSOCIATED WITH WAR-RELATED MEDICAL AND PSYCHOLOGICAL ILLNESSES

Symptoms	U.S. Civil War, Da Costa Syndrome	World War I, Effort Syndrome	World War II, Combat Stress Reaction	Vietnam, Agent Orange Exposure	Vietnam and Other Conflicts, Posttraumatic Stress Disorder	Persian Gulf, Unexplained Illnesses
Fatigue or exhaustion	+	+	+	+	+	+
Shortness of breath	+	+	+		+	+
Palpitations and tachycardia	+	+	+		+	+
Headache	+	+	+	+	+	+
Muscle or joint pain			+	+	+	
Diarrhea	+		+	+	+	
Excessive sweating	+	+				
Dizziness	+	+		+	+	
Fainting	+	+				
Disturbed sleep	+	+		+	+	+
Forgetfulness	+	+		+	+	+
Difficulty concentrating		+		+	+	+

+ sign indicates a commonly reported symptom
Adapted from Hyams, Kenneth C., M.D., F. Stephen Wignall, M.D., and Robert Roswell, M.D. "War Syndromes and Their Evaluation: From the U.S. Civil War to the Persian Gulf War." *Annals of Internal Medicine* 125, no. 5 (September 1, 1996).

symptoms and other names given to the same or similar conditions, such as COMBAT STRESS REACTION and effort syndrome. As the chart shows, whether the disorder was called PTSD (as during the Vietnam War and today), Da Costa syndrome, effort syndrome, or combat stress syndrome reaction, in all cases fatigue and exhaustion were symptoms, as were headaches. In most cases, other symptoms included shortness of breath, heart palpitations and rapid heart beat (tachycardia), disturbed sleep, forgetfulness, and difficulty concentrating.

World Wars I and II   During World War I, soldiers exhibiting behavior similar to that described by Da Costa were said to have Da Costa syndrome. However, in World War I, the British Army used the term SHELL SHOCK or combat fatigue to describe individuals who were traumatized by their combat experience. At that time, experts believed that being hit with artillery shells resulted in tiny hemorrhages of the brain, causing a variety of both physical ailments and psychiatric symptoms.

It was thought that the percussive waves from the explosive shells and bullets produced actual physical damage to the hearing, the brain, and the spinal column, resulting in hysteria-like symptoms (e.g., loss of function), such as blindness, AMNESIA, hearing loss, muteness, paralysis, and seizures. It was later discovered that soldiers did not have to be around exploding shells to exhibit this same type of behavior, and it was also learned that the true underlying problem was that the soldiers were responding to the severe psychological stress of warfare. Based on this new understanding, the term *shell shock* was later replaced by *war neurosis* and then was called battle fatigue.

In World War II, *convoy fatigue* was a term used for a particular combat stress reaction. At that time, the United States was using about 6,000 ships manned by merchant marines for trade. This fleet was commissioned by President Roosevelt as part of the country's economic recovery program. However, these ships were defenseless against predators and enemies, and they were often sunk or boarded. The merchant marines on board were demoralized, and they were said to experience convoy fatigue.

After the end of World War II, the Veterans Administration developed its own diagnostic manual to describe the symptoms and syndromes observed in soldiers during wartime. This led the American Psychological Association to create its own manual, *DIAGNOSTIC AND STATISTICAL MANUAL of Mental Disorders* (*DSM-I*), that covered victims of stress under the term GROSS STRESS REACTION.

Concentration camp syndrome, or KZ SYNDROMET, the German name for a concentration camp syndrome, described a phenomenon that was exclusive to World War II. It was a trauma syndrome related to wartime, although not all concentration camp members were soldiers or sailors. The earliest publications describing and labeling this particular syndrome were by Danish psychiatrists Herman and Thygesen in 1954. The *KZ* is an abbreviation of *Konzenstrationlager,* or concentration camp. The authors started a comprehensive evaluation of former prisoners in a concentration camp, and they found that 75 percent of all expatriated prisoners suffered from "neurotic" symptoms. Both brutal treatments and undernourishment contributed substantially to long-term dullness, intellectual impairment, apathy/depression, memory loss, emotional irritability, and instability, as well as a loss of a sense of the future.

Freudian Views on Trauma   Austrian psychiatrist Sigmund Freud dominated the views on causes of trauma in the late 19th century, and some argue that his views proliferated in the United States until the end of the Vietnam War in 1974. According to Wilson in his analysis of Freud's views in the *Journal of Traumatic Stress,* Freud initially postulated that traumatic experiences in childhood could cause extreme distress such that the individual regressed into an earlier stage of development. Neurotic behaviors and symptoms would then ensue. Freud's views later shifted, however, and he came to believe that fantasy and imagery were more dominant in their effects than actual child abuse. However, Freud clearly understood the nature of trauma. In his *Introductory Lectures on Psychoanalysis,* published in 1917, Freud said:

"The closest analogy to this behavior of our neurotics is afforded by illnesses which are being produced with special frequency precisely at the present time by the war—what are described as traumatic neurosis. Similar cases, of course, appeared before the war as well, after railway collisions and other alarming accidents involving fatal risks. . . . The traumatic neurosis gives a clear indication that a fixation to the traumatic accident lives at their root. These patients regularly repeated the traumatic situation in their dreams; where hysteriform attacks occur that admit of an analysis, we found that the attack corresponds to a complete transplanting of the patient into the traumatic situation. [This is a description of a flashback.] It is as though these patients had not yet finished with the traumatic situation, as though they were still faced by it as an immediate task which has not been dealt with, and we take this view quite seriously."

The Vietnam War Many reluctant individuals were drafted into the military during the Vietnam War, and some served in combat conditions. Similar to their cohorts in earlier wars, some of the soldiers experienced the emotional consequences of the alternate stress and boredom of wartime conditions; this was referred to by some experts as POST-VIETNAM SYNDROME and by others as PTSD. By 1980, PTSD became the official nomenclature of the disorder.

According to experts such as Alan Peterson and colleagues in their 2008 article in *Perspectives in Psychiatric Care,* it is generally believed that 500,000 individuals still suffer from PTSD that originally developed when these individuals served in Vietnam.

According to the National Center for Posttraumatic Stress Disorder, the lifelong prevalence for PTSD among Vietnam combat veterans is 30.9 percent, and nearly half of all male combat veterans as well as half of all female veterans who served in Vietnam have experienced "clinically serious stress reaction symptoms."

Helmus and Glenn say in their monograph *Steeling the Mind: Combat Stress Reactions and Their Implications for Urban Warfare* that the rate of PTSD for those with high levels of war-zone exposure was 35.8 percent of men and 17.5 percent of women who met the criteria when data on the National Vietnam Veterans' Readjustment Study was published in 1990. In contrast, according to the National Center for Posttraumatic Stress Disorder, the estimated lifetime prevalence of PTSD for all adults in the United States is 6.8 percent.

The National Vietnam Veterans Readjustment Survey (NVVRS), which was conducted from 1986 to 1988, found that almost half of all Vietnam combat veterans with PTSD had been arrested or were in jail at least once, and more than a third (34.2 percent) were arrested or in jail more than once. In addition, 11.5 percent had been convicted of a felony.

Researchers Schnurr, Lunney, and Sengupta (2004) reanalyzed the data from the NVVRS and found that several key risk factors for the development of PTSD among Vietnam combat veterans were family instability, severe punishment during childhood, and depression. Military risk factors for PTSD were war zone exposure, PERITRAUMATIC DISSOCIATION (immediate dissociation at the time of the traumatic event), and depression. Some risk factors for PTSD maintenance (continuation) were serious injury during the Vietnam war, war-zone exposure, and peritraumatic exposure, as well as recent stressful life events in the individual's post-military life.

The researchers found that social support was a protective factor against the development of PTSD. Social support for veterans was not common during the Vietnam War, when many people opposed to the war often blamed the soldiers, most of whom were drafted, and ridiculed and scorned them when they returned home. Other protective factors against the development of PTSD included a high school or college education, an older age upon the entry to war, a higher socioeconomic status, and a positive paternal relationship. Social support upon coming home and continued social support were also protective factors against the development of PTSD.

Afghanistan, Iraq, and Beyond Although all those who join the military now are volunteers, it is inevitable that some will become distressed and dismayed by the experience of combat, and some will develop PTSD. It is believed that at least 20 percent of soldiers and airmen returning from combat in Afghanistan or Iraq suffer from mental health symptoms immediately, and more than 40 percent of returning National Guard and Reservists who served in Iraq suffer from mental health symptoms as of this writing, according to Peterson and colleagues in their 2008 article for *Perspectives in Psychiatric Care.* It is unknown how many individuals specifically suffer from PTSD, but it is believed to be a substantial portion of the estimated 2 million individuals who were deployed to military combat in Afghanistan or Iraq.

Efforts are being made for service members returning from deployment to receive information on what to expect when returning from a war zone and to help them reintegrate successfully to home life. There are hotlines and family support information through toll-free telephone numbers for both the serviceman and his or her family describing the effects of war zone stress and PTSD.

Civilian Trauma throughout History

Of course, soldiers under combat conditions were not and are not the only individuals to react to severe trauma. BRIQUET'S SYNDROME, named after French physician Paul Briquet, who wrote about hysteria in 1859, is an example of a traumatic stress disorder. Briquet's syndrome was believed to be most common among chronically ill women who may have had multiple surgeries. These individuals also had a higher rate of having suffered past CHILD PHYSICAL ABUSE and CHILD SEXUAL ABUSE than those without the disorder. Today, Briquet's syndrome is known as SOMATIZATION DISORDER in the *Diagnostic and Statistical Manual of Mental Disorders, Fourth Edition, Text Revision (DSM-IV-TR)*.

Women with Briquet's syndrome (or somatization disorder) often had additional psychiatric problems, such as DEPRESSION and ANXIETY DISORDERS. Men with Briquet's syndrome were more likely than women to have antisocial personality disorder and to engage in excessive drinking and the commission of criminal acts. Briquet's syndrome was very difficult to treat because individuals with this syndrome were usually completely convinced that they were truly, physically ill and that physicians, for unknown reasons, had not yet found the true cause of their illness. Sometimes treating secondary disorders such as depression seemed to improve the primary disorder of Briquet's syndrome.

Another trauma diagnosis identified in the 19th century was DEMENTIA PRAECOX, which was first described in 1896 by Emil Kraepelin, a German physician. Many of the symptoms Kraepelin included in dementia praecox were later redefined by Bleuler as schizophrenia.

GANSER SYNDROME is another disorder stemming from trauma, identified in 1898 by German psychiatrist Sigbert J. Ganser to describe prisoners who sought to avoid prosecution. The *Diagnostic and Statistical Manual (DSM)* currently categorizes Ganser syndrome as a dissociative disorder, not otherwise specified. Ganser syndrome is a pseudodementia often associated with prison conditions and environments of torture, and many experts also consider it to be a form of malingering (faking illness). However, some experts believe that a TRAUMATIC BRAIN INJURY could lead to the symptoms of Ganser syndrome, while others believe organic dementia may cause the symptoms. The syndrome may occur subsequent to a stressful or traumatic experience, such as problems in the sexual, domestic, or financial areas of life. It is believed to occur as a result of an event that is intolerable to the individual. Symptoms may include hysterical seizures, paralysis, visual and olfactory hallucinations, a disorientation of time and place, and amnesia. One unique symptom is that, when questioned, individuals with Ganser syndrome can give only approximate answers to questions with clear right and wrong answers; for example, if the person is shown a glove and asked what the item is, he or she may state that it is a hand. The answer is wrong but it approximates the correct answer. Ganser syndrome is difficult to treat, and generally only accompanying psychiatric disorders such as depression can be treated. However, experts report that often the syndrome resolves on its own.

Another traumatic syndrome discovered in the nineteeth century was *SCHRECKNEUROSE* (fright neuroses). Emile Kraeplin wrote that this syndrome consisted of multiple nervous and psychic phenomena that arose from severe emotional upheaval or a sudden fright, such as experienced through serious accidents and injuries, particularly fires, railroad derailments, or collisions. It is known today that startle responses and exaggerated reactivity are characteristic of people prone to develop posttraumatic stress disorder.

Stockholm syndrome is a concept that was introduced in the 1970s after the seemingly inexplicable behavior of four bank employees who were taken hostage by an escaped convict in Stockholm, Sweden, in 1973. The captives were held in the bank vault for five days. After the hostages were released, they reported no ill feelings toward the convict and his accomplice who arrived later, and instead said that they were more afraid of the police than the convicts. This behavior, which startled many people, was subsequently named Stockholm syndrome.

Many people have used the case of heiress Patti Hearst as another example of Stockholm syndrome. Hearst was kidnapped in 1974 by the Symbionese Liberation Army (S.L.A.), a guerilla warfare group that considered itself a revolutionary army. This group committed bank robberies, two murders, and other acts of violence between 1973 and 1975, and Hearst assisted the group in some of their illegal activities. However, she later alleged that she had been held in close confinement and was sexually assaulted and brainwashed. The underlying assumption is that she was not fully in control of her acts, although some authorities have disputed this.

Treatment for Stockholm syndrome involves reversing the conditions that led to the victim's identification with his or her captors. According to a 1999 article in the *FBI Law Enforcement Bulletin*, Stockholm syndrome is much less common than believed, and most hostages are unsympathetic to their captors.

Behavior similar to that of Stockholm syndrome can be seen among children who have been victimized by CHILD ABUSE AND NEGLECT at the hands of their parents. Despite sometimes horrific abuse, children usually strongly resist being removed from their parents, even when their own safety will clearly be at risk if they remain.

Battered women often return to their abuser, and if, for example, they are told by a judge that they must leave the abuser or they will lose custody of their children, they will often remain with the abuser anyway. Members of cult groups may react in a similar slavishly devoted way, as may incest victims. The common denominators among all these groups appear to be several key factors, including a fear that the abuser will harm them; the presence of small acts of kindness by the abuser to the victim; physical isolation of the victim from other people and perspectives than that of the

abuser, and the inability or the belief of an inability to escape the situation.

A more recent concept of trauma DENY, ATTACK, AND REVERSE VICTIM AND OFFENDER (DARVO), was introduced by Jennifer Freyd in 1997. Freyd's concept was that perpetrators, especially those guilty of sexual offenses, often deny the behavior and attack the person who has accused them. The perpetrator attempts a role reversal, claiming that it is he or she who is really the victimized person.

Another concept described by Freyd was betrayal trauma theory (BTT), which refers to trauma induced at least in part by the abuse of trust. In essence, the theory describes the situation of children who trust their caregivers (usually their parents), who then subsequently betray the child's trust with sexual, physical, or emotional abuse. Because such a betrayal is so psychologically painful, the victimized child represses the memories of the abuse and develops amnesia of the incident(s), which may be remembered at a later time.

According to Freyd's betrayal trauma theory, children abused by their caretakers are more likely to experience amnesia following child sexual abuse than are children abused by noncaretakers. Children abused by their caregivers face a senseless situation, as the perpetrator is the same person whom they rely on for food and shelter and ultimately survival. BTT maintains that to resolve this conflict, children continue to bond with the perpetrator and to block memories of sexual abuse.

Freyd says that children abused by a parent or other close caregiver may react with adaptive blindness or PSYCHIC NUMBING. They are attached to the individual providing them with care, and if they accused that individual of sexual abuse, then the care would end and the children would feel physically and mentally threatened. Thus, the memory of the abuse is blocked, and the relationship continues. Unfortunately, the abuse often continues as well.

New understandings of trauma continue to develop. In the 21st century, the SEPTEMBER 11, 2001, terrorist attack traumatized many people. At 8:45 A.M., the first hijacked airliner crashed into the north tower of the World Trade Center building in New York City. Eighteen minutes later, a second airliner crashed into the south tower. Both towers collapsed after burning for less than 90 minutes as news cameras captured this horrific TRAUMATIC EVENT in real time. Millions of horrified viewers around the world watched this on television.

As part of the coordinated attack on the United States, at 9:37 A.M., a third hijacked airliner was crashed into the U.S. Department of Defense Pentagon in Arlington County, Virginia. At 10:03, a fourth airliner crashed into a field in Somerset County, Pennsylvania, 80 miles southeast of Pittsburgh, when the passengers resisted the hijackers. The hijackers' original target was believed to be either the U.S. Capitol or the White House in Washington, D.C.

At the World Trade Center, more than 2,900 people died in the attack, 125 died at the Pentagon, and 256 died on the four airliners. In the aftermath of the attack, the United States declared a war on terrorism and also resolved to bring Osama bin Laden and Islamic Al Qaeda to justice, with the invasion of Afghanistan by U.S.-led coalition forces in October 2001.

The attacks on the World Trade Center frightened and traumatized many people in the United States. While terrorism occurs in every country in the world to some extent, the suddenness of the attacks, the scope of the damage, the loss of life, and the fact that this event represented a concerted assault by a terrorist organization against the Untied States made the aftermath even more frightening. The United States responded with the creation of the government agency called Homeland Security, laws that restrict the rights of individuals, an attack on Afghanistan, and use of dogs and heightened security in airports. These things have become examples of new symbols of anticipated danger arising out of insecurity and recognition of the lack of safety in the world.

Treatment of Trauma through History

Treatments for severe reactions to trauma have evolved over the last century and a half. For example, soldiers diagnosed with Da Costa's syndrome (also known as soldier's heart) during the Civil War were treated with drugs such as digitalis, since the problem was often perceived as heart-related. During World War I, when soldiers exhibited symptoms of shell shock (such as shortness of breath, heart palpitations, headaches, diarrhea, and for-

getfulness) they were given supportive treatment rather than drugs.

Soldiers with battle fatigue or combat exhaustion in World War II and the Korean War were also treated with psychological support rather than medication. In addition, during World Wars I and II, it was considered very important to return the traumatized soldier to the battlefield as soon as possible. In World War I, the proximity, immediacy, expectancy, simplicity (PIES) method was considered the most desirable tactic—the principles of proximity to battle, immediacy of treatment, expectation of a full recovery, and simplicity of treatment. Thus, soldiers with shell shock were treated close to the front lines as soon as possible with food, sleep, and exercise for two to six weeks (the simplicity of treatment) and were assured that they would recover.

According to Moore and Reger in their discussion of the historical and contemporary perspectives of combat stress, during World War I the U.S. Army provided several echelons of care for traumatized soldiers. "The first-echelon of care consisted of a psychiatrist positioned within the division. The job of the psychiatrist was to screen for those susceptible to combat stress, consult with command on the prevention of combat stress casualties, triage cases just behind the front so that soldiers with simple exhaustion were rested by their units, and personally treat more symptomatic cases while supervising medical personnel in the division rear."

The second echelon of care included a psychiatrist and other mental health professionals who provided "neurological hospitals" in old buildings in France to specifically treat individuals who could not return to duty right away. Most soldiers were able to return to duty after one to three weeks. The third echelon of care was a rear hospital that provided care for weeks or months, as needed. Some of these soldiers returned to combat but fewer than with the first and second echelons.

Combat stress teams were also used in subsequent wars. The Army created the Division Mental Health Section during the Korean War. At this time, mobile psychiatric detachments were also formed and have continued to exist to the present. Treatment today is often umbrellaed under the doctrine of brevity, immediacy, centrality, expectancy, proximity, and simplicity, or BICEPS (similar to PIES). Brevity refers to treatment that is as brief as needed, while immediacy refers to intervention in the early stages of a problem. Centrality refers to providing a central place to care for the soldier so he or she maintains his or her warrior identity. Expectancy means that the solider is expected to get better. Proximity refers to treating the soldier as close to his or her unit as possible. Simplicity refers to the level of complexity of the problem; for example, many soldiers will improve with rest, food, water, and restored confidence.

Before the Vietnam War, it was assumed that most soldiers would recover, unless they had some inherent psychological defect or earlier life trauma. The delayed stress of some soldiers in the Vietnam War, however, showed that stress from wartime conditions could cause chronic long-term problems.

In the military environment in the 21st century in Iraq, military members in combat environments who may be at risk for combat stress are informally assessed by mental health specialists, according to Moore and Reger. As with past wars, sometimes a key problem is simple sleep deprivation, which is readily treated. For example, they described two mental health specialists in a preventive team who traveled throughout units and talked to the soldiers.

In one case, a soldier said that she had witnessed the death of someone in her unit a month previously when she was driving a five-ton truck that rolled over. She was not sleeping well and had significantly less confidence. The team emphasized her strengths to her and offered her advice on how to get more restful sleep. They also offered her further assistance if she needed it. After following their suggestions, she reported feeling better. Of course, in other cases, more intensive treatment may be required. Antidepressants and therapy may be important components of treatment for the traumatized soldier, although each case is assessed differently.

Carver, Joseph M. "Love and Stockholm Syndrome: The Mystery of Loving an Abuser." Available online at http://www.mental-health-matters.com/articles/article.php?artID=469. Accessed August 12, 2008.

Fuselier, G. Dwayne. "Placing the Stockholm Syndrome in Perspective." *FBI Law Enforcement Bulletin* (July 1999). Available at URL: http://www.au.af.mil/au/awc/awcgate/fbi/stockholm_syndrome.pdf. Downloaded March 19, 2007.

Helmus, Todd C., and Russell W. Glenn. *Steeling the Mind: Combat Stress Reactions and Their Implications for Urban Warfare.* Santa Monica, Calif.: RAND Corporation, 2005.

Jones, Edgar, and Simon Wessely. "Psychological Trauma: A Historical Perspective." *Psychiatry* 5, no. 7 (2006): 217–220.

Moore, Bret A., and Greg M. Reger. "Historical and Contemporary Perspectives of Combat Stress and the Army Combat Stress Control Team." In *Combat Stress Injury: Theory, Research, and Management*, edited by Charles R. Figley and William P. Nash, 161–181. New York: Routledge, 2006.

Peterson, Alan L., Monty T. Baker, and Kelly R. McCarthy. "Combat Stress Casualties in Iraq: Part 1: Behavioral Health Consultation at an Expeditionary Medical Group." *Perspectives in Psychiatric Care* 44, no. 3 (July 2008): 146–158.

Schnurr, P. O., C. A. Lunney, and A. Sengupta. "Risk Factors for the Development Versus Maintenance of Posttraumatic Stress Disorder." *Journal of Traumatic Stress* 17 (2004): 85–95.

Wilson, John P. "The Historical Evolution of PTSD Diagnostic Criteria: From Freud to DSM-IV." *Journal of Traumatic Stress* 7, no. 4 (1994): 681–698.

hostage identification/response syndrome See STOCKHOLM SYNDROME.

hydrocortisone See CORTISOL.

hyperventilation syndrome A condition brought on by rapid, shallow breathing with attenuated outbreath. Hyperventilation syndrome depletes the blood of carbon dioxide, enabling receptors that normally bond to carbon dioxide to bond with oxygen instead, thus depriving all body organs of oxygen.

Symptoms and Diagnostic Path

Hyperventilation syndrome causes many symptoms, ranging from shortness of breath to dizziness, trembling, sweating, and dry mouth. Hyperventilation itself is the most common cause of dizziness in the general population. It can also produce many symptoms in different systems of the body and in puzzling combinations, as in cardiovascular symptoms (such as a rapid heart rate), neurological symptoms (slurred speech) and respiratory symptoms (chest pain). Hyperventilation syndrome is diagnosed based on the symptoms.

The mechanism by which hyperventilation develops is unknown. Hyperventilation may have organic or physiological causes but it usually is associated with emotional triggers. Studies by Bass (1997) have shown that hyperventilation is not a cause for panic symptoms, and instead, the link between hyperventilation and panic may be cognitive: panic attacks occur when the body/mental sensations accompanying hyperventilation are interpreted as signs of impending catastrophe. However, once hyperventilation begins, stresses from everyday life in combination with new hyperventilation symptoms can create a self-perpetuating cycle of chronic hyperventilation.

Treatment Options and Outlook

Relaxation training is the best approach to treating hyperventilation, specifically breath training. Proper breath training for hyperventilation involves learning to take slow outbreaths. By slowing the outbreath, the body begins to absorb more carbon dioxide into the bloodstream and thereby change the body chemistry from acidic to alkaline. Alkaline biochemistry is associated with relaxed states and activates vagal nerve calming responses.

There are many breathing techniques that can be used to manage hyperventilation syndrome, but the most effective will incorporate slow outbreathing. Diaphragmatic breathing also facilitates long outbreath.

See also BREATHING RETRAINING; PROGRESSIVE RELAXATION.

Bass, C. "Hyperventilation Syndrome: A Chimera?" *Journal of Psychosomatic Research* 42, no. 5 (1997): 421–426.

hypothalamic-pituitary-adrenal (HPA) axis   The connections between the three endocrine glands of the hypothalamus, pituitary, and adrenal glands, leading to the release of hormones or the inhibition of the release of hormones. The HPA axis is the main pathway for the stress system and stress response. STRESS activates two body systems; the AUTONOMIC NERVOUS SYSTEM (ANS) and the HPA axis, which reacts more slowly. When the hypothalamus is activated, it induces the pituitary gland to secrete ADRENOCORTICOTROPHIC HORMONE (ACTH), which in turn stimulates the adrenal cortex to secrete CORTISOL.

According to experts, the outer portion of the adrenals, the adrenal cortex, produces GLUCOCORTICOIDS, which are released during stress and act on all cells of the body. The central portion of the adrenals, the adrenal medulla, secretes the hormones EPINEPHRINE and NOREPINEPHRINE (also called adrenaline and noradrenaline), which act on the internal organs.

It has been reported that lower levels of norepinephrine stimulation in monkeys increase the efficiency of the brain, while higher levels render the brain more inefficient. In addition, animals that are exposed to stressors over a lifetime have shown an exaggerated norepinephrine response.

Norepinephrine plays a crucial role in the human stress response. Individuals have increases in blood pressure, breathing rate, and subjective sensation of anxiety after injections of norepinephrine. Additionally, the stimulation of the norephineprine systems recreates the symptoms of POSTTRAUMATIC STRESS DISORDER (PTSD), which include FLASHBACKS, excessive arousal, and hypervigilance, as well as an increased startle response. Epinephrine stimulates the heart to beat more rapidly and squeeze more vigorously with each contraction. The increase in blood pressure stimulates blood flow and the delivery of oxygen and glucose, which are essential actions for the body to cope with the increased demand.

New research shows that the HPA axis controls virtually all of the hormones, nervous system activity, and energy expenditure in the human body, as well as modulating the immune system.

Any stressor that persists for a period of time (often minutes) activates the paraventricular nucleus (PVN), which is deep in the brain and a part of the hypothalamus. The presence of PVN releases corticotrophin-releasing hormones (CRH) into the bloodstream, which act on the pituitary gland located above the roof of the mouth's bony structure. The pituitary gland has many functions and effects, but when CRH is present, the pituitary is forced to release adrenocorticotrophic hormone (ACTH), which travels to the adrenal gland located on the kidneys.

The adrenal gland has a top section or cortex and a main section or medulla. The cortex of the adrenal gland secretes cortisol, an activating but wide-ranging hormone that is associated directly with the stress response. ACTH causes the release of cortisol, which is slowly metabolized or used up by the body, so its effects may last for 15 to 20 minutes. This is the slower stress reaction or activation in the body and most people have experienced this effect of prolonged agitation and anxiety-like symptoms.

There is also a fast-track pathway for activation when stressors appear that are threatening. It is neurological. The vagus nerve backs off resulting in activation of the heart and lungs and other sympathetic responses. Neurological activation is immediate and intense but diminishes quickly when the stressor is removed or neutralized. For example, a car coming upon a person in an intersection might stimulate an immediate neurological activation and the driver would stamp on the gas pedal. The car misses the person, and both the driver and the pedestrian are relieved. But if the HPA axis is engaged by this incident, the individual might feel shaky for some time, and relive the incident in his or her mind until the cortisol is metabolized.

In addition to cortisol, the adrenal cortex releases dexamethasone (DHEA), a precursor to sex hormones, which helps to maintain blood volume and pressure under activation conditions. An interesting aspect of this situation is that the ratio of cortisol to DHEA is reflective of conditions of stress versus those of warm and compassionate feelings; high DHEA levels relative to cortisol are indicative of feelings of warmheartedness, whereas low ratios correspond to feeling stressed. A DEXAMETHASONE SUPPRESSION TEST determines deficiencies of DHEA and concurrent DEPRESSION or posttraumatic stress disorder.

See also BRAIN.

hypothalamus   See BRAIN.

hysteria   A term describing the behavior of a highly emotional person who reacts to many situations with intense emotion that is out of proportion to the situation itself. People like this are called hysterics or hysterical personalities. It is thought that the difficulty modulating emotions seen in the hysteric comes from two sources. The first is a mother who is not modulated herself and therefore cannot help the infant modulate. Frequently, there is a lack of psychological bonding with the infant. The second is possible small "t" traumas that come from an environment that is emotional and chaotic. The developing child experiences emotional traumatic reactions at a subclinical level and takes on a life of emotional ups and down.

At one extreme is the hysterical personality disorder, currently known as histrionic personality disorder. People with histrionic personality disorders always seem to be "on stage" with exaggerated gestures, mannerisms, and grandiose language. They manipulate others for attention to satisfy their dependence on others, and can even use SUICIDE as a manipulative device. They may dress outlandishly in style, color, and body exposure. Their relationships are shallow and much less intimate than they perceive them to be.

The development of histrionic personality disorder seems to be fixed at a young teenage level. The teenager affected fears loss of dependency, is flirtatious, demonstrates a lack of intimacy, and experiences a deep level of unhappiness.

These individuals are difficult to treat because of their high levels of self-attention, seductiveness, and dependency and because they often "change" superficially just to please the therapist. Even though it has been recognized for many decades, this type of disorder has not changed except in its diagnostic name.

On the other hand, hysterical disorder, or within current usage hysterical somatoform disorder, is very different. It includes those with changes in or an actual loss of physical functioning without any actual physical damage. Common hysterical disorders are blindness (in the absence of any damage to the optic mechanism or brain), paralysis, deafness, anesthesia, and pain perception loss. In the current diagnostic system, there are three types of hysterical somatoform disorder: conversion disorder,

SOMATIZATION DISORDER, and pain disorder associated with psychological factors.

Conversion disorder is the most relevant to this discussion. In conversion disorder, there are two or more symptoms that are indicative of deficits in the voluntary motor or sensory functions (see above). These deficits are psychologically caused, and they are not intentional or faking in nature. Often these deficits remove the individual from a stressful situation under the guise of a medical problem. The conversion disorders are equivalent to the older terminology of *hysteria* or *hysterical personality disorder*.

The most thorough and in-depth early work with hysteria was that of Pierre Janet (1859–1947), and his interest in traumatic experience was transformed into psychopathology. Janet influenced the work of Charcot, Pinel, Freud, Rush, and William James. Unfortunately, Janet's more psychologically based theories were displaced by the biological approach that emphasized genetics (constitutional factors) and medical factors over more psychological approaches.

By the turn of the 20th century, psychoanalysis offered an alternative explanation to many medically based theories. Freud postulated that traumatic experience was isolated from the rest of experience and personality. Eventually, Freud concluded that sexual wishes formed an unconscious and unacceptable impulse that produced "symptoms" of shutdown or hysterical dysfunction. Janet's theories and observations languished under Freud's relentless pursuit of early fantasized sexual trauma.

Janet argued that hysteria (conversion disorder) was a mode of adaptation to frightening, traumatic experiences that were separately stored and that had the effect of narrowing consciousness. Feelings were dissociated, as were memories of these frightening experiences. Hysteria (loss of function) could develop or psychasthenia (what is known as obsessive-compulsive disorder today) would occur, leading to obsessions, ruminations, and phobias, as well as a decreased capacity for creativity and fluidity. DISSOCIATION was the crucial psychological process to deal with overwhelming experience (trauma), but stored traumatic events would be expressed in sensory perceptions, affective states, and behavior reenactments. Janet showed the interdependence of memory processes, state-dependent learning, dissociative reactions, and posttraumatic psychopathology.

While Janet emphasized the interdependence of dissociation and hysteria, today these two processes are divided into separate diagnostic categories, and mental health professionals no longer view them as interrelated: dissociation is a diagnostic category by itself, hysteria is a separate category, and the relationship is lost.

Society owes a debt to Janet for connecting dissociation, memory, and state-dependent learning, all of which form the basis for traumatic reactions. His legacy is the observation of how the mind can dissociate in the face of overwhelming threat, fragmenting the mental process and producing physiological, behavioral, cognitive, and emotional residue that will follow the individual for the rest of life if untreated. His science was observation, just as the astronomer is able only to observe. Psychopathology was the result of weakened, dissociated, and fragmented ways of functioning in traumatized individuals.

Janet, P. *Psychological Healing.* 1919. Reprint, New York: Macmillan, 1925.

I

iconic memory   See VISUAL MEMORY.

image habituation therapy (IHT)   A form of exposure therapy that was developed by Vaughan and Tarrier to treat survivors of TRAUMA suffering from POSTTRAUMATIC STRESS DISORDER (PTSD). IHT exposes the patient to self-evoked images of the trauma in order to produce habituation or decreased response of anxiety. This involves the patient's creating a verbal description of the traumatic event on an audiotape and then using the tapes in self-directed homework assignments, maximizing his or her exposure to cognitive events.

The key benefit of IHT is the limited use of time for the clinician by using audiotapes to facilitate the self-directed exposure to traumatic-related images. For the client, the benefit is that the treatment sessions can be carried out in his or her home, thus decreasing problems with anticipatory anxiety (reactions to the "idea" about an event). Vaughan and Tarrier showed that there were significant decreases in anxiety between and within homework sessions, suggesting that habituation did occur and that it was responsible for improvement.

See also THERAPY, TYPES OF.

Vaughan, K., and N. Tarrier. "The Use of Image Habituation Therapy." *British Journal of Psychiatry* 161 (1992): 658–664.

imagery rehearsal therapy (IRT)   A brief, well-tolerated treatment that is used to decrease chronic NIGHTMARES in survivors with POSTTRAUMATIC STRESS DISORDER (PTSD). With imagery rehearsal therapy, the participants are encouraged to select a recent nightmare, to write it down, and then to change the nightmare any way that they wish by altering scenes of the original nightmare so that it becomes less distressing. Next, the participant uses imagery to rehearse the "new dream" scenario, without writing it down from this point forward, and to rehearse it as a mental process.

IRT does not involve imaginal exposure to the nightmare or traumas associated with the nightmare. The participant engages in rehearsing the "new dream" at least five to 20 minutes per day for seven days or until the nightmare ends. IRT can also be provided by a therapist in small group formats over several sessions.

Krakow et al. studied 114 sexual assault survivors with nightmares and a diagnosis of PTSD, of whom 54 received IRT during a three-week period. The women who received IRT in small groups of four to eight women in two three-hour sessions reported not only a reduction of their nightmares but also a reduction of their PTSD symptoms ranging from intrusive thoughts to emotional arousal.

See also THERAPY, TYPES OF.

Krakow, B., et al. "A Controlled Study of Imagery Rehearsal for Chronic Nightmares in Sexual Assault Survivors with PTSD." *Journal of the American Medical Association* 286, no. 5 (2001): 537–545.

imagery rescripting (IR)   An imagery-focused treatment for individuals with symptoms of POSTTRAUMATIC STRESS DISORDER (PTSD) and TRAUMA-related beliefs. Imagery rescripting (IR) was developed as a schema-focused information processing treatment for the recurrent traumatic cognitions of sexual, physical, and emotional abuse, although other IR applications to disturbing, repetitive images have been researched as well.

The goals of IR are to (1) decrease physiological arousal; (2) eliminate intrusive PTSD symptoms that are related to the targeted trauma; and (3) facilitate cognitive change in the meaning of the event and in the pathogenic schemas associated with the trauma.

In IR, the patient accesses the entire fear network of his or her traumatic memory through the use of imaginal exposure and then uses imaginal rescripting to change fearful images and challenge trauma-based beliefs. He or she modifies the helplessness/powerlessness schema, replacing it with mastery imagery. Mastery images that are developed include coping strategies in which the patient visualizes himself or herself taking control. Since the patient, not the therapist, is in control and directs changes, IR encourages active and creative "new" images to produce change in self-appraisal and self-perception.

See also THERAPY, TYPES OF.

Rusch, M., and B. Grunert. "Imagery Rescripting for Recurrent, Distressing Images." *Cognitive and Behavioral Practice* 7 (2000): 173–182.

Smucker, M. R., and J. Niederee. "Treating Incest-Related PTSD & Pathogenic Schemas Through Imaginal Exposure & Rescripting." *Cognitive and Behavioral Practice* 2, no. 1 (1995): 63–92.

Impact of Event Scale (IES)   See ASSESSMENT AND DIAGNOSIS; INSTRUMENTS/SCALES/SURVEYS THAT EVALUATE POSTTRAUMATIC STRESS DISORDER (PTSD).

Impact of Event Scale, Revised (IES-R)   See ASSESSMENT AND DIAGNOSIS; INSTRUMENTS/SCALES/ SURVEYS THAT EVALUATE POSTTRAUMATIC STRESS DISORDER (PTSD).

implicit memory   Refers to memories of tasks, reflexive action, or classically conditioned responses. Implicit memory is sometimes called non-declarative or procedural memory and is basically unconscious and not part of one's awareness. Traumatic "memories" are usually held in implicit memory in the form of body sensations, feelings and fear reactions that can subtly control behavior related to traumatic events.

Implicit memory can best be described as procedural or "how to" knowledge, such as the ability to ride a bike or shuffle cards. Implicit memory is best represented in learning and improving tasks. It is non-declarative because the individual is unable to verbalize or "declare" these step-by-step processes. Driving a car is an example in which the processes are largely unconscious and nonverbal. Conditioned emotional responses to a traumatic situation are unconscious and automatically elicited by particular triggers that are unconscious and nonverbal and therefore fall into the category of implicit memories.

The AMYGDALA plays a crucial role in the long-term storage of implicit memories that are traumatic or conditioned. Brain damage to the cerebellum and basil ganglia appears to affect implicit memory. Furthermore, the HIPPOCAMPUS seems to be necessary for the acquisition of implicit conditioned emotional responses, while the amygdala is crucial for long-term implicit memory storage and retrieval.

See also BRAIN; MEMORY.

implosive therapy   Developed by Stampfl and Levis (1967), implosive therapy involves FLOODING techniques with a variation, in that all procedures are done by having the individual imagine the anxiety-producing situations as if they were conscious distorted memories. The imagined scenes are often exaggerated to the extreme in order to elicit as much anxiety as possible, and these scenes include hypothesized sources of the anxiety, such as anxiety toward parental figures, sex, rejection, or a death wish. The individual is asked to imagine alternative ways of responding to the anxiety to make it more bearable. After several sessions, the goal is to extinguish the anxiety. Stampfl has a strong Rogerian (Carl Rogers) background, which emphasized compassionate understanding, empathetic regard, and nondirectiveness in dealing with clients. Ironically, he chose to engage in a therapy that is excessively confrontational and anxiety-provoking. Psychological research indicates that implosive therapy has short-term positive effects that diminish over the long term.

See also THERAPY, TYPES OF.

Stampfl, T. C., and D. J. Levis. "Essentials of Implosive Therapy: A Learning-theory Based Psychodynamic Behavioral Therapy." *Journal of Abnormal Psychology* 72 (1967): 496–503.

Injury Severity Score (ISS) Introduced in 1974, the Injury Severity Score (ISS) is the most widely used scoring method to assess the severity of injury for patients with multiple injuries. The index is used to assess severity of injury for purposes of insurance and treatment. Furthermore, it can be used to monitor treatment progress and outcome prediction of survivability. Multiple injuries are frequently associated with traumatic experience or events due to the life-threatening nature of bodily injury. Sometimes the severity of an injury is enhanced by previous trauma to the body and flashing back to a time and place where a horrific memory is embedded. Each injury is allocated to one of six body regions (the head and neck, face, chest, abdomen, extremity, and external) and is assigned an abbreviated injury scale score (AIS). Only the three most severe AIS scores are squared and added together to produce the ISS. The limitation of this method is that it accounts for only one injury per body region, and it underscores the severity in trauma victims who have multiple injuries to one body region. The ISS score values range from 0 to 75, when 75 is unsurvivable.

In 1997, a New Injury Severity Score was introduced to improve outcome prediction in trauma victims by adding scores for the three most severe injuries, regardless of body region. The use of the New ISS to replace the ISS is still being studied. In 2002, Husum and Strada found no significant differences for the predictive power of the two scoring methods when studying the predictive accuracy for victims of penetrating trauma.

Husum, H., and G. Strada. "Injury Severity Score versus New Injury Severity Score for Penetrating Injuries." *Prehospital and Disaster Medicine* 17, no. 1 (2002): 27–32.

insomnia: early, middle, and late Inability to sleep, which may be caused by severe STRESS and TRAUMA. Individuals with insomnia may also suffer from other sleep disorders, such as frequent NIGHTMARES.

Early insomnia (also known as initial insomnia) occurs when it takes a person longer than about a half hour to fall asleep. Early insomnia is often associated with the presence of ANXIETY DISORDERS. Middle insomnia occurs when, after falling asleep, a person wakes up at least a half hour before he or she needs to wake up. In addition, the individual may wake up many times during the night. In general, middle insomnia is associated with DEPRESSION or with pain syndromes. Late insomnia (also known as terminal insomnia) refers to waking up consistently before a person has slept for at least six and half hours. Late insomnia is often linked to depression.

All forms of insomnia may be caused by medical problems, such as endocrine changes caused by pregnancy, menopause, or hyperthyroidism. Gastrointestinal conditions such as gastroesophageal reflux disease may cause or contribute to insomnia. The use or abuse of stimulants or narcotics may lead to insomnia, as well as the use of drugs such as corticosteroids or decongestants. Antipsychotic medications can impair sleep, as can some antidepressants.

Problems with daily life such as BEREAVEMENT or work stress can cause insomnia, as can POSTTRAUMATIC STRESS DISORDER (PTSD).

Symptoms and Diagnostic Path

Many people with insomnia know that they have a problem although they may minimize the extent of the problem to themselves. They may walk around all day yawning and may have trouble concentrating at work. If the sleep deficit is severe, the person may find himself or herself nodding off while driving a car or operating heavy equipment, and some individuals have been injured or killed from car crashes or other accidents as a result of falling asleep while operating a motor vehicle or dangerous machinery.

Once the insomnia problem has been presented to a physician, the doctor should run basic laboratory tests, such as a complete blood count and thyroid function tests. In addition, it may be advisable to run a toxicology screen for alcohol and drugs. Sleep studies may be ordered in some cases, to measure the individual's blood oxygen levels and determine if the patient may have obstructive sleep apnea, a disorder in which the person stops breathing for brief periods of time. The doctor may also order the patient to keep a sleep journal for several weeks, noting the number of hours slept each night and how many times that he or she woke up as well as when each awakening occurred. The sleep journal can provide important information to both the patient and the doctor.

Treatment Options and Outlook

Any identified medical problems causing or contributing to the insomnia, such as hyperthyroidism or other disorders, should be treated. If no medical problems are identified, psychotherapy is often highly beneficial for the patient with chronic insomnia, who may suffer from depression, an anxiety disorder, or PTSD. Many patients with insomnia have a combination of psychiatric problems, such as PTSD and depression.

The person with insomnia may need medications to normalize the sleep cycle. BENZODIAZEPINE drugs are often used to treat insomnia. Newer medications such as zaleplon (Sonata) and zolpidem (Ambien) are short-term hypnotics that help individuals fall asleep. These drugs are scheduled drugs (that is, they can be prescribed only in limited quantities) because they carry a risk of drug dependence. A newer medication, ramelteon (Rozerem), is not a scheduled drug, and it is believed to help create a normal sleep-wake cycle. This drug is recommended primarily for those with early insomnia.

In severe cases, such as with individuals who suffer from chronic sleep disruption caused by PTSD, the antipsychotic olanzapine (Zyprexa) may provide relief. But there are recognized side effects, which may include:

- akathisia (an inability to remain still)
- dry mouth
- dizziness
- sedation
- insomnia
- urinary retention (the inability to pass urine), which can lead to catheterization if treatment is not stopped
- orthostatic hypotension
- weight gain (90% of users experience weight gain)
- increased appetite
- runny nose
- low blood pressure
- impaired judgment, thinking, and motor skills
- impaired spatial orientation
- impaired responses to senses
- seizure
- trouble swallowing
- dental problems and discoloration of teeth
- missed periods
- problems with keeping body temperature regulated
- apathy, lack of emotion

In one case review of seven individuals with PTSD as well as other psychiatric problems and severe chronic insomnia, reported by States and St. Dennis, the patients' insomnia resolved with treatment with olanzapine after other medications had failed. In another case the patient had trauma, PTSD, depression, and anxiety. She could not sleep for more than 45 minutes and suffered from severe nightmares when she finally did fall asleep. Antidepressants did not improve her condition, whereas olanzapine enabled her to sleep without nightmares.

In another case, the patient had PTSD, which began when she was sexually assaulted at the age of 10. She also had depression and both early and middle insomnia. Previous trials with a variety of medications had not helped improve her insomnia or other symptoms. She was treated with a combination of olanzapine and the antidepressant venlafaxine (Effexor), and her sleep problems were resolved.

Noted the authors, "The importance of recognizing and treating chronic sleep disruption in potential PTSD patients cannot be overemphasized. This symptom may be the only symptom patients will volunteer, and it should trigger a more in-depth PTSD workup on the part of the clinician."

Risk Factors and Preventive Measures

In general, women are more likely to suffer from insomnia than men, possibly because of hormonal fluctuations. Age is also a risk factor, and individuals older than age 50 are more likely to suffer from insomnia than younger people are. In some cases, medications may cause or contribute to sleep disorders such as insomnia.

Individuals with all forms of insomnia should avoid consuming products with caffeine from four to six hours before they go to bed. They should avoid using nicotine after the late afternoon because of its stimulating effect. In addition, they should avoid heavy exercise for several hours prior to sleep, as well as consuming heavy meals late in the evening. It is best to avoid daytime naps. Most physicians advise patients to avoid watching television in bed and to use their beds only for sleep and sex.

If the person with insomnia is unable to sleep, rather than worrying about when he or she will finally fall asleep and trying to compel sleep to occur (which is usually futile), the person should get out of bed and perform nonstimulating activities, such as reading. When tired, then he or she should return to bed.

See also PARASOMNIAS.

Bonds, Curley L., M.D., and Michael A. Lucia, M.D. "Sleep Disorders," eMedicine, updated April 3, 2006. Available online. URL: http:www.emedicine.com/med/topic609.htm.

States, James H., M.D., and Clarke D. St. Dennis. "Chronic Sleep Disruption and the Reexperiencing of Post-traumatic Stress Disorder Symptoms Are Improved by Olanzapine: Brief Review of the Literature and a Case-Based Series." *Primary Care Companion Journal of Clinical Psychiatry* 5, no. 2 (2003): 74–79.

instruments/scales/surveys that evaluate post-traumatic stress disorder (PTSD) Evaluative measures that offer items that help counselors and others determine whether a person either currently has or is at risk for developing POSTTRAU-MATIC STRESS DISORDER (PTSD). In general, since 1980 when PTSD was officially recognized as a psychiatric disorder, a myriad of successful assessment measures have been developed. A comprehensive assessment strategy includes gathering information about the person's life context, symptoms, beliefs, strengths and weaknesses, and ability to cope. The challenge is to combine appropriate measures to distinguish which individuals develop PTSD once exposed to potentially traumatic events.

It is also important to note that there is a great deal of evidence to show that criteria in the DIAG-NOSTIC AND STATISTICAL MANUAL-IV reflect the conceptions of Western cultures and should not be generalized to non-Western cultures. In contrast to the rigid *DSM-IV* criteria for PTSD, there are test instruments that have been shown to be reliable and valid in non-Western cultures. Among those instruments are the Harvard Trauma Questionnaire, the Clinician Administered PTSD Scale and the Impact of Event Scale-Revised.

In 2005, Jon Elhai and his colleagues surveyed experts in traumatic stress and compiled the following most commonly used instruments to query for general traumatic exposure, posttraumatic stress or ACUTE STRESS DISORDER, and event-specific exposure (such as combat), using self-report or interviewer-administered formats. These instruments are listed below in alphabetical order.

Clinician-Administered Instruments

Acute Stress Disorder Interview
Anxiety Disorders Interview Schedule—Revised—
  PTSD Module
Child Maltreatment Interview Schedule
Clinician-Administered PTSD Scale
Clinician-Administered PTSD Scale for Children
  and Adolescents
Composite International Diagnostic Interview—
  PTSD Module
Diagnostic Interview Schedule—PTSD Module
Mini International Neuropsychiatric Interview—
  PTSD Module
National Women's Study PTSD Module
Structured Clinical Interview for *DSM-IV*—PTSD
  Module
Structured Interview for PTSD

Self-Report Instruments

Combat Exposure Scale

Conflict Tactics Scale

Davidson Trauma Scale or Self-Rating Traumatic Stress Scale

Deployment Risk and Resilience Inventory

Detailed Assessment of Posttraumatic Stress

Distressing Events Questionnaire

Harvard Trauma Questionnaire

Impact of Event Scale

Impact of Event Scale, Revised

Life Events Checklist

Life Stressor Checklist

Los Angeles Symptom Checklist

Minnesota Multiphasic Personality Inventory-02-Keane PTSD Scale

Minnesota Multiphasic Personality Inventory-2-Schlenger PTSD Scale

Mississippi Civilian PTSD Scale

Mississippi Combat PTSD Scale

Modified PTSD Symptom Scale—Self Report

Personality Assessment Inventory-PTSD Scale

Posttraumatic Cognition Inventory

Posttraumatic Stress Diagnostic Scale

PTSD Checklist

PTSD Reaction Index (or UCLA PTSD Index)

PTSD Symptom Scale

Sexual Abuse Exposure Questionnaire

Stanford Acute Stress Reaction Questionnaire

Symptom Checklist-90-PTSD Scale

Trauma Assessment for Adults—interview or self-report version

Trauma Related Guilt Inventory

Trauma Symptom Checklist for Children

Trauma Symptom Checklist-40

Trauma Symptom Inventory

Traumatic Life Event Questionnaire

Clinician Administered Posttraumatic Stress Disorder (PTSD) Scale (CAPS)   The Clinician Administered Posttraumatic Stress Disorder Scale (CAPS) is a 30-item structured interview tool used by therapists with individuals who may have posttraumatic stress disorder. CAPS has specific requirements for both the intensity and frequency of symptoms and can address an individual who has occasional symptoms as well as the individual who has more frequent but less intense symptoms.

Each item has a behavioral reference rating scale for both intensity and frequency of behaviors described in the scale, with a time frame of one month for current symptoms. The CAPS is used to make a current or lifetime diagnosis of PTSD by using the worst ever one-month period to measure and eliminate the possible inflated reporting of multiple lifetime rates.

CAPS also includes questions to rate the individual's social and occupational functioning and the overall PTSD severity. It has excellent test reliability with combat veterans, but lacks validation with nonveterans. Otherwise, CAPS is an excellent choice for use in research and clinical settings.

The CAPS was designed to be given by clinicians, research clinicians, and paraprofessionals familiar with traumatic stressors and PTSD. It can be given in 45–60 minutes. CAPS has a children and adolescent version, CAPS-CA.

Davidson Trauma Scale   The Davidson Trauma Scale (DTS) is a 17-item self-report instrument used to measure the presence, frequency, and severity of symptoms that are characteristic of individuals who develop posttraumatic stress disorder. The Davidson Trauma Scale measures three categories of symptoms that are associated with PTSD: intrusive reexperiencing, avoidance and numbing, and hyperarousal. The intrusive score is the cumulative score of the frequency and severity scores for five questions relating to this category. The avoidance and numbing score is the cumulative score for six corresponding questions, and the hyperarousal score is the cumulative score for four corresponding questions.

The DRS is not a diagnostic instrument; however, it is useful to make a preliminary determination as to whether the symptoms meet the *Diagnostic and Statistical Manual-IV* criteria for PTSD.

Harvard Trauma Questionnaire (HTQ)   The Harvard Trauma Questionnaire is an interview checklist to assess a variety of trauma events cross-culturally. It was developed by the Harvard Program in Refugee Trauma. The Harvard Trauma Questionnaire was first used with Indochinese refugees in three languages: Laotian, Cambodian, and Vietnamese. Later versions added a checklist in Japanese after the 1995 Kobe earthquake, and there are also a Croatian veterans' version for soldiers from the Balkan war and a Bosnian version for civilian survivors of these wars.

The Harvard Trauma Questionnaire has four sections, beginning with the interviewer's assessment of traumatic life experiences. Section II includes open-ended questions about the worst experience of trauma for the population being assessed. Section III asks questions about experiences that may have led to a head injury (this part was eliminated for the Japanese version). Section IV asks about specific trauma symptoms. In the most recent versions of the Bosnian and Croatian veterans' versions, section IV focuses on the impact of trauma on the individual's perception of how well he or she functions in day-to-day life activities.

Impact of Event Scale (IES) The Impact of Event Scale was developed by Mardi Horowitz, Nancy Wilner, and William Alvarez in the 1970s in order to assess psychological stress reactions after any major life event, such as BEREAVEMENT, rape, war, and MOTOR VEHICLE ACCIDENTS. The Impact of Event Scale is the most widely used self-report questionnaire to assess the frequency of intrusive and avoidant phenomena after a variety of traumatic experiences. Sundin and Horowitz describe the IES as being "anchored in its instructions to a particular event and measur[ing] two categories of responses: intrusive experiences and avoidance of thoughts and images associated with that event."

Intrusions comprise intrusive thoughts, NIGHT-MARES, intrusive feelings, and visual imagery of the traumatic event. These intrusions can disrupt the individual's daily life and interfere with normal functioning while he or she attempts to integrate and process the trauma into a meaningful context. Avoidance behaviors try to block out intrusive images. Examples of avoidance are numbing of responsiveness, loss of interest, and avoidance of situations or locations of the traumatic event. Although maladaptive, these responses are coping strategies.

The IES contains 15 items that are added into two subscales: IES intrusion (seven items) and IES avoidance (eight items). In a self-report format, the subject is asked to report the frequency in the past seven days of symptoms on a four-point measurement scale, with 0 indicating not at all, 1 indicating rarely, 3 indicating sometimes, and 5 indicating often.

The questionnaire has been able to show good reliability on the subscales of avoidance and intrusion. A third dimension, hyperarousal, is not addressed in the IES, but is included in the Impact of Event Scale, Revised, developed by Daniel S. Weiss and Charles R. Marmar. The IES was developed prior to the adoption of posttraumatic stress disorder as a legitimate diagnosis in the *Diagnostic and Statistical Manual* in 1980.

The strength of the IES lies in its short and easily administered and scored questionnaire. It can be used repeatedly with the subjects to gauge progress. Its limitation remains as a screening tool and not a comprehensive test for recent traumatic events. The IES has been translated into several languages, including Arabic, Hebrew, Dutch, German, Swedish, and Croatian.

According to an analysis of 12 studies reported in 2002 in the *British Journal of Psychiatry*, this scale "is a useful measure of stress reactions after a range of traumatic events, and it is valuable for detecting individuals who require treatment." Some examples of the traumatic events evaluated in relation to the scale were the death of a parent, an earthquake, an alcoholic-induced blackout, combat exposure, psychiatric illness, exposure to violent acts, political imprisonment, accidents, and illness.

Impact of Event Scale, Revised (IES-R) The Impact of Event Scale, Revised is a self-report scale that was developed by Daniel S. Weiss and Charles Marmar in 1997 to help evaluate an individual's current distress over a severe life event and addresses the third major symptom cluster of PTSD and persistent hyperarousal.

There are 22 items in the Impact of Event Scale, Revised (IES-R). Individuals rate items on the scale based on events in the past seven days from 0 (not at all) through 4 (extremely).

Two examples of items that individuals respond to and rate on the Impact of Event Scale, Revised are: "My feelings about it were kind of numb" and "Reminders of it caused me to have physical reactions, such as sweating, trouble breathing, nausea, or a pounding heart."

Only minimal changes were made to the original intrusion and avoidance items of the IES. Seven items were added to the 15 original items. Six new hyperarousal items target anger and irritability, concentration, hypervigilance, startle response, physiological arousal and FLASHBACK experience. The seventh item split the original sleep item into two: "I had trouble staying asleep" and "I had trouble falling asleep."

The instructions were revised to ask the respondent to rate the distress caused by symptom, rather than by frequency. The format was modified to a five-point scale response range: 0 (not at all), 1 (a little bit), 2 (moderately), 3 (quite a bit) and 4 (extremely), according to the past seven days.

Baumert et al. found that reliability and construct validity for the intrusion and avoidance subscale proved to be high, but was only sufficient for the hyperarousal subscale. Weiss and Marmar, in their study of four different population samples, reported that the internal consistency or reliability of the three subscales was very high. The IES-R is available in several languages including Spanish, Japanese, and Chinese and is one of the most widely used instruments to assess PTSD, partly because of its reliability, construct validity, and ease of administration.

Posttraumatic Stress Diagnostic Scale   The Posttraumatic Stress Diagnostic Scale is a 49-item self-report instrument developed by Edna Foa to assist in the diagnosis of PTSD. The Posttraumatic Stress Diagnostic Scale (PSDS) is used to screen for the presence of PTSD in large groups and gauge the symptom severity and functioning of individuals who have been already identified with PTSD features.

The PSDS breaks down the technical language of the *Diagnostic and Statistical Manual-IV* criteria of PTSD to an eighth-grade reading level for respondents. The PSDS asks respondents to check any traumatic event that they have witnessed or experienced and to briefly describe the event. The PSDS is not intended to bypass a structured diagnostic interview. It can be used as a paper and pencil test or can be taken online in 10 to 15 minutes.

Symptom Checklist (SCL)-90-Revised   The Symptom Checklist (SCL)-90-Revised measures psychiatric distress within the past week on several dimensions of pathology. The scales are: SOMATIZATION (SOM), obsessive-compulsive (O-C), interpersonal sensitivity (I-S), depression (DEP), anxiety (ANX), hostility (HOS), phobic anxiety (PHOB),

paranoid ideation (PAR), psychoticism (PSY), and additional items, such as the global severity index (GSI), the positive symptom distress index (PSDI), and the positive symptom total (PST). The SCL-90 Revised replaces some test items on the anxiety and the obsessive-compulsive dimensions of the original SCL-90 that were psychometrically flawed.

The SCL-90-R is a self-report 90-item symptom inventory that uses ratings on a five-point scale from 0 (not at all) to 4 (extremely distressed). It provides a global score as a best single indicator of stress. Its uses include symptom assessment upon intake evaluations and measurement of progress during and after treatment.

There is a Chinese version of the SCL-90-R that was used as a screening device for measuring symptoms of anger/hostility or interpersonal sensitivity in a study by Huang et al. in 2006 of 471 Hunan female prisoners who experienced at least one traumatic event.

Trauma Symptom Inventory   The TRAUMA SYMPTOM INVENTORY is a 100-item test used to evaluate acute and chronic posttraumatic symptomatology of the psychological effects of rape, spousal abuse, CHILDREN AND TRAUMA, child physical assault, combat and war experiences and natural disasters. The Trauma Symptom Inventory (TSI) has 10 clinical subscales to assess the broad symptoms that are related to posttraumatic stress disorder and acute stress disorder and additional intra- and interpersonal difficulties associated with chronic psychological trauma over a six-month period. The 10 clinical scales assessed in the TSI are: anxious arousal, depression, anger/irritability, intrusive experience, defensive avoidance, dissociation, sexual concerns, dysfunctional sexual behavior, impaired self-reference, and tension reduction behavior.

There is an 86-item alternate version, the TSI-A, that does not contain sexual concerns or dysfunctional sexual behavior scales.

Trauma Symptom Checklist/Trauma Symptom Checklist for Children/Traumatic Stress Schedule   The Trauma Symptom Checklist-40 (TSC-40) was developed by John Briere and Marsha Runtz as a research instrument to evaluate symptomatology in adults with childhood or adult traumatic experiences. The Trauma Symptom Checklist, Trauma

Symptom Checklist for Children, and Traumatic Stress Schedule help determine the presence of traumatic reactions in adults and children.

The TSC-40 is a 40-item self-report instrument with six subscales: anxiety, DEPRESSION, DISSOCIATION, sexual abuse trauma index (SATI), sexual problems, and sleep disturbances. The TSC-40 should not be used to validate a psychological diagnosis of posttraumatic stress disorder since it does not measure all 17 criteria of PTSD. The TSC-40 requires only 10 to 15 minutes to complete and five to 10 minutes to score.

The Trauma Symptom Checklist for Children (TSCC) is a self-report instrument measuring posttraumatic stress and related psychological symptomatology in children ages eight to 16 years who have experienced traumatic events such as CHILD PHYSICAL ABUSE OR CHILD SEXUAL ABUSE or have witnessed a violent act or natural disasters. The 54-item measure can be given individually or in a group within 15 to 20 minutes. The TSCC contains six clinical scales: anxiety, depression, anger, posttraumatic stress, dissociation, and sexual concerns. There is an alternate 44-item version (TSC-A) which is identical to the TSCC except it makes no reference to sexual issues. The TSCC was developed by John Briere and is standardized on a large sample of diverse children in urban and suburban environments.

Briere has also developed the Trauma Symptom Checklist for Young Children (TSCYC), for children ages three to 12 years, as a 90-item caretaker report of children's trauma. Both the TSCC and the TSCYC have good reliability and are associated with exposure to childhood sexual abuse, physical abuse, and the witnessing of domestic violence.

Traumatic Stress Schedule The TRAUMATIC STRESS SCHEDULE is a short instrument for measuring the occurrence and impact of traumatic events that can be administered by a lay interviewer. The event categories assessed by the Traumatic Stress Schedule (TSS) are: robbery, physical assault, sexual assault, the tragic death of a friend or family member, a motor vehicle accident, military combat, loss through fire, natural disaster, and hazard or danger, as well as one unspecified event. Once the respondent reports an event, there are 12 addi-

tional detailed closed and open-ended questions pertaining to the scope, threat to life, blame, physical injury, and range of symptoms.

The TSS functions well as a screening device for many purposes and may be used for clinical and research purposes, but may result in a lack of standardization.

Traumatic Life Event Questionnaire (TLEQ) The TRAUMATIC LIFE EVENT QUESTIONNAIRE (TLEQ) is a 23-item self-report questionnaire assessing 22 types of childhood and adulthood traumatic events including natural disasters, exposure to war, robbery involving a weapon, physical and sexual abuse, and stalking. The TLEQ asks the respondent to provide the number of times exposed to such traumatic events from "never" to "more than 5 times." The questionnaire assesses subjective reactions of terror, horror, and threat to life, as well as the presence of injury, characteristics of the perpetrator (stranger), and identifying what event "causes you most distress."

A sample item from the TLEQ is: "Were you involved in a motor vehicle accident for which you received medical attention or that badly injured or killed someone?"

The TLEQ is a beneficial screening measure for clinical and research purposes.

Structured Interviews Structured interviews use the diagnostic criteria in an interview format that is standardized across interviewees. These structured interviews tend to improve diagnostic accuracy and often aid in planning treatments. The structured interviews also carry good reliability and validity. The STRUCTURED CLINICAL INTERVIEW for DSM (SCID) is the most widely used diagnostic interview schedule and has the added advantage of having subscales that help differentiate anxiety, affective disorders, substance abuse disorders, and psychosis from PTSD.

The PTSD Interview, developed by Watson and colleagues (1991), has excellent psychometric properties, has a schedule that the interviewee reads during the interview, and uses intensity ratings for each endorsed question. There is also the Structured Interview for PTSD (SI-PTSD), developed by Davidson, Smith, and Kudler (1989), that focuses on identifying symptom severity and more in-depth probe of symptoms experiences.

Blake et al. (1990) suggest another structured clinical interview, the Clinician-Administered PTSD Scale (CAPS) for use by trained and experienced clinicians. The CAPS assesses all 17 possible symptoms of PTSD along with social and occupational functioning. It has separate ratings for frequency and intensity of each symptom with behavioral samples.

Finally, there is the PTSD Symptom Scale Interview (PSS-I) developed by Foa, Riggs, Dancu, and Rothbaum (1993) for clinical and research purposes. It is brief and has good psychometric properties. However, it was developed for use with female sexual assault victims and has some limitations outside of that population.

Self-Report Instruments   The next category of assessment is the self-report measure. These assessments do not require any interaction with an examiner, which has a limitation in terms of follow-up questions. On the other hand, self-report measures are economical, less time-consuming, and good for screening purposes. The Impact of Event Scale, Revised (IES-R) by Horowitz, Wilner, and Alvarez (1979) is the most widely used self-report measure in research and clinical work.

The Mississippi Scale for Combat-Related PTSD by Keane, Caddell, and Taylor (1988) is a 35-item scale designed to measure combat-related PTSD. This scale has excellent psychometric properties and its scores are highly correlated with more in-depth interview measures.

The Keane PTSD Scale of the Minnesota Multiphasic Personality Inventory-2 is derived from MMPI responses and benefits from the MMPI validity indexes, which attempt to measure the respondent's willingness to be honest. It shows good reliability but has not had sufficient validation with nonveteran populations.

Hammerberg (1992) states that the Penn Inventory for Posttraumatic Stress is a 26-item questionnaire that can be used across diverse populations (but mostly male populations). The Penn Inventory was an early scale that is often not used today, owing to its inadequate gauge of PTSD symptoms in the female civilian population. Therefore, it is not listed in our catalog of instruments. The 17-question Posttraumatic Stress Diagnostic Scale (PTDS) developed by Foa, Cashman, Jaycox, and Perry (1997) is taken directly from the *DSM* criteria. It

provides a 12-item checklist of possible trauma situations and then asks for the most troublesome events of those within the past month. It has good correspondence with the SCID.

The PTSD Checklist (PCL) has a military and a civilian version and rates the 17 diagnostic criteria for PTSD on an intensity scale. It has strong correlations with other measures of PTSD. The Los Angeles Symptom Checklist (LASC) consists of 43 intensity-rated items and has been standardized on various populations, ages, and both sexes. It has good internal reliability and is as sensitive as most instruments.

All these self-report instruments are sensitive and have good psychometric properties. They are most useful for research and clinical screening and have limitations only around populations they were validated against and the potential bias produced by self-evaluations.

Psychophysiological Measures   This is a category of PTSD assessment that requires a good deal of time to administer as well as specialized equipment. This category of assessment reduces measures to physiological indexes. Although these measures are valid and useful, they do not reflect the actual behavioral criteria of PTSD.

The most promising measure is that of reactivity to audio and audiovisual presentations that attempt to introduce stimuli similar to the trauma. Imagery is also used for this purpose. Heart rate, blood pressure, heart rate coherence, galvanic skin response (GSR), and electromyogram are usually measured during audio-type presentations. Arousal and reactivity measures correlate adequately with the self-report and interview instruments previously described. Psychophysiological measures offer great promise as preventive and diagnostic assessments in children.

In general, since 1980, when PTSD was officially recognized as a psychiatric disorder, a myriad of successful assessment measures have been developed. A comprehensive assessment strategy includes gathering information about the person's life context, symptoms, beliefs, strengths, weaknesses, and ability to cope. The challenge is to combine appropriate measures to distinguish which individuals develop PTSD once exposed to potentially traumatic events.

See also ASSESSMENT AND DIAGNOSIS; CHILD ABUSE AND NEGLECT.

Baumert, J., H. Simon, H. Gundel, G. Schmitt, and K. H. Ladwig. "The Impact of Event Scale-Revised: Evaluation of the Subscales and Correlations to Psychophysiological Startle Response Patterns in Survivors of a Life-Threatening Cardiac Event: An Analysis of 129 Patients with an Implanted Cardioverter Defibrillator." *Journal of Affective Disorder* 82, no. 1 (October 1, 2004): 29–41.

Blake, D. D., F. W. Weathers, L. M. Nagy, D. G. Kaloupek, G. Klauminzer, D. S. Charney, and T. M. Keane. "A Clinical Rating Scale for Assessing Current and Lifetime PTSD: The CAPS-1." *Behavior Therapist 18* (1990): 187–188.

Briere, J. *Trauma Symptoms Inventory Professional Manual.* Odessa, Fla.: Psychological Assessment Resources, 1995.

Briere, J., et al. "The Trauma Symptom Checklist for Young Children (TSCYC): Reliability and Association with Abuse Exposure in a Multi-Site Study." *Child Abuse & Neglect* 25, no. 8 (2001): 1,001–1,014.

Davidson, J., R. Smith, and H. Kudler. "Validity and Reliability of the DSM-III Criteria for Posttraumatic Stress Disorder: Experience with a Structured Interview." *Journal of Nervous and Mental Disease 177* (1989): 336–341.

Elhai, J. D., M. G. Gray, T. B. Dashdan, and C. L. Franklin. "Which Instruments Are Most Commonly Used to Assess Traumatic Event Exposure and Posttraumatic Effects?: A Survey of Traumatic Stress Professionals." *Journal of Traumatic Stress* 18, no. 5 (October 2005): 541–545.

Foa, E. B., L. Cashman, L. Jaycox, and K. Perry. "The Validation of a Self-report Measure of Posttraumatic Stress Disorder: The Posttraumatic Diagnostic Scale." *Psychological Assessment* 9 (1977): 445–451.

Foa, E. B., D. S. Riggs, C. V. Dancu, and B. O. Rothbaum. "Reliability and Validity of a Brief Instrument for Assessing Post-traumatic Stress Disorder." *Journal of Traumatic Stress* 6 (1993): 459–473.

Hammerberg, M. "Penn Inventory for Posttraumatc Stress Disorder: Psychometric Properties." *Psychological Assessment* 4 (1992): 67–76.

Horowitz, M. J., N. Wilner, and W. Alvarez. "Impact of Event Scale: A Measure of Subjective Distress." *Psychosomatic Medicine* 41 (1979): 209–218.

Huang, G., et al. "Prevalence and Characteristics of Trauma and Posttraumatic Stress Disorder in Female Prisoners in China." *Comprehensive Psychiatry* 47, no. 1 (January–February 2006): 20–29.

Keane, T. M., J. M. Caddell, and K. L. Taylor. "Mississippi Scale for Combat-Related PTSD: Three Studies in Reliability and Validity." *Journal of Consulting and Clinical Psychology* 56 (1988): 85–90.

Kubany, E. S., S. N. Haynes, M. B. Leisen, J. A. Owens, A. S. Kaplan, S. B. Watson, and K. Burns. "Development and Preliminary Validation of a Brief Broad-spectrum Measure of Trauma Exposure: The Traumatic Life Events Questionnaire." *Psychological Assessment* 12 (2000): 210–224.

Newman, E., D. Kaloupek, and T. Keane. "Assessment of Posttraumatic Stress Disorder in Clinical and Research Settings." In *Traumatic Stress,* edited by B. Van der Kolk, A. McFarlane, and L. Weisaeth. New York: Guilford Press, 1996.

Norris, F. "Screening for Traumatic Stress: A Scale for Use in the Genera Population." *Journal of Applied Social Psychology* 20 (November 1990): 1,704–1,718.

Renner, W., I. Salem, and K. Ottomeyer. "Cross-Cultural Validation of Measures of Traumatic Symptoms in Groups of Asylum Seekers from Chechnya, Afghanistan, and West Africa." *Social Behavior and Personality* 34, no. 9 (2006): 1,101–1,114.

Sundin, Eva C., and Mardi J. Horowitz. "Horowitz's Impact of Event Scale Evaluation of 20 Years of Use." *Psychosomatic Medicine* 65, no. 5 (September/October 2003): 870–876.

Sundin, Eva C., and Mardi J. Horowitz. "Impact of Event Scale: Psychometric Properties." *British Journal of Psychiatry* 180 (2002): 205–209.

Watson, C., M. P. Juba, V. Manifold, T. Kuccala, and P. E. Anderson. "The PTSD Interview: Rationale, Description, Reliability and Current Validity of a DSM-III-based Technique. *Journal of Clinical Psychology* 47 (1991): 179–188.

Weiss, D., and C. Marmar. "The Impact of Event Scale-Revised." In *Assessing Psychological Trauma and PTSD,* edited by J. Wilson and T. Keane. New York: Guilford, 2004.

intergenerational trauma   Refers to the passing on of trauma from one generation to the next. The phenomenon of transgenerational trauma is a real one, and has been shown to manifest itself in a number of documented mass traumas, such as the Holocaust of the Jews in World War II, the genocide of Armenians by the Turks, the experience of Cambodian refugees or of those engaged in combat in Vietnam, and in many other large-scale culturally traumatic events.

Symptoms and Diagnostic Path

The common symptomology found in research studies involving children of the survivors of mass trauma are as follows: DEPRESSION, anxiety, insecure attachment, GUILT and separation problems, health problems, and acting-out behaviors. Often the children of survivors feel a need to succeed, and they seek to avoid failure and carry on the culture as a way to please their parents, especially if there has been a threat to the culture and a displacement of their parents. Evidence from physiological studies indicates that the effects of intergenerational trauma may appear as far out as three generations from the original survivors.

Treatment Options and Outlook

There are no specific treatments for transgenerational trauma. The effects show up in various ways and inconsistently within subsequent generations. For example, second generation immigrant Jews to the United States experienced a sense of alienation from their parents because their parents wanted to integrate these children rapidly within the culture and hence kept a distance from them and did not teach them the "old country" ways. The sense of loss and separation from their parents had a profound effect on this generation.

Risk Factors and Preventive Measures

The 2001 tsunami in Southeast Asia, mass genocides in Somalia and Darfur, and floods, hurricanes and other natural disasters have produced large numbers of victims affected with POSTTRAUMATIC STRESS DISORDER (PTSD). Development of PTSD depends on many variables, including but not limited to, support, past trauma and depression, degree of safety to survivors, and coping mechanisms.

International Classification of Disease-10 (ICD-10)

The tenth version of an international classification code of diseases that is published by the World Health Organization in Geneva, Switzerland, and which delineates the type of disease or disorder that is diagnosed in an individual, including psychiatric disorders as well as all other disorders. This coding system is used by many countries worldwide, including the United States.

The ICD codes were first developed in the late 19th century, when they were known as the International List of Causes of Death. The World Health Organization took over management of these medical codes when they began to include disease (morbidity) in 1948, at the time of the sixth revision of the codes.

The ICD-10 code is used on death certificates and by doctors when submitting claims to insurance companies. In addition, ICD-10 information is used to gather data for compiling national and international information on the epidemiology of diseases. As of this writing, there are 12,420 codes in the ICD-10. Mental and behavioral disorders are covered in Chapter V of the ICD-10; for example, behavioral syndromes associated with physiological disturbances and physical factors are encompassed in blocks F50–F59. A list of the types of classifications is available online at http://www3.who.int/icd/currentversion/fr-icd.htm.

The ICD-10 classifications and diagnostic criteria often differ from those same categories in the DIAGNOSTIC AND STATISTICAL MANUAL published by the American Psychiatric Association.

International Society for Traumatic Stress Studies (ISTSS)

A clearinghouse for information on POSTTRAUMATIC STRESS DISORDER (PTSD). One of the organization's functions is to track empirical studies demonstrating effective treatments for PTSD. They use a grading system of A through E as a guideline for the degree of empirical support that an approach has received. The guidelines are updated yearly, and they generally confirm recommendations from other practice-related bodies, such as the Veterans Administration (VA) and the American Psychiatric Association.

The treatments in the A category have the highest level of empirical support. These include: PROLONGED EXPOSURE THERAPY (a therapist-guided gradual recall or IN VIVO THERAPY), COGNITIVE PROCESSING THERAPY (CPT) (deals with erroneous thinking often with exposure), STRESS INOCULATION TRAINING (another form of COGNITIVE BEHAVIORAL THERAPY that is oriented to prevention and management), EYE-MOVEMENT DESENSITIZATION AND REPROCESSING (accelerated information processing),

and the use of medications (such as SELECTIVE SERO-
TONIN REUPTAKE INHIBITORS [SSRIs]).

The ISTSS also tracks new drug and psychotherapy approaches as well as comorbidity studies
and maintains information on its Web site (www.
istss.com).

See also THERAPY, TYPES OF.

interoceptive exposure therapy (IE) One of the
most effective methods for reducing anxiety sensitivity. Individuals undergoing IE therapy are
given behaviorally induced tasks to arouse bodily
sensations so that the person can learn that exposure to the sensations has no harmful effects upon
the body. For example, the individual is asked to
hyperventilate for several minutes, inducing dizziness and increased heartbeats, in order to learn
that these sensations do not cause medically catastrophic consequences.

IE is widely used to treat PANIC DISORDERS.
Whether IE is effective with individuals diagnosed
with POSTTRAUMATIC STRESS DISORDER (PTSD) is
still a question in the early investigative stages.
Wald and Taylor (2005) used interoceptive exposure therapy as one component of treatment and
combined it with trauma-related exposure therapy
(imaginal exposure or IN VIVO THERAPY) to show
results of significant reduction in the severity of the
PTSD and anxiety sensitivity at the one-month and
three-month follow-ups.

See also THERAPY, TYPES OF.

Wald, J., and S. Taylor. "Interoceptive Exposure Therapy
Combined with Trauma-related Exposure Therapy for
Posttraumatic Stress Disorder: A Case Report." *Cogni-
tive Behaviour Therapy* 34, no. 1 (2005): 34–40.

in vivo therapy A form of EXPOSURE THERAPY in
which the clinician asks individuals to overtly face
their situations that are associated with trauma,
physically confronting the feared situation in a
realistically safe environment over an extended
period of time. Examples of such stimuli that are
related to trauma and are appropriate for use with
in vivo exposure are the sites of traumatic events,
the clothing worn during trauma, the weapons
used during an attack (guns, knives, duct tape),
or the experience of sitting in a car after a MOTOR
VEHICLE ACCIDENT.

During an in vivo exposure, the individual is
asked to focus on the stimuli or event fully for
30 to 45 minutes or until their discomfort level
decreases by 50 percent. In vivo exposure therapy
combines both cognitive psychology and behavioral therapy.

See also FLOODING; INTEROCEPTIVE EXPOSURE
THERAPY; THERAPY, TYPES OF.

Istanbul Protocol See TORTURE.

kindling   A descriptive term that refers to an external stimulus that triggers the FIGHT OR FLIGHT RESPONSE in the BRAIN and sets up a resulting self-perpetuating circuitry where such defensive activity occurs. For example, an auto accident can represent an external event that is experientially life threatening. Arousal and procedural memory circuitries are part of this traumatic kindling effect. The arousal and memory circuits are linked to sensory organs of the head and neck (or other damaged areas of the body) and will cause a cyclical repetition of the sensations experienced at the time of TRAUMA. This repetitive cycle of sensation and brain reactions, most often associated with DISSOCIATION and avoidance, is the kindling effect that perpetuates the trauma.

KZ Syndromet/Syndrome   The German name for a concentration camp syndrome that was exclusive to World War II. The earliest publications describing and labeling this syndrome were by Hermann and Thygesen (1954), who wrote about this syndrome eight years after the liberation.

The *KZ* is an abbreviation of *Konzenstrationlager* or concentration camp. Danish medical doctors who had been in concentration camps started a comprehensive evaluation of five groups of former prisoners: (1) 566 expatriated prisoners who were given detailed self-report questionnaires and interviews; (2) 52 intensively examined prisoners; (3) 710 police officers confined in a "very severe" Nazi camp; (4) 67 former inmates examined in 1949 (two years later); and (5) ex-prisoners who had been arrested but not deported to camps outside Denmark.

The researchers found that 75 percent of all expatriated prisoners suffered from "neurotic" symptoms caused by individual predispositions, war factors other than deportation, conditions of repatriation, and psychological and physical stress.

The Thygesen, Hermann, and Willaugar follow-up of former concentration camp prisoners in Denmark helped to identify some of the long-term PTSD effects on individuals exposed to severe traumatic stress. These observations were incorporated into the European diagnostic system (ICD-10). Brutal treatment and undernourishment contributed substantially to long-term dullness, EMOTIONAL NUMBING, intellectual impairment, apathy/DEPRESSION, MEMORY loss, emotional irritability and instability, and a loss of a sense of the future.

See also COMBAT STRESS REACTION; POSTTRAUMATIC STRESS DISORDER (PTSD).

Thygesen, P., Hermann, K., & Willaugar, R. "Concentration Camp Survivors in Denmark: Persecution, Disease, Disability Compensation: A 23-Year Follow-up." *Danish Medical Bulletin* 17 (1970): 65–108.

learned helplessness An imposed feeling of incapacity and inevitable failure that initially occurs when individuals seek to act in some normal way, but they are (or feel that they are) coerced or otherwise prevented from attempting actions which they are fully capable of performing. After repeated incidents of being prevented from acting, the individual gives up and ceases trying to perform these actions, allowing others to take over many actions they formerly accomplished themselves and allowing others to make decisions for them, internalizing the overall belief that they are incapable and cannot recover. Feelings of helplessness are common when faced with a traumatic event. Individuals who maintain a state of "learned helplessness" will react to trauma in an even more helpless manner than those who do not have that learning.

Both adults and children may be affected by learned helplessness. Some battered women have allegedly "snapped" after years of abuse and learned helplessness, only to kill their abusers (usually their spouses or partners), using the BATTERED WOMAN SYNDROME as a defense. Some experts have actively challenged this defense.

Elderly people sometimes experience learned helplessness when well-meaning individuals, such as their adult children or spouses, take over tasks that the older person could still perform, such as preparing meals, caring for pets, paying bills, and so forth. Such a situation may happen after an elderly person recovers from an injury, and family members may decide to take over, thinking that they are being helpful. Eventually the elderly person may lose all interest in most activities and his or her health may decline as a result.

When individuals accept that they are no longer capable of performing tasks that they can actually perform, an unnecessary and often harmful helplessness ensues. Affected individuals may develop lethargy and DEPRESSION, as they generalize the helpless feeling to the extent that they feel that there is nothing that they accomplish anymore. They become emotionally numb.

The concept of learned helplessness was initially developed by Martin Seligman in 1968 in relation to animals. In 1971, he expanded the concept to humans.

Life Events Checklist (LEC) A checklist developed by Bhagat et al. in 1985, which is used to determine an individual's level of stress based on major events that have occurred in the past year. Individuals rate themselves from -3 to +3 for whether the stress was negative or positive. The Life Events Checklist (LEC) includes items that are related to work, children, family, health, marriage, financial issues, legal issues, love, and home.

In general, the more major events that have occurred, and the more negatively they are perceived, the higher the probability that the individual is experiencing stress. Some examples of life events include moving, getting a new job, getting married, having a new baby, getting divorced or separated, having financial problems, experiencing the injury or death of a loved one, and being the victim of a crime.

The Life Events Checklist is a variation on Holmes and Rahe's SOCIAL ADJUSTMENT SCALE that also rates the respondent on the number and intensity of "life change units" (LCUs) in the recent past. The Social Adjustment Scale has been the standard measure of stress since 1967 when it was first developed.

LIFE EVENTS CHECKLIST

Place a check mark in the column labeled "Happened" for those events that occurred in the past 12 months. Now record your score with the event value for each. Total the score. The items are ranked according to the average magnitude of the stressful impact for most people. Research indicates there is a connection between the number of major life events a person experiences in a year and the likelihood of illness. The people who scored highest (over 300) on this questionnaire experienced the highest amount of physical illness in the year following the test. *Notice that many of these stressors are things we often consider desirable events.*

Happened	Rank	Value	Event
	1	100	Death of a spouse
	2	73	Divorce
	3	65	Marital separation
	4	63	Detention in jail or other institution
	5	63	Death of close family member
	6	53	Major personal injury or illness
	7	50	Marriage
	8	47	Being fired at work
	9	45	Marital reconciliation
	10	45	Retirement from work
	11	44	Major change in the health or behavior of a family member
	12	40	Pregnancy
	13	40	Sex difficulty
	14	39	Gaining a new family member through birth, adoption or remarriage
	15	39	Major business readjustments
	16	38	Major change in financial state
	17	37	Death of close friend
	18	36	Change to a different line of work
	19	35	Major increase in the number of arguments with spouse
	20	31	Taking on a mortgage
	21	30	Foreclosure on a mortgage or loan
	22	29	Major change in responsibilities at work (promotion, demotion, transfer)
	23	29	Son or daughter leaving home
	24	29	In-laws trouble
	25	28	Outstanding personal achievement
	26	26	Spouse beginning or ceasing work outside the home
	27	26	Going back to school
	28	25	Major change in living condition (building, remodeling or deterioration of home)
	29	24	Revision of personal habits
	30	23	Troubles with supervisor, boss, or superiors
	31	20	Major change in working hours or conditions
	32	20	Change in residence
	33	20	Change to a new school
	34	19	Major change in type or amount of recreation
	35	19	Major change in church activities
	36	18	Major change in social activities
	37	17	Purchase of a car or other big purchase
	38	16	Major change in sleeping habits
	39	15	Major change in the number of family get-togethers
	40	15	Major change in eating habits
	41	13	Vacation
	42	12	Christmas or holiday observances
	43	11	Minor violations of the law (traffic tickets)

TOTAL =

Source: Holmes, T. H. and R. H. Rahe. "The Social Readjustment Rating Scale," *Journal of Psychosomatic Research,* 11 (1967): 213–218.

Lifton's Characteristics of a Survivor Characteristics named by Robert Jay Lifton in his book *Death in Life: Survivors of Hiroshima*, published in 1967. These characteristics included the death imprint, DEATH GUILT, PSYCHIC NUMBING, conflicts around nurturing and contagion, and finally, the survivor's struggle to formulate/find meaning from the experience.

With regard to the death imprint, Lifton listed three key characteristics that were present, including first, the sudden awareness of the deaths of the people around the individual and the shock and realization of the ultimate finality of death. The second aspect of the death imprint was the specter of death that was related to the nuclear bomb that was dropped on Hiroshima. The third aspect was a fear of the end of the entire world, caused by a nuclear war.

Death guilt referred to the guilt that the living people felt about others who had died, such as the guilt of parents who had survived their children. Psychic numbing was perceived as a form of AMNESIA about the event that occurred as a protective mechanism.

Conflicts around nurturing and contagion refers to a condition identified by Lifton to describe feelings of the survivors of the Hiroshima bombing and their subsequent conflicted feelings, causing difficulties in their relationships with other people. The conflict around nurturing was related to the survivors' belief that others could never understand their feelings and thus, any aid was not valid. The conflict around contagion also referred to the societal (and the survivors') belief that the Hiroshima survivors were somehow invisibly tainted by the bombing. The public also feared that something bad would happen with individuals with whom the Hiroshima survivor interacted. As a result, the survivor would isolate himself or herself from others to avoid pain.

Formulation of meaning referred to a survivor's search to make sense of a traumatic event and its aftermath. The meaning is a cognitive way of describing or looking at the event in memory. Meaning by itself does not resolve a traumatic experience, but resolving a traumatic experience will change and affect its meaning to the individual. In the struggle to find meaning, the survivor

of the atomic blast may seek to make sense of it through blaming others (scapegoating).

Many of the attitudes and beliefs of individuals affected by the Hiroshima bombing were driven by the loss of a sense of the future, which was an outcome of the traumatic experience of shock, devastation, and the grotesqueness of the atom bomb attack. The sense of "futurelessness" is common in cases of severe POSTTRAUMATIC STRESS DISORDER (PTSD).

See also SURVIVOR GUILT.

Lifton, Robert Jay. *Death in Life: Survivors of Hiroshima.* New York: Random House, 1967.

limbic system The area of the BRAIN that is responsible for its emotional responses and the formation of memories. The prominent brain structures that comprise the limbic system include the hypothalamus, HIPPOCAMPUS, AMYGDALA, and cingulate gyrus.

The limbic system is one of the oldest areas of the brain in evolutionary terms. It was once referred to as the rhinencephalon or nose brain because of its importance to the sense of smell. It was not until 1937 that neurologist James Papez proposed an anatomical mechanism of emotion, after studying people with problems in the limbic system. He concluded that emotion was stored in the hippocampus, then relayed via the thalamus to the cingulate gyrus and hypothalamus, where it could be subjectively experienced. This pathway came to be known as the Papez circuit.

The Papez circuit is only a part of the limbic system. The survival of the species depends upon the amygdala's ability to react to a fearful situation when confronted with danger.

The amygdala and hippocampus are responsible for storing the "danger" memory for future recall. Imagine early in the evolution of humans a man encountering a wild hungry tiger; he would either have been killed or survived by escape to live another day with this knowledge stored in his brain. When that man and a tiger cross paths again, his brain's ability to search for this information and recall it immediately would certainly increase his chances of survival over those of another member of the tribe who did not have previous tiger memory and might end up as the tiger's meal. The fastest limbic response allows for this quality to be passed on for generations to come.

Although the limbic system is essential to our survival, it also controls emotions such as love and laughter.

See also AUTONOMIC NERVOUS SYSTEM; BRAIN; CENTRAL NERVOUS SYSTEM; FIGHT OR FLIGHT RESPONSE; SYMPATHETIC NERVOUS SYSTEM.

locus coeruleus (LC)   A cluster of neurons in the brain stem and also the major source of the NOREPI-NEPHRINE NEUROTRANSMITTER. STRESS activates the locus coeruleus to deliver norepinephrine to major parts of the CENTRAL NERVOUS SYSTEM through long neuron projections. The locus coeruleus seems to be a focal area in panic attacks. The locus coeruleus projects norepinephrine throughout the cerebral cortex, HIPPOCAMPUS, thalamus, midbrain, brain stem, cerebellum, and spinal cord.

Rats exposed to an uncontrollable stressor will produce behavioral and vegetative changes that bear a resemblance to the changes that are associated with human DEPRESSION, such as weight loss, a decreased intake of food and water, a decreased ability to compete with other animals, the loss of normal aggressiveness, decreased grooming and play activity, decreased response to appetite rewards, decreased response to rewarding brain stimulation, deficits in the ability to make corrective choices in an intentional situation, and decreased sleep behavior.

Symptoms that are reminiscent of anxiety are observed in rats exposed to uncontrollable stress. This condition is also seen conjunctively with clinical depression. Clinical depression has been linked with altered levels of norepinephrine in the central nervous system (CNS). Thus, research has been done to determine whether changes in CNS norepinephrine levels are responsible for the behavioral depression produced by uncontrollable shock in experimental animals. Findings indicate that stress-induced depression is correlated with a depletion of norepinephrine in the brain, and in particular, in the nucleus LC located in the brain stem.

In rats, the LC is located underneath the fourth ventricle and contains the largest cluster of norepi-nephrine-containing neurons in the CNS. Through its scattered projection system, it gives rise to more than 50 percent of all norepinephrine-containing nerve terminals in the CNS.

To explain how exposure to uncontrollable stress decreased the norepinephrine levels in the LC of the rats, experts have suggested a hypothetical mechanism. During uncontrollable stress, depolarization is more frequent and causes more norepinephrine to release than under normal conditions. Eventually there is a decrease in the norepinephrine levels in the LC region as degeneration exceeds synthesis. This presumption is that there is a "bottleneck." That is, the alpha 2 receptors are normally stimulated by norepinephrine in the LC. The result of exposure to uncontrollable stress is a decreased stimulation or a "functional blockade" of alpha 2 receptors. This blockade of alpha 2 receptors has been proposed as a mediating step in the development of behavioral depression.

It was hypothesized that exposure to uncontrollable stress while receiving pharmacological blockade of alpha 2 receptors should imitate exposure to uncontrollable stress that would occur without the drug. Researchers found behavioral depression could be produced in unstressed animals via the pharmacological blockade of alpha 2 receptors. Moreover, they also found that behavioral depression could be eliminated after exposure to a stressor by stimulating the alpha 2 receptors in the LC region.

See also BRAIN.

locus of control   A concept and line of research that was originally developed by Julian Rotter in the 1950s as part of the social learning theory of personality at that time. Locus of control refers to a perceived generalized expectancy for reinforcement of behavior to be either from internal or external sources. Individuals who are internals tend to attribute the outcomes of events to their own control, whereas those who are externals attribute outcomes to external circumstances such as luck or chance. This theory has implications for trauma acquisition and treatment. Internals will have less tendency to acquire a traumatic reaction than externals, according to this theory. On the other hand, externals generally make better psychotherapy clients and are more willing to focus on internal change and self-improvement. Consequently, they should make better progress in resolving traumatic responses. For example, Brown, Mulhern, and Joseph (2002) found that external locus of control was in fact associated with trauma acquisition from incident-stressors. But these external control subjects tended to use avoidance rather than self-exploration as a coping mechanism. Part of these results may be because subjects were firefighters and "being tough" is a value in that culture.

To Rotter, internals tend to show high levels of achievement motivation and low levels of outer directedness, as determined by scales that were developed to measure this dimension. Internals were more able than externals to resist coercion, to adjust their goals or expectations based on their performance, to delay gratification, and to tolerate ambiguous situations. Externals, on the other hand, were less willing than internals to take risks, to work on self-improvement, or to do remedial work.

Brown, J., G. Mulhern, and S. Joseph. "Incident-Related Stressors, Locus of Control, Coping and Psychological Distress among Firefighters in Northern Ireland." *Journal of Traumatic Stress* 15, no. 2 (2002): 161–168.

looping A term from EYE MOVEMENT DESENSITIZATION AND REPROCESSING (EMDR) therapy that refers to a type of blocking during ABREACTION (emotional release) that blocks the continuation of the associative chain and resolution of the affective reaction. Steady progress is stopped, and the client, according to Francine Shapiro, founder of EMDR therapy, then "cycles around the same plateau of information." The same set of emotions, images, sensations, etc. keep recurring in each set of eye movements. Typically, the EMDR therapist will change the direction or method of bilateral stimulation (e.g., eye movements) or offer a suggestion or interweave to help get past the blockage. Looping is not a form of pathology nor a resistance mechanism but tends to occur naturally when there are competing ideas about the situation. For example, an adult client might start looping when thinking of being beaten in the home. The client might claim that he should have defended himself. The therapist might insert a statement like "But you were only a child" to bring the client into the reality of the situation where defense might not have been possible against a grown parent.

See also THERAPY, TYPES OF.

Shapiro, F. *Eye Movement Desensitization and Reprocessing.* 2nd ed. New York, Guilford Press, 2001.

major depression Major depression is one of the most serious and frequently occurring forms of mental illness, and it is often the result of a traumatic experience. Furthermore, POSTTRAUMATIC STRESS DISORDER (PTSD) itself usually carries a strong depressive element that includes a persistently low or high level of depression. In a given year, approximately 5 percent of the population has experienced a major depression. Unlike sadness, worry, or a passing mood, major depression is persistent and insidious. It invades all aspects of the person's functioning and can have profound effects on health.

Major depression is also known as unipolar depression. Its moderate or lesser disorder is called dysthymia.

There is no clearly identified cause of depression. Brain chemicals undoubtedly contribute to the onset or maintenance of major depression, but it is unknown if this is a cause or a result of the depression. Generally, there is a family history of depression, so it appears that the individual's biological makeup plays a role. Life events also contribute, usually in the form of a loss. The loss can be of a significant relationship, such as the loss of a friend, spouse, or even a pet, or it can be a loss of esteem, an important job, and so on. Chronic stress is often present, but does not usually trigger depression by itself.

Symptoms and Diagnostic Path

The symptoms of depression, at any age, are quite dramatic and often elicit concern in significant others. Although depression was thought to be an adult disorder only, recent clinical and research evidence indicates that children and teenagers also can experience depression. Children and teenagers will usually seclude themselves, often in their rooms, so the symptoms are not so apparent. Sadness, crying, drug use, sleep difficulties, concentration problems, lack of motivation, suicidal ideation, loneliness, self-condemnation, and low self-esteem are signs of a depressive episode. Parents should be alert to these signs, because frequently the child or teenager will try to hide their despair and not want others to know. Certainly they do not want intervention by parents or professionals. However, consultation with a professional therapist, particularly those who deal with pre-adult clients, can help structure an approach to the child or teenager that is likely to be effective in bringing them into treatment.

The adult symptoms of major depression include the following:

- deep persistent sadness and/or irritable negative mood
- profound changes in sleep, appetite, and energy levels
- difficulty with thinking or concentrating
- a slowing down or behavioral agitation
- a lack of interest in formerly pleasurable activities
- feelings of guilt, worthlessness, hopelessness, and emptiness
- recurrent thoughts of SUICIDE or death

Often symptoms are accompanied by pain symptoms (headaches, body discomfort, etc.), digestive disorders (constipation, stomachaches, etc.), low energy levels, and headaches. These symptoms profoundly affect all aspects of the person's functioning and interpersonal behavior.

Treatment Options and Outlook

Major depression is usually first treated with anti-depressive medications to improve the individual's mood and functioning. Most people will get better over time, so any treatment is facilitated by time itself. Research has shown that 50 percent of those with major depression will recover within six months, another 25 percent will recover within one year, and the remaining 25 percent will take over one year to recover without any intervention. Medications, therapeutic contact, and social support can improve these recovery rates somewhat.

Medications for depression were first introduced in the 1950s. There are several major classes of medications for major depression: the tricyclic antidepressants (Tofranil, Elavil, Norpramin, etc.), monoamine oxidase inhibitors (Nardil, Parnate), which are used with atypical depression, a subtype of dysthymia, and major depression, and SELECTIVE SEROTONIN REUPTAKE INHIBITORS (SSRIs) (Prozac, Zoloft, Paxil, Celexa and Lexapro). Bupropion (Wellbutrin) is categorized as an atypical antidepressant with some tranquilizing qualities. There are also SEROTONIN NOREPINEPHRINE REUPTAKE INHIBITORS (SNRIs), antidepressants that inhibit the reuptake of both serotonin and norepinephrine to elevate mood. They include such drugs as venlafaxine (Effexor) and duloxetine (Cymbalta).

Generally, the antidepressant takes two to three weeks to become fully effective. Energy levels improve first, and later mood begins to improve. Most antidepressants have side effects that often prevent sufferers from getting up to clinically effective levels or they complicate the use of the drug, and thus the person discontinues them. The most common are dizziness and disorientation, lightheadedness, and sometimes stomachaches.

The COGNITIVE BEHAVIORAL THERAPIES (CBT) have proven to be the most effective form of treatment for major depression, and they exceed the effects of medications or any other therapeutic forms. CBT focuses on irrational thoughts or beliefs that produce depressive mood and helps the client identify them. Then comes the work on ways to modify these internal triggers. Methods focus on switching thoughts once the deviant ones are identified by the client in life situations. The client must be aware, motivated, and willing to practice in order to be successful at CBT.

Interpersonal therapy (IPT) is a relatively new form of treatment that focuses on assisting the individual by learning nondepressive behaviors in interpersonal situations, for example, learning to focus on others rather than one's self, being responsive interpersonally rather than withdrawn, activating one's self rather than being sluggish and dull, etc. Electroconvulsive therapy (ECT) is another form of therapy that is used with excessive, severe, and often psychotic forms of depression. Here, electrical shocks (at the level of volts, whereas the brain works at micro-volt levels) are administered to the brain via electrodes while the client is anesthetized and protected against seizures. The mechanism for ECT effectiveness is not known, but there is evidence that brain damage and memory loss may be associated with the use of ECT.

Risk Factors and Preventive Measures

More than twice as many women experience depression as men, and depression can occur at any age, from childhood to adulthood, in any racial, ethnic, or socioeconomic group. Most people who do develop major depression will experience two or more episodes of the disorder in their lifetimes. If untreated, major depression will last for up to a year, and the risk for suicide is considerably greater during this time.

Men and women returning from a war zone, both military and civilians, often have painful memories of their experience, loss of family and friends, guilt, and regrets during the war and may have a difficult time adjusting to normal life. This can lead to depression and numbing feelings of not connecting to the day-to-day activities in a community, including forming new relationships.

The best preventive measure against major depression is evaluation by a mental health professional. There is considerable evidence that depression (1) runs in families and (2) is preceded by self-defeating, negative, depressing thoughts. The expert can help individuals struggling with suicidal ideas and provide treatment that could be life-changing as well as life-extending. Chronic negative self-talk is almost always associated with eventual depression.

mania   See BIPOLAR DISORDER.

manic-depressive illness   See BIPOLAR DISORDER.

Marshall Type Debriefing Samuel Lyman Atwood Marshall was the chief combat historian of the U.S. armed forces during World War II and the Korean War. A proponent of oral historical truth, he would gather soldiers immediately after combat in a warm and supportive environment to discuss their experiences. He focused more on the events and less on emotional "feelings." This became known as the Marshall Type Debriefing, a method of reviewing the details of the event without addressing the psychological impact of combat, even though the expressions of feelings were respected.

The one advantage of this type of debriefing is the presentation of facts and firsthand accounts of the event, where soldiers were able to share the same combat situation and hear different perspectives of the same experience. The goal of the Marshall Type Debriefing is to promote group functioning and morale through cohesion and leadership and minimize any conflicts of not seeing the whole picture.

See also NATURAL DEBRIEFINGS.

media Television, radio, and other broadcast outlets that provide information and entertainment to the public. In a disaster, the media can provide critically important information to viewers or listeners; however, at the same time, the media's presentation of the disaster to the public can strongly affect how it perceives the disaster and may have a negative impact. This is especially true of children. In some cases, reporters take an almost breathlessly excited view of disasters, and they may report the disaster as more ominous than it actually is in order to build up the number of their viewers or the listening audience. In other cases, information is not readily available, so reporters speculate on the circumstances, sometimes speculating wildly. This speculation can be harmful to their audiences.

In a study reported in the *Journal of Anxiety Disorders* in 2007 by M. W. Otto and colleagues, the researchers studied the effect on children and their mothers of watching television coverage at the time of the SEPTEMBER 11 bombing of the Twin Towers in New York City. The researchers found that the presence of POSTTRAUMATIC STRESS DISORDER (PTSD) symptoms in children and their mothers who were not present at the September 11 disaster but did view the incident on television was 5.4 percent in the children and 1.2 percent in the mothers. They also found that for younger children particularly, the amount of television viewing of the 9/11 events directly correlated to a greater risk for PTSD. The researchers suggested that parental monitoring of the exposure to media was important, particularly in the case of young children. It is also important for parents to respond to children's questions and to reassure the children that they are safe.

See also STIGMATIZATION.

Otto, M. W., et al. "Posttraumatic Stress Disorder Symptoms Following Media Exposure to Tragic Events: Impact of 9/11 on Children at Risk for Anxiety Disorders." *Journal of Anxiety Disorders* 21, no. 7 (2007): 888–902.

medical illness–related psychological distress The trauma that is sometimes induced by an individual who receives a serious medical diagnosis, such as the diagnosis of cancer or another life-threatening disease or disorder. Studies in this area also include parents who receive frightening diagnoses for their children, such as cancer, diabetes, and so on.

According to the National Child Traumatic Stress Network, medical events may lead to traumatic stress for the following reasons:

- The events challenge the individual's view about the world as a safe place and remind the individual of his or her vulnerability.
- There may be a valid sense of threat to life.
- Medical treatment can be frightening or terrifying to a child or a parent.
- There may be uncertainty about the potential outcome of the medical event, with the worst outcome being death.
- Often the individual has pain or severe pain. This is very hard for a parent to cope with.
- While they are under severe distress, the family is often required to make quick decisions about medical treatment that are very difficult to make quickly.

Symptoms and Diagnostic Path

Receiving this diagnosis may lead to symptoms that are similar to those seen with POSTTRAUMATIC STRESS DISORDER (PTSD), causing reactions of fear and horror and feelings of helplessness and hopelessness, mainly for parents but also for children. Some studies have indicated that when a child has cancer, the rates of posttraumatic stress symptoms are higher in the parents than in the children; for example, according to Kazak et al., among 150 teen cancer survivors an average of five years after treatment, about 14 percent of their mothers had posttraumatic stress symptoms, as did about 10 percent of their fathers, compared to about 4 percent of the teens with PTSD who actually had had the cancer. Nearly 20 percent of the families had at least one parent with current PTSD years later.

Treatment Options and Outlook

Medical illness–related psychological stress is a problem that requires more information and a plan of action. It is vital that the individual with this problem talk about his or her feelings and gain reassurance and support. If death is part of the picture, then acceptance is important in order to maintain a good quality of life in the meantime. Since the focus is frequently on the child or teen being treated, parents may neglect their own feelings or hold them in abeyance until a clear path of recovery or course of illness is determined. Unfortunately, the medical establishment also focuses on the designated patient and frequently neglects the state of the parents. If the medical facility has an ombudsman or social worker, then parental care is possible. Otherwise, it is up to the parents themselves to seek professional treatment. Grief counseling is available in most cities. Likewise, most psychotherapists are skilled at working with traumatized or potentially traumatized parents. The stress of a child in danger can also put a great deal of strain on the marriage relationship and may require some form of marriage counseling.

Risk Factors and Preventive Measures

The range of risk factors starts with the vulnerability of the child, behaviorally and emotionally, and includes the following from the National Child Traumatic Stress Network.

- has had severe early traumatic stress reactions
- has experienced more severe levels of pain
- is exposed to scary sights and sounds in the hospital
- is separated from parents or caregivers
- has had previous traumatic experiences
- has had prior behavioral or emotional problems
- lacks positive peer support

According to the National Child Trauma Stress Network, "Early childhood disorders are rare, and often little information or treatment resources are available in the local area." A proper medical examination and a quick response to complaints of children or changes in their behavior or appearance are important to note. Local resources can be obtained from the phone book or online in your local living area.

See also BATTERED CHILD SYNDROME; CHILD ABUSE AND NEGLECT; CHILD PHYSICAL ABUSE; CHILDREN AND TRAUMA; MEDICAL STRESSORS.

Center for Pediatric Traumatic Stress, The Children's Hospital of Philadelphia. "Medical Events and Traumatic Stress in Children and Families." National Child Trauma Stress Network. Available online. URL: http://www.nctsnet.org/nctsn_assets/pdfs/edu_materials/MedicalTraumaticStress.pdf. Accessed December 5, 2008.

Kazak, Anne E., et al. "Posttraumatic Stress Disorder (PTSD) and Posttraumatic Stress Symptoms (PTS) in Families of Adolescent Childhood Cancer Survivors." *Journal of Pediatric Psychology* 29, no. 3 (2004): 211–219.

medical stressors The study of POSTTRAUMATIC STRESS DISORDER (PTSD) for nearly forty years has focused on populations of combat veterans and disaster victims. However, in recent years, studies have investigated more commonly occurring sources of trauma, to include MOTOR VEHICLE ACCIDENTS, violent assaults, learning of an unexpected life-threatening illness of a child, or being diagnosed with a life-threatening disease. Research on the effects of life-threatening medical diagnoses on patients is ongoing with major illnesses such as cancer, heart disease, the human immunodeficiency virus (HIV), and acquired immunodeficiency syndrome (AIDS).

A medical diagnosis can create a situation of extreme fear, helplessness, and horror, a criterion for PTSD in the DIAGNOSTIC AND STATISTICAL MANUAL of Mental Disorders, IV. Medical stressors share the same characteristics as traumatic stressors by the presence of life-threatening events that are mostly unexpected, sudden, and unavoidable, such as a myocardial infarction (heart attack). Despite these similarities, however, there are also important differences in the relative incidence of PTSD and the development of psychopathology, which is generally lower for medical patients.

In contrast to conventional traumatic stressors, medical stressors focus on future-oriented life events, with fears and anxiety about treatment and survival time, and concerns about a possible recurrence of illness, as well as fears about the unknown dangers of the disease. Understanding one's illness and the potential for its recurrence can produce greater PTSD symptoms compared to the initial diagnosis if the degree of the life threat is more intense. According to Mundy and Baum, a persistent life threat is ongoing in the case of cancer, acquired immunodeficiency syndrome (AIDS), and other chronic diseases, and it is one major difference in medical and nonmedical stressors.

Children and adolescents are sometimes impacted by medical stressors due to the sudden onset of a physical illness or injury. At least 10 percent of children with chronic illness have conditions serious enough to affect their daily lives. Hospital systems are now more aware of how medical stressors affect children, and medical providers are addressing this issue from a biological, social, and psychological approach, assessing the medical and psychosocial interplay.

See also MEDICAL ILLNESS–RELATED PSYCHOLOGICAL DISTRESS; PEDIATRIC MEDICAL TRAUMATIC STRESS.

Mundy, E., and A. Baum. "Medical Disorders as a Cause of Psychological Trauma and Posttraumatic Stress Disorder." Current Opinion Psychiatry 17, no. 2 (2004): 123–128.

medications used with trauma   Medications are often used to treat traumatized individuals, along with psychotherapy, in order to reduce the numerous symptoms (intrusive FLASHBACKS, NIGHTMARES, depressed moods, and anxiety) of traumatic stress that impair the daily functioning of trauma survivors. Often medications are used when symptoms are so severe as to block the therapy process. The response to pharmacotherapy with POSTTRAUMATIC STRESS DISORDER (PTSD) is relatively slow, with maintenance periods of a year or longer for the stabilization of symptoms. Since there is no absolute predictor of the response to medications, a psychiatrist who is familiar with trauma-related illnesses should be consulted rather than a family physician.

The medications that are generally prescribed for trauma are antidepressants, mood stabilizers, antianxiety drugs (BENZODIAZEPINES), and antipsychotics.

Antidepressants

Specific medications in the SELECTIVE SEROTONIN REUPTAKE INHIBITOR (SSRI) class are used as the first line of treatment for PTSD, as well as for the DEPRESSION that is a common result of suffering from trauma. Examples of SSRIs include citalopram (Celexa), fluoxetine (Prozac), paroxetine (Paxil), and sertraline (Zoloft). SSRIs have been shown to influence impulse control, sleep regulation, and hyperarousal symptoms through the increased availability of SEROTONIN to the BRAIN.

Tricyclics, the second line of drug therapy, are older antidepressants that include such drugs as amitryptiline (Elavil) and clomipramine (Anafranil). The tricyclics help reduce hyperarousal, intrusive recollections, flashbacks, and traumatic nightmares but do not necessarily decrease symptoms of depression. The third line of drug therapy, even older antidepressant drugs including monoamine oxidase inhibitors (MAOIs) such as phelzine (Nardil), can cause extreme side effects particularly with yeast and fermented products and cheese. The side effects of SSRIs are usually less problematic than those of MAOIs, except for possible gastrointestinal and sexual problems, which can limit their use.

Clinical research has shown that SSRIs are very helpful in treating PTSD by reducing core symptom clusters, such as hyperarousal, avoidance, and the reexperiencing of trauma. Due to fewer problematic side effects that occur with SSRIs, this category of drug should be the first line of pharmacotherapy for PTSD symptoms. It is important to note that medications should be discontinued when the response to psychotherapy is robust and maintained.

Mood Stabilizers

Mood stabilizer medications may help reduce hyperarousal and hyperreactivity symptoms such as INSOMNIA, angry outbursts, mood swings, or irritability. Some examples of mood stabilizers are lithium (Lithobid), carbamazepine (Tegretol), valproate (Depakene), and lamotrigine (Lamictal), an anticonvulsant with mood-stabilizing properties. The mood stabilizers may prevent the development of sensitization (a response) and KINDLING in the first few hours or days after exposure to traumatic events; however, results are mixed.

Monoamine Oxidase Inhibitors (MAOIs)

Monoamine oxidase inhibitors (MAOIs) are antidepressants that are used infrequently because they require a very rigid adherence to dietary controls as well as an avoidance of some common medications. Drugs in this class indirectly inhibit the use of the hormone NOREPINEPHRINE, which results in an elevated mood and higher anxiety threshold. The MAOIs reduce symptoms of panic, anxiety, insomnia and intrusive symptoms. They require strict compliance in abstaining from alcohol, opiates, and other drugs.

Dangerous reactions, such as sudden increase in blood pressure, may occur when MAOIs are taken with some foods. Those taking an MAO inhibitor must avoid the following foods:

- aged cheese
- yogurt
- caffeine in large amounts (in soft drinks or chocolate)
- pickled, smoked, or aged meat
- some types of beans
- liver

The patient taking an MAO inhibitor must also avoid taking over-the-counter nasal decongestants and cough and cold medicines unless they are first approved by the physician. Patients taking MAO inhibitors should check with their physicians before taking any new medication to avoid a medication interaction.

If a patient's doctor recommends an antidepressant other than an MAO inhibitor, the patient usually must wait one to two weeks before beginning the new medication to make sure the MAO inhibitor is completely out of his or her system.

Antianxiety Medications

Benzodiazepines (minor tranquilizers) can relieve anxiety and PANIC ATTACKS, but they are controversial because of their addictive nature and the withdrawal symptoms that may occur when use is discontinued. Although an ANTIANXIETY MEDICATION may be a logical choice for survivors following a traumatic event, more research is needed to determine their therapeutic value for the treatment of PTSD.

The benzodiazepines that are commonly used are diazepam (Valium), alprazolam (Xanax), clonazepam (Klonopin), and lorazepam (Ativan). The benzodiazepines are effective in calming arousal and lowering norepinephrine in several areas of the body.

Antipsychotics

Antipsychotics, also known as neuroleptics, are generally not used for the treatment of PTSD. Only if antidepressants and other drugs are not effective to control extreme anger or self-destructive suicidal behavior are antipsychotics such as clozapine (Clozaril) or thorazine prescribed. Although hallucinatory flashbacks do occur with PTSD, they are consistent with DISSOCIATION and not with a psychotic episode.

See also THERAPY, TYPES OF; TREATMENT: PSYCHOTHERAPY PSYCHOPHARMACOLOGY AND ALTERNATIVE MEDICINE.

Albucher, R. C., and I. Liberszon. "Psychopharmacological Treatment in PTSD: A Critical Review." *Journal of Psychiatry Research* 36 (2002): 355–367.

Hageman, I. M., H. S. Anderson, and M. B. Jergensen. "Posttraumatic Stress Disorder: A Review of Psychobiology and Pharmacotherapy." *Acta Psychiatric Scandinavica* 104 (2001): 411–422.

memory In simple form, information is coded in the BRAIN, stored by the creation of new synapses, and then recalled as memory. Memories are classified as short-term or long-term. The difference between the two may be in how memories are coded and stored for permanent representation. Long-term memory can be divided into declarative, or explicit, memory and procedural, or IMPLICIT MEMORY. It is widely accepted that EXPLICIT MEMORY undergoes a constructive process called MEMORY CONSOLIDATION. This theory assumes that a new memory is integrated into the existing mental experiences and is no longer a separate, permanent entity, but undergoes changes and distortions by associated experiences and the emotional state at the time of recall.

Implicit or procedural memory refers to memories of implicit or sensory learning and not conscious or imaginal recall. These are memories of motor skills, habits, reflexive actions, and conditioned responses and are retrieved unconsciously by accessing these learned experiences, such as driving a car.

A unique feature of traumatized patients is that the trauma memory exists in a highly charged and distressing psychological state. Patients diagnosed with POSTTRAUMATIC STRESS DISORDER (PTSD) may have extremes of retention and forgetfulness and AMNESIA, and their TRAUMATIC MEMORIES exist in partial or completed FLASHBACKS. They may have normal recall or fading of expectable experiences, whereas traumatic memories appear to be fixed and unaltered by the passage of time.

With the research in the past century, the observations of traumatic memories indicate that memories for ordinary events are coded differently than are those of trauma. Memories, particularly for traumatic events, are stored in the body as conditioned responses that can recur intensely if triggered by ongoing events or visual memories. The body experience is the most important resource for treatment of the trauma.

See also BODY MEMORY; CELLULAR MEMORY; ECHOIC MEMORY; FALSE MEMORY SYNDROME; MEMORY RECOVERY THERAPIES.

van der Kolk, B. A., and R. Fisler. "Dissociation & the Fragmentary Nature of Traumatic Memories: Overview & Exploratory Study." *Journal of Traumatic Stress* 8, no. 4 (1995): 505–525

memory consolidation Memory first involves encoding a sensation or an idea into a neural pattern that lasts a few minutes. Consolidation involves the process of moving a memory pattern from short-term to long-term memory storage. The memory in short-term storage is unstable and can be lost quickly. Through a series of processes (consolidation) of NEUROTRANSMITTER release and neural growth, the memory takes on a stable, long-term quality. Memory retrieval (decoding) is a reconstructive process in the sense that stored memory must be reconstructed in the nervous system. Some experts think this process may actually change the memory as it is consolidated back into long-term memory.

The HIPPOCAMPUS plays a vital role in the memory process. The hippocampus is involved in the recognition of place or context. Some research suggests that the hippocampus may participate only in consolidation processes. Of course, the hippocampus is also involved in trauma memories. There is, however, some evidence that the hippocampus can be involved in older memories—perhaps when they are particularly traumatic.

The entorhinal cortex, through which all information passes on its way to the hippocampus, handles incremental learning, or learning that requires repeated experiences. Episodic learning—memories that are stored after only one occurrence—might be mainly stored in the hippocampus. This may help explain the persistence of some vivid trauma memories in the hippocampus. Traumatic memories tend to be vivid and persistent, and they are retained in a single trial.

See also MEMORY; MEMORY RECOVERY THERAPIES.

memory recovery therapies Therapies that actively encourage the client to seek out repressed memories that are traumatic. The risk with this therapy is that through misinterpretation of past memories, a therapist could lead or even implant memories in a client. In past years, memory recovery techniques were used to recover memories of CHILD SEXUAL ABUSE. Subsequent research revealed that some patients did *not* experience childhood abuse that in their therapy sessions they were led to believe had occurred. Serious family damage often resulted in such cases, with false accusations, lawsuits, and permanent family repercussions and separations. Memory recovery therapies that rely upon suggestion and/or hypnosis are no longer used by most therapists.

See also FALSE MEMORY SYNDROME; MEMORY; MEMORY CONSOLIDATION.

Montgomery-Asberg Depression Rating Scale (MADRS)

A rating scale used to evaluate patients' DEPRESSION that was developed by British and Swedish researchers S. A. Montgomery and M. Asberg in 1979. Depression is a common symptom of POSTTRAUMATIC STRESS DISORDER (PTSD), and the rater has to evaluate whether trauma is involved in the depressive reaction. The rating is based on the clinician's interview of the patient and may be used for any time intervals, weekly to monthly. This scale is used subsequent to the administration of antidepressants to help physicians determine whether the medication has been effective in reducing depression. With this scale, patients are rated on the following 10 items:

1. apparent sadness
2. reported sadness
3. inner tension
4. reduced sleep
5. reduced appetite
6. concentration difficulties
7. lassitude
8. inability to feel
9. pessimistic thoughts
10. suicidal thoughts

For example, with regard to suicidal thoughts, a *0* is given when a patient "Enjoys life or takes it as it comes," while a *2* is given if a patient is "Weary of life. Only fleeting suicidal thoughts." A *4* is given if the patient has suicidal thoughts indicating that he or she is "Probably better off dead. Suicidal thoughts are common, and SUICIDE is considered as a possible solution, but without specific plans or intention." Last, a *6* is given if the patient has "Explicit plans for suicide when there is an opportunity. Active preparations for suicide." The rater (physician) must decide if the rating lies on the

defined scale of *0, 2, 4, 6* or between them (*1, 3, 5*) which are not defined on the scale.

After the scores are added on all 10 items on the MADRS, it has been suggested that a score of 35 or more indicates severe depression, although a study reported in the *Journal of Psychiatry & Neuroscience* indicated that a cutoff of 30 was more realistic.

The most widely used rating scales to measure the range of depressive symptoms with patients diagnosed with major depression are the MADRS, the Hamilton Depression Rating Scale, and the Beck Depression Inventory.

Benazzi, Franco, M.D. "Severity Gradation of the Montgomery Asberg Depression Rating Scale (MADRS) in Outpatients." *Journal of Psychiatry & Neuroscience* 24, no. 1 (1999): 51–52.

Montgomery, S. A., and M. Asberg. "A New Depression Scale Designed to Be Sensitive to Change." *British Journal of Psychiatry* 134 (April 1979): 382–389.

motor vehicle crash/accident (MVC)/(MVA)

A car crash often engenders enormous anxiety, even when it is a minor accident, and most people consider such a circumstance to be a form of traumatic event. The level of trauma is based on the individuals involved as well as the severity of injuries that they suffer. "MVA in the United States in 2006" illustrates the number of fatalities and injuries from MVAs in 2006 in the United States.

Motor vehicle accidents represent one of the most common forms of traumatic events in civilian populations. There are frequent soft tissue injuries to muscle and ligaments with immediate pain, swelling, and tenderness. Whiplash accounts for many of these injuries and often involves delayed spinal myofascial (soft tissue) pain and slow recovery. Concussions represent another form of injury and can produce dizziness, headache, blurred vision, irritability, and sleep disturbance. At the trauma level, MVAs typically produce DISSOCIATION and freezing responses without opportunities for the subsequent neuromuscular discharge of energy.

If trauma occurs, MVAs usually produce an acute traumatic disorder, which, after one month turns into POSTTRAUMATIC STRESS DISORDER (PTSD) for most acute victims. Acute traumatic stress disorder is a relatively new diagnostic category that

MVA IN THE UNITED STATES IN 2006

Police-Reported Motor Vehicle Traffic Crashes

Fatal	38,588
Injury	1,746,000
Property Damage Only	4,189,000
Total	**5,973,588**

Traffic Crash Victims	Killed	Injured
Occupants	31.986	2,375,000
Drivers	22,830	1,666,000
Riders	9,156	709,000
Motorcycle Riders	4,810	88,000
Nonoccupants	5,740	112,000
Pedestrians	4,784	61,000
Pedacyclists	773	44,000
Other/Unknown	183	7,000
Total	**42,536**	**2,575,000**

Other National Statistics

Vehicle Miles Traveled	3,014,116,000,000
Resident Population	299,398,484
Registered Vehicles	251,422,509
Licensed Drivers	202,810,438
Economic Cost of Traffic Crashes (2000; estimate for reported and unreported crashes)	$230.6 billion

National Rates: Fatalities

Fatalities per 100 Million Vehicle Miles Traveled	1.41
Fatalities per 100,000 Population	14.24
Fatalities per 100,000 Registered Vehicles	16.96
Fatalities per 100,000 Licensed Drivers	21.03

National Rates: Injured Persons

Injured Persons per 100 Million Vehicle Miles Traveled	85
Injured Persons per 100,000 Population	860
Injured Persons per 100,000 Registered Vehicles	1,024
Injured Persons per 100,000 Licensed Drivers	1,269

Sources: Crashes, Fatalities, Injuries, and Costs—National Highway Traffic Safety Administration
Population—U.S. Bureau of the Census
Vehicle Miles Traveled—Federal Highway Administration
Registered Vehicles—R. L. Polk & Co. and Federal Highway Administration

identifies people who exhibit posttraumatic symptoms and some dissociation but soon after a traumatic event. If the symptoms persist for more than one month, then these people are rediagnosed as having PTSD.

Mowrer's Two-Factor Theory A theory that combined both classical conditioning theory (sign or cue learning) and operant conditioning (instrumental behavior) to explain why some responses remain strong over time. Mowrer argued for nonmagical (reality-based rather than imaginary) explanations of human conditioning phenomena. His two-factor theory helped to unify behavior therapy and explain human responses that failed to extinguish (end), even after many trials. Phobias or fear reactions to particular triggers are cases in point. Classical conditioning postulates that autonomic fear reactions can become conditioned to particular stimuli if the presentation of that stimulus is associated with a fear-inducing event (such as a painful shock or in the case of humans, a traumatic event).

Presumably, the continued presentation of the pain-producing stimulus would eventually lead to extinction or reduction of the fear response. However, operant or instrumental behavior that terminates the pain-fear response will be reinforced or strengthened in its likelihood of occurring. The instrumental response is called AVOIDANCE, and avoidance is reinforcing because it reduces or eliminates pain-fear reactions. In this way, avoidance responses lead to preservation of the conditioned pain-fear reaction by preventing extinction from occurring.

In this sense, exposure therapies that are used with POSTTRAUMATIC STRESS DISORDER (PTSD) are essentially preventing the avoidance response, thus allowing the extinction of the conditioned fear reaction to occur. Furthermore, since words can be substitutes for the conditioned stimuli that lead to pain, words and images can be used in therapy to assist in the extinction process. In fact, images are the main source of therapeutic focus in SYSTEMATIC DESENSITIZATION—a potent form of treatment for phobias and fear reactions.

See also THERAPY, TYPES OF.

multigenerational trauma See TRANSGENERA-
TIONAL TRAUMA.

multiple-channel exposure therapy (M-CET) A
therapy that was adapted from COGNITIVE PRO-
CESSING THERAPY and PANIC DISORDER treatment to
reduce the physiological, cognitive, and behavioral
symptoms of people suffering from POSTTRAUMATIC
STRESS DISORDER (PTSD) and panic attacks. M-CET
is used for both individuals and groups to provide
cost-effective treatment.

M-CET was developed to address the high
levels of physiological arousal and intense fear
sensations that individuals reported with panic
attack and PTSD when talking about their traumatic memories. By the therapist's first providing exposure through physiological channels,
followed by cognitive and behavioral channels
treatment by M-CET, trauma-related cues are not
emphasized and the degree of reaction is thereby
reduced. These cues by themselves are not dangerous but they become linked at the time of the
trauma.

Exposure exercises focus on physiological channels, and they are conducted through INTEROCEP-
TIVE EXPOSURE to physiological reactions based on
treatment methods of panic disorder. To bring
the panic-like sensations as a point of focus, the
individual is asked to perform such exercises as
spinning in a chair, hyperventilating, or breathing through a straw. The treatment aim is to
reduce fearful preoccupation to physical sensations, thereby reducing fearful reactions to trauma
reminders.

Exposure to cognitive channels is organized
through writing assignments about the individual's
traumatic experience. Writing provides a mechanism for individuals to describe the traumatic event
in detail while still maintaining confidentiality
among group members. Exposure through behavioral channels is accessed through IN VIVO THERAPY
using conditioned cues of trauma.

M-CET also provides education about PTSD and
panic attack symptoms to help prevent individuals
from catastrophizing (making a situation worse
than it really is). M-CET further allows individuals to challenge distorted beliefs by relying on facts

about the trauma in order to process the traumatic
experience.

See also THERAPY, TYPES OF.

Falsett, S. A., H. S. Resnick, J. Davis, and N. G. Gallagher. "Treatment of Posttraumatic Stress Disorder with
Comorbid Panic Attacks: Combining Cognitive Processing Therapy with Panic Control Treatment Techniques." *Group Dynamics: Theory, Research, and Practice*
5, no. 4 (2001): 252–260.

multiple personality disorder (MPD) See
DISSOCIATION.

multiple stressor debriefing model (MSDM) A
modification by Armstrong, O'Callahan, and Marmar (1991) of Jeffrey Mitchell's CRITICAL INCIDENT
STRESS DEBRIEFING (CISD) model for Red Cross personnel who were engaged in long-term relief operations following the 1989 San Francisco earthquake.
The multiple stressor debriefing model (MSDM)
accounts for the fact that major disasters can last
for days, weeks, or even months, as in the Katrina
hurricane disaster of 2005 and Hurricane Ike in
Texas in 2008. Debriefings are scheduled near the
end of the disaster response, and all relief personnel
involved are invited to attend, not only those who
are showing signs of symptomatic stress. The four-
phase MSDM debriefing model is as follows:

1. The first phase is the disclosure of events. It
   allows participants to talk about their experiences, both positive and negative. Group
   facilitators communicate the importance of confidentiality and emphasize that a debriefing is
   neither psychotherapy nor an operations critique of the emergency response.
2. The second phase is feelings and reactions.
   Group participants are encouraged to talk
   about their feelings and thoughts associated
   with troubling aspects of the disaster, and
   facilitators help them to normalize their stress
   reactions.
3. Coping strategies are discussed in the third phase.
   Group facilitators educate individuals about
   effective coping strategies and self-destructive

responses to stress. It is an opportunity for group members to identify their effective coping skills and begin using them.

4. The fourth and final phase is termination. Participants prepare for their departure from the disaster site by reflecting on the positives of their experience, anticipating their return home, saying good-bye to coworkers, and receiving additional support for counseling, if it is needed.

There has been no research to evaluate the effectiveness of MSDM for relief personnel other than reports of participants' satisfaction.

See also NATURAL DEBRIEFINGS.

Armstrong, K. R., P. E. Lund, L. T. McWright, and V. Tichenor. "Multiple Stressor Debriefing and the American Red Cross: The East Bay Hills Fire Experience." *Social Work* 40 (1995): 83–90.

narrative memory Memory that is constructed from both semantic (words) and symbolic (pictures) memories, is adaptive, changes over time, and is influenced by the individual's sense of self. Narrative memory can be condensed or expanded depending upon the social contexts. It appears that as people become more aware of their traumatic experience, they construct a narrative memory to explain what happened to them.

B. van der Kolk and R. Fisler found critical differences between the ways that people experience traumatic memory versus narrative memory. The researchers state that the very nature of traumatic memories are dissociative, and they are initially stored as sensory fragments and images that do not have a stable coherent semantic (explanation) component. Transcribing intrusive traumatic memories into a personal narrative does not match up to a one-to-one correspondence of what actually happened.

The process of forming the narrative out of disparate sensory elements of a life experience is probably much like how people construct narrative memory out of ordinary conditions to understand themselves or the events of their lives. However, when people have day-to-day non-TRAUMATIC EVENTs, the sensory elements of these events are not registered in the brain separately but rather are automatically integrated into the personal narrative.

See also MEMORY; MEMORY CONSOLIDATION.

van der Kolk, B., and R. Fisler. "Dissociation and the Fragmentary Nature of Traumatic Memories: Overview and Exploratory Study." *Journal of Traumatic Stress* 8, no. 4 (1995): 505–525.

National Crime Victimization Survey (NCVS) An annual survey of information that is collected by the U.S. Census Bureau for the Bureau of Justice Statistics within the Justice Department on the victims of serious crimes, including assault, theft, burglary, rape, motor vehicle theft, purse snatching, pocket picking, and crimes that occur in school to children ages 12 to 18 years. The information is drawn from Ohio, Michigan, and West Virginia, and the data is generalized to the United States for a national estimate. Victims of such crimes are often severely traumatized and some experience POSTTRAUMATIC STRESS DISORDER (PTSD).

The most recent data from the National Crime Victimization Survey as of this writing was published in September 2006 for the year 2005. According to this report, in 2005, there were 23 million violent and property crimes, including 5.2 million violent crimes (rape, sexual assault, robbery, aggravated assault, and simple assault) and 227,000 personal thefts (purse snatching and pocket picking).

The rates for most crimes reported by the National Crime Victimization Survey for 2005 were similar to previous years. However, the rate of firearm violence increased from 1.4 victimizations per 1,000 persons age 12 and older in 2004 to 2.0 victimizations in 2005. In addition, the number of robberies increased from 501,820 in 2004 to 624,850 in 2005. The number of other crimes, such as rape/sexual assault, motor vehicle theft, and theft, decreased from 2004 to 2005. (SEE TABLE ON PAGE 179.)

Demographics of Victims of Crime

According to the demographic data on crime victims, males were more likely to be victimized by strangers (54 percent of all violence was against males), while females were more likely to be victimized by people they knew (64 percent). There were

CRIMINAL VICTIMIZATION, NUMBERS, AND RATES, 2004 AND 2005

Type of crime	Number of victimizations		Victimization rate (per 1,000 persons age 12 or older or per 1,000 households)	
	2004	2005	2004	2005
All crimes	24,061,120	23,440,710	—	—
Violent crimes*	5,182,660	5,173,710	21.4	21.2
Rape/sexual assault	209,880	191,670	0.9	0.8
Robbery	501,820	624,850	2.1	2.6
Assault	4,470,960	4,357,190	18.5	17.8
Aggravated	1,030,080	1,052,260	4.3	4.3
Simple	3,440,880	3,304,930	14.2	13.5
Personal theft	224,070	227,070	0.9	0.9
Property crimes	18,654,400	18,039,930	161.1	154.0
Household burglary	3,427,690	3,456,220	29.6	29.5
Motor vehicle theft	1,014,770	978,120	8.8	8.4
Theft	14,211,940	13,605,590	122.8	116.2

* The data is based on interviews with victims and therefore cannot measure murders. The total population ages 12 or older was an estimated 241,703,710 in 2004 and 244,493,430 in 2005.
Source: Bureau of Justice Statistics, "National Crime Victimization Survey: Criminal Victimization, 2005," *Bureau of Justice Statistics Bulletin* (September 2006): 2.

also racial and age differences among crime victims. In 2005, those of two or more races or blacks and individuals age 24 and younger had the greatest risk of being victims of crime. In 2005, Hispanics were more likely to be victimized than were non-Hispanics. "Violent Victimization Rates for Selected Demographic Groups, 2004–2005" illustrates information about gender, race, and income.

In addition, some categories of individuals had a higher rate of victimization than others; for example, never-married individuals had the highest rate of victimization (followed by those who were divorced or separated), as did those who lived in either urban or rural areas. Individuals with a household income of less than $7,500 were more likely to be robbed or assaulted than were those with incomes of $35,000 or more; however, individuals in all income categories were almost equally likely to be raped or sexually assaulted. (SEE TABLE ON PAGE 180.)

See also RAPE TRAUMA SYNDROME.

Bureau of Justice Statistics. "National Crime Victimization Survey: Criminal Victimization, 2005." *Bureau of Justice Statistics Bulletin* (September 2006): 1–12.

VIOLENT VICTIMIZATION RATES FOR SELECTED DEMOGRAPHIC GROUPS, 2004–2005

Demographic characteristic of victim	Number of violent crimes per 1,000 persons age 12 or older	
	2004	2005
Gender		
Male	25.0	25.5
Female	18.1	17.1
Race		
White	21.0	20.1
Black	26.0	27.0
Other race	12.7	13.9
Two or more races	51.6	83.6
Hispanic origin		
Hispanic	18.2	25.0
Non-Hispanic	21.9	20.6
Annual household income		
Less than $7,500	38.4	37.7
$7,500–14,999	39.0	26.5
$15,000–24,999	24.4	30.1
$25,000–34,999	22.1	26.1
$35,000–49,999	21.6	22.4
$50,000–74,999	22.1	21.1
$75,000 or more	17.0	16.4

Source: Adapted from Bureau of Justice Statistics, "National Crime Victimization Survey: Criminal Victimization, 2005," *Bureau of Justice Statistics Bulletin* (September 2006): 6.

RATES OF VIOLENT CRIME AND PERSONAL THEFT, BY HOUSEHOLD INCOME, MARITAL STATUS, REGION, AND LOCATION OF RESIDENCE OF VICTIMS, 2005

Demographic characteristic of victim	Population	All	Rape/ sexual assault	Robbery	Assault Total	Assault Aggravated	Assault Simple	Personal theft
Household income								
Less than $7,500	8,367,490	37.6	2.2	5.6	29.8	9.7	20.1	3.2
$7,500–14,999	14,798,200	26.5	0.6	4.9	21. 0	6.8	14.2	1.6
$15,000–24,999	22,414,530	30.1	1.4	3.5	25 .2	6.4	18.8	1.1
$25,000–34,999	22,504,200	26.1	1.7	2.8	21 .6	5.2	16.4	1.0
$35,000–49,999	30,575,740	22.4	0.9	2.5	19 .0	4.3	14.7	1.1
$50,000–74,999	35,692,930	21.1	0.5	1.8	18 .8	4.3	14.5	0.6
$75,000 or more	52,979,190	16.4	0.6	2.1	13.7	2.6	11.1	1.0
Marital status								
Never married	79,664,210	37.4	1.4	4.8	31.2	7.7	23.5	1.5
Married	122,198,090	10.3	0.2	1.0	9.0	2.4	6.6	0.5
Divorced/separated	26,079,910	31.7	1.5	3.8	26.4	5.2	21.2	1.1
Widowed	14,312,360	6.1	0.8	1.4	4.0	0.5	3.6	0.8
Region								
Northeast	43,951,390	19.3	0.6	2.4	16.3	3.6	12.7	0.9
Midwest	57,895,360	22.8	0.7	3.2	18.9	4.7	14.2	0.9
South	88,262,190	18.5	0.9	2.1	15.5	3.8	11.7	1.1
West	54,384,500	25.2	0.9	2.7	21.6	5.2	16.4	0.7
Location of residence								
Urban	67,484,160	29.8	1.5	4.7	23.6	6.0	17.6	1.6
Suburban	120,424,060	18.6	0.7	1.9	16.0	3.6	12.4	0.6
Rural	56,685,220	16.4	0.1	1.4	14.9	3.8	11.0	0.9

Note that because data was drawn from personal interviews, data on murders are not included in this table.
Source: Bureau of Justice Statistics, "National Crime Victimization Survey: Criminal Victimization, 2005," *Bureau of Justice Statistics Bulletin* (September 2006): 8.

natural debriefings Formal debriefings by trained professionals following a TRAUMATIC EVENT allow survivors/victims to talk about their experience in a safe environment. In a similar model of intervention, natural debriefings use the resources of peers, friends, family, and in the case of the military, buddies in the battlefield, to provide interpersonal communication about the trauma. Naturally occurring discussions of "what happened" to "how are you feeling" may be universal responses following a devastating traumatic event. Done informally, natural debriefings provide a supportive environment in response to stressful times by talking with family and peers.

Fullerton et al. report that the potential advantage of a natural debriefing over a formal debriefing is that mental health professionals have generally believed that survivor groups need to find their own resources of emotional and practical support, both at work and at home. The mutuality of helping each other is the potential resource in the target of disaster intervention.

See also CRITICAL INCIDENT STRESS DEBRIEFING.

Fullerton, C. S., R. J., Ursano, K. Vance, and L. Wang. "Debriefing following Trauma." *Psychiatric Quarterly* 71, no. 3 (2000): 259–276.

natural disasters   Naturally occurring hazardous events (sometimes referred to as acts of God) that result in devastating damage to the landscape and populated cities. Human loss depends on the magnitude of the destructive force of the natural disaster. An example of a natural disaster was the 2004 Indian Ocean tsunami when a 9.3 magnitude earthquake hit the northeast area of Sumatra, killing more than 250,000 people and possibly up to a million in related deaths due to the tsunami. Listed below are other types of natural disasters and varied numbers of fatalities:

- avalanche—snow sliding down a mountainside often mixing with air to form a cloud known as powder snow. Avalanches can reach speeds of 200 miles per hour (mph). Worldwide, an average of 150 people are killed by avalanches each year.
- blizzard—a severe winter storm with strong winds resulting in low visibility (usually less than one-fourth of a mile). The Great Blizzard of 1888 in the eastern United States and Canada led to 400 deaths.
- cyclone—a violent tropical storm in which the wind moves in a circular pattern. Cyclones are also referred to as hurricanes and typhoons, depending on the geographical area of the world in which the storm originates. In the Indian Ocean or Southern Hemisphere, these storms are called cyclones. In 2008, in Myanmar (Burma), Cyclone Nargis caused an estimated 79,000–120,000 deaths.
- hurricane—a severe storm fed by warm ocean waters with winds over 74 mph developing in the Northeast Pacific basin or Atlantic Ocean. In 2004, Hurricane Katrina off the Gulf Coast led to 1800 deaths and vast amounts of property damage.
- typhoon—storm with winds reaching hurricane strength (74 mph) developing in the Northwestern Pacific region. The Great Hong Kong Typhoon of 1937 caused 11,000 deaths.

- drought—a period of unusually dry weather where rainfall is absent for long periods of time and crops are damaged by the lack of water. Drought in India resulted in tens of millions of deaths over the course of the 18th, 19th, and 20th centuries.
- earthquake—movement of the earth's upper layer of plates that collide or slide against each other, causing great damage in populated areas by shaking and torquing. Measured on the Richter scale, a 4 magnitude would be a mild earthquake and a 7 a major destructive one. In 2008, in Sichuan, China, there were 69,000–90,000 deaths from a 7.9 magnitude earthquake.
- flood—occurs when water overflows rivers or levees or dams break, or in flash floods, an overabundance of rain in a very short period. The 1993 Midwest Flood in the United States caused damage or destruction to 50,000 homes and businesses.
- hailstorm—hail is made of lumps of ice that form from super cold water droplets in storm clouds. Their size can vary from a few millimeters to 150 mm (5.9 inches) in diameter. In 1986, in Munich, Germany, a hailstorm felled thousands of trees and caused extensive property damage.
- heat wave—an extended time of extremely hot weather lasting from a few days to a few weeks. The heat wave in Europe in 2003 led to 37,451 deaths.
- tornado—a violent, vertical funnel of spinning air moving at 40 to 100 mph and in contact with land. In 1936, Gainsville, Georgia, had 203 deaths from tornadoes.
- tsunami—a series of huge waves, usually generated by underwater earthquakes or volcanic eruptions, that send water up to 100 feet onto land with destructive force. In Messina, Italy, there were 70,000–100,000 deaths from a tsunami in 1908.
- volcano—the result of highly explosive energy that is released when thick magma and gas from deep in the earth's crust vent in a volcanic eruption. In 1883, Mt. Krakatoa in Indonesia erupted, killing some 36,000 residents.
- wildfire—uncontrolled fire fed by dry brush and winds that consumes large areas of land within

a short period of time. The Tasmanian Fires in Australia in 1969 resulted in 62 deaths.

Disaster preparedness starts with each individual in his or her community. It is the preparation that occurs prior to a possible catastrophic natural disaster and involves organizing available resources and using every governmental aid available. In the United States, following a natural disaster, the Federal Emergency Management Agency (FEMA) provides resources to mitigate the ongoing impact of the disaster upon people and property by providing food, water, and shelter, as well as financial assistance to rebuild a community. In other countries, such as Tajikistan, there is no formal government agency, but local volunteers maintain an emergency resource center to teach people how to react and behave before, during, and after a natural disaster. The goal is to lessen the impact of a traumatic event (hurricanes to floods) on the people who are in the direct path of such horrendous danger.

One such intervention or psychological first aid is CRITICAL INCIDENT STRESS DEBRIEFING (CISD). CISD is a group process, led by a mental health professional, that is designed to mitigate acute symptoms of stress, assess the need for follow-up, and provide a sense of post-crisis closure.

Natural disasters can be traumatic, especially for children. A sense of helplessness often pervades these events. The devastation of their homes and surroundings can leave a lifetime of horrific memories with lasting distress, such as POSTTRAUMATIC STRESS DISORDER (PTSD), acute traumatic stress disorder, ANXIETY DISORDERS, and DEPRESSION. Common symptoms include INSOMNIA, FLASHBACKS, GRIEF, and despair. Every case of survival will rely on family members to cope and lessen the emotional impact of the trauma, and teaching children to use effective coping techniques will help them understand their reactions. It is typical for parents, grandparents, and guardians to prioritize caring for their children at the expense of their own mental health needs.

After Hurricane Katrina hit the Gulf Coast in 2005, federal and local disaster relief efforts underestimated mental health needs as compared to physical health needs. Mitigating the long-term emotional effects on children and adults is dependent upon restoring people to pre-disaster level of functioning, which is essential to community resilience and recovery. Following Katrina, it became evident that family reunification was the most important factor to begin the process of healing for children and adults. When mental health becomes an integral part of disaster planning response and recovery, risks are minimized to the vulnerable population facing natural disasters.

Grant, R., and P. Madrid. "Meeting Mental Health Needs Following a Natural Disaster: Lessons From Hurricane Katrina." *Professional Psychology: Research and Practice* 39, no. 1 (2008): 86–92.

negative cognition A term that is used in EYE MOVEMENT DESENSITIZATION AND REPROCESSING (EMDR) therapy to denote an irrational, self-referencing (referring to oneself) belief that is currently held regarding a TRAUMATIC EVENT that the individual experienced. The negative cognition is viewed as a statement that reflects stored affective reactions regarding the memory. It is a manifestation (or self-evaluation) from the memory, but it is not itself the cause of pathology. To the contrary, it is a symptom or a byproduct of the trauma. A negative cognition can generalize to related events or to the person's life experience. It is not an emotion.

Negative cognitions are organized around four belief-themes. The first is Responsibility: Shame-based, and these negative cognitions are self-worth statements that are shame-driven, such as "I am unlovable," "worthless/invisible," "bad," "defective," or "incompetent." The second type of negative cognition is Responsibility: Action-based, and examples include "I should have done something," "I did something wrong," and "I should have known better." Note that it is mainly guilt that is a part of the Responsibility: Action-based category, arising from individuals' perceptions about their actions or inactions in the situation.

The third negative cognition has to do with issues of Safety/Vulnerability. Negative cognitions here have to do with "not trusting anyone," feeling they cannot "protect" themselves, being in "danger" and "not safe." In other words, there is danger in the environment and individuals see themselves as unsafe.

The fourth area is Control and Choices, in which individuals feel that they were "weak" or "powerless" or that they "failed" to perform or take action or succeed. This category centers on lacking self-efficacy in the situation.

Negative cognitions can have an organizing effect on current behavior but, more importantly, they are a guide to the stored affect or emotional aspects of the trauma and help access the memory of the situation. The negative cognition is not the cause of the situation but rather a symptom or effect of the situation on the individual.

See also NEGATIVE COPING ACTION; THERAPY, TYPES OF.

negative coping action Coping actions are behavioral tools that an individual uses to counter adversity, stress, or traumatic situations. Negative coping actions may reduce distress in the short term, but they also perpetuate the problems; for example, people suffering from POSTTRAUMATIC STRESS DISORDER (PTSD) symptoms may turn to alcohol and drugs for immediate relief, only to become dependent or addicted to drugs. Alcohol dependence can cause problems in relationships with family and friends and place the person at risk for suicidal or violent behaviors.

Other negative coping actions are avoidance, isolation, high risk behaviors (e.g., unsafe sex), overeating, anger, and compulsive behaviors (e.g., gambling). Negative coping behaviors perpetuate negative emotions such as irritability, fear, depression, and anger. Fewer positive activities lead to fewer opportunities for success and positive emotions. People who try desperately to avoid thinking about the trauma may keep distress at a distance, but this behavior prevents progress on coping with their problems.

See also NEGATIVE COGNITION; THERAPY, TYPES OF.

neurocirculatory asthenia See COMBAT STRESS REACTION (CSR).

Neuropeptide Y (NPY) There are 50 known peptide NEUROTRANSMITTERS, including opioids, insulin, gastric, enkephaline, and pancreatic. The neuropeptides serve also as communication devices throughout the body. Trauma exposure and reaction are therefore being communicated to many locations in the body via this communication system. Neuropeptides consist of short chains of amino acids that are bonded together and very slowly recreated in the cell's DNA. They have an enormous range of purpose in the nervous system including serving as hormones, facilitating learning and cognitive activity, regulating eating and drinking, and helping regulate pleasure and pain.

Neuropeptide Y, found abundantly in the BRAIN, is an extremely potent stimulator of feeding behavior and affective reactions and disorders. Studies with animals show that antidepressant medication and lithium will increase the action and amount of Neuropeptide Y in the HIPPOCAMPUS. Likewise, stress situations also increase its presence and, in turn, affect the tendency to intake foods.

neurotransmitters Any one of numerous chemicals produced in each neuron and released at the terminal end of the neuron when an electrical signal discharges the neurotransmitter into the synaptic gap, the space between two adjacent neurons. Neurons in the BRAIN communicate with each other through an electrochemical process. The transmission of the signal from one neuron to another is completed when the neurotransmitter attaches to the receptor sites of the adjacent neuron, referred to as a key fitting the lock. Not all neurotransmitters can bind to all receptors, but when the specific neurotransmitter locks onto a specific receptor site it is described as becoming activated, and information can pass from neuron to receptor site.

There are hundreds of neurotransmitters; the first was discovered in 1921 by Otto Loewi and by Henry Dale in 1914. Then known as *vagusstoff*, it is now known as ACETYLCHOLINE and is important in the stimulation of muscle tissue. Other well-studied neurotransmitters and their actions are:

- ENDORPHINS—modulation of pain
- SEROTONIN—role in mood, memory, sleep

- EPINEPHRINE and NOREPINEPHRINE—arousal and prepares body for rapid energy; released for FIGHT OR FLIGHT RESPONSE

- dopamine—voluntary movement, attention, motivation and reward

- GAMMA-AMINOBUTYRIC ACID (GABA)—inhibitory action on neurons

Neurotransmitter production, particularly the production of epinephrine, norepinephrine and GABA, is affected by traumatic experiences. Early childhood neglect, abuse, poor parental attachment, and trauma can disrupt the brain's production of neurotransmitters such as GABA. People with POSTTRAUMATIC STRESS DISORDER have more reactive neurotransmitter effects, as too much norepinephrine and epinephrine induces hypervigilance, autonomic arousal, FLASHBACKS, and intrusive memories. Imbalanced serotonin levels in the brain may play a role in depression and anxiety with trauma victims.

See also BRAIN.

nightmares   Extremely unpleasant dreams that can cause severe stress and that often cause the dreamer to wake up. They are usually triggered by anxiety, extreme STRESS, DEPRESSION, or a combination of these conditions. Some individuals suffer from chronic and/or recurring nightmares as a result of past or recent traumatic events and unresolved conflicts. Studies have shown that patients with chronic nightmares have a higher rate of psychiatric disorders than those without frequent nightmares. Nightmares are common among individuals with POSTTRAUMATIC STRESS DISORDER (PTSD), such as rape victims or soldiers who have been in combat. An estimated 50 percent of the survivors in the Oklahoma City bombing in 1995 had nightmares up to six months after this traumatic event.

Some dreams are replicative dreams in which the individual relives terrifying events of the past. Such dreams cause a hyperarousal of the body, and the dreamer wakes up with a pounding heart and is often drenched with sweat. Such dreams are similar to the night terrors of children, and the response to them is akin to that of a panic attack. Some individuals with chronic nightmares must

sleep separately from their partners because their frequent terrified wakenings disturb the other person's sleep.

According to Peretz Lavie in his 2001 article on sleep disturbances in the wake of traumatic events,

Trauma-related anxiety dreams appear to be the most consistent problem reported by patients with PTSD. Studies involving veterans of combat, survivors of Japanese imprisonment during World War II, and Holocaust survivors indicate that such dreams persist, sometimes for more than 40 years after traumatic events.

In some cases, a fear of nightmares inhibits an individual's ability to get to sleep, leading to chronic insomnia. In this case, the affected individual cannot get to sleep because of his or her anticipatory fears. This is considered a case of early insomnia. Middle and late insomnia refer to waking after falling asleep.

Treatment for chronic nightmares includes psychotherapy and medications. Specific therapeutic interventions may include IMAGERY REHEARSAL THERAPY, which teaches patients that nightmares are often caused by traumatic yet uncontrollable events; however, after months, these nightmares no longer serve a psychological purpose, and learned behaviors can control them.

A study reported by Krakow et al. in 2001 indicated that imagery rehearsal therapy was effective in decreasing chronic nightmares in a significant number of study subjects, as well as in decreasing the overall symptom severity of PTSD. In this study, 88 subjects were randomly assigned to the treatment group and 80 subjects were randomly assigned to the control group. The researchers found that PTSD symptoms decreased in 65 percent of the treatment group, while symptoms remained unchanged or were worse in 69 percent of the control group.

Progressive muscle relaxation therapy may be useful for some patients with frequent nightmares, while others may benefit from EXPOSURE THERAPY. Medications such as BENZODIAZEPINES may be helpful, both in calming anxiety and sedating patients. Other drugs such as TRICYCLIC ANTIDEPRESSANTS or clonidine may be used to suppress nightmares. These drugs also reduce the length of rapid eye movement (REM) sleep, the time during which dreams occur. SELECTIVE SEROTONIN REUPTAKE INHIBITORS (SSRIs) are also used.

See also INSOMNIA: EARLY, MIDDLE AND LATE; MEDICAL ILLNESS–RELATED PSYCHOLOGICAL DISTRESS; MEDICAL STRESSORS; PARASOMNIAS; PROGRESSIVE RELAXATION; THERAPY, TYPES OF.

Krakow, Barry, M.D., et al. "Imagery Rehearsal Therapy for Chronic Nightmares in Sexual Assault Survivors with Posttraumatic Stress Disorder: A Randomized Controlled Trial." *New England Journal of Medicine* 286, no. 5 (August 1, 2001): 537–545.
Lavie, Peretz. "Sleep Disturbances in the Wake of Traumatic Events." *New England Journal of Medicine* 345, no. 25 (December 20, 2001): 1,825–1,832.
Schreuder, B. J. N., V. Igreja, J. van Dijk, and W. Kleijn. "Intrusive Re-Experiencing of Chronic Strife or War." *Advances in Psychiatric Treatment* 7 (2001): 102–108.

non-accidental trauma (NAT) Non-accidental trauma (NAT) is currently called child abuse or BATTERED CHILD SYNDROME, and it refers to the intentional infliction of pain, injury or humiliation on a child. Such abuse tends to occur when some individuals are under stress and almost always occurs with alcohol and/or drug use. Many perpetrators were themselves abused as children, and they often do not realize that abuse is not a form of discipline and that it is harmful to children both physically and psychologically.

The incidence of child abuse (25.2 per 1,000 children) in the United States is alarming with 5.7 per 1,000 subject to physical abuse, 2.5 per 1,000 victims of sexual abuse, 3.4 per 1,000 emotionally abused, and nearly 16 per 1,000 neglected. These categories overlap but still represent a growing American problem that will not only affect the children who are growing into adulthood but also the adults who have been severely affected in their own functioning and life success by previous abuse. NAT occurs across all religions, socioeconomic classes, and races. It is a national problem.

NAT takes many forms. Some categories that physicians look for are:

- infant or child shaking by caretaker(s)
- falls
- chronic subdural hematomas (bruises, cuts, abrasions, broken bones, etc.)
- fatal head injuries
- retinal hemorrhages

Differentiating accidental from non-accidental trauma to a child is sometimes difficult, but examining personnel consistently note certain signs including social isolation, unrealistic expectations of the child, a pattern of increased severity of injury over time, the use of multiple hospitals or providers, and a history of abuse in siblings of the abused child. Any of these signs would represent red flags to inquiring professionals and lead to a more thorough investigation.

See also CHILD ABUSE AND NEGLECT; CHILD PHYSICAL ABUSE; CHILD SEXUAL ABUSE; CHILDREN AND TRAUMA.

norepinephrine Also known as noradrenaline. Norepinphrine is a CATECHOLAMINE and a NEUROTRANSMITTER located mainly in the brain stem in the area known as the LOCUS COERULEUS that transports signals within the synaptic brain. It is also a hormone released by the adrenal glands. As a stress hormone, along with epinephrine, norepinephrine affects the FIGHT OR FLIGHT RESPONSE through the SYMPATHETIC NERVOUS SYSTEM by increasing the heart rate and releasing energy to the muscle and brain. Panic and anxiety attacks are associated with norepinephrine.

See also BRAIN; CORTICOSTEROID; EPINEPHRINE; GLUCOCORTICOIDS; SELECTIVE SERATONIN REUPTAKE INHIBITORS.

numbing The attempt by traumatized people to avoid distressing memories, intrusive thoughts, or feelings of the trauma by shutting down their internal sensations. Much of this is an automatic physiological response and is a naturally occurring mechanism to avoid painful experiences, much like pulling your hand away from a flame. Energies are spent internally on controlling the distress; thus the individual does not attend to external environmental cues.

Numbing is a common symptom of POSTTRAU-MATIC STRESS DISORDER (PTSD). The survivors of trauma tend to lose satisfaction in the daily activities that once gave them pleasant feelings, and they may find themselves feeling "dead to the world." This emotional numbing is expressed as DEPRESSION or as a dissociative state. There is a lack of motivation to engage with the environment, and numbing becomes the baseline functioning of the survivor. Many traumatized people stop feeling pleasure and just "go through the motions" of daily living. Emotional numbness interferes with their recovery in therapy and they give up on imaging a future for themselves.

Numbing is seen in children who have been involved in school shootings, those witnessing parental assault and murder, or those who were sexually abused. These children become less playful, and they withdraw from social interaction and isolate themselves.

See also LEARNED HELPLESSNESS; PSYCHIC NUMBING.

van der Kolk, Bessel A., Onno van der Hart, and Jennifer Burbridge. "Approaches to the Treatment of PTSD." In *Extreme Stress and Communities: Impact and Intervention,* edited by S. Hobfoll and M. de Vries. Norwell, Mass.: Kluwer Academic, 1995.

obsessional ruminations　An obsession is a great preoccupation with particular thoughts and fears. Ruminations are repetitive thoughts or images that are usually highly positive or highly negative that seem to repeat on their own in one's waking experience. This phrase is an oxymoron, in that obsessions are ruminations and ruminations are obsessions. But ruminations are common among people as a way to work out their concerns and fears for anticipated events, past mistakes, or distressing events. One might ruminate over a girlfriend who jilted him, a job that he or she did not get, or the effects of an examination in school. Ruminations may cause some individuals to stay up at night and be unable to sleep. They may also be preoccupied during the day for a while and find it difficult to concentrate. With time, however, the rumination will fade and one's regular life will return.

Obsessions, on the other hand, reflect intense worry about something from the past or in the future that might be harmful to the individual or others. Obsessions produce fear and keep it going unless or until the obsession is dealt with. At a clinical level, obsessions usually take the form of excessive washing and checking thoughts that are related to danger. Washing obsessions usually have to do with possible contamination from substances that are real or imaginary. The fear is of contamination, getting sick, or dying. Unfortunately, at clinical levels, obsessions are usually irrational or totally out of proportion to reality. Compulsions develop in order to reduce anxiety from the obsessions.

Another obsession category is checking behavior, which involves the fear of making an error that will harm the individual or others. Worries about whether something is locked are common—front doors, car doors, and safes might be checked over and over to be sure that they are locked. Checking occurs not just once or twice but multiple times, often leading to hours of checking.

This level of obsessive behavior is one that interferes with one's life in that it takes excessive time and focus, and the individual lives and plans his or her life around the irrational concern. Obsessions can lead to obsessive-compulsive disorder, which is one form of ANXIETY DISORDER. Obsessions are chronic, prolonged, engaging, and fear inducing. It is the individual's own thoughts turned against himself or herself, so that the obsession is difficult to stop, difficult to treat, and difficult to erase.

See also ANTI-ANXIETY MEDICATION; BENZODIAZEPINE; THERAPY, TYPES OF.

obsessive-compulsive disorder (OCD)　Obsessive-compulsive disorder (OCD) involves worried thoughts, anxiety, and an effort to undo or diminish this anxiety. About 3.3 million adults have OCD in the United States.

Symptoms and Diagnostic Path

Obsessions are persistent, worrisome, and unwelcome thoughts or images that intensify anxiety that the individual cannot seem to control. These thoughts could be of contamination, errors, sexual ideas, religious preoccupations, medical/disease-oriented thoughts, or vague thoughts of harming oneself or others. Compulsions are rituals that are aimed at reducing or eliminating the obsessively driven anxiety. These rituals are stereotypical to the individual but usually fall into the two broad categories of either washing or checking.

Washing rituals or compulsions involve efforts to remove perceived dangerous outside or inside triggers by individuals' washing themselves excessively or washing the environment or both. Excessive hand washing is common. The individual may lose sight of time and scrub areas of his or her body that have previously been scrubbed. Washing can take many repetitions and even hours. Likewise, cleaning the living space in order to separate it from the perceived outside contaminated world usually takes hours.

As with washing, checking that occurs with OCD is far more than routine checking. Checking for the OCD sufferer will persist for many repetitions that occur over long periods of time. Doubt and "forgetting" set in so that the compulsion must be completed again and again until a calmer state occurs. Individuals with OCD often repeatedly check to make sure locks are secured and stoves and electrical appliances are turned off. In addition, these individuals are compulsive about checking and rechecking details related to their jobs. Sometimes an individual with OCD might be consumed with the fear that he or she has accidentally run over someone with his or her car and will return to the location to make sure no one has been hurt. Almost any preventive situation can become extremely ritualized.

The obsessions and compulsions of OCD are usually seen as distressing, senseless, unpleasant, and seemingly out of the control of the sufferer.

Treatment Options and Outlook

Treatment of OCD is often difficult, because it usually involves response prevention (not allowing the individual to perform the compulsive behavior) and exposure to the triggering events (such as dirt, errors, etc.) over several weeks at a concentrated level. As with all anxiety disorders, medications do not cure the problem but they may make behavioral treatment somewhat more effective.

Risk Factors and Preventive Measures

About a third of those with OCD experienced their reactions in childhood. Men and women have similar rates of OCD, and the condition tends to get worse with age, often leading to restricted lives and work.

panic attack   Panic attacks are an extreme form of anxiety in which the individual experiences, usually out of the blue, intense arousal or terror. Heart rate increases rapidly; respiration is intense and often difficult; the sense of groundedness begins to diminish; dizziness, shock, and an overwhelming desire to escape are all present. The panic attack can be precipitated by drug effects (usually withdrawal) but usually comes from a gradual increase in overall stress in the body leading to an increased tension, arousal, and vulnerability to anxiety attacks. Thus, overall stress may take years to reach a critical level where panic is likely. Often there is a suppression of emotions that creates and adds to the stress level. The triggers for panic may be subtle and often involve body sensations that are read as dangerous by the individual, in the sense that the person may subconsciously think that he or she is having a heart attack or stroke or going crazy.

Frequently, situations where the individual feels trapped will trigger panic. This could be as innocuous as waiting in a left turn lane, being in a crowded elevator, or riding in the back seat of a car. Panic attacks have great shock and trauma value. Usually the location or situation in which panic occurs is avoided in the future, and this may generalize to similar situations with time. In the more complicated case, agoraphobia, panic usually leads to a gradual withdrawal from places distant from the "safe place." The safe place is usually one's home, and distance from home represents distance from the feeling of safety. Consequently, the area of functioning becomes restricted with the agoraphobic and can shrink to just being able to stay in the house and not venture out at all. Usually the individual will experience a few panic attacks, and then there are no more, but the shock and fear of having another one can control his or her life forever.

Medications, particularly the use of SELECTIVE SEROTONIN REUPTAKE INHIBITORS have proven helpful, but stress management, cognitive behavioral work with catastrophic thoughts, and exposure are the most effective treatment options.

panic control treatment (PCT)   Panic control treatment or therapy (PCT) was initially developed to work with agoraphobic individuals who typically experienced or anticipated experiencing panic attacks when they went beyond their perceived "safe area" of functioning. PCT is a brief, structured, COGNITIVE BEHAVIORAL THERAPY that has been successfully applied to a wide range of anxiety-related problems that frequently involve panic attacks. The therapy consists of an array of cognitive and behavioral components, including education, cognitive restructuring, breathing retraining, relaxation, and exposure to internal sensation, for example, by having the person hyperventilate or engage in exerting exercise.

The cognitive component involves identifying and correcting maladaptive thoughts and behaviors that lead to, maintain, or exacerbate anxiety and panic attacks. A three-component model is used that emphasizes physical, cognitive, and behavioral contributions to anxiety. The physical component includes body system changes that are due to neurological changes and hormonal and cardiovascular and their associated somatic sensations (such as shortness of breath, palpitations, lightheadedness, and so on).

The critical focus of PCT, however, is on cognitive consequences to these sensations in the form of maladaptive thoughts (such as thoughts of dying, losing control, running, and so on). The behavioral component points out actions that people do when they are anxious, such as pacing, leaving or avoiding situations, seeking help, carrying safe objects, taking drugs, and so on. The three components interact to create the panic/anxiety problem for the person.

PCT teaches skills for controlling each of these three components. Anxiety sufferers usually do not feel in control, and they lose sight of the things that might be helpful in their attempts to flee the experience and the situation. Breathing and relaxation techniques and behavioral controls are taught and practiced in graduated exposure sessions that usually produce panic attacks. During EXPOSURE THERAPY, clients deliberately provoke physical sensations in order to practice and eventually enter actual anxiety-provoking situations in a graded manner for in vivo practice.

PCT has empirically proven efficacy above that of relaxation alone, as well as with anxiety medications, no treatment, or placebo conditions. Furthermore, while a large proportion of clients refuse medications (around 33 percent), PCT has less than a 1 percent (0.3 percent) refusal rate. Promising results have also been reported with PCT with self-help treatments, drug withdrawal effects (from anxiety medications particularly), and with schizophrenics with panic attacks.

See also ANXIETY DISORDERS; PANIC DISORDER; THERAPY, TYPES OF.

Hoffman, S. G., and D. A. Spiegal. "Panic Control Treatment and Its Application." *Journal of Psychotherapy Practice and Research* 8, no. 1 (1999): 3–11.

panic disorder   A form of ANXIETY DISORDER that causes sudden "out of the blue" feelings of terror along with physical symptoms, called a PANIC ATTACK. Note, however, that not everyone who has panic attacks will develop panic disorder. Individuals with panic disorder are debilitated by the problem to the point that they change their lives, and as many as a third of those with panic disorder are housebound at some time because of their fear of having a panic attack should they go out. (Panic disorder that progresses this far is also called agoraphobia.)

Many people who are suffering from a panic disorder mistakenly believe that they are experiencing a heart attack or dying. People with repeated untreated panic attacks often dread the onset of an attack, and they avoid triggers, such as places where panic has occurred in the past. Panic attacks often begin in late adolescence or early adulthood. Many people with panic disorder have other forms of anxiety disorders as well as DEPRESSION. They may also have problems with SUBSTANCE ABUSE/DEPENDENCE.

An estimated 6 million adults in the United States suffer from panic disorder. According to Dr. Wayne Katon in his 2006 article for the *New England Journal of Medicine*, individuals with panic disorder represent 3–8 percent of the patients seen by primary care physicians. Says Katon, "Panic disorder may result from an abnormally sensitive fear network, which includes the prefrontal cortex, insula, thalamus, AMYGDALA and projections from the amygdala to the locus coeruleus, hypothalamus, periaqueductal gray substance, and parabrachial nucleus." In other words, all the parts of the brain involved in producing fear or anxiety may be oversensitized and vulnerable to quick, intense reactions, setting off a whole chain of reaction within the brain.

Symptoms and Diagnostic Path

Common symptoms of a panic disorder are:

- increased sweating
- pounding heart
- weakness
- faintness and sometimes a brief lapse of consciousness
- dizziness
- nausea
- feelings of impending doom

The inevitable effect of panic attacks is to create conditioned reactions of anxiety when the individual subsequently revisits or thinks about places or situations in which the attacks occurred. Avoidance and escape immediately reduce anxiety in a particular evoking situation and become a first-line protective measure. However, avoidance can also spread so that individuals with panic disorder gradually limit their areas of function and at worst, can become housebound. The restriction of one's area or boundaries of safety is usually called panic disorder with agoraphobia. When a significant restriction does not occur but the individual experiences panic attacks, it is panic disorder without agoraphobia.

To diagnose panic disorder, physicians take a medical and psychiatric history to rule out any other medical or psychiatric problems. Medical problems that may mimic the symptoms of panic disorder include hypothyroidism, hyperthyroidism, asthma, cardiac arrthythmias, an excessive intake of caffeine, alcohol withdrawal, and temporal lobe epilepsy. Laboratory tests and imaging tests, if necessary, can rule out most disorders that have mimicking symptoms.

Note that almost all of the symptoms of a panic attack are also those of hyperventilation. David Clarke, a British psychological researcher, has shown that breath retraining by itself can actually prevent further panic attacks.

Treatment Options and Outlook

Panic disorder is highly treatable with psychotherapy and medications. Antidepressants may be helpful, such as SELECTIVE SEROTONIN REUPTAKE INHIBITORS (SSRIs), SEROTONIN NOREPINEPHRINE REUPTAKE INHIBITORS (SNRIs), tricyclic antidepressants, and monoamine oxidase inhibitors (MAOIs). Most physicians choose a medication from the SSRI class first. Many physicians do not prescribe MAOIs because of the strict dietary adherence required with these drugs and the many drug interactions that could occur. BENZODIAZEPINES (ANTIANXIETY MEDICATIONS) may also be used to treat panic disorder.

COGNITIVE BEHAVIORAL THERAPY (CBT) is often helpful to patients with panic disorder. Patients may receive 12 to 16 sessions over three to four months. With CBT, clients are assessed for the triggers that produce an anxiety or panic reaction, the irrational thoughts associated with these triggers (i.e., "I am helpless and having a heart attack or stroke, or going crazy," "People will laugh at me if I ask for help," "No one will help me," etc.) and a program will be developed to expose the client to these triggers gradually and with avenues of escape. Along with the exposure, the CBT therapist will help guide the introduction of new thoughts that are more coping and constructive and less fear-inducing. This is a somewhat subjective process but has proven to be more effective than drugs alone.

Risk Factors and Preventive Measures

Panic disorder is twice as common in women as in men. There is a higher prevalence of panic disorder among some families, suggesting a psychological and perhaps a genetic vulnerability to the disorder.

Panic attacks almost always start under conditions of stress as the precipitating or underlying condition. Panic disorder is also comorbid with (occurs along with) other conditions, such as depression, drug abuse, alcoholism, and STRESS. In some situations, a panic attack can quickly become a conditioned behavior and, as a result, anxiety or panic will be elicited on subsequent similar occasions. For example, if a person has a panic attack on an airplane or highway or in an elevator, these situations will usually induce another panic response when repeated.

Anticipatory anxiety will also occur with memories of the original situation, and this will heighten tension and vulnerability to anxiety as the person moves into the real conditioned situation. Sometimes, generalization occurs from the original situation to other situations. Panic that occurs on one freeway, for example, leads to anticipatory anxiety and actual anxiety when the individual is on other freeways. If the anxious individual avoids freeways altogether, then generalized avoidance or agoraphobia may begin. Because agoraphobia leads to a greater restriction of range and activities, it is usually much more debilitating than panic disorder without agoraphobia.

Depression and low self-esteem are highly characteristic of agoraphobia. Both panic disorders, with and without agoraphobia, are very treatable in motivated people.

See also LOCUS COERULEUS; PANIC CONTROL TREATMENT; THERAPY, TYPES OF.

Doctor, Ronald M., and Ada P. Kahn with Christine Adamec. *The Encyclopedia of Phobias, Fears, and Anxieties.* 3rd ed. New York: Facts On File, Inc., 2008.
Katon, Wayne J., M.D. "Panic Disorder." *New England Journal of Medicine* 354, no. 22 (June 1, 2006): 2,360–2,367.

parasomnias Nocturnal behaviors occurring during sleep, such as sleepwalking, binge eating, moving objects about, sleep driving, or even manipulating weapons and harming others while in a sleep state. In children, parasomnias include night terrors and nocturnal enuresis (bedwetting). There is no memory of these acts the next day. Individuals who have experienced severe trauma may experience parasomnia. The clear-cut distinction between sleep and wakefulness that is present in most people is not present among those with parasomnia.

Symptoms and Diagnostic Path

The diagnosis of a parasomnia is initially based on reports from the patient and others who live in the home, followed by an evaluation at a sleep disorder center. The most common form is sleepwalking. The patient answers questions about his or her medical history, use of drugs and alcohol, and psychiatric history. The patient undergoes overnight polysomnographic monitoring, which records any epileptiform activity. Imaging studies are helpful to determine if there is any brain damage that is causing the behavior. The Mental Status Exam of Sleep can help determine indications of a parasomnia or another sleep disorder.

Treatment Options and Outlook

BENZODIAZEPINE medications are usually ordered for many parasomnias because they have been found to be effective not only with sleepwalking and night terrors but also with other forms of parasomnias. Sometimes antidepressants are effective as well. With sleep-related eating that is associated with sleepwalking (which usually is the core problem), physicians may order antidepressants such as fluoxetine (Prozac) or bupropion (Wellbutrin), in addition to a benzodiazepine.

Patients with nocturnal DISSOCIATIVE DISORDERS need long-term psychotherapy. Benzodiazepines are not given because they can exacerbate nocturnal dissociative disorder. These disorders are associated with nighttime anxiety or night terrors, and anything that enhances the dissociative feelings (such as tranquilizers) can make it more difficult to sleep or relax at night. Long-term therapy is needed in order to focus on the dissociative process and trauma-related precipitants.

Risk Factors and Preventive Measures

Night terrors are most common among children but they may occur among adults as well, particularly those who suffer from POSTTRAUMATIC STRESS DISORDER (PTSD).

Sleepwalking is most common among children ages 6–12, but it can also occur in people of any age. Aside from the behavior itself, there are often secondary reinforcers to sleepwalking in the form of more parental attention the next day. Sleepwalking may also be triggered by sleep deprivation, menstruation, or pregnancy. Sleepwalking in which the sleepwalker is injured is more common among males than females, while noninjurious sleepwalking occurs at about the same incidence in both genders.

Some parasomnias may be triggered by other disorders, such as obstructive sleep apnea, seizures, and neurological disorders. Alcohol abuse may trigger parasomnia in some individuals. Some medications, such as lithium carbonate (used to treat bipolar disorder), may cause parasomnia in some individuals.

There appears to be a familial risk factor for parasomnias, such that if biological relatives have the disorder, their offspring may inherit it.

Sleepwalking

Sleepwalking (somnambulism) is a sleep disorder, evident in some adults and children, in which the individual leaves the bed to move about the home and, in some cases, even leaves the home. This disorder may stem from a traumatic event. Somnambulism frequently occurs when the individual is under stress. It is common in the teenage years and usually declines in frequency with age.

Sleepwalking is a form of parasomnia that occurs during non-rapid eye movement (REM) sleep. (REM sleep occurs when people are dreaming.) Patients who sleepwalk do not see anyone who may be present and generally stare straight ahead, as if in a trance. It is difficult or impossible to communicate with a sleepwalking person, although it is a myth that it is dangerous to talk to a sleepwalker. In the morning, sleepwalkers do not remember what happened.

Unusual Parasomnias

Some individuals have sleep-related eating, which is barely remembered or not remembered at all on the next morning. This eating is usually done in a binge fashion.

Some individuals experience nocturnal dissociative disorders, another form of parasomnia, and they may re-enact episodes of abuse that have occurred to them in the past, such as being choked. They may also exhibit sexual behavior, such as pelvic thrusting, coupled with defensive acts of apparently trying to push a person off them. Such acts are usually in relation to sexual abuse that has occurred in the past.

There also some individuals who exhibit violent behavior, ostensibly during a state of parasomnia. This is probably the most controversial form of parasomnia, and it is also the most difficult to prove.

In their comprehensive article on parasomnias, Elser and Schenck describe unusual cases of individuals with parasomnias, such as a 19-year-old man with elaborate episodes during which he acted like a jungle cat during sleep. Said the authors,

> These episodes typically began 1–2 hours after falling asleep, when he would leave his bed while growling, hissing, crawling, leaping about, and biting objects, for as long as one hour. He then would collapse abruptly on the floor, perspiring profusely, and be completely unresponsive.

The man would not remember his behavior the next day but did recall a dream of being a tiger or lion being let out of his cage at a zoo. The dream ended with him being shot with a tranquilizer gun. (This is the only known case of such behavior.)

According to his family, the man exhibited super-human strength during his episodes of parasomnia, such as raising a mattress with his jaws and dragging it across the room. He had injured his gums and lips several times while asleep. The man was studied in a sleep laboratory, where he exhibited the behavior and where the findings indicated a normal wakeful electroencephalogram rather than a sleep pattern during the behavior. He was diagnosed with multiple personality disorder (now called dissociative identity disorder).

See also INSOMNIA: EARLY, MIDDLE AND LATE; NIGHTMARES.

Elser, A. S., and C. H. Schenck. "Dreaming: A Psychiatric View and Insights from the Study of Parasomnias." *Schweizer Archives für Neurologie und Psychiatrie* 156 (2005): 440–470.
Schenck, Carlos H., M.D., and Mark W. Mahowald, M.D. "Parasomnias." *Postgraduate Medicine* 107, no. 3 (2000): 145–156.

parasympathetic nervous system One of two parts of the AUTONOMIC NERVOUS SYSTEM; the other is the SYMPATHETIC NERVOUS SYSTEM. The parasympathetic nervous system returns the organism to homeostasis (a state of stability) and works in the opposite direction of the sympathetic nervous system. Consider the state where the body accelerates the heart rate, constricts blood vessels, and increases glucose for energy in order to immediately run away when faced with a barking dog when walking down the sidewalk. Once we realize the dog is behind a tall, locked fence, we breathe a sigh of relief and slow down to a walk again while the parasympathetic nervous system puts on the brakes. The PNS slows down the heart rate, and we begin to relax and maybe even think about lunch as our gastric juices secrete and prepare for digestion. This balance is always working—whether we feel threatened or at rest and relaxing—to maintain normal internal functions of the body. Generally ACETYLCHOLINE has inhibiting (parasympathetic) effects and NOREPINEPHRINE has stimulating (sympathetic) effects.

See also BRAIN; CENTRAL NERVOUS SYSTEM.

pediatric medical traumatic stress Stress reactions for both children and their families that are caused by traumatic experiences in children who have a medical illness or injury. Pediatric medical traumatic stress is the response seen in children and their families to pain, injury, serious illness, and frightening medical procedures. These are all subjective responses to the experiences of the medical event itself, rather than to its objective severity.

In the field of traumatic stress related to children with medical illness or injury, there is a problem of understanding trauma with medical professionals, as "trauma" to this profession means physical injury. For the disciplines of pediatric psychology, which include child psychologists and social workers, treating traumatic stress symptoms and other psychological distress with the child extends to the immediate family and the interplay of how traumatic stress responses affect family functioning.

Pediatric medical stress can disrupt the basic functioning of the child and families. Statistics on childhood injury and illness show:

- Five out of 100 American children are hospitalized for major acute or chronic illness, injury, or disability each year.
- Twenty million children in the United States suffer unintentional injuries every year.
- One thousand children per year have organ transplants.
- More than 11,000 children are diagnosed with new cancers each year in the United States, and today there are approximately 250,000 survivors of childhood cancer.

The key symptoms of pediatric medical traumatic stress are the core ACUTE STRESS DISORDER (ASD) symptoms of arousal, fear, shock, denial, and avoidance. In families where the child is diagnosed with cancer, the rates of ASD are often higher in the parents than in the child. In pediatric injury cases, one in five injured children and their parents develop POSTTRAUMATIC STRESS DISORDER (PTSD) symptoms lasting more than four months.

See also MEDICAL ILLNESS–RELATED PSYCHOLOGICAL DISTRESS; MEDICAL STRESSORS.

peritraumatic dissociation (PD) A form of DISSOCIATION (a psychic disconnection from self, body, or environment) that occurs just before the onset of a traumatic event or immediately afterward. Peritraumatic dissociation helps the individual who is about to experience a trauma separate from time and from his or her body sensations and to become "mechanical" in his or her behavior. Peritraumatic dissociation also helps the bystander deal with the event. Peritraumatic dissociation is, therefore, a coping mechanism for preparing for trauma and tends to occur in anticipatory situations, such as impending auto accidents, natural catastrophes, sexual assaults, incidents of domestic violence, and violent civilian and military encounters. Peritraumatic dissociation is of great interest to researchers because people who experience it are highly likely to eventually develop POSTTRAUMATIC STRESS DISORDER (PTSD).

There is some evidence that people who experience peritraumatic dissociation have developed dissociation as a coping mechanism to tolerate abuse during their development, but the relationship is not one-to-one. Children that are physically and sexually abused, in extreme cases, develop dissociative disorders, and studies have shown that abused children demonstrate more dissociation than nonabused children.

Symptoms and Diagnostic Path

The term *peritraumatic dissociation* (an early dissociation just preceding a traumatic event or just following its occurrence) was first described by Charles Marmor in 1997 when he was looking at natural disasters, but it has since become evident in many trauma situations. For example, Ursano et al. found that 78.7 percent of victims of MOTOR VEHICLE ACCIDENTS who were sampled had at least one peritraumatic dissociative symptom, the most common of which was a feeling of a change in their sense of time (with time seeming to speed up or slow down). Other symptoms include feeling like a spectator, outside of oneself watching what is happening, feeling disoriented, losing track of time or where you are, and feeling disconnected from one's body. Of these people, 34.4 percent developed PTSD one month later, and 25.3 percent still showed PTSD symptoms three months after. Peritraumatic dissociation is identified in people who have experienced a traumatic event when they report dissociative symptoms (experiencing a moment of blanking out) and also by giving the person a Peritraumatic Dissociative Experiences Questionnaire (self-report) that measures and assesses dissociative phenomena.

Treatment Options and Outlook

Some emergency room personnel try to directly treat peritraumatic dissociative reactions among admitted patients by using beta-blockers and other drugs to minimize the dissociative symptoms. There has been some small success with this approach, which may have limited success in preventing PTSD. Psychotherapy is highly recommended, with a supportive therapeutic alliance with the therapist to reconstruct traumatic memories and work through perceived threats of the trauma without resorting to dissociation. Some researchers have suggested the use of hypnosis as an adjunct to other treatments to provide a way to create a safe, calm environment where the patient has more control over his or her traumatic memories.

Risk Factors and Preventive Measures

Previous trauma and dissociation are common risk factors. In addition, the intensity of the traumatic event and the associated shock value contribute.

Peritraumatic dissociation has also been linked to the development of acute traumatic stress following an event. While its role may have short-term beneficial effects in terms of shielding an individual from the full emotional and physical impact of a traumatic event, it also has many negative long-term consequences.

Ursano, R. J., et al. "Peritraumatic Dissociation and Post-traumatic Stress Disorder Following Motor Vehicle Accidents." *American Journal of Psychiatry* 15 (1999): 1,808–1,810.

phase-oriented treatment   See ELABORATED POST-TRAUMATIC STRESS DISORDER; STAGE-ORIENTED/PHASE-ORIENTED TREATMENT.

physiology of trauma   When a person experiences a major and severe traumatic event, he or she usually responds with all or nearly all of the body, including the key parts of the BRAIN, such as the AMYGDALA, the cerebral cortex, the CORPUS CALLOSUM, the hypothalamus, the HIPPOCAMPUS, and the LOCUS COERULEUS. In addition, the CENTRAL NERVOUS SYSTEM, the LIMBIC SYSTEM, the AUTONOMIC NERVOUS SYSTEM, the SYMPATHETIC NERVOUS SYSTEM and the PARASYMPATHETIC NERVOUS SYSTEM all work actively in the basic survival mode to keep the individual aware and alive.

Neurotransmitters are chemicals produced by the brain and the adrenal glands, and in many cases, their production is in full alert status during a crisis, including such chemicals as EPINEPHRINE (also known as adrenaline), as well as ACETYLCHOLINE, hydrocortisone, dopamine, GAMMA-AMINO-BUTYRIC ACID (GABA), glutamate, NOREPINEPHRINE, SEROTONIN, NEUROPEPTIDE Y, ADRENOCORTICOTROPIC HORMONE (ACTH), and CORTISOL.

The heart rate/response of the individual speeds up in crisis. The person may also sweat more to cool down the body so that he or she can act or leave the scene (which is also known as the FIGHT OR FLIGHT RESPONSE). When the crisis is over, the body returns to its normal state. However, in a severe or a sustained crisis, a BODY MEMORY of the trauma may remain, along with an overall hyperarousal of the system. In some cases, a chronic state such as HYPERVENTILATION SYNDROME may occur, which is a condition that may be present along with POST-TRAUMATIC STRESS DISORDER (PTSD).

Trauma and the Brain

The brain is intimately involved in responding to all aspects of a traumatic event; for example, the amygdala, in the limbic system within the brain, is a key area for the generation of core primitive emotions, such as fear, aggression, and sexual responses. The amygdala can rapidly place the body into a level of complete alertness in times of perceived danger, and it is a vital brain center when trauma occurs. The amygdala is key to the processing, interpretation, and integration of emotional functioning, and it is also the command center of the brain's fear system. It receives input from other parts of the brain, such as the thalamus, hypothalamus, and hippocampus. The amygdala judges the emotional value of input from both the outside and the inside world (including the imagination), and when needed, it activates a body-wide emergency response. The amygdala also plays a key role in terms of a person's emotional reactions to both memory and experience. In addition, the amygdala activates the autonomic system and the cortex to respond to both sensations and perceptions of threat.

The cerebral cortex is the most complex part of the brain, containing more than 50 percent of all the neurons in the entire brain. The cerebral cortex mediates all conscious activity, including planning, problem-solving, language, and speech. It is also involved in perception and voluntary motor behavior. The cerebral cortex has five main parts: the frontal lobes, the temporal lobes, the parietal lobes, the occipital lobes, and the corpus callosum. The corpus callosum consists of a large bundle of nerves that connect the right and left hemispheres (sides) of the brain. It is fully developed after about age four.

Childhood abuse and neglect can actually affect the development of parts of the brain; for example, a study in a 2004 issue of *Biological Psychiatry* of 26 abused or neglected children compared to nonabused healthy subjects found that a magnetic resonance imagery (MRI) scan revealed that the corpus callosum of the brain was 17 percent smaller among the abused children than among the control subjects. It was also 11 percent smaller than the corpus callosum in psychiatric patients who had not been neglected or abused. The researchers found that in most cases, neglect was a stronger predictive factor for smaller brain size than abuse, and neglect was associated with a 15 to 18 percent reduction in the corpus callosum regions. However, sexual abuse was the strongest factor for the reduced size of the corpus callosum in girls.

The hippocampus is another important area of the brain. The hippocampus, located between the brain stem and the cortex, plays a major role in memory, particularly episodic or body memory for stressful events. Reexposure to previously stressful or traumatic events or events that are similar to those in the past will then trigger a hippocampal response, which will then result in an arousal/anxiety reaction in both the brain and the body.

The hypothalamus is a small area near the base of the brain, just ventral to the thalamus. It is said that this structure is "the door from the brain to the body." It is here that neurons interface with neuropeptides that travel to the pituitary gland and stimulate the release of hormones throughout the body. These hormones regulate body temperature, appetite, sexual behavior, levels of fear and aggression, and the sleep cycle.

The hypothalamus also serves as a gateway for the brain to stimulate stress responses in the body,

such as an increased heart rate, an elevated blood pressure, and the divergence of energy to the muscles and the brain. The hypothalamus is crucial in signaling the pituitary glands to release stress hormones when an individual perceives threatening situations. The adrenal glands are signaled by the hypothalamus to release cortisol, epinephrine, and norepinephrine into the bloodstream. The immediate reaction to this release is the speeding up of the heart rate, the breathing rate, the overall body metabolism, and the blood pressure. In response to physical or mental stress, corticotrophin-releasing hormone (CRH) is released from the hypothalamus, which in turn triggers the production of adrenocorticotropic hormone (ACTH). It is ACTH itself which stimulates the release of cortisol and GLUCOCORTICOIDS.

The HYPOTHALAMIC-PITUITARY-ADRENAL (HPA) AXIS is also involved with the hypothalamus. The connections between the hypothalamus, pituitary, and adrenal glands lead to the release or the inhibition of hormones. The HPA axis is the main pathway for both the stress system and stress response.

The locus coeruleus is a cluster of neurons in the brain stem and the major source of norepinephrine. Stress activates the locus coeruleus to deliver norepinephrine to major parts of the central nervous system through long neuron projections. The locus coeruleus also seems to be a focal area in panic attacks.

Studies of rats exposed to an uncontrollable stressor showed that they produced behavioral and vegetative changes that bore a resemblance to changes associated with human depression, such as weight loss, a decreased intake of food and water, a decreased ability to compete with other animals, the loss of normal aggressiveness, deficits in the ability to make correction choices in an intentional situation, and decreased sleep behavior. Research findings indicate that stress-induced depression is correlated with a depletion of norepinephrine in the brain, and in particular, in the nucleus locus coeruleus located in the brain stem.

The thalamus is the neurological center in the brain that acts as a sensory gateway to other parts, processing sensory information from the outside world and relaying it to the cortex. During times of stress, the thalamus works with the hippocampus and amygdala to filter sensory input and coordinate the relay of this information. Virtually all sensory input goes through the thalamus, except smell, which goes directly to the limbic system.

Trauma and the Nervous Systems

The autonomic nervous system (ANS) helps regulate blood pressure and also controls the constriction and dilation of blood vessels, the size of the pupils of the eyes, the heart's electrical activity, and the contraction and relaxation of smooth muscles. In addition, the ANS also regulates the movement of the stomach, intestines, and the salivary glands. Another part of the ANS, called the enteric nervous system, acts to regulate the digestive organs and is thought to be a very early form of the brain.

The sympathetic nervous system (SNS) activates the sympathetic adrenal response, which is commonly known as the fight or flight response. It prepares the body for the response of fear, fight, and escape during a period of very high stress. The sympathetic preganglionic fibers originate in the spinal cord and end in the adrenal medulla. It is here where acetylcholine is secreted, a chemical which triggers the release of both epinephrine (adrenaline) and norepinephrine. This response acts directly on the cardiovascular system and diverts blood flow from the skin to muscle, brain, and heart. The sympathetic nervous system also raises blood pressure, dilates the pupils of the eyes, stimulates heartbeat, and converts glycogen in the liver to glucose used for energy.

The parasympathetic nervous system (PNS) works to save energy, and as a result, it is often referred to as the "rest and digest" response. The PNS works to slow down the heart rate, lower blood pressure, and return the function of digestion to a calm resting state. The PNS and SNS work together to bring body functions back to normal. In times of danger, the body prepares itself for either fight or flight through the SNS, and when the danger or emergency is over, the PNS works to reverse these actions.

Neurotransmitters and Stress Hormones A
variety of chemical actions serve to propel the body into full alertness or calm the body down when the crisis is over. For example, CATECHOLAMINES are chemical compounds in the body that act as both hormones and NEUROTRANSMITTERS. The three most common catecholamines are epinephrine, norepinephrine, and dopamine. A catecholamine responds to traumatic stress by preparing the body for fight or flight responses. However, in general, they prepare the body to act rather than to flee.

Epinephrine is released by the adrenal medulla. In times of stress, this catecholamine increases the heart rate, dilates the pupils, and constricts the small capillaries in the skin while also dilating the arteries in muscles.

Norepinephrine is a neurotransmitter located in the locus coeruleus. It is also a hormone released by the adrenal glands in times of trauma. Norepinephrine affects the fight or flight response of the individual through the sympathetic nervous system by increasing the heart rate and releasing needed extra energy to the muscle and brain.

Dopamine is a precursor (forerunner) of adrenaline. As a neurotransmitter, dopamine is similar to adrenaline, and it affects the brain areas that control movement, emotional response, and the ability to experience pleasure. Addiction-prone people refer to dopamine as the "gusto" brain chemical, as it results from naturally rewarding experiences such as sex and food.

Serotonin is a neurotransmitter that helps relay messages from one area of the brain to another, modulating anger, aggression, body temperature, sleep, appetite, and mood. Serotonin is important for adequately coping with stress, as low serotonin functioning is implicated in depression and ANXIETY DISORDERS.

Cortiocosteroids are produced in the cortex of the adrenal gland. The two main groups of corticosteroids are glucocorticoids, which are essential in carbohydrate, fat, and protein metabolism and are involved in the body's stress response system, and mineralocorticoids, which regulate the electrolyte and salt-water balance within the body. The main hormone produced by the adrenal cortex that seems to be indicative of posttraumatic stress disorder (PTSD) is cortisol. This substance is associated with chronic stress reactions and seems to be involved in sustained autonomic arousal.

Cortisol acts to increase blood sugar levels for energy, heightens memory functioning, increases pain threshold, and increases immune function.

Cortisol also brings the body back to homeostasis once the stress reaction passes. Immune dysfunction results from chronic, long-term stress on the body, as higher levels of cortisol in the bloodstream have negative effects on health. Excessive cortisol can also interfere with how neurotransmitters function for memory retrieval, resulting in confusion or the mind going "blank" during a crisis situation. This substance is associated with chronic stress reactions and also is apparently involved in a state of sustained autonomic arousal. If arousal remains chronic, cortisol will atrophy the hippocampal structure over time. Atrophy to parts of the hippocampus create problems with memory and learning and tend to fire up the arousal system too easily.

Some studies have shown that survivors of CHILD SEXUAL ABUSE have abnormally suppressed levels of cortisol in the DEXAMETHASONE SUPPRESSION TEST, years after the abuse had occurred. A study of pregnant women near the World Trade Center at the time of the SEPTEMBER 11, 2001, attacks found that nearly half of the mothers who developed PTSD had higher levels of cortisol than mothers who did not develop PTSD. Mothers who had PTSD also rated their babies as having greater distress to loud noises, new foods, and unfamiliar people than mothers without PTSD. Another study showed prenatal stress to be related later to more difficult infant behavior and emotional problems, such as more crying and negative facial expressions.

A subtle but pervasive source of trauma is what is also called TRANSGENERATIONAL TRAUMA. This type of trauma occurs in children of traumatized individuals, but it is usually subliminal or less obvious. For example, second generation survivors of the Holocaust (Yehuda et al., 1995) and of the Armenian genocide show significantly lowered cortisol levels, indicating a stress component in their lives. Similar effects are evident in the children of World War II veterans, of tsunami victims, and of victims of other civilian catastrophes.

Acetylcholine is a neurotransmitter that stimulates both the peripheral and central nervous system nerves in humans and in most organisms. In the peripheral system, acetylcholine's presence stimulates muscle contractions and tension. In the brain, it causes excitatory actions. Glands that receive impulses from the parasympathetic nervous system are also stimulated by this chemical. Nerve gas agents (such as Sarin) inhibit the enzyme that breaks down acetylcholine, resulting in the continuous stimulation of muscles, glands, and the central nervous system. Acetylcholine is important in mediating parasympathetic responses in the body, resulting in calming effects.

Gamma-aminobutyric acid (GABA) is an inhibitory neurotransmitter in the brain associated with anxiety, DEPRESSION, PANIC DISORDER, and posttraumatic stress disorder. GABA carries messages to inhibitory neurotransmitters that, once received, cause the neuron to stop firing. It is hypothesized that excitability or anxiety states involve generalized arousal or excitability throughout the brain, and GABA release is part of a feedback system to reduce the level of excitability.

Some researchers believe that malfunctions of this feedback system can cause increased anxiety, generalized anxiety, or the chronic arousal states seen in PTSD. Increased GABA levels in the brain can bind with GABA receptors to produce sedation. Likewise, drugs that also bind with these receptors, such as anesthetics, BENZODIAZEPINES, sedatives, or alcohol, will typically have relaxing and antianxiety effects. GABA, discovered in 1950, and glycine seem to be the most important inhibitory neurotransmitters in the brain. Unfortunately, research on GABA effects has been conducted mainly on animal subjects, and generalization to humans seems rather simplistic.

Glutamate is a major excitatory neurotransmitter in the brain. Together with GABA, it serves crucial purposes in controlling cognitive functions and stress responses in humans with probable roles in the physiopathology of posttraumatic stress disorder. When a person is faced with a stressful event, there is a therapeutic window where increased GABAergic activity can block the adverse cognitive effects of glutamate and norepinephrine that are associated with both acute stress and PTSD.

Neuropeptide Y is one of 50 known peptide neurotransmitters including natural opioids, insulin, enkephalin, and gastric and pancreatic neurotransmitters. They consist of short chains of amino acids bonded together and recreated in the cell's DNA very slowly. They have an enormous range of purpose in the nervous system, including serving as hormones, facilitating learning and cognitive activity, regulating eating and drinking, and helping regulate pleasure and pain. Neuropeptide Y is abundantly found in the brain and is an extreme potent stimulator of feeding behavior and affective reactions and disorders. Studies with animals show that antidepressant medication and lithium will increase the action and amount of Neuropeptide Y in the hippocampus. Stress situations also increase its presence and, in turn, affect the tendency to intake foods.

Body Memories of Trauma

Subsequent to the resolution of the trauma, the body returns to its former state of a significantly lowered alert level. The crisis is over, so the heart rate slows down, and the neurochemicals, hormones, and brain functions all return to the level that is needed to manage normal body functions. This does not mean that the person remains entirely unaffected by the trauma, particularly if it was an extreme one. Both the brain and the body retain a body memory of the trauma, and depending on how intense the trauma was, this memory may remain vivid for months, years, or even for the rest of the person's life.

Adults who suffered from CHILD ABUSE AND NEGLECT may have a body memory that causes them to be more likely than others to suffer from such chronic muscle disorders as fibromyalgia in adulthood. Body memories that cause significant problems in an individual's daily life may be diagnosed as SOMATOFORM DISSOCIATION.

A body memory may also cause a person to unconsciously resist physical intimacy in adulthood, as with women who were sexually abused when they were children or women who were raped as adults. They may experience severe pelvic pain when they attempt to have intercourse with a partner whom they love at a later point in life, possibly as a result of unconsciously tightening the pelvic muscles to keep out the rapist—or anyone else. This is largely or solely an unconscious act on the part of the traumatized woman. Treatment is crucial to overcome this problem.

Overreaction and Prolonged Reaction to Trauma

Sometimes the brain and body overreact or react too long to trauma. When stress continues for a prolonged period, sometimes the body continues to produce stress hormones and chemicals beyond when they are needed, as with hyperventilation syndrome, a condition which causes rapid, shallow breathing with an attenuated outbreath.

Hyperventilation syndrome depletes the blood of carbon dioxide, enabling receptors that normally bond to carbon dioxide to bond with oxygen, depriving all body organs of oxygen. The individual may also have shortness of breath, dizziness, trembling, sweating, and dry mouth. Hyperventilation is the most common cause of dizziness in the general population. It can also produce many symptoms in different body systems in puzzling combinations, as in cardiovascular (rapid heart rate), neurological (slurred speech), and respiratory (chest pain). It is diagnosed based on the symptoms.

Hyperventilation usually is associated with emotional triggers. Studies have shown that hyperventilation is not a cause for panic symptoms. Instead, the link between hyperventilation and panic may be cognitive: panic attacks occur when the body/mental sensations accompanying hyperventilation are interpreted as signs of impending catastrophe (Bass, 1997). However, once hyperventilation begins, stresses from everyday life in combination with new hyperventilation symptoms can create a self-perpetuating cycle of chronic hyperventilation.

Relaxation training is the best approach to treating hyperventilation, specifically breath training. Proper breath training for hyperventilation will involve learning to take slow outbreaths. By slowing the outbreath, the body begins to absorb more carbon dioxide into the blood stream and thereby changes the body chemistry from acidic to alkaline. Alkaline is associated with relaxed states and activates vagal nerve calming responses. There are many breathing techniques, but the most effective will incorporate slow outbreathing. Diaphragmatic breathing also facilitates a longer outbreath.

Teicher, Martin H., et al. "Childhood Neglect Is Associated with Reduced Corpus Callosum Area." *Biological Psychiatry* 56, no. 1 (July 2004): 80–85.

PIES See PROXIMITY, IMMEDIACY, EXPECTANCY, SIMPLICITY.

post torture syndrome Distinguished from POST-TRAUMATIC STRESS DISORDER (PTSD) because both the traumatic events and the effects of the TORTURE produce posttraumatic stress symptoms.

Symptoms and Diagnostic Path

Victims of torture manifest several of the following symptoms that are associated with PTSD in that they may develop anxiety, DEPRESSION, feelings of resignation, guilt, apathy, fear, suspiciousness, aggressiveness, sudden weeping, intensive rage, irritability, SUICIDE attempts, introversion, drowsiness, exhaustion, MEMORY difficulties, lack of concentration, disorientation, sleeping difficulties, paresthesia (of "pins and needles" or of a limb being "asleep"), or sexual and psychosomatic disturbances.

Torture effects are particularly acute and severe because torture is administered by another individual who acts against the victim, and human-against-human trauma is typically much more traumatic than an impersonal trauma, such as an accident or a natural event. Furthermore, torture will produce PTSD or similar symptoms but not the complete diagnostic picture without the need for vulnerability on the victim's part. Almost anyone tortured will develop these symptoms described, whereas most people exposed to traumatic events will not develop PTSD.

Treatment Options and Outlook

Torture survivors are difficult to treat and require great care, as well as caring and understanding. Torture victims are not prone to describe their torture to others because most people cannot understand what they have been through physically, psychically, and emotionally. Torture is aimed at breaking down the individual's will to resist. Sometimes people torture just to see a victim in physical and psychological pain, and almost always these are torturers with psychosis, usually for political purposes. Restoring faith in a benevolent world, one's self-value, the importance of the individual with others, and the ability to take initiative are critical to the therapy process. A skilled and knowledgeable therapist is essential.

Risk Factors and Preventive Measures

Countries that seek to dominate their populace use torture as a political control device to immobilize politically active citizens and make them useless to political causes. Others at risk of developing post torture syndrome include individuals who are refugees, political prisoners, and prisoners of war.

See also WATERBOARDING.

posttraumatic amnesia (PTA) A phenomenon or reaction that causes the inability to store or retrieve new information after a TRAUMATIC BRAIN INJURY. There are an estimated 1 million individuals with brain injuries that require hospitalization, and of these, 70 percent of patients will develop posttraumatic amnesia. In addition, of those developing PTA, a third will experience the condition for more than 30 days.

People who are in recovery post trauma are considered to be "in PTA" when their time frame of memory lasts from a few minutes to a few hours and they remember nothing that occurred after the brain injury. This condition of disorientation and impaired memory may last a few days to a few months, by which time the person comes "out of PTA" and he or she can maintain day-to-day memories. Most people with PTA will experience frustration, agitation, and a lack of impulse control prior to emerging from this condition.

See also AMNESIA; POSTTRAUMATIC EPILEPSY; POST-TRAUMATIC PSYCHOSIS.

posttraumatic embitterment disorder (PTED) PTED is the result of a single negative life event, a psychological process of experiencing injustice, humiliation, or a violation of an individual's basic beliefs. Unlike with POSTTRAUMATIC STRESS DISORDER (PTSD), posttraumatic embitterment disorder is not a result of a particularly stressful event.

Symptoms and Diagnostic Path

The symptoms of PTED are severe, chronic, and life-threatening (such as suicidal thoughts), resulting in the impairment of daily functioning to the point of disability and often job loss. The term PTED was first described by Michael Linden as a compound emotion that includes despair, aggression against oneself or other persons, hopelessness, and mental blocks.

Risk Factors and Preventive Measures

A person can be "stricken" with PTED by such events as a job dismissal, a separation from a loved one, or even a quarrel that leads to intrusive memories of the occurrence and agitation due to the hurt that the individual experiences in important areas that define his or her life.

In a pilot study by Linden et al. in 2004, the authors found negative life events to be a job loss in 38 percent of the cases, conflict at work in 24 percent, the death of a loved one in 14 percent, familial strain in 14 percent, and other events in 10 percent. When reminded of the negative life event, patients reported feelings of embitterment (85.7 percent), sadness (81.0 percent), anger (76.2 percent), or helplessness (75.0 percent).

See also THERAPY, TYPES OF.

Linden, M., B. Schippan, K. Baumann, and R. Spielberg. "Posttraumatic Embitterment Disorder (PTED). Differentiation of a Specific Form of Adjustment Disorders." *Nevenartz* 75, no. 1 (2004): 51–57.

posttraumatic epilepsy (PTE)   A complication of TRAUMATIC BRAIN INJURY (TBI), in which seizures most often occur in patients with a critical injury, such as subdural or epidural hematomas. People who experience a TBI from any type of war wound are significantly at high risk for epilepsy. There is a basic division of "early" and "late" posttraumatic epilepsy: early seizures are those that occur during the first week after the trauma, and late posttraumatic epilepsy refers to those seizures that commence after the first week.

In some people, grand mal seizures are easily diagnosed. They will lose consciousness, fall to the ground, and start shaking their arms and legs that are stiff and rigid. For others, the seizures are mild and subtle, and their behavior may appear odd, including staring off into space, memory difficulty,

and unexplained emotional outbursts that doctors sometimes believe are a result of TBI and not seizures.

In a study by Gottesman and colleagues (2003) of traumatic brain injury in Minnesota, the incidence for posttraumatic epilepsy in patients with nonfatal TBI and without a prior history of epilepsy was 2.1 percent with mild TBI, 4.2 percent with moderate TBI, and 16.7 percent for patients with severe TBI. Why this happens to the brain is not clear. As the brain tries to repair itself by compensating for the injured part and making new connections, the new connections are more susceptible to seizures than the original connections. There is no known way to block this process, but focused research continues in this area.

See also POSTTRAUMATIC AMNESIA; POSTTRAUMATIC PSYCHOSIS.

Gottesman, R., R. Komotar, and A. Hillis. "Neurologic Aspects of Traumatic Brain Injury." *International Review of Psychiatry* 15, no. 4 (2003): 302–309.

posttraumatic growth   The recognition that life after a trauma can foster positive growth on a personal level is a concept that has been studied in recent years. Posttraumatic growth is sometimes referred to as positive change. Tedeschi et al. state that positive changes fall into three main areas: the perception of self, the approach to interpersonal relationships, and the philosophy of life.

Following a traumatic event, people may accept their vulnerabilities, but they may also see themselves as stronger. Interpersonal relationships can bring stronger bonds as people put more value on their family and friends, becoming more open and compassionate for each other. Changes in life philosophy may come through greater spirituality, as individuals begin appreciating that life is precious and reviewing their life priorities.

The core of posttraumatic growth can also be found in world religions that view suffering as having an important positive role in personal growth and development of wisdom. This was noted by Shaw and his colleagues (2005) in their review article.

See also SPIRITUALITY AND TRAUMA.

Shaw, A., S. Joseph, and P. A. Linley. "Religion, Spirituality and Posttraumatic Growth: A Systematic Review." *Mental Health, Religion & Culture* 8, no. 1 (March 2005): 1–11.

Tedeschi, R. G., C. L. Park, and L. G. Calhoun. "Posttraumatic growth: Conceptual issues." In Posttraumatic Growth: Positive Changes in the Aftermath of Crisis, edited by R. G. Tedeschi, C. L. Park, and L. G. Calhoun, 1–22. Mahwah, N.J.: Lawrence Erbaum, 1998.

posttraumatic psychosis There are two meanings of posttraumatic psychosis. First, in a TRAUMATIC BRAIN INJURY (TBI), posttraumatic psychosis is a rare complication that may occur after injury. The individual may experience psychotic symptoms, such as delusions and hallucinations, characterized with the flight of ideas, thought blocking, speaking in nonsense words or neologisms (making up words), and the psychosis associated with schizophrenia, causing great distress to the individuals and their family members and friends.

McAllister and Ferrell (2002) concluded that disorders of both thought content, or bizarre thoughts disconnected from reality and often fragmentary, and thought processes occur in TBI patients at greater rates than in the non-TBI population. The more severe the brain injury, the greater is the likelihood of psychosis.

The second meaning of posttraumatic psychosis is a reference to POSTTRAUMATIC STRESS DISORDER (PTSD) with psychotic symptoms. In the histories of people with psychosis, there is a high incidence of physical and sexual abuse, and there is also a high incidence of PTSD in people who have a primary diagnosis of psychosis. The view that psychosis is trauma-induced is supported by research that childhood trauma is a risk factor for psychotic experiences.

Symptoms and Diagnostic Path

Kilcommons and Morrison pointed out that PTSD and psychosis are characterized by intrusion and avoidance, and they highlighted the similarity of cognitive models of psychosis and PTSD. Negative beliefs and dissociation are factors that may implicate the development of PTSD and psychosis after traumatic life experiences.

Risk Factors and Preventive Measures

Unfortunately, as with most psychosis, there is no "cure" in the pure sense and while there are some predictive indicators, basically nothing can prevent the onset of psychosis, particularly that caused by traumatic events. Early indicators are bizarre or strange thinking and behavior, isolation, interpersonal difficulties, and sometimes hallucinations and/or delusions.

See also CHILDREN AND TRAUMA; THERAPY, TYPES OF.

Kilcommons, A., and A. Morrison. "Relationships Between Trauma and Psychosis: An Exploration of Cognitive and Dissociative Factors." *Acta Psychiatric Scandinavica* 112 (2005): 351–359.

McAllister, T., and R. Ferrell. "Evaluation and Treatment of Psychosis after Traumatic Brain Injury." *NeuroRehabilitation* 17, no. 202: 357–368.

Posttraumatic Stress Diagnostic Scale See INSTRUMENTS/SCALES/SURVEYS THAT EVALUATE POSTTRAUMATIC STRESS DISORDER (PTSD).

posttraumatic stress disorder (PTSD) Posttraumatic stress disorder (PTSD) was first recognized as a psychiatric disorder in 1980 by the American Psychiatric Association in its third edition of the *DIAGNOSTIC AND STATISTICAL MANUAL of mental disorders* (DSM-III). At that time, PTSD was classified under the category of ANXIETY DISORDERS because anxiety/panic and chronic tension were major diagnostic characteristics of the condition. An estimated 5.2 million American adults ages 18 to 54, or approximately 3.6 percent of people in this age group in a given year, have PTSD.

This classification created a conceptual framework in which to study trauma and its residual effects upon the individual. Lasiuk and Hegadoren (2006) pointed out that since it stipulated that an external TRAUMATIC EVENT was critical to the development of PTSD rather than an internal inherent weakness of the individual, PTSD became the first psychiatric diagnosis to have an external rather than internal cause.

Symptoms occurring within the first four weeks of experiencing a traumatic event are diagnosed as

ACUTE STRESS DISORDER. These are essentially similar to symptoms of PTSD (with the added symptoms of dissociation being present in some form) that last for up to one month, after which they are renamed PTSD.

PTSD develops from the experience of an overwhelming or traumatic event. Traumatic events that may cause PTSD are generally life-threatening events such as natural disasters (earthquakes, hurricanes, floods), violent personal attacks (physical and sexual abuse, kidnapping, rape, violent crime), terrorist incidents (SEPTEMBER 11), military combat, or accidents (plane, train, MOTOR VEHICLE ACCIDENTS). However, it appears that cumulative small "t" trauma, or not so dramatic events, can also cause PTSD. For example, just living in a dysfunctional family or viewing disturbing scenes in movies or on television can also lead to PTSD. For this reason, the more liberal definition of a traumatic event is to say that it is any event that produces posttraumatic reaction.

Furthermore, among people who experience PTSD are rescue workers involved in the aftermath of 9/11 and military personnel serving in the Vietnam War, Gulf Wars, and more recently in Afghanistan and Iraq. Survivors from war-torn countries such as Rwanda, Bosnia, or Iraq may experience PTSD even though these people may have not had direct exposure to the traumatic event(s).

Victims can be of any age, gender, or race, but there seem to be some predisposing conditions that make people more vulnerable to developing PTSD. These include early psychiatric problems, DEPRESSION and/or anxiety, previous traumatic reactions or symptoms, and lack of personal support. There is also a cultural concern that people living in poverty and in high-crime areas will develop anxiety and panic related to PTSD.

PTSD symptoms may occur soon after the traumatic event or they may occur several years later in both adults and children and other family members of surviving victims.

Symptoms and Diagnostic Path

The symptoms of PTSD include reexperiencing the trauma as FLASHBACK episodes, memories, somatic (body) sensations, and NIGHTMARES. Reminders of the trauma, including anniversary dates, can trigger symptoms of reliving the tragedy. PTSD is diagnosed if symptoms are present one month after a traumatic event.

Sufferers of PTSD say that they cannot feel emotions toward their loved ones, and they begin to feel distant, cold, and preoccupied. This lack of emotion and empathy leads to poor relationships at home and work and a decline in work performance. Avoiding the places and the people that remind them of the traumatic events can create isolation from others, depressed affect, lack of initiative, sleep disturbances, depression, and anxiety.

Another set of symptoms can be described as hypervigilance, when the person feels like he or she is on guard all the time and is easily startled. War veterans may have an exaggerated startle response; for example, upon hearing a low-flying helicopter or fireworks, they may feel that they are back in a battlefield. Feelings of intense guilt are common among individuals who have survived a trauma while others did not, such as in SURVIVOR GUILT. For combat veterans, guilt can result from witnessing or participating in wartime behavior that was necessary for survival yet which is unacceptable in normal society. This may contribute to the individual's feelings of low self-worth and the development of depression.

PTSD can interfere with normal social and family functioning. For example, there is a much higher than average incidence of SUICIDE and DIVORCE among PTSD sufferers than among nonsufferers.

It is generally agreed that the symptoms of posttraumatic stress disorder (PTSD) fall into six major clusters or criterion categories. These are listed in the *Diagnostic and Statistical Manual-IV (DSM-IV)*, published by the American Psychiatric Association. The first criterion, (A), is that the individual has experienced or was confronted with a major traumatic event that was life-threatening or that threatened serious injury to the self or to others. Terror and intense fear/horror combined with helplessness are usually present. What constitutes a life-threatening or horrific event is an individual matter, defined by the reaction itself and not necessarily by the characteristics of the event. Also, multiple exposures to an event can accumulate into a traumatic stimulus.

The second criterion, (B), is the reexperiencing of the traumatic event(s) by recollection (images, thoughts, perceptions), dreams, feelings (as if the event were recurring), or distress or physiological reactions triggered by internal or external symbolic cues or reminders of the traumatic event. Many of these reactions may be automatic or subconscious.

The third criterion, (C), is characterized by avoidance and NUMBING of general responsiveness in order to avoid thoughts, feelings, or conversations associated with the trauma. Also avoidance and numbing can be associated with places or situations that could be reminders. A markedly diminished memory for the event(s) also commonly occurs. Other effects that are associated with avoidance and numbing include a diminished interest in activities, feelings of estrangement and detachment from others, repressed and restricted affect (i.e., sexual and loving feelings), and a foreshortened sense of the future. Major depression can be the result of these reactions if intense enough.

Criterion (D) involves a pervasive and persistent increase in physiological arousal to the extent that sleep difficulties appear and anger, irritability, and poor management of emotions occur. There are also difficulties with concentrating, learning, and recall, as well as with hypervigilance and exaggerated startle reactions.

Criterion (E) is that these symptoms must be present for more than one month for a diagnosis of PTSD. Criterion (F) is that the symptoms of A–D must be of such intensity and degree of distress that they impair the individual's social, occupational, or other important areas of functioning.

While PTSD is usually viewed as arising from a single external threatening incident, it can also result from accumulated small events. Horrific scenes, such as accidents, fires, terrorist attacks, etc., endured by emergency personnel or by indirect observation via film or video can trigger PTSD reactions. Repeated direct or indirect involvement in dealing with crimes against others, particularly children, where there is pain and suffering can also lead to PTSD in observers or with interventionists.

Loss and BEREAVEMENT are now seen as a major source of traumatic reactions. Regular intrusions and boundary violations such as harassment, stalking, bullying, and domestic violence can be contributors to PTSD, particularly if the target is relatively helpless and unsupported in coping with these intrusions and violations. Verbal, physical, and sexual abuse, of course, can lead to PTSD reactions.

Where the symptoms are the result of a series of events rather than one horrific experience, they may be categorized as prolonged duress stress disorder (PDSD) or more commonly, COMPLEX PTSD. Complex PTSD is the preferred term, but is unofficial in that it is not included in the *DSM-IV* or the INTERNATIONAL CLASSIFICATION OF DISEASES-10 (ICD-10). Its use is preferred over such terms as "rolling PTSD," PDSD, and "cumulative stress," all of which have been used in the past.

Physiological studies have identified specific brain areas (mostly in the midbrain and forebrain) that are affected by traumatic exposure, causing dysregulation and dysfunction and creating many of the symptoms noted earlier. A common side effect of PTSD is the experience of not feeling safe. Victims will invariably report that they do not feel safe or that they feel safe in only well-circumscribed areas or with certain people.

DELAYED POSTTRAUMATIC STRESS DISORDER is the appearance of PTSD six months or longer after the traumatic event. Delayed PTSD, while common, has not been studied in the research literature. The dynamics of delayed PTSD are poorly understood due to the question, "Is it delayed onset of symptoms or delayed presentation of symptoms?"

Treatment Options and Outlook

PTSD treatment includes a variety of psychotherapy techniques and pharmacological agents. Some of the best treatments are COGNITIVE BEHAVIORAL THERAPIES including cognitive restructuring, EXPOSURE THERAPY, and EYE MOVEMENT DESENSITIZATION AND REPROCESSING (EMDR). The aim of therapy is to help traumatized individuals move from the reexperiencing of the past to being fully engaged in the present.

B. van der Kolk and colleagues (1996) point out that typically therapists address two fundamental aspects of PTSD: "(1.) deconditioning of anxiety and (2.) altering the way victims view themselves and their world by reestablishing a feeling of personal integrity and control."

In order for these two aspects to occur, traumatized individuals need to regain control over their emotional responses and be able to place the trauma in its historical place in the timeline, and not in the present. For this to occur, the individual must take control of his or her life by integrating the terror, the incomprehensible, into his or her present life, which includes self-beliefs and self-concepts about who he or she is today. They must come to accept this trauma as a part of their past life that makes up who they are and something that cannot be avoided.

Risk Factors and Preventive Measures

The National Center for PTSD, Department of Veterans Affairs states that the risk for developing PTSD increases if people:

- were directly exposed to the traumatic event as a victim or a witness
- were seriously injured during the trauma
- experienced a trauma that was long lasting or very severe
- saw themselves or a family member as being in imminent danger
- had a severe negative reaction during the event, such as feeling detached from one's surroundings or having a panic attack
- felt helpless during the trauma and were unable to help themselves or a loved one
- have experienced an earlier life-threatening event or trauma
- have a current mental health issue
- have less education
- are younger
- are women
- have recent, stressful life changes

Most people exposed to a traumatic event recover without any long-term mental health problems. Of those exposed to trauma, the prevalence rate for developing PTSD in their lifetime is 7 to 8 percent of the total population. In the United States, about 5 million people are suffering from PTSD, and twice as many women (more than 10 percent) as men (more than 5 percent) experience PTSD in the population as a whole. Why the rates in women are higher can be speculated, as possibly women are more apt to report trauma (sexual attack) than men. Also, studies of Vietnam veterans with PTSD indicate that approximately 15 percent are men and 9 percent are women. We know that in Vietnam men were in combat roles, while most women were nurses; others included physical therapists, air traffic controllers, and intelligence and language specialists.

Some factors that make people more vulnerable or at risk for PTSD following a traumatic event include:

- the magnitude or severity of the trauma
- prior trauma
- post-trauma social support
- pre-trauma VULNERABILITY

Magnitude or severity of the trauma War and combat conditions represent strong risk factors for PTSD, especially for military personnel. The intensity of torture and traumas that include severe injury to the self are highly predictive of PTSD, compared to those who are not injured. Being directly involved in a traumatic event and exposed to seeing dead bodies or grotesque remains can be an overwhelming experience and is associated with acute and chronic PTSD, as in the September 11, 2001, terrorist attack on the United States.

Prior trauma A history of early childhood abuse or family trauma is a risk factor for chronic PTSD following exposure to subsequent trauma, and adult women were more likely than men to develop PTSD following childhood trauma. According to Yehuda et al. there is evidence that a family psychiatric history for Holocaust parents constitutes a high risk group for their children. An epidemiological study by Breslau et al. (2008) found that prior trauma alone did not predict PTSD in subsequent trauma. The risk of developing PTSD increases only among individuals who developed PTSD in response to a prior trauma. A sample of civilian bus drivers with symptoms of PTSD (not the actual disorder) and who reported a prior trauma were at increased risk of a high level of PTSD symptoms from the subsequent trauma. To explain why this is, without direct evidence, Breslau wrote that other factors should be considered, such as "(1) PTSD cases identified at baseline might already have been sensitized by early childhood traumas, which were undetected in our study, and (2) PTSD from subsequent trauma among respondents with prior PTSD might have been a continuation of chronic, unremitted PTSD."

Posttraumatic stress disorder—full remission/ posttraumatic stress disorder—partial remission Posttraumatic stress disorder has a specific course of development, with severe psychosocial impairment defined by the symptom clusters of the *Diagnostic and Statistical Manual-IV.* Johnson et al. studied 1,300 patients who met the criteria for lifetime posttraumatic stress disorder. They were divided into three groups: (1) patients with current PTSD; (2) individuals with a history of PTSD and with clinically significant residual symptoms, or the partial remission group (PTSD-PR); and (3) those in full remission (FR) with no clinically significant residual PTSD symptoms. The researchers found that the PTSD-PR group met the criterion for reexperiencing (criterion B in the *DSM-IV* definition) but not for avoidance (criterion C) as support for partial remission specifier for PTSD.

Post-trauma social support Social support facilitates recovery from trauma as victims are exposed to additional stressors during recovery. Without social support, families living with a member with PTSD can easily burn out. Support groups, virtual communities on the Internet for online PTSD discussion groups, church fellowships, and extended family can lend practical as well as moral support. On the other hand, following an individual's exposure to a traumatic event, disapproval and rejection from both family and social environment (work settings) is related to higher PTSD symptoms. Think about the rape victim who is blamed, shamed, and rejected by her husband, or the returning soldiers from Vietnam who were not supported once they returned to the states and felt isolated. One reason that military groups need a supportive environment is to not feel a stigma (weakness) in asking for help or treatment for their chronic PTSD.

Factors operating at the time of trauma and immediately after the trauma such as a lack of social support, trauma severity, and additional life stress proved to contribute to high risk for PTSD in Brewin's meta-analysis of the literature. These studies argue the relevance of social environmental processes to individual trauma recovery.

Pre-trauma vulnerability The study of risk factors and vulnerability has a role in understanding the development of PTSD. Shalev (1996) and Brewin (2000) identified numerous pre-trauma vulnerability predictors such as family history of mental illness, gender, genetic factors, personality traits, early traumatization, negative parenting experiences, and lower education.

An individual's risk factor for developing PTSD increases with a history of mental disorders. Following exposure to traumatic events, these individuals also develop other forms of psychiatric disorders, such as depression, anxiety or substance abuse, according to King et al.

Individual personality and unique characteristics such as a pattern of negative or pessimistic thoughts or the inability to express emotions and cope with difficult situations are risk factors. If an individual, due to negative parenting as a child, is predisposed to shame, guilt, distrust, and secrecy and not able to reach out for help, all this points to vulnerability for PTSD symptoms. Genetics may play a role in biology in which certain individuals have an overreactive nervous system, do not deal with stress with healthy coping behaviors and may go for "quick fixes" such as the use and abuse of alcohol and drugs.

Depression, alcohol or other substance abuse, or other anxiety disorders frequently co-occur with PTSD. The likelihood of treatment success is increased when these other conditions are appropriately diagnosed and treated as well. Substance abuse most likely occurs after the trauma or life-threatening event as a way to cope, even if is not recommended. Early intervention is critical since the longer the individual with PTSD tries to mask the symptoms of recurring memories, flashbacks, and panic attacks, the more complicated his or her recovery becomes; the use of drugs and alcohol must be controlled or eliminated in order for treatment to begin in addressing PTSD symptoms.

Some prescribed medications, such as Zoloft, have been shown to be helpful with PTSD and substance abuse disorders as well as with major depression and anxiety disorders.

See also CIRCUMSCRIBED POSTTRAUMATIC STRESS DISORDER; COMBAT-RELATED POSTTRAUMATIC STRESS DISORDER; ELABORATED POSTTRAUMATIC STRESS DISORDER; MEDICAL ILLNESS–RELATED PSYCHOLOGICAL DISTRESS; MEDICAL STRESSORS; PANIC DISORDER; PEDIATRIC MEDICAL TRAUMATIC STRESS; POST-VIETNAM SYNDROME; RESILIENCE TO STRESS; THERAPY, TYPES OF.

American Psychiatric Association. *Diagnostic and Statistical Manual of Mental Disorders.* 4th ed. Washington, D.C., 2000.

Brewin, C. R., B. Andrew, and J. D. Valentine. "Meta-analysis of Risk Factors for Posttraumatic Stress in Trauma Exposed Adults." *Journal of Consulting and Clinical Psychology* 68, no. 5 (2000): 748–766.

Johnson, D. M., C. Zlotnick, and M. Zimmerman. "The Clinical Relevance of a Partial Remission Specifier for Posttraumatic Stress Disorder." *Journal of Traumatic Stress* 16, no. 5 (October 2005): 515–518.

King, D., D. Vogt, and L. King. "Risk and Resilience Factor in the Etiology of Chronic Posttraumatic Stress Disorder." In *Early Intervention for Trauma & Traumatic Loss,* edited by B. T. Litz. New York: Guilford Press, 2004.

Lasiuk, G. C., and K. M. Hegadoren. "Posttraumatic Stress Disorder Part I: Historical Development of the Concept." *Perspectives in Psychiatric Care* 42, no. 1 (February 2006): 13–20.

van der Kolk, Bessel, Alexander McFarland, and Onno van Der Hart. "A General Approach to Treatment of Posttraumatic Stress Disorder." In *Traumatic Stress: The Effects of Overwhelming Experience on Mind, Body and Society,* edited by B. A. van der Kolk, A. C. McFarland, and L. Weisaeth. New York: Guilford Press, 1996.

Yehuda, R., et al. "Low Cortisol & Risk for PTSD in Adult Offspring of Holocaust Survivors." *The American Journal of Psychiatry* 157, no. 8 (2000): 1,252–1,259.

posttraumatic stress disorder—full remission/posttraumatic stress disorder—partial remission See POSTTRAUMATIC STRESS DISORDER; THERAPY, TYPES OF.

Posttraumatic Stress Disorder (PTSD) Model

Clinicians and researchers have used the term Posttraumatic Stress Disorder (PTSD) Model to explain the effects of traumatic stress on individuals based on the *DIAGNOSTIC AND STATISTICAL MANUAL of Mental Disorders,* currently in its fourth edition. It is a framework to explain the full range of symptoms to account for long-term effects and treatment course of those who are survivors of traumatic events.

However, using a model does not always fit nicely into the PTSD box. Using childhood sexual abuse, for example, the PTSD model enables an understanding of its impact on the child, a syndrome with a core etiology rather than just a list of symptoms. Sexual abuse causes a wide range of survivor symptoms, such as DEPRESSION, GUILT, sexual problems, and self-destructive and suicidal behaviors, and the model allows for broader similarities to other traumatic experiences. Yet at the same time, many of the diagnostic criteria for PTSD are not met. Sexual abuse is not always a threat or accompanied by danger or violence, but may be more of an ordeal resulting in years of abuse rather than a single traumatic event. COMPLEX PTSD is the term used to include prolonged exposure to account for social and interpersonal trauma. Complex PTSD is now under consideration for inclusion in the fifth edition of the *DSM.*

Finkelhor, D., and A. Browne. "The Traumatic Impact of Child Sexual Abuse: A Conceptualization." *American Journal of Orthopsychiatry* 55, no. 4 (1985): 530–541.

post-Vietnam syndrome (PVS) The Vietnam War that ended in April 1975 brought the psychological problems of many combat veterans to the forefront of U.S. media when many former soldiers suffered from INSOMNIA, DEPRESSION, NIGHTMARES, alienation, apathy, and mistrust. In addition to the cultural negativity of the war in the 1960s, many veterans felt uprooted from their communities and restless, fell prey to drug addiction, and were unable to reenter accepted societal jobs or careers. This became known as post-Vietnam syndrome.

To understand the impact of war on veterans of the Vietnam War, the U.S. Congress mandated the National Vietnam Veterans Readjustment Study (NVVRS) in the mid-1980s and found that 15.2 percent of male and 8.9 percent of female Vietnam veterans were found to have POSTTRAUMATIC STRESS

DISORDER (PTSD). This study confirmed that for many veterans PTSD was a chronic condition. Fourteen years later, in 1998, researchers at Harvard School of Public Health, Columbia University, and State University of New York found that almost three decades after the Vietnam War many veterans continued to show problems with PTSD. At the initial interview, the NVVRS reported a 12 percent rate of PTSD, and the 1998 study reported a slight decrease (to 11 percent). These veterans continued to have serious psychological and social problems. There were also high levels of DIVORCE and SUICIDE among these veterans. These problems were identified as related to their combat experience, and although still known as post-Vietnam syndrome in the 1970s, by 1980 these symptoms were categorized under posttraumatic stress disorder in the *DIAGNOSTIC AND STATISTICAL MANUAL of Mental Disorders (DSM)*.

See also COMBAT-RELATED POSTTRAUMATIC STRESS DISORDER; COMBAT STRESS REACTION.

potentially traumatizing event (PTE) An event that has a high likelihood of causing trauma in an individual, such as a medical diagnosis of cancer or the diagnosis of severe illness in one's spouse or partner. The severe illness of a child is particularly traumatizing, and some studies have demonstrated that parents (especially mothers) are at risk for POSTTRAUMATIC STRESS DISORDER (PTSD) years after the event, even when their child has already survived a major medical problem, such as cancer. Other potentially traumatizing events are severe natural disasters such as hurricanes, storms, earthquakes, floods, and so on.

Generally the more severe the natural catastrophe, the more PTSD is reported afterward. The most likely events for traumatizing are those inflicted by another human, such as violence, shaming, or humiliation. Rape is a major category for PTSD due to its violent nature. Shootings, stabbings, random assaults, and similar events are also highly likely to produce PTSD in their victims. In terms of social violence, victims of shaming and humiliation are often candidates for PTSD. The younger the victim, the more likely these events will traumatize him or her.

See also MEDICAL ILLNESS-RELATED PSYCHOLOGICAL DISTRESS; MEDICAL STRESSORS; PEDIATRIC MEDICAL TRAUMATIC STRESS.

Potential Stressful Events Interview (PSEI) A 62-item interview that was designed to identify POSTTRAUMATIC STRESS DISORDER (PTSD) and stressful civilian- and combat-encountered events within the criteria of the *Diagnostic and Statistical Manual IV (DSM-IV)* published by the American Psychiatric Association. The Potential Stressful Events Interview was developed in 1996 by Resnick and colleagues to provide descriptive data on the prevalence of traumatic events as well as of PTSD. The interview includes gaining information on demographics, low-magnitude stressors (e.g., job-related issues, illness, etc.), and high-magnitude stressors (such as combat, witnessing serious injuries, etc.).

Objective and subjective assessments are also made on the high- and low-magnitude events reported. Finally, respondents are asked about 15 emotional responses to events in their lives and 10 physical/bodily reactions, such as hyperventilation and palpitations. There is also an independent subsection for women to provide detailed information on sexual and physical assaults.

PSEI is a comprehensive interview with five parts: (1) demographics; (2) low-magnitude stressors in the last year, such as job loss and serious illness; (3) high-magnitude stressors, such as combat or military experience or witnessing someone being seriously injured; (4) objective characteristics of the prominent high- and low-magnitude events; and, (5) subjective characteristics of these prominent events. The final part (5) is a self-report that examines 15 emotional responses, such as "surprised" or "ashamed," and 10 physical reactions, such as shortness of breath and rapid heart rate. PSEI can be used for both research and clinical purposes.

See also INSTRUMENTS/SCALES/SURVEYS THAT EVALUATE POSTTRAUMATIC STRESS DISORDER (PTSD).

Resnick, H. S., S. A. Falsetti, D. G. Kilpatrick, and J. R. Freedy. "Assessment of Rape and Other Civilian Trauma-Related Post-traumatic Stress Disorder: Emphasis on Assessment of Potentially Traumatic

Events." In *Stressful Life Events,* edited by T. W. Miller, 231–266. Madison, Wis.: International Universities Press, 1996.

power spectral density (PSD) A mathematical method for transforming HEART RATE VARIABILITY (HRV) measures in order to discriminate between and quantify the contributions of parasympathetic and sympathetic activity. This is important in trauma research and treatment because trauma disorders result in excessive sympathetic activity. By being able to monitor the balance of sympathetic and parasympathetic activity, it is possible to roughly measure the effects of any intervention on the traumatized individual. Power spectral analysis reduces the HRV signal into three main frequency components: very low frequency, low frequency, and high frequency. The very low frequencies are associated with sympathetic activity, while high frequencies are an index of parasympathetic activity. Low frequency characterizes the baroreceptor or blood pressure feedback signals that are sent from the heart to the brain, and it is a more complex measurement.

primary/secondary stressors Primary stressors occur during the initial impact of POTENTIALLY TRAUMATIZING EVENTS, such as the destruction of personal property, experiencing serious accidents, witnessing the violent deaths of others, or exposure to a sudden unexpected death.

Secondary stressors (such as relocation, isolation, the loss of social support, feeling uncared for, or experiencing humiliation) can also significantly contribute to the occurrence of stress disorders among survivors. Secondary stressors violate a basic biosocial habit of humans. Loss affects social bonding. Relocation attacks people's territorial habits, and isolation violates the need for human contact. Humiliation and degradation leave psychological scars that go deeper than the immediate threat, such as in the case of group rape. The management of secondary stressors is paramount, and it should be a primary goal in early therapeutic intervention.

See also STRESS.

Shalev, A. Y. "Acute Stress Reactions in Adults." *Biological Psychiatry* 51 (2002): 532–543.

primary/secondary/tertiary traumatic stress disorders Primary traumatic stress disorder is a term that was first used by Charles Figley in 1992 to describe individuals whose symptoms resulted from a direct exposure to a traumatic event. Secondary traumatization refers to people who care for individuals who are directly traumatized or who are involved with them. Secondary traumatization is also referred to as VICARIOUS TRAUMATIZATION or COMPASSION FATIGUE, which sometimes occurs due to caring, empathizing, and having an emotional investment in helping those who are suffering.

Secondary traumatic stress (STS) disorder is the direct result of listening to emotionally troubling or shocking experiences of survivors, such as when mental health professionals engage empathetically with their clients. It is also seen in wives of combat veterans and nontraumatized children who play with traumatized children. The symptoms of STS are nearly identical to those of POSTTRAUMATIC STRESS DISORDER (PTSD), including re-experiencing traumatic memories, avoiding or experiencing numbing of the reminders of the event, as well as persistent arousal, as in sleep disturbance and hypervigilance. Figley suggests that STS symptoms lasting more than 30 days should be classified as secondary traumatic stress disorder.

Tertiary traumatization is a term that is less frequently used, and it refers to those individuals who support the supporters and who are vicariously traumatized. This includes the family members of first responders to traumatic events, such as what followed the destruction of the World Trade Center and the Pentagon on SEPTEMBER 11.

See also THERAPY, TYPES OF.

Figley, Charles R., and Rolf J. Kleber. "Beyond the 'Victim': Secondary Traumatic Stress." In *Beyond Trauma: Cultural and Society Dynamics,* edited by Rolf J. Kleber, Charles R. Figley, and Berthold P. R. Gersons, 75–98. New York: Plenum Press, 1995.

Professional Quality of Life Scale (ProQol) A self-test that was devised by Beth Hudnall Stamm in 1997 that allows users to measure their levels of compassion satisfaction, burnout, and trauma/COMPASSION FATIGUE. The most recent version of the test as of this writing is Revision IV. The Professional

Quality of Life Scale (ProQol) is the most widely used measure of SECONDARY TRAUMATIZATION.

Individuals using this scale respond with numbers ranging from 0 (Never) to 5 (Very Often) to such questions as "I am preoccupied with more than one person I help" and "I am losing sleep over traumatic experiences of a person I help." Responses are based on how the individual has felt over the past 30 days. The ProQol has largely replaced an earlier test, the COMPASSION SATISFACTION AND FATIGUE TEST.

See also COMPASSION FATIGUE; VICARIOUS TRAUMATIZATION.

progressive relaxation   The method or procedure for progressive relaxation therapy is quite simple, and involves two basic steps: tension and release. First the individual is instructed to apply tension to each muscle group, one at a time. Generally, the major muscle groups that are "progressively" tensed are the feet, lower legs, full legs, hands, forearms, entire arms, abdomen, chest, neck and shoulders, forehead, and face. About eight seconds of tension is followed by release and a rest for about 20 seconds. Tension is demonstrated by clenching and contracting the muscles. For the hands, one closes the hands and squeezes them very tightly. The face can be tensed by clenching teeth, closing eyes tightly, and squeezing lips closely. Breathing is important, as are calming thoughts and intentions. Once the tension is stopped or released, the muscle group begins to relax.

Progressive relaxation was developed by Edmund Jacobson, M.D., in the first part of the 20th century to help reduce or alleviate what he called "tension states." In 1929 the University of Chicago Press published Jacobson's book, *Progressive Relaxation: A Physiological and Clinical Investigation of Muscular States and Their Significance in Psychology and Medicine.* In 1934, Jacobson published a similar book entitled *You Must Relax.*

Progressive Relaxation detailed Jacobson's clinical observations on the role of tension in the development of diseases, particularly chronic diseases. Since the term *relaxation* had so many varied meanings and connotations, he preferred the term "tension control," which he felt more accurately described his clinical approach. Jacobson was one of the founders of the American Association for the Advancement of Tension Control in 1974, an organization that later evolved into the International Stress and Tension Control Society (ISTCS).

Jacobson developed progressive relaxation from his knowledge of physiology, and he taught it to his nurses, who in turn taught progressive relaxation to patients with a very wide range of diseases, based on the idea that tension was related to these diseases. The results were astonishing, and many case histories were presented in the appendix of the progressive relaxation book to justify Jacobson's contention. Today, after much empirical research, progressive relaxation seems to be the most potent form of "tension control," and it is superior to medications, hypnosis, and massage. The method (described below) takes some months to master, but the user, once competent, can actually consciously reduce muscle tension and prevent its effects from developing. It is in the area of anxiety reduction where progressive relaxation has been extensively used.

Through repetitive practice over a period of months, the practitioner can learn to discriminate tension from relaxation and can voluntarily release tension where tension is present. Jacobson used many more muscle groups (even the tongue), but research and practice has shown that relaxation of the major groups over time will produce the same result and does not take the time that Jacobson's procedure required.

A variation of the Jacobson technique is "cue-controlled" relaxation, in which breath control becomes important. The individual breathes in while tensing each major muscle group, and breathes out with release, using a cue word such as "relax." Gradually, the word used at release becomes associated with tension reduction and can be used in the natural environment for the conscious release of tension in particular muscle groups.

Joseph Wolpe popularized the use of progressive relaxation with anxiety and panic problems, and it became a central part of his SYSTEMATIC DESENSITI-

ZATION therapy. Subsequently, progressive relaxation has been used with POSTTRAUMATIC STRESS DISORDER (PTSD) as a mode of self-control of body tension associated with the PTSD.

See also THERAPY, TYPES OF.

prolonged exposure therapy   A brief form of COGNITIVE BEHAVIORAL THERAPY that has been shown to be effective in the treatment of POSTTRAUMATIC STRESS DISORDER (PTSD). Individual therapy consists of eight to 12 sessions of psychoeducation, or education on psychological illness imaginal exposure, or revisiting the trauma through imagination, and in vivo exposure, or real life-based exposure, to anxiety-provoking traumatic events or feared objects to reduce or extinguish intrusive thoughts, fear, anxiety, and the startle response. Presenting anxiety-provoking material over a long enough period reduces the intensity of emotional reactions to triggering traumatic memories.

EXPOSURE THERAPY is a safe treatment method, although some individuals may find high levels of anxiety disturbing during the exposure treatment process. To help reduce this anxiety the therapist teaches the patient relaxation techniques, such as PROGRESSIVE RELAXATION, prior to beginning treatment. Progressive relaxation involves tightening and relaxing muscle groups throughout the body to release tension and stress.

Prolonged exposure therapy is generally used with adults, although it has also been used with children and adolescents under the care of a very skilled therapist. More than 20 years of research has proven the effectiveness of prolonged exposure therapy in reducing PTSD symptoms in cases of rape, CHILD SEXUAL ABUSE, combat, MOTOR VEHICLE CRASH/ACCIDENTS, and criminal assaults.

See also EXPOSURE THERAPY; THERAPY, TYPES OF.

proximity effect   The closer that an individual is to a TRAUMATIC EVENT, such as a natural disaster, robbery, or war, the greater the likelihood that symptoms of POSTTRAUMATIC STRESS DISORDER (PTSD) will occur.

In a study following the destruction of the Twin Towers on SEPTEMBER 11, 2001 by Blanchard et al., students in Albany (150 miles away) showed greater levels of stress symptoms than did students in Augusta, Georgia (800 miles away). In addition, the students in Georgia showed more symptoms than did students in Fargo, North Dakota, which was 1,500 miles away. Another study reported by the authors found an overall prevalence of posttraumatic stress disorder of 7.5 percent in New York City within 5–9 weeks after September 11 and they found a rate of 20 percent for those living closest to the World Trade Center, a site specified as south of Canal Street.

Violante et al. found a high SUICIDE risk group among police officers who worked in proximity to the World Trade Center following the September 11 attack, compared to the suicide risk for officers prior to September 11. This data was gathered for a period of four years (2001–2004) through a telephone hotline that was specifically for police officers.

See also SEPTEMBER 11.

Blanchard, E. G., D. Rowell, E. Kuhn, R. Rogers, and D. Wittrock. "Posttraumatic Stress and Depressive Symptoms in a College Population One Year after the September 11 Attacks: The Effect of Proximity." *Behavior Research and Therapy* 43 (2005): 143–150.
Violante, J., C. Castellano, J. O'Rourke and D. Paton. "Proximity to the 9/11 Terrorist Attack and Suicide Ideation in Police Officers." *Traumatology* 12, no. 3 (2006): 248–254.

proximity, immediacy, expectancy, simplicity (PIES)   The concept of psychological intervention and DEBRIEFING for soldiers was first used during World War I for SHELL SHOCK or COMBAT STRESS REACTIONS. Observations made by medical officer Thomas Salmon argued for intervention as close to the front lines as possible with rest and nutrition and empathizing with the psychologically wounded soldier that, with time, he will get better.

As soldiers are deployed to war-zone areas such as Afghanistan and Iraq they are faced with many stressors from fear of death or injury to discomforts such as fatigue, hunger, being far from home, and the feelings of loneliness. More severe symptoms may be self-destructive behaviors, depression, body tremors, and paralysis. In the face of WAR-ZONE STRESS REACTIONS, there are two factors (push and pull) that determine if a soldier will break down or not. "Pull" factors are instinctual to everyone such as self-preservation, and the need for food and water and tend to pull the soldier back out of harm's way. However, there is the "push" factor, which counterbalances the pull factor and keeps the soldier motivated to continue fighting due to his or her sense of duty, to not let down his or her fellow soldier, and the support received from family and country. Given this fine balance between pull and push factors, the soldier in a stressful situation will feel guilty about thoughts of abandoning the combat unit and want to defy feelings of cowardice, but may think he or she is "sick." The military psychologist/psychiatrist will intervene at this point to let the soldier know he or she is not sick and that he or she has suffered through an extremely stressful situation and is in need of rest and recuperation. Therein lie the principles of combat PSYCHOLOGICAL FIRST AID also known as PIES.

- proximity—treatment is carried out close to the battlefields or front lines
- immediacy—treatment as soon as possible after onset of symptoms
- expectancy—with full expectation that they will return to duty
- simplicity—food, drink, rest

PIES has been used successfully in all U.S. armed forces since World War I and has shown that managing the symptoms of combat stress reaction casualties can result in 60 percent of soldiers returning to military duty within 72 hours.

Singapore Armed Forces Medical Corps, "Minds in War." Available online. URL: http://www.mindef.gov.sg/imindef/mindef_websites/atozlistings/safmc/publications/articles/MindsinWar.html. Downloaded September 16, 2008.

psychic numbing Loss of emotional affect in the face of trauma, such as with the death of a loved one in combat experience or an assault such as rape. Psychic numbing is also known as emotional numbing, and it occurs as a form of "emotional anesthesia" when the person cannot cope with the distress from a problem any further. The individual may be nonresponsive or have a flat affect when communicating with others and may shut him or herself off from others. Some experts believe that psychic numbing is a symptom of POSTTRAUMATIC STRESS DISORDER (PTSD), while others believe that it is a predictor for the development of PTSD.

The term *psychic numbing* was originally developed by Robert J. Lifton in the 1980s to explain some of the reactions of survivors to the bombing of Hiroshima. Psychic numbing was later extended to encompass other severe trauma, and some experts use the term to describe the reactions of individuals who fear an impending severe trauma.

According to John P. Wilson in his chapter on PTSD in *Assessing Psychological Trauma and PTSD,*

Manifestations of psychic numbing take many forms, including a loss of normal capacity to experience emotions, diminished sensuality and sexuality, a loss of spirituality, and the outward appearance of being emotionally flat, nonresponsive, vapid, unfeeling, indifferent, cold, and lacking in vitality. These emotional states can be considered as coping efforts to control the level of HYPERAROUSAL inherent in PTSD as a dysregulated stress-response syndrome.

In essence, the person "shuts down" emotionally because he or she cannot cope with the distressing issue anymore.

In some cases, victims who testify in court exhibit behavior that stems from psychic numbing, and jury members may mistakenly believe that the victim has not suffered, since he or she is not crying or showing any emotion. This may be especially true of children who have been abused for years, particularly by sexual abuse. These children may shut down their emotions with regard to the abuse as a means of coping with it.

See also COMPASSION FATIGUE; COMPLEX POST-TRAUMATIC STRESS DISORDER; LEARNED HELPLESSNESS; PRIMARY/SECONDARY/TERTIARY TRAUMATIC STRESS DISORDER.

Wilson, John P., "PTSD and Complex PTSD: Symptoms, Syndromes, and Diagnoses." In *Assessing Psychological Trauma and PTSD*, 2nd ed., edited by John P. Wilson and Terence M. Keane, 7–44. New York: Guilford Publications, 2004.

psychoanalysis   See ABREACTION; TREATMENT: PSYCHOTHERAPY, PSYCHOPHARMACOLOGY, AND ALTERNATIVE MEDICINE; TYPES OF THERAPY.

psychogenic death   Death that results either from an intense belief that death is impending, such as when a person believes that a curse has been placed upon him or her, or when the individual is diagnosed with a serious illness.

In the case of disasters and trauma, psychogenic death may occur when some individuals fail to act adaptively and either deny imminent danger or assume that death will occur anyway and there is no point to taking any action. This is an irrational response that is evinced by a tiny minority of individuals. Those individuals who respond in this manner cling to their beliefs. An example is when a volcanic eruption is deemed imminent and almost everyone evacuates except for some individuals who refuse to accept that the volcano will erupt or who think that they should stay in the area because that is where they "belong."

See also PSYCHOGENIC FUGUE.

psychogenic fugue   In the latter part of the 18th century medical and disease theories of mental illness began to shift to a "psychogenic" perspective, a view that abnormal functioning could be caused by an individual's past psychological history and emotional factors. The advent of psychoanalysis strengthened this view, particularly with its emphasis on unconscious phenomena as causes of neuroses. Fugue states are conditions in which there is a sudden alteration or confusion in one's identity, leading to distress and dysfunction. These states may last for minutes or hours or, in more extreme cases, they may produce a long-term separation from one's identity and the acquiring of another identity, such as with dissociative identity disorder.

Dissociative fugues are associated with extreme STRESS and trauma, and they represent an effort of individuals to distance themselves and cope with the traumatic experience and the personal distress that it generates. Often these individuals will suddenly "awaken" in a strange place, not knowing who they are or how they got to that place. Some adolescent runaways experience fugue states, but most often it is an adult who tends to repress his or her traumatic experience and not have ways to deal with arousal and distressful feelings and experiences.

Alterations in identity that do not involve escape are present in multiple personality or dissociative identity disorders. In a sense, the dissociative identity disorders (DID) are an internal form of fugue, except that the different identities have been present for some time, probably beginning in early childhood when abuse was present.

Treatment for dissociative fugue is usually psychotherapy, with an emphasis on current stressors, and often supplemented with medications. Hypnosis often helps patients recall memories. The dissociative state usually diminishes quickly once trusted people find the person in the fugue state and therapy begins. The rare nature of these disorders, however, makes systematic research difficult because patient populations are so small.

See also PSYCHOGENIC DEATH; DISSOCIATION/DISSOCIATIVE DISORDERS.

psychological debriefing   See DEBRIEFING.

psychological first aid (PFA)   Practical and immediate crisis intervention actions that are taken to help or treat victims of severe trauma who either exhibit symptoms of or appear to be at risk for an ACUTE STRESS DISORDER or who fit categories of individuals at risk for mental health problems. For example, according to Bruce H. Young in his chapter on psychological first aid in *Following Mass Violence and Disasters: Strategies for Mental Health Practice*, individuals with extreme acute stress reactions may evidence excessive anxiety resulting in dissociative symptoms, detachment, depersonalization, and a "dreamlike interpretation of their surroundings." Such individuals also may have prolonged and uncontrollable distressful emotions and may have a prolonged inability to sleep or eat. They may also exhibit poor concentration, confusion, and poor decision making.

Psychological first aid is meant to counter and deflect such emotional problems in the early stages. Says Young.

The principal objective of PFA can be stated as aiding the adaptive coping and problem-solving processes of survivors who appear at risk for being unable to regain sufficient functional equilibrium on their own. Problems may be related to safety and security, extreme acute stress reactions, and connecting survivors to resources that are restorative and better address respective problems through more in-depth services.

Some predisaster risk factors that are relevant to those who may need psychological first aid include

- low income
- female gender
- ages 40–60 years
- a past psychiatric history

Some within-disaster factors include

- injury
- bereavement
- panic
- horror
- threat to life

Some postdisaster risk factors for those who may need psychological first aid include

- relocation
- loss of home and/or property
- deterioration of social support
- exaggerated view of the risk of future trauma
- a perceived decline in social support

In some cases, medication can help, such as a low dose of a TRICYCLIC ANTIDEPRESSANT such as imipramine, or a SELECTIVE SEROTONIN REUPTAKE INHIBITOR (SSRI). Providing information to survivors is also an important aspect of psychological first aid, such as telling them where they can get shelter, medical care, water, food, and so forth. It may be necessary to provide transportation to necessary resources since often survivors have lost their means of transportation.

Those providing psychological first aid also need to talk to distressed survivors and whenever possible, offer empathic reactions. Often, teaching others how to reframe their distressing thoughts can help considerably. For example, according to Young, such negative thoughts as "I was a coward. Because of me, other people died" can be reframed with such statements as "Many factors beyond your control resulted in the deaths that occurred and it's unfair to you to take any blame in this."

Experts can also advise survivors when they should seek further treatment, such as when they exhibit a phobic avoidance of reminders of the disaster, when they suffer from extreme sleep deprivation and frequent NIGHTMARES, or when they exhibit symptoms of clinical DEPRESSION.

See also COMPASSION FATIGUE; PRIMARY/SECONDARY/TERTIARY TRAUMATIC STRESS DISORDER.

Young, Bruce H. "The Immediate Response to Disaster: Guidelines for Adult Psychological First Aid." In *Interventions Following Mass Violence and Disasters: Strategies for Mental Health Practice,* edited by Elspeth Camaron Ritchie, et al. New York: Guilford Press, 2006.

psychosocial trauma History has shown that humans can carry out extremely harmful acts upon each other that result in suffering and long-lasting painful memories. POSTTRAUMATIC STRESS DISORDER (PTSD) has been the model to explain the emotional, behavioral, and physical symptoms an individual experiences following traumatic events. The use of the term psychosocial trauma introduces the social context of people into trauma diagnosis resulting from political violence and terrorism.

As an example, trauma from the military dictatorship in Chilean society was not the same for everyone. Individuals in some social classes were subjected to extreme violence while others fled the country with fear and uncertainties. To explain their different traumatic experiences it must also be acknowledged that the range of effects go beyond the medical, psychological, and psychosocial processes. These experiences include the pervasive fear of those in power, as well as such factors as poverty, hatred against others, and the disruption to the social fabric of the community that is well beyond the initial conflicts or war. Psychosocial trauma is a process that affects the entire society over time.

Psychosocial trauma also refers to events such as natural catastrophes and the social consequences of the traumatic event.

Madariaga, C. "Psychosocial Trauma, Posttraumatic Stress Disorder, and Torture." Paper presented at the First Latin American and Caribbean Seminar "Models to Work with People that have Suffered Torture and Other Violations of Human Rights," Antigua, Guatemala, April 2000.

psychotherapy See ABREACTION; COMPASSION FATIGUE; PRIMARY/SECONDARY/TERTIARY TRAUMATIC STRESS DISORDER; TREATMENT: PSYCHOTHERAPY, PSYCHOPHARMACOLOGY, AND ALTERNATIVE MEDICINE; THERAPY, TYPES OF.

psychotraumatogenesis Refers to factors or vulnerabilities within the individual that will lead to the development of trauma disorders if they are exposed to a traumatic stressor. This point of view emphasizes key psychological variables that support or enhance trauma reactions. Beliefs are the core source of potential traumatization. Everly, Lating, and Jeffrey have identified five such core beliefs that they believe make a person vulnerable to develop trauma if these beliefs are involved in one or more traumatic events.

First, the belief that the world is just and fair can be attacked by outside events to the contrary. Second, the belief that all people can be trusted can be violated by betrayal, treachery, abandonment, and rejection, especially if perpetrated by a trusted person or institution. Third, the belief that people are physically safe can be violated by threats to personal safety, especially if perpetrated by another human. Fourth, the belief that one must have a positive self-identify can be contradicted by others. Fifth, the belief that there is an overarching order to life, a spiritual or unifying paradigm, can be affected or violated. In essence, there is a dark side to life, people, institutions, and so on, and this dark side can attack or violate these human core beliefs, causing an event to be perceived as traumatic. This results in two psychological or existential effects: a sense of betrayal from life and a sense of being alienated, separate, and disconnected from others, of being alone. Successful trauma treatment has to address these two factors.

Everly, G., and J. M. Lating. "Personality Psychology." In *Personality-Guided Therapy for Posttraumatic Stress Disorder*, edited by G. Everly, J. M. Lating, and J. R. Lating, 33–51. Washington D.C.: American Psychological Association, 2003.

PTSD See POSTTRAUMATIC STRESS DISORDER.

PTSD Checklist (PCL) A 17-item self-report measure of POSTTRAUMATIC STRESS DISORDER (PTSD) that takes a short time to administer. The 17 items parallel diagnostic criteria B (the traumatic event is re-experienced), C (persistent avoidance of reminders associated with trauma) and D (persistent symptoms of increased arousal) for PTSD in the *Diagnostic and Statistical Manual of Mental Disorders, Fourth Edition* (*DSM-IV*). The PCL appears to be one of only a few self-report instruments that are constructed along the diagnostic criteria of *DSM-IV*, a symptom-driven screening tool, rather than a trauma-based screen, and may yield greater predictive validity on PTSD diagnosis.

Respondents are asked on a 5-point scale (1=not at all to 5=extremely) to rate the extent to which symptoms bothered them in the past month.

PTSD CHECKLIST—CIVILIAN VERSION (PCL-C)

Patient's Name:

Instruction to patient: Below is a list of problems and complaints that civilians sometimes have in response to stressful life experiences. Please read each one carefully, put an "X" in the box to indicate how much you have been bothered by that problem *in the last month.*

No.	Not at all (1)	A little bit (2)	Moderately (3)	Quite a bit (4)	Extremely (5)
1. Repeated, disturbing *memories, thoughts,* or *images* of a stressful experience from the past?					
2. Repeated, disturbing *dreams* of a stressful experience from the past?					
3. Suddenly *acting* or *feeling* as if a stressful experience *were happening again* (as if you were reliving it)?					
4. Feeling *very upset* when *something reminded* you of a stressful experience from the past?					
5. Having *physical reactions* (e.g., heart pounding, trouble breathing, or sweating) when *something reminded* you of a stressful experience from the past?					
6. Avoid *thinking about* or *talking about* a stressful experience from the past or avoid *having feelings* related to it?					
7. Avoid *activities* or *situations* because *they remind you* of a stressful experience from the past?					
8. Trouble *remembering important parts* of a stressful experience from the past?					
9. Loss of *interest in things that you used to enjoy?*					
10. Feeling *distant* or *cut off* from other people?					
11. Feeling *emotionally numb* or being unable to have loving feelings for those close to you?					
12. Feeling as if your *future* will somehow be *cut short?*					
13. Trouble *falling* or *staying asleep?*					
14. Feeling *irritable* or having *angry outbursts?*					
15. Having *difficulty concentrating?*					
16. Being *"super alert"* or watchful on guard?					
17. Feeling *jumpy* or easily startled?					

Weathers, F. W., Huska, J. A., Keane, T. M. *PCL-C for DSM-IV.* Boston: National Center for PTSD—Behavioral Science Division, 1991.

The PCL is one of the most widely used measures of PTSD in clinical and research settings, and has excellent reliability and validity with both civilian and military populations.

The PCL was developed by researchers at the National Center for PTSD in 1991. The civilian and military versions are both in the public domain.

PTSD CHECKLIST—MILITARY VERSION (PCL-M)

Patient's Name:

Instruction to patient: Below is a list of problems and complaints that veterans sometimes have in response to stressful life experiences. Please read each one carefully, put an "X" in the box to indicate how much you have been bothered by that problem *in the last month*.

| No. | Response: | | | | |
---	Not at all (1)	A little bit (2)	Moderately (3)	Quite a bit (4)	Extremely (5)
1. Repeated, disturbing *memories, thoughts,* or *images* of a stressful military experience?					
2. Repeated, disturbing *dreams* of a stressful military experience?					
3. Suddenly *acting* or *feeling* as if a stressful military experience *were happening again* (as if you were reliving it)?					
4. Feeling *very upset* when *something reminded* you of a stressful military experience?					
5. Having *physical reactions* (e.g., heart pounding, trouble breathing, or sweating) when *something reminded* you of a stressful military experience?					
6. Avoid *thinking about* or *talking about* a stressful military experience from the past or avoid *having feelings* related to it?					
7. Avoid *activities* or *situations* because *they remind* you of a stressful military experience?					
8. Trouble *remembering important parts* of a stressful military experience?					
9. Loss of *interest in things that you used to enjoy?*					
10. Feeling *distant* or *cut off* from other people?					
11. Feeling *emotionally numb* or being unable to have loving feelings for those close to you?					
12. Feeling as if your *future* will somehow be *cut short?*					
13. Trouble *falling* or *staying asleep?*					
14. Feeling *irritable* or having *angry outbursts?*					
15. Having *difficulty concentrating?*					
16. Being *"super alert"* or watchful on guard?					
17. Feeling *jumpy* or easily startled?					

Weathers, F. W., Huska, J. A., Keane, T. M. *PCL-C for DSM-IV.* Boston: National Center for PTSD—Behavioral Science Division, 1991.

Ruggiero, K., K. Del Ben, J. Scotti and A. Rabalais. "Psychometric Properties of the PTSD Checklist-Civilian Version." *Journal of Traumatic Stress* 16, no. 5 (October 2003): 495–502.

Published International Literature on Traumatic Stress (PILOTS)   An electronic index to articles on POSTTRAUMATIC STRESS DISORDER (PTSD) and traumatic stress worldwide. It is produced and updated by the National Center for PTSD in Vermont. There is no charge to access the database, and although it is sponsored by the U.S. Department of Veterans Affairs, it is not limited to literature on veterans.

Each PILOTS record provides the following information:

1. Bibliographic citation with author, title, and source needed to locate the document
2. A brief description or abstract of the article's content

To access PILOTS contact the National Center for PTSD at www.ncptsd.va.gov.

rape trauma syndrome (RTS)   A cluster of behaviors that occurs in many rape victims who have been traumatized by sexual assault. Some experts consider rape trauma syndrome (RTS) to be a subset of POSTTRAUMATIC STRESS DISORDER (PTSD).

The syndrome was initially named by Ann Wolbert Burgess and Lynda Lytle Holmstrom in their article in the *American Journal of Psychiatry* in 1974. The authors interviewed and followed up 146 rape victims in Boston, including 109 adult women, 34 female children, and 3 male children. They then analyzed their results from 92 adult female rape victims. According to the authors,

> Rape trauma syndrome is the acute phase and long-term reorganization process that occurs as a result of forcible rape or attempted forcible rape. This syndrome of behavioral, somatic, and psychological reactions is an acute stress reaction to a life-threatening situation.

Symptoms and Diagnostic Path

Wolbert Burgess and Lytle Holmstrom found that the syndrome occurred in two phases: an acute phase and a long-term phase. In the acute phase of the syndrome, the women expressed fear, anxiety, and anger, although some women exhibited masked or hidden feelings. The authors found that in the acute phase, sleep disturbances were common, and women who had been awakened from sleep by their assailant found themselves later waking up at the same time that the rape had occurred.

Many of the women also experienced stomach pains and appetite loss, as well as gynecological symptoms and general pain throughout the body.

Emotional reactions included self-blame, fear, humiliation, embarrassment, anger, and a desire for revenge.

In the long-term phase, which the authors called "reorganization," the women had mild to moderate symptoms. Most women changed their telephone numbers and many sought help from family members, particularly family members who lived in distant locations. Others turned to close friends. Many experienced distressing dreams, including severely frightening NIGHTMARES.

Some of the women became phobic as a result of the rape and feared being inside. Conversely, women who had been attacked outside of their homes feared being outside. Nearly all victims feared being alone and many developed a fear of crowds. Some of the victims developed a fear of people walking behind them. Sexual difficulties were common among the rape victims.

According to the authors, there are two primary types of rape trauma syndrome: compounded reaction and silent reaction. Compounded reactions were experienced by women with psychiatric, social, or physical problems that occurred before the rape. According to the authors, "It was noted that this group developed additional symptoms such as DEPRESSION, psychotic behavior, psychosomatic disorders, suicidal behavior, and acting-out behavior associated with alcoholism, drug use, and sexual activity."

The silent reaction refers to the reaction of the women who had never reported the rape to the authorities or to anyone else and who, consequently, suffered from attempts to repress the memories of the rape and their feelings about it. Some of the rape victims interviewed by the researchers had been raped as children. According to the authors,

> The current rape reactivated their reaction to the prior experience. It became clear that because they had not talked about the previous rape, the syndrome had continued to develop, and these

women had carried unresolved issues with them for years. They would talk as much of the previous rape as they did of the current situation.

Treatment Options and Outlook

Rape is an act of violence against another person. Rape counselors and therapists must be very understanding, patient, and supportive while bringing the victim back into their self-esteem. Studies show that some 94 percent of rape victims experience ACUTE STRESS DISORDER and many of these move into PTSD after one month. Victims typically continue to have higher levels of anxiety, suspiciousness, depression, self-esteem problems, self-blame, FLASHBACKS, sleep disorders, and sexual dysfunction.

The immediate treatment must be provided by medical experts. Examination and blood tests for sexually transmitted diseases are necessary as well as pregnancy tests. Victims suffer from long-term health problems even years after assaults. Clinicians use insight or traditional forms of verbal or talk therapy and COGNITIVE BEHAVIORAL THERAPY as treatment modalities. SOMATIC EXPERIENCING THERAPY and EYE MOVEMENT DESENSITIZATION AND REPROCESSING (EMDR) therapy are exceptionally useful in treating the traumatic psychological and somatic (bodily) reactions to rape. Rape is an act of violence usually against women. Constraint, suddenness, helplessness, humiliation and threat of one's life are all part of the experience. The psyche and the body are assaulted or injured and both carry scars of that injury or harm. At the psychological level there are often feelings of self-blame, anger-revenge and degradation. At the somatic level resistance and often fears develop around intimacy or sometimes the victims may feel soiled or dirty and acts that out by being promiscuous.

Risk Factors and Preventive Measures

Studies have shown that rape victims are often unsuspecting and lack caution. They most frequently have a victim-type appearance and gait. Preventive measures to avoid rape include avoiding unsafe areas, walking with others, and using self-protective training and measures (such as Mace). Preventive measure to avoid development of RTS include the victim's willingness to step forward and seek out the perpetrator (who is often known to the victim), take legal recourse, seek medical assistance, and find and participate in counseling and psychotherapy resources. The support of family and friends is also important if there is true understanding and no blame or humiliation in those supportive resources.

Prison Rapes

Most victims of rape trauma syndrome (RTS) are females but males are raped as well, often through anal abuse. For example, the rape of male prison inmates by other inmates is a common problem that, until recently, was often ignored. There was also a belief that prisoners deserved to be assaulted as part of their prison experience. Some experts estimate that as many as 25 percent of male inmates are sexually assaulted. Males who are raped are often psychologically and physically traumatized.

According to Robert W. Dumond in his article in the *Journal of the American Academy of Psychiatry and the Law* (2003), male prisoners are highly vulnerable to sexual assault by other inmates, particularly those who are young, weak, mentally ill, or developmentally disabled, disliked by the staff or other inmates, or homosexual. Among female inmates, women who are young, first-time offenders, and mentally disabled are the most likely to suffer from sexual assaults. According to Dumond,

> The mental health consequences of prisoner sexual assault are catastrophic. Male and female victims often experience posttraumatic stress disorder, anxiety, depression, and exacerbation of preexisting psychiatric disorders, and most victims are at risk of committing SUICIDE to avoid the ongoing trauma.

According to Dumond, the Prison Rape Elimination Act of 2003 resulted in the development of standards and created an accountability among prison officials that was absent in the past. Prison officials are now responsible for the safety of their prisoners.

See also CHILD SEXUAL ABUSE; THERAPY, TYPES OF.

Dumond, Robert W. "Confronting America's Most Ignored Crime Problem: The Prison Rape Elimination Act of

2003." *Journal of the American Academy of Psychiatry and the Law* 31, no. 3 (2003): 354–360.

Wolbert Burgess, Ann, and Lynda Lytle Holmstrom. "Rape Trauma Syndrome." *American Journal of Psychiatry* 131, no. 9 (September 1974): 981–986.

Rapid Assessment of Mental Health Needs of Refugees, Displaced and Other Populations Affected by Conflict and Post-Conflict Situations Available Resources (RAMH)   A technical document that was produced by the World Health Organization (WHO), the International Red Cross and Red Crescent Societies, the Disaster Mental Health Institute, and the University of South Dakota. RAMH was endorsed at the International Consultation on Mental Health of Refugees and Displaced Populations in Conflict and Post-Conflict Situations conference in Geneva, Switzerland, in October 2000.

RAMH is a tool that is intended for use by mental health professionals and nonhealthcare personnel involved in mental and psychosocial community support. It is intended to help workers at the first level of contact with displaced people in any post-conflict situation to assess mental health needs in emergency situations.

The purpose of RAMH is to describe the conflict and how it affects the population by identifying demographic data, the leading cause of mortality, the nature of the traumatic event, and coping mechanisms of individuals and families. It also identifies mental health professionals available in the area of conflict and makes recommendations to respond to the needs of vulnerable groups of people and overall affected communities.

The RAMH document is clear in its intent to respond to extraordinary violent events with adequate mental health resources in order to limit the impact of these events, speed up coping responses, and return individuals to their normal functioning.

recovered memory   For over a century, it has been understood that painful memories can be forgotten and later recovered. After each world war, soldiers reported forgetting traumatic combat experiences and later recovering and remembering them. This came to be known as combat neurosis and was never considered controversial. By the 1980s, people began claiming that sexual abuse memories, once forgotten, were recovered. The debate and controversy that followed focused on false memories. The question became "How could recovered memories remain intact and accurate?"

Psychotherapists began asserting that some individuals who had been abused as children had not remembered it until years later, as adults, when something triggers images that are suggestive of childhood traumatic events. Therapeutic techniques called Recovered Memory Therapy (RMT) arose to recover repressed memories of abuse. Unfortunately, it was discovered that, through RMT, and presumed social pressures within the therapy, one group of individuals "recovered" memories for events that never happened. This created great concern by the legal community, researchers, and the public that the strong influence of therapists working with individuals could lead to the creation of false beliefs about childhood trauma.

Trying to answer the question of how accurate were traumatic memories, Allen (1995) points out that trauma can wreck havoc on memory because traumatic memories can be stored in fragmentary form, which works against meaningful recall. Self-protective dissociation during trauma can blur the memory, creating a sense of unreality, and if the memory is not clearly coherent, it cannot be clearly retrieved. Traumatized persons may have too much memory, high emotional arousal, and burned-in images. They are vulnerable to creating "memories" to "explain" their discomfort and distress as most humans seek reasons to intellectually justify their situations.

See also FALSE MEMORY SYNDROME.

relational trauma   See COMPLEX POSTTRAUMATIC STRESS DISORDER.

repetition compulsion   A concept developed by Freud and discussed in his essay "Beyond the Pleasure Principle" (1920) to describe behavior that he interpreted as an attempt to master or resolve a traumatic experience. The behavior may be some form of reenacting the event overtly in another situation (e.g., marrying another abusive spouse), or engaging in activities with a high probability of repeating the trauma (e.g., drinking and being raped again) or reliving the event through fantasy or dreams.

Interestingly, studies of rape victims who had been asked to suppress memories or thoughts of the rape found even more memories or more frequent memories occurred under these conditions. One common form of repetition compulsion is when terrifying childhood events become an adult attraction to be acted out; for example, being spanked as a child may result in accepting spanking during sexual activity. Psychoanalysts see this as an attempt to master the childhood experience unconsciously, without the negative consequences that resulted in childhood.

Freud, S. *Jenseits Des Lustprinzips, 2. Durchgesehene Auflage,* Leipzig, Germany: Internationaler Psychoanalytischer Verlag, 1920, excerpted in Laplanche, J., and J. B. Pontalis. *The Language of Psycho-Analysis.* New York: Norton, 1974.

resilience to stress   A term usually applied to the phenomenon of *not* developing a disorder under conditions when others might and also of recovering quickly if a disorder does develop. Resilience is a very general term that can apply to different ages, situations, and physiologies.

Resilience and Posttraumatic Stress Disorder (PTSD)

Apparently resilience can be taught and because of this, experts think of resilience as having a strong learned component. For children, resilience is taught in specially designed psycho-educational groups that focus on cognitive flexibility (being able to include other views of meanings), a sense of self-mastery (a sense of personality power or responsibility in making cognitive changes), self-regulation (having a standard of balance and calmness in the body), and positive self-definition (valuing oneself) or self-regard. Skills are taught in these areas, but exposure to adversity is the true test of effectiveness, and this comes only through life experiences. It is an empirical question as to whether resilience training will reduce the incidence of PTSD but since

most people do not develop PTSD when exposed to a severe stressor, it is presumed that resilience training will have a positive effect on the incidence of PTSD.

Study of Vietnam Veterans

One of the most intense and dramatic laboratory studies of POSTTRAUMATIC STRESS DISORDER (PTSD) in adults was with veterans of the Vietnam War. The National Vietnam Veterans Readjustment Study tracked 1,632 female and male war veterans. Family instability, psychiatric symptoms at a younger age, and age of exposure to war trauma were predictive of PTSD symptom development. The researchers used a multi-method assessment approach (i.e., with questionnaires, self-reports, interviews, etc.), and grouped participants according to the degree of their involvement in the Vietnam War. Vietnam veteran responses were compared to other veterans who did not serve in Vietnam and with nonveterans of a similar age and background to the test sample.

The results showed that 15.2 percent of male Vietnam veterans and 8.5 percent of female Vietnam veterans met the criteria for a full diagnosis of PTSD. If the veterans were exposed to war zones, the percentages increased to 35.8 percent of males and 17.5 percent of females who had developed full PTSD. Overall, 26 percent of the 830,000 men and women who served in Vietnam developed PTSD impairment.

Protective factors, or what might be called resilience, were also found among the Vietnam veteran study subjects. These protective factors decreased the odds of developing PTSD, and included

- Japanese-American ethnicity
- a high school degree or higher
- an older age at entry to the war
- a higher socioeconomic status
- a more positive paternal relationship.
- positive social support

It is evident that given a potentially traumatic event, the majority of individuals exposed to the event do not develop PTSD, or if they do develop it, they recover quickly. Level of adjustment, support, socioeconomic status, and a history free of psychopathology strengthen the levels of resilience. On the other hand, these factors only correlate with resilience, and very few personal or physiological variables have been isolated, leaving experts with the conclusion that resilience is as much the result of outside resources and upbringing as it is an internal state of personality. As research begins to move toward the study of physiological assessment and variables, perhaps more objective measures will emerge.

Torture Victims

Torture is the infliction of severe pain and suffering, a perverted form of interaction between the torturer and the victim, and can include any unacceptable human standards of treatment characterized by degradation, humiliation, and cruel punishment. In a study of torture victims and PTSD, experts found that social support in exile, political commitment, and prior knowledge of confinement and torture were insulating factors against the development of PTSD and anxiety problems.

New Yorkers and the September 11 Attack

Studies of New Yorkers living near the World Trade Center towers six months after the terrorist attacks on SEPTEMBER 11, 2001, found widespread resilience rates. The total sample (n=2,752) included only 6 percent with probable PTSD after six months. Almost 29 percent had recovered from their traumatic symptoms and 65 percent had never developed symptoms of trauma.

People developed PTSD symptoms in proportion to their PROXIMITY to the event. For example, of people in the general public who were physically injured in the event, 33 percent did not develop symptoms, while 41 percent did develop symptoms but had recovered by the six-month assessment. Thus, 26 percent had developed PTSD. Interestingly, 11.8 percent of the rescuers had PTSD at six months, and 37 percent had developed trauma symptoms but recovered. Fifty-one percent of the rescuers remained resilient in not developing PTSD at all.

Abused Children and Resilience

Among abused children, the key factor that seems to enhance resilience is having a person in their life on whom they felt they could depend. In general, females are more resilient than males. Other factors related to resilience include a child's temperament (easygoing children are more resilient than others), the ability to not blame themselves for the abuse they suffer, and the ability to avoid abusive parents.

In addition, key characteristics of child resilience were discussed in *Promoting Resilience: A Review of Effective Strategies for Child Care Services*, a publication in the United Kingdom. The following traits were key characteristics among resilient children: a sense of humor, positive peer relationships, personal attractiveness to others, feelings of empathy, problem-solving abilities, academic success, membership in a faith group, involvement in extracurricular activities, and good social skills.

Resilience and Brain Circuitry

Studies are ongoing to locate and identify the brain areas that are associated with the experience of the capacity of resilience. A study reported in the *Journal of Neuroscience* in 2006 found a brain area, the prefrontal cortex, that responds (sometimes by shutting down) to a traumatic experience. By training rats to control their responses during traumatic events, researchers were able to condition the prefrontal cortex to remain active during noncontrollable traumatic events. This activation turned off the mood-regulating cells of the AMYGDALA and prevented panic and avoidance. In other words, the prefrontal cortex remained active as if it had control of the situation, which was resilience in action.

Resiliency Assessments

Questionnaire (self-report) instruments that are used to assess the baseline or current levels of resilience. Resiliency is a capacity that can be learned, given the right learning environment. The first step in any learning situation, however, is to assess the level or degree of the capacity of the individual at the onset so that progress can be monitored along the way. There are many types of resiliency assessment tools. One such resource is the Resiliency Map, a program that provides a questionnaire, score grid, and interpretation guide.

See also ASSESSMENT AND DIAGNOSIS; CHILD ABUSE AND NEGLECT; CHILD PHYSICAL ABUSE; CHILD SEXUAL ABUSE; CHILD SEXUAL ABUSE ACCOMMODATION SYNDROME; INSTRUMENTS/SCALES/SURVEYS THAT EVALUATE

POSTTRAUMATIC STRESS DISORDER (PTSD); STRESS; VULNERABILITY.

Miller, Laurie, M.D., with Christine Adamec. *The Encyclopedia of Adoption*, 3rd ed. New York: Facts On File, 2007.

Newman, Tony. *Promoting Resilience: A Review of Effective Strategies for Child Care Services*, prepared for the Centre for Evidence-Based Special Services, University of Exeter, U.K., 2002.

resistance In psychology and the trauma area, resistance is a personal and active attempt to *not* listen to the therapy, *not* explore experience with negative emotions or traumatic events, or an unwillingness to take medications, or to practice what the therapist proposes. Resistance can take many forms, and overcoming and dealing with resistance is a major focus in any form of therapy.

The term *resistance* actually originated in psychoanalysis, where resistance was seen as a natural tendency to keep traumatic unconscious material or experience unconscious and not let it emerge into conscious awareness. It was thought to be held in the unconscious state by repression, a force to prevent aversive or scary material from emerging into consciousness. Free association was developed as a method for getting around resistances, as were dreams and slips of the tongue. Working resistance can be seen as the focus of psychoanalytic or other dynamic therapies because, whether conscious or unconscious, it prevents movement, insight, and healing within those approaches. Unfortunately, PTSD victims naturally seek to avoid thoughts, emotions, and reminders of a traumatic event, so psychotherapy, if they even try it, is usually unsuccessful or, if they stick it out, very long term due to resistance.

Restorative Retelling Group (RRG) Close family members are vulnerable to trauma distress after the violent death of a loved one from an accident, suicide, or homicide. The family's preoccupation with the final thoughts and feelings of the victim at the time of death recur as intrusive thoughts, FLASHBACKS, or dream patterns. Only 5 percent of family members actually witness the violent death of their loved one. For most survivors, the reenacted story of the violent death will subside within weeks, but mothers and small children are at greater risk from suffering a dysfunctional fixation. There is no final continuity or transformation to be found after the violent death unless the retelling comes from our commitment to live beyond the story. The transformation occurs when the fixation and preoccupation of the violent death moves to acceptance.

Rynerson, et al., developed a systematic community-based support program for family members after a violent death. Time-limited interventions consist of 10 weekly two-hour sessions with a closed-group format limited to 10 members.

The first 10-session group is called the criminal death support group. The objective of this intervention during the early period of spotlighted media exposure (whether local or national), the raw recounting of events and the judicial findings are to provide reasons for clarification and advocacy for the demands resulting from public retelling of the victim's death.

The second 10-session group is called restorative retelling. It is offered after the investigation and trial are completed. The objective of this intervention is to moderate the internalized trauma of the violent death experience. When factual and imaginary retelling becomes prolonged and obsessive, the recounting can be reframed to include the resilient reconnection with positive life memories of the deceased. It is this reconnection with vital imagery that is the basis for restorative retelling. The group focuses on commemorating the vital living memory of the deceased followed by writing and drawing exercises allowing the survivors to restore meaning and purpose in life beyond the violent death.

Restorative retelling groups were used with family members bereaved by SEPTEMBER 11 events of the World Trade Center.

See also TESTIMONY THERAPY; THERAPY, TYPES OF.

Rynerson, E., J. Favell, and M. Saindon. "Group Intervention for Bereavement After Violent Death." *Psychiatric Services* 53 (October 2002): 1,340.

retraumatization Experiencing the same traumatic impact as suffered in the past, such as when the victim of rape is raped again or when the victim of a robbery is robbed again. Retraumatization is extremely difficult for the victim, who often needs therapy. Some retraumatized individuals, such as those who were sexually assaulted, have never reported the initial rape to anyone. Yet studies have indicated that it is as acutely active in their minds as the subsequent assault, even with the passage of many years between the rapes.

Interestingly, retraumatization often occurs in therapy itself when patients are led through therapy to describe, in detail, a traumatic event. The act of telling about the event can cause retraumatization and symptoms of regression. Skilled and competent therapists are very cautious before asking a patient to relive an event. Containment, the ability to tolerate intense emotional states, and a strong working relationship with the therapist, are essential prerequisites when working with retraumatized victims.

Retelling itself, even with proper containment, is usually not totally therapeutic or healing.

See also ABREACTION.

revictimization   Experiencing the same type of trauma from victimization that has occurred in the past, such as when a victim of sexual assault is again assaulted or when a victim of robbery or burglary experiences yet another theft. Revictimization usually causes severe trauma and may lead to the development of POSTTRAUMATIC STRESS DISORDER (PTSD). Freud pointed out that traumatized people often reproduce their trauma in present-day events. For example, unresolved Oedipal events will be acted out in adulthood with a spouse. This unconscious process is called REPETITION COMPULSION and, in Freud's eyes, was an effort to resolve the original trauma. Ironically, revictimization can occur in trauma therapy when the therapist's effort to have the client face or examine a traumatic experience can be perceived as a form of victimization or abuse by the client.

See also RETRAUMATIZATION.

rewind technique   A safe, nonintrusive psychological method for desensitizing the traumatic experience developed by Dr. David Muss. The aim of the technique is to return the feeling of control to the trauma survivor when he or she recalls the traumatic event, and to eliminate FLASHBACKS, NIGHTMARES, and emotional distress. The control

allows the emotions not to be overpowered when a reminder of the trauma is accidentally brought up in conversation or heard in a news story. The steps involved in the rewind technique take approximately 10 to 15 minutes to explain to the client and two to three minutes for the client to perform.

The experienced practitioner first teaches the client to reach a deep state of relaxation. In this relaxed state, the client is asked to imagine sitting alone in a room with a television screen in front of them, with a remote control. The rewind technique is explained as pretending to watch a film of the traumatic event, first forward, then backward. Before the screen comes into view, the client is asked to "float" out of his or her body and to watch himself or herself sitting in front of the television screen.

The client is asked to watch himself or herself watching the film with all the sounds and details as if someone who had filmed them during the traumatic event is now showing the film. The film of the traumatic event starts before the traumatic event and ends at a point of safety or when the images fade.

The second film is called the rewind. The client is asked to see himself or herself *in* the film, not watching as in the first film. The client is asked to hit the rewind button on the remote control in his or her mind and watch the film go backwards in every detail and stop at the starting point before the traumatic event occurs. The rewind must be done quickly. If the forwarded film runs one minute, then the rewind runs 15 seconds.

Both films are repeated back and forth, with the client controlling the speed of the film until the films evoke little or no emotion. The rewind technique is a powerful desensitization technique with simple and easy instructions.

See also THERAPY, TYPES OF.

Muss, D. A. "A New Technique for Treating Post-Traumatic Stress Disorder." *British Journal of Clinical Psychology* 30 (1991): 91–92.

ripple effect   The study of secondary trauma or the vicarious acquisition of a traumatic experience from another. The sexual assault field has been an area of intense study of the ripple effect. Here, the effects of a rape are widespread and include mental health workers, the victim's family and intimate relationships, his or her coworkers, and the culture as a whole. Emotional energy spreads to others, whether positive or negative, because people have a general capacity for compassion and empathy and can identify with the response of another based on how they would feel in a similar situation.

Some evidence regarding the ripple effect indicates that fetuses can become victims of their mothers' trauma through hormonal influences and perhaps through other sources of transmission.

The term and concept of the ripple effect was introduced by Jacob Kounin in 1970, in his book *Discipline and Group Management in Classrooms,* where

he pointed out that teacher praise in the classroom as well as teacher reprimands influenced nearby students. Kounin went on to study the ripple effect in other group settings, including industrial and corporate settings.

Kounin, J. S. *Discipline and Group Management in Classrooms.* New York: Holt, Rinehart and Winston, 1970.

Rosenberg Self-Esteem Scale This early self-esteem scale (1965) was developed by Morris Rosenberg and is now in the public domain. It has

---

THE ROSENBERG SELF-ESTEEM SCALE

Below is a list of statements dealing with your general feelings about yourself.

If you STRONGLY AGREE circle SA, if you AGREE with the statement circle A.

If you DISAGREE, circle D. If you STRONGLY DISAGREE, circle SD.

	Strongly Agree	Agree	Disagree	Strongly Disagree
1. I feel that I'm a person of worth, at least on an equal plane with others.	SA	A	D	SD
2. I feel that I have a number of good qualities.	SA	A	D	SD
3. All in all, I am inclined to feel that I am a failure.	SA	A	D	SD
4. I am able to do things as well as most other people.	SA	A	D	SD
5. I feel I do not have much to be proud of.	SA	A	D	SD
6. I take a positive attitude toward myself.	SA	A	D	SD
7. On the whole, I am satisfied with myself.	SA	A	D	SD
8. I wish I could have more respect for myself.	SA	A	D	SD
9. I certainly feel useless at times.	SA	A	D	SD
10. At times I think I am no good at all.	SA	A	D	SD

Scores are calculated as follows:
For items 1, 2, 4, 6, and 7

Strongly agree	3
Agree	2
Disagree	1
Strongly Disagree	0

For items 3, 5, 8, 9, and 10 (which are reversed valence)

Strongly agree	0
Agree	1
Disagree	2
Strongly Disagree	3

Your score on the Rosenberg self-esteem scale is:

The scale ranges from 0 to 30. Scores between 15 and 25 are within normal range; scores below 15 suggest low self-esteem.

The Rosenberg Self Esteem Scale may be used without explicit permission from the Rosenberg Foundation. However, the family of the author would like to be kept informed of its use, at The Morris Rosenberg Foundation, c/o Department of Sociology, University of Maryland, 2112 Art/Soc Building, College Park, Md. 20742.

been translated into French and Norwegian for use as an educational and research tool. The scale is a global unidimensional measure of self-esteem that was originally developed for use with adolescents. It measures overall feelings of self-worth and self-acceptance. Answers are given on a four-point intensity scale that can also be administered through an interview. Scores range from 0 to 30 with higher scores indicating higher self-esteem. It is usually identified as the SES or Self-Esteem Scale and has good reliability and validity across a wide range of sample groups.

Rosenberg, Morris. *Society and the Adolescent Self-Image.* Rev. ed. Middletown, Conn.: Wesleyan University Press, 1989.

S

SAFER Model   See TREATMENT: PSYCHOTHERAPY, PSYCHOPHARMACOLOGY, AND ALTERNATIVE MEDICINE.

Schreckneurose **(fright neuroses)**   A fearful fright response following a traumatic experience such as an actual threat against life. A syndrome consisting of "multiple nervous and psychic phenomena arising as a result of severe emotional upheaval or sudden fright, which would build up great anxiety. It can be observed after serious accidents and injuries, particularly fires, railroad derailments or collisions," according to Emil Kraeplin, the famous turn-of-the-century nosologist and developer of the first commonly used diagnostic system. In this case, Kraeplin's early 1900s system (translated by Jablensky, 1985) formed the basis for the first *Diagnostic and Statistical Manual (DSM)*, which, in turn, influenced subsequent editions of the *DSM* to varying degrees.

It must be remembered that at the turn of the century when Kraeplin studied these disorders, railroad accidents were numerous and horrific, fires were intense and rapidly destructive, and collisions were unexpected and often quite bloody (safety glass had yet to be invented). Today we know that startle responses and exaggerated reactivity are characteristic of people who are prone to develop POSTTRAUMATIC STRESS DISORDER.

Saigh, P. A., and J. D. Bremmer. *Posttraumatic Stress Disorder: A Comprehensive Text.* Needham Heights, Mass.: Allyn & Bacon, 1999.

script-driven imagery   A well-established technique for test subjects to listen to a script about a stressful or traumatic scene and measure increases in physical and emotional symptoms (symptom provocation paradigm) in POSTTRAUMATIC STRESS DISORDER (PTSD) research. In studies, subjects listen to their own trauma script tape recording, which triggers intense, vivid FLASHBACK memory that begins at the beginning of the script and continues well after the tape ends. Subjects report that after the 30-second script has ended, the trauma script elicits memories of their traumatic experience that are a typical recall for them. Script-driven imagery has been used to investigate psychophysiological responses in PTSD measuring physiological arousal such as heart rate, electrical skin conductance, electromyogram (muscle tension), and facial muscle movement.

Construction of the scripts begins with the subjects providing written descriptions of two neutral autobiographical events and two very stressful autobiographical traumatic events (e.g., sexual abuse or military combat). The subjects' visceral and muscular reactions are written into a 30-second script by a research investigator. Each 30-second script portrays each experience in the second person, present tense, and incorporates as many bodily sensations as the subject recalls.

See also THERAPY, TYPES OF.

Orr, S., R. Pitman, N. Lasko, and L. Herz. "Psychophysiological Assessment of Posttraumatic Stress Disorder Imagery in World War II and Korean Combat Veterans." *Journal of Abnormal Psychology* 102, no. 1 (1993): 152–159.

secondary symptoms   The term commonly used to highlight the side effects of medications that can usually produce quite distressing and disturbing "symptoms." The side effects usually prevent or discourage users from continuing their regime. There is also high incidence of drug resistance or withdrawal when side effects begin to appear after many months of continuous use.

Secondary symptoms also reflects the adult damage that can result from CHILD ABUSE AND NEGLECT. Frequently, survivors go to counselors or therapists with these secondary issues rather than the initial and causative abuse. These behaviors and issues are called the secondary symptoms of abuse. Listed below are common secondary symptoms. This list is not comprehensive, nor do all abuse survivors manifest all of these behaviors. However, many of the following symptoms are present in older teens and adults

- anger issues
- isolation and loneliness
- depression
- eating disorder
- body dysmorphic reactions
- Type A personality
- substance abuse
- sexual dysfunction
- sleep disorders
- hypervigilence
- anxiety
- fear and panic
- dysfunctional relationships
- spiritual void and emptiness
- concentration difficulties
- trust issues
- intimacy problems
- poor self image
- stress
- poor parenting skills

secondary traumatic stress (STS)/secondary traumatic stress disorder (STSD) Secondary traumatic stress (STS) refers to a syndrome that affects those professionals, as well as the general population, who are helping or supporting people who are suffering from a traumatic event. STS and STSD are natural consequences of caring between

two people; one who experienced a horrific event and the other who is affected by the very nature of the person who has been traumatized. Charles Figley calls this a natural by-product of caring for traumatized people. Figley has previously described STS/STSD as COMPASSION FATIGUE. STS/STSD is not recognized as a formal disorder in the *DIAGNOSTIC AND STATISTICAL MANUAL of Mental Disorders* fourth edition, text revision (DSM-IV-TR).

Some of the symptoms of STS are fatigue, exhaustion, avoidance, a hypersensitive startle response, numbing, intrusion, and avoidance. STS is not a cognitive phenomenon, but is one of experience that is directly linked by being involved with those who have been exposed to trauma. The emotional cost of caring can be considerable, whether the exposure to victims is short (such as by rescue workers who are exposed to the trauma of disaster victims), or longer (as seen in psychotherapists treating victims of sexual abuse). STSD symptoms are nearly identical to POSTTRAUMATIC STRESS DISORDER (PTSD) symptoms, except that STSD is associated with knowledge of a traumatic event through the victims, while PTSD sufferers are directly connected to the traumatic event.

A close and intense relationship with those suffering from PTSD may challenge the caregiver's or significant other's basic faith in loyalty, creating a vulnerability to escape the relationship. A strong ongoing support system is needed to deal with these disruptive reactions. Open communication can lessen the impact of feeling "burned out" and provide ways to lessen the arousal "stress" state and to process this state of distress.

Secondary traumatic stress disorder (STSD) may develop if the identification with the victims is too strong or intense and the coping strategies are inappropriate, or the helpers/rescuers are unable to execute their own survivor strategies adaptively.

See also THERAPY, TYPES OF.

Figley, Charles R., ed. *Compassion Fatigue: Coping with Secondary Traumatic Stress Disorder in Those Who Treat the Traumatized.* New York: Brunnzer/Mazel, 1995, 1–8.

secondary traumatization Exposure to traumatic events by the accounts of events from others or the media. This is a very common phenomenon among mental health professionals who work with trauma victims and are exposed to stories, re-accounts, and descriptions of traumatic experiences involving horror, suffering, helplessness, and fear. The term was first used by Rosenheck and Nathan in 1985 to describe their observations that the children of trauma survivors displayed symptoms of trauma but to a lesser degree than the parents' symptoms.

POSTTRAUMATIC STRESS DISORDER (PTSD)-type symptoms may develop from exposure to traumatic events through the media and involve recurrent thoughts, hyperarousal, and avoidance, along with DEPRESSION, anxiety, and other disturbing emotions. Secondary traumatization has also been called COMPASSION FATIGUE and VICARIOUS TRAUMATIZATION.

Secondary traumatization has not been studied very much, so little is known about its dynamics. Furthermore, there is a controversy in the clinical literature by detractors who claim that labeling clinicians with secondary PTSD pathologizes (casts in a negative light) what is a normal reaction and not a disorder. They argue that clinicians will recover from their "reactions" unless a trauma that the clinician has not resolved is stimulated. A meta-analysis was done by Everly et al. (1999) that also discusses the prevention and treatment of secondary traumatization. He, and others, found that insufficient training and the trauma history of the therapist were the leading causes of secondary traumatization among therapists.

See also SECONDARY TRAUMATIC STRESS (STS)/ SECONDARY TRAUMATIC STRESS DISORDER (STSD).

Everly, G. S., S. H. Boyle, and J. M. Lating. "The Effectiveness of Psychological Debriefing with Vicarious Trauma: A Meta-Analysis." *Stress Medicine* 15, no. 4 (1999): 229–233.
Rosenheck, R. "Secondary Traumatization in the Children of Vietnam Veterans with Posttraumatic Stress Disorder." *Hospital Community Psychiatry* 36 (1985): 538–539.

selective serotonin reuptake inhibitor (SSRI) A type of ANTIDEPRESSANT that inhibits the reuptake of SEROTONIN (an essential brain hormone and chemical messenger), thus allowing for greater levels of serotonin and leading to an enhanced mood

state if the antidepressant is effective. The effect of SSRIs on traumatized people is to relieve some of the depression or anxiety associated with PTSD and ASD. Medications in the selective serotonin reuptake inhibitor (SSRI) class are often effective in treating DEPRESSION, and they usually do not cause the sedation or weight gain that is often seen with TRICYCLIC ANTIDEPRESSANTS. However, SSRIs may cause sexual side effects in some people, such as delaying orgasm.

There are many different brands of SSRIs. Some examples of SSRIs approved by the Food and Drug Administration (FDA) are citalopram (Celexa), escitalopram (Lexapro), fluoxetine (Prozac), fluvoxamine (Luvox), paroxetine (Paxil), and sertraline (Zoloft).

It should be noted that the risk for SUICIDE in severely depressed individuals does not immediately abate with the use of antidepressants, and individuals exhibiting signs of suicide attempts should be referred for emergency treatment. Many antidepressants have a cumulative effect and must "build up" in the system, so that their full effect is often not felt for weeks. In addition, some antidepressants are not effective in some individuals. However, if one SSRI does not help a depressed individual, this does not mean that no SSRI could be helpful. Sometimes the second medication that is tried (or the third) is the most effective.

Medication treatment with antidepressants is largely a trial and error effort, since there are no laboratory tests that measure either depression or a remission from depression, and the patient and the physician work together to seek the right treatment.

It should also be noted that many studies have shown that a combination of behavior therapy and medications is the most effective treatment for depressive symptoms.

See also DEPRESSION; MONOAMINE OXIDASE INHIBITORS; SEROTONIN NOREPINEPHRINE INHIBITORS; TRICYCLIC ANTIDEPRESSANTS.

self-efficacy A concept that was developed and elaborated on by Albert Bandura in the 1990s. It refers to the perceived belief in one's capacity to produce levels of performance that affect events in one's life. It is reflected in how one feels, thinks, motivates oneself and behaves in relationship to those events. Self-efficacy permeates four major aspects of functioning: cognition, motivation, affect, and selection processes. For example, people with a strong sense of self-efficacy approach difficult tasks as challenges to deal with rather than as aversive events to be avoided. Their outlook displays interest and involvement. Failure is not regarded as personal but rather as an outcome caused by insufficient effort or deficient knowledge and skills that one can acquire. Such individuals have a success-oriented outlook, reduced stress, and no or little depression.

People with low self-efficacy see difficult tasks as threatening; they aspire to little and have weak commitments. They are more self-involved than performance-involved and are set back by failure rather than motivated to succeed. They can feel like victims and can become depressed easily with failure.

Self-efficacy seems to be built on earned successes, observation, and motivation from others (vicarious models), positive social persuasion that one has the capabilities to succeed, and an energized sense of affective arousal.

COMPLEX TRAUMA or single incident trauma can severely damage one's sense of self-efficacy and undermine behavior throughout the life cycle. Motivation and initiative are affected. One's sense of body and emotions feels dysregulated and, in turn, the ability to take initiative and trust one's instincts is clouded. Trauma is the great killer of self-efficacy because the external and internal worlds are no longer trustworthy and safe.

See also SELF-ESTEEM MODEL.

Bandura, A. *Self-Efficacy: the exercise of control.* New York: Freeman, 1997.
———. "Self-efficacy: toward a unifying theory of behavior change." *Psychological Review* 84: 191–215.

self-esteem model   The feeling one has about one's ability to accomplish or master events and tasks in life. It is usually defined as an individual's sense of his or her value or worth, or the extent to which an individual values, approves of, appreciates, and prizes or likes him or herself. It is generally considered an evaluative or affective component of self-concept.

Self-esteem has been related both to socioeconomic status and to various aspects of health and health-related behavior, as has a similar construct, SELF-EFFICACY. Self-efficacy, a term associated with the work of Bandura, refers to an individual's sense of competence or ability in general or in particular domains.

See also ROSENBERG SELF-ESTEEM SCALE (SES).

self-trauma model   An integrative theoretical model or approach to the concept, study, and treatment of trauma. The self-trauma model was developed by John Briere at the Keck School of Medicine at the University of Southern California in the early 1990s. It focuses on the effects of early abuse by omission (neglect) or commission (sexual, physical, or emotional abuse). Abuse helps form core or essential beliefs in the victim that are often carried into adulthood. The model draws from psychodynamic theory (the unconscious role of emotion and behavior), attachment theory (bonding with mother), cognitive-behavioral (role of thoughts and beliefs in behavior) and psychophysiological (physiological processes and their behavioral correlates development), and classical conditioning (associative learning).

The self-trauma model suggests that stored subconscious trauma affects the cognitive, sensory, emotional, and self-evaluative/identity levels during development. It also disrupts normative functioning, particularly at the affect (mood) regulation level. These stored experiences create interpersonal difficulties and bias the individual's development toward defensive strategies, such as AVOIDANCE, DISSOCIATION, distorted cognitive schema, and exaggerated or inappropriate emotional reactions. These defensive strategies slow or arrest development, leading to a poorly integrated self-concept, and they often create "characterological" or personality difficulties. This negative information stored in the nervous system becomes self-traumatizing and creates pervasive and enduring distress.

Briere, J. *Child Abuse Trauma: Theory and Treatment of the Lasting Effects.* Newbury Park, Calif.: Sage, 1992.

sensate experience   In the trauma field, the term *sensate experience* usually refers to the bodily sense of a past experience or the body sensations linked or conditioned to a particular experience. These body sensations such as tingling, tension, electricity, numbness, and so on, are the direct result of a traumatic experience and represent the body "memory" of an event. Eugene Gendlin (in his book *Focusing*) referred to these sensations as the FELT SENSE of what is troubling or traumatic. They tell a story, not at a visual or verbal level, but rather at the sensory level.

These sensations are usually more subtle than "feelings" and involve perceptions that are (1) kinesthetic (muscle tension, movement impulses, etc.), (2) proprioceptive (the position as sensed through position of joints), (3) vestibular or inner ear perceptions (which integrate kinesthetic and proprioceptive cues to help individuals know where they are in relation to gravity, uprightness, and balance), and (4) autonomic (arousal experiences like temperature, digestion sensations, heart rate changes and other involuntary functions).

Becoming aware of and "tracking" sensations is a key part of SOMATIC EXPERIENCING (SE) THERAPY developed by Peter Levine as described in his book *Waking the Tiger*. Levine points out that humans, like other animals, have a natural healing mechanism for releasing traumatic experience and his therapy is built on that basic premise.

Gendlin, Eugene T. *Focusing*. New York: Bantam, 1982.
Levine, Peter, *Waking the Tiger: Healing Trauma: The Innate Capacity to Transform Overwhelming Experience*. Berkeley, Calif.: North Atlantic Books, 1997.

Sensation, Imagery, Behaviors, Affect, and Meaning (SIBAM)

An acronym from SOMATIC EXPERIENCING (SE) THERAPY. Each of these five areas of human functioning contributes, in some way, to the trauma constellation. Each part is active in any given experience. For example, a simple intact memory can be found in the following statement:

I still have a clear visual image from yesterday when I rode on the biggest roller coaster ever [behavior] and it nearly scared me to death [sensation]. Afterwards I felt courageous and proud [affect]. It was good to overcome my fears and have some fun [meaning].

The relationship of these parts is important in healing traumatic reactions. For example, some traumatic reactions tend to split or separate these parts, so that the experience is diluted. Or, in somatic experiencing terms, they are "undercoupled." In undercoupling, the parts are separated and do not represent a coherent whole. Therapy must recombine the parts in order for healing to occur. Feelings and images should go together, as an example. The therapist might work at joining them into a coherent felt experience.

Likewise, "overcoupling" can occur among parts so that one part can trigger a reaction in other parts, setting off a chain reaction of suddenly re-experiencing the traumatic event from one element (such as thinking about it or feeling it). By assessing the relationship among parts, the therapist can work to recombine these essential elements by containing, releasing, pendulating or moving between positive and negative affect, and allowing felt experience to guide healing.

See also THERAPY, TYPES OF.

sense of coherence (SoC)   The concept of sense of coherence (SoC) was proposed and developed by Aaron Antonovsky in 1979 as a mediating variable to explain the occurrence of illness under stress. Antonovsky defined the concept as "The extent to which one has a pervasive, enduring though dynamic feeling of confidence that one's environment is predictable and that things will work out as well as can reasonably be expected." In other words, SoC is a mixture of optimism and control. He saw SoC as a combination of understanding a situation or comprehensibility, feelings of SELF-EFFICACY in managing it, and a sense of meaning derived from experiences. A strong sense of SoC was associated with less pain and DEPRESSION and less likelihood of developing POSTTRAUMATIC STRESS DISORDER (PTSD).

Antonovsky A. *Health Stress and Coping*. San Francisco: Jossey-Bass, 1979.

———. "The Structure and Properties of the Sense of Coherence Scale." *Social Science & Medicine* 36 (March 1993): 725–733.

———. *Unraveling the Mystery of Health. How People Manage Stress and Stay Well.* San Francisco: Jossey-Bass, 1987.

September 11   Refers to September 11, 2001, also known as 9/11. This was a clear and sunny Tuesday morning when suicide terrorists seized four commercial U.S. airliners to attack the United States. At 8:45 A.M., the first hijacked airliner crashed into the north tower of the World Trade Center building in New York City. Eighteen minutes later, a second airliner crashed into the south tower. Both towers collapsed after burning for less than 90 minutes as news cameras captured this horrific TRAUMATIC EVENT in real time, and as millions of horrified viewers watched these events on television around the world.

As part of the coordinated attack on the United States, at 9:37 A.M., a third hijacked airliner crashed into the U.S. Department of Defense, in the Pentagon building, in Arlington County, Virginia. At 10:03 A.M., a fourth airliner crashed into a field in Somerset County, Pennsylvania, 80 miles southeast of Pittsburgh, when the passengers resisted the hijackers. The hijackers' original target was believed to be either the U.S. Capitol or the White House in Washington, D.C.

The death toll of September 11 was significant: more than 2,900 people died at the World Trade Center, 125 people died at the Pentagon, and 256 people on the four airliners. This total includes the 19 Arab terrorists who used the four planes as guided missiles with more than 10,000 gallons of jet fuel on board. In the aftermath of the attack, the United States declared a war on terrorism and resolved to bring Osama bin Laden (the suspected mastermind of the attack) and Islamic Al Qaeda (the radical Middle Eastern insurgency group that claimed responsibility for the attack) to justice through the U.S.-led coalition force invasion of Afghanistan, where bin Laden was reportedly hiding, in October 2001.

The attacks on the World Trade Center towers frightened and traumatized many people in the United States. While terrorism occurs in every country in the world to some extent, the suddenness, extent of the damage, and senseless loss of life, and the fact that this event represented a concerted attack by a terrorist organization against the United States made the aftermath even more frightening.

It is known that attacks by people against other people often produce the greatest trauma. It is also known that unexpected, random attacks are more frightening than predictable or anticipated attacks. Organized attacks by groups intent on hurting and killing others is another factor in producing traumatic reactions. When all three of these factors are present, the likelihood of widespread traumatic reactions is the greatest, which is why the attack on September 11 had such an impact on people all over the world. Traumatic events produce a feeling of lack of safety in one's environment and these effects were seen throughout the United States.

In response to the attacks of September 11, a new government agency called the Department of Homeland Security (DHS) was established in November 2002. According to the Homeland Security Act of 2002, the mission of DHS is to prevent terrorist attacks within the United States, reduce the vulnerability of the United States to terrorism, minimize the damage, and assist in the recovery from terrorist attacks that do occur within the United States.

Feeling unsafe can intensify traumatic reactions and symptoms, and may lead to paranoia and suspiciousness. Deep, widespread changes in the way of life in the United States resulted from the events of September 11, and some of these changes, such as enhanced security and surveillance and color-coded threat-level warnings, induced a state of low-level fear in some people. The vigilance and fear arising from such sources, while mostly subliminal, creates a low level of arousal that may persist for years, even for lifetimes. In a survey by the New York City Department of Health and Mental Health of 11,000 residents living in Manhattan at the time of the September 11 attack, researchers found that two to three years later, the prevalence of probable PTSD was 12.6 percent, a rate three to four times higher than the general population. Another study found that 7.5 percent of New York City area residents had probable PTSD one to two months after September 11, compared to a rate of 4 percent for the rest of the country.

See also AVOIDANCE/AVOIDANCE BEHAVIOR; TERRORISM; TORTURE.

Digrande, L., M. Perrin, L. Thorpe, L. Thalji, J. Murphy, D. Wu, M. Farfel, and R. Brackbill. "Posttraumatic Stress Symptoms, PTSD, and Risk Factors among Lower Manhattan Residents 2–3 Years after the September 11, 2001, Terrorist Attacks." *Journal of Traumatic Stress* 21, no. 3 (June 2008): 264–273.

Galea, S., J. Ahern, H. Resnisk, D. Kilpatrick, M. Bucuvalas, J. Gold, and D. Vlahov. "Psychological Sequelae of the September 11 Terrorist Attacks in New York City." *New England Journal of Medicine* 346 (2002): 982–987.

The 9/11 Commission. *The 9/11 Commission Report.* National Commission on Terrorist Attacks upon the United States. Washington, D.C., 2004.

U.S. Department of Homeland Security. "Homeland Security Act of 2002." Available online. URL: http://www.dhs.gov/xabout/laws/law_regulation_rule_0011.shtm. Accessed December 4, 2008.

sequential traumatization Traumas that appear one after the other, such as a death in the family, which is immediately followed by a natural disaster. Multiple or "pile-on" tragic events are not only difficult for an individual to cope with but also take a long time to process and resolve. Furthermore, they can lead to symptoms of POSTTRAUMATIC STRESS DISORDER (PTSD) that persist for those people who are vulnerable to developing PTSD and for those who are less vulnerable but are hit with many traumas at the same time.

Events that are the most likely to have lasting effects are early separation from or loss of parents and early traumatizations, such as surgeries, isolation, and accidents. Sequential or multiple traumas that occur early in life have the most profound effect on adult behavior and the development of some or all PTSD symptoms.

As adults, individuals who were traumatized in a sequential manner at an early age have difficulties in bonding closely with others and have high DIVORCE rates. They also often show evidence of interpersonal problems centered around trust. Sequential traumas that occur to an adult can also produce PTSD-like symptoms, such as DEPRESSION, withdrawal, anxiety, etc. Usually each event must

be dealt with in treatment in order for the individual to restore well-being.

serotonin A monoamine NEUROTRANSMITTER that is produced in the BRAIN and found in blood platelets and the intestines. The disruption of the metabolism or the uptake mechanism of serotonin in the brain has been shown to affect mood, learning ability, and sleep. Serotonin has a key role in DEPRESSION, and much research has targeted the serotonin uptake mechanism in the brain in the development of antidepressant drugs called SELECTIVE SEROTONIN REUPTAKE INHIBITORS (SSRIs). These drugs include Prozac (fluoxetine), Paxil (paroxetine), and Zoloft (sertraline). The serotonin reuptake inhibitors have been shown to be effective pharmacological agents in the treatment of POSTTRAUMATIC STRESS DISORDER (PTSD).

See also BRAIN; DEPRESSION; NOREPINEPHRINE; SEROTONIN NOREPINEPHRINE REUPTAKE INHIBITORS.

serotonin norepinephrine reuptake inhibitor (SNRI) A type of ANTIDEPRESSANT medication that inhibits the reuptake of both SEROTONIN and NOREPINEPHRINE, thus allowing for greater levels of these neurochemicals in the blood. With trauma victims, this medication can help relieve some of the depressive and anxiety symptoms and improve cognition and motivation to get better. In addition to treating DEPRESSION, medications in this class of drugs may also be effective in treating symptoms of anxiety, and they are sometimes used to help treat chronic pain. Some examples of SNRIs are duloxetine (Cymbalta) and venlafaxine (Effexor, Effexor XR). It is still too early to determine the range of conditions and effectiveness of these forms of antidepressant and antianxiety medications.

See also DEPRESSION; SELECTIVE SEROTONIN REUPTAKE INHIBITORS; TRICYCLIC ANTIDEPRESSANTS.

shame A painful self-evaluation of the feelings of worthlessness, humiliation, and powerlessness. Research is now beginning to show traumatized individuals with POSTTRAUMATIC STRESS DISORDER

(PTSD) suffer from symptoms of shame seen as the feeling of doubting their right to exist.

Shame diminishes the person's sense of self and sense of value. This may cause a desire to hide from others or from community activities or to isolate themselves so as not to be seen, resulting in a debilitating affective disorder. In public, shamed people may force a smile, look downward, bite their lips, or hide their faces, common indicators of a severely shamed person.

Shame can impede the recovery process by keeping the victims of trauma in an immobile state, unable to forgive themselves for the outcome of a traumatic event. According to Leskeda and his colleagues (2002), veterans with PTSD scored higher on measures of shame than nonshamed veterans and were more likely to turn to SUBSTANCE ABUSE or DEPRESSION.

See also GUILT; SURVIVOR GUILT.

Leskeda, J., M. Dieperink, and P. Thuras. "Shame and Posttraumatic Stress Disorder." *Journal of Traumatic Stress* 15, no. 3 (2002): 223–226.

shell shock   A term used in World War I by the British army, when experts believed that artillery shells caused tiny hemorrhages of the BRAIN, resulting in a variety of physical ailments (headaches, fatigue) and psychiatric symptoms (disconnect from surroundings, panic attacks). It was later discovered that soldiers did not have to be around exploding shells to exhibit these symptoms of shell shock and, instead, the soldiers were responding to the stress of warfare. The term *shell shock* was later changed to *war neurosis* and then to *battle fatigue*. The most recent term for the same behavior is *combat stress reaction*.

Over 80,000 combatants from England and Canada suffered diagnosed forms of shell shock in World War I. Faithful to the prevailing biological/constitutional view of mental illness at the time, it was thought that percussive waves from explosive shells and bullets produced actual physical damage to hearing mechanisms, the brain, and the spinal column, resulting in hysteria-like symptoms (e.g., loss of function) such as blindness, AMNESIA, hearing loss, muteness, paralysis, and seizures.

Officers seemed to suffer more from anxiety states, whereas enlisted soldiers suffered more hysteria-like symptoms. This differential effect seemed to rule out organic explanations. Sigmund Freud countered this assumption by postulating that these war or combat neuroses were due to internal conflicts between self-preservation and the sense of honor and duty to one's comrades—in other words, a clash in opposing values within the person. The conflict differed between enlisted men and officers. Cowardice and malingering (faking) were also diagnostic considerations, and examiners used many "tricks" to distinguish between those with true reactions and fakers trying to avoid combat and potential death. For example, someone might yell out, "Hit the deck" behind a supposedly deaf-afflicted combatant to see if he reacted.

See also COMBAT-RELATED POSTTRAUMATIC STRESS DISORDER.

situationally accessible memory (SAMS)   See DUAL REPRESENTATION THEORY OF POSTTRAUMATIC STRESS DISORDER.

sleep disorders   See INSOMNIA: EARLY, MIDDLE, AND LATE; NIGHTMARES; PARASOMNIAS.

sleepwalking   See PARASOMNIAS.

small "t" trauma   See EYE MOVEMENT DESENSITIZATION AND REPROCESSING (EMDR).

Social Adjustment Scale (SAS)   A self-report (and interview version) form used to assess a two-week period on a broad range of social functioning. There are 42 questions rated on a scale from 1 to 5 (a higher number signifies greater impairment). There are six subscales, and each subscale falls into four major categories: the respondent's performance at expected tasks, the amount of friction with people, interpersonal behavior, and feelings and satisfaction. The six subscales are

1. Work-impaired performance
2. Social and leisure activities—decreased activities with friends, relationships
3. Relationships with extended family—parents, in-laws, siblings, adult children
4. Marital role as a spouse—sexual problems, impaired communications
5. Role as a parent—lack of involvement or attention with children
6. Role as a member of the family—economic inadequacies, resentment, guilt

Some sample questions are: "Have you found your work interesting in the last 2 weeks?" or "Have you had open arguments with your partner in the last 2 weeks?"

The SAS has been used with a variety of populations of patients ranging from those with DEPRESSION to patients with TRAUMATIC BRAIN INJURY. Head-injured patients report social and behavioral problems as long as five years post-trauma. The impact of the social network is substantial, says Burton (1993), developer of this scale, with the changes in the role of the head-injured person, with the greatest impairment seen in the areas of work, extended family, and parental roles.

Volpe, Bruce. "Social Adjustment Scale Assessments in Traumatic Brain Injury." *Journal of Rehabilitation* 59, no. 4 (October–December 1993): 34–37.

social anxiety disorder   Social anxiety disorder, also known as social phobia, involves generalized situations (such as being in any group of people) and specific situations (such as urinating in public restrooms, signing one's name in public, public speaking, and so forth). Each situation, however, involves other people and produces anticipatory and situational anxiety; hence the term *social anxiety disorder*. An estimated 5.3 million adults in the United States, or 6.8 percent of the adult population, have social anxiety disorder.

Symptoms and Diagnostic Path

People with social phobias usually have a persistent and intense fear of being watched and judged by others. They often fear feeling embarrassed or humiliated by others for their actions. Obviously workplace and social situations are significantly affected by these fears, and worry, dread, and avoidance are commonplace. Furthermore, there are often uncontrollable, overt signs of their distress that add further fuel to the fears. These overt signs include blushing, trembling, sweating, difficulty talking or thinking, and so on.

A fear of public speaking is the most common form of social anxiety, and it is estimated that 50–70 percent of people have some anxiety in public speaking situations. The individual may function well in all other situations, but feels fearful when having to speak in a public setting. Other specific fears are urinating in public restrooms (confined to males) when others are present.

Signing one's name in public can be a problem for some individuals. Walking through a room full of people with their eyes on the individual is a commonly fearful situation. Almost any situation in which people are watching an individual—or in which the individual perceives he or she is being watched—can develop into a specific social phobia.

The generalized form of this disorder consists of anxiety in almost any social situation. This can be very debilitating to the individual and it has pervasive effects in all aspects of the lives of those who are affected. The specific form is usually limited to one or several situations. For example, some people have difficulty signing their name on a credit slip if they feel that someone is watching them.

Embarrassment and humiliation are the feared outcomes to their behavior among those with social phobia, suggesting a past trauma history around these situations.

Treatment Options and Outlook

Treatments for social phobias have improved recently due to a greater understanding of the condition. Specifically, treatment must not only address the social fears but also the social deficits that need attention. Individuals with social phobias often lack the ability or skill to start conversations, communicate their needs, or to meet the needs of others. Skill building must focus on these limitations, since they create a vicious cycle of social failure and anxiety. Well-designed exposure therapy and skill training are very helpful therapeutic tools for the individual with this type of anxiety disorder.

Antidepressant medications can be helpful in lowering the anxiety that is associated with social phobia, but effective treatment combines medication with cognitive-behavioral skill building, usually in a group setting. Assertiveness and social skills training are the key components in recovery.

Risk Factors and Preventive Measures

Social phobias of a narrow or generalized nature usually begin in late childhood or adolescence and continue into adulthood. Early shyness is frequently a precursor, although classically conditioned fear reactions in specific social situations (e.g., public speaking, signing one's name in public, urinating in public restrooms, and so on) seem to lead to the specific and limited forms of social phobias. Research has shown that 12 percent of people report having a social phobia in their lifetimes, while 6.8 percent report experiencing a social phobia in any given year. Substance abuse is a common form of self-medication for those afflicted with social anxiety.

social perspectives on trauma   An array of social attitudes among the public often directly shapes how individuals respond to traumatic events, as well as their ability or inability to cope with them and the speed of their recovery. For example, how people in varying groups generally perceive individuals who are mentally ill will affect their regard toward those with traumatic stress disorders. If individuals in a group believe that people with psychiatric symptoms are mostly "faking" their illness (to obtain disability benefits, medications, pity, or for other reasons) or lack the "willpower" to overcome their trauma reactions, then they may also believe that traumatized individuals are actually malingering or weak-willed and consequently treat them with disdain.

In another example, if a social group believes that mentally ill people are dangerous individuals who are likely to harm others, then they may also believe that traumatized individuals are a threat, and consequently, that they should be shunned by members of the group. The mentally ill as a group are usually perceived as violent and unpredictable and often avoided or rejected for that reason, although most studies show that the mentally ill are more likely to be victims than victimizers, according to Stephen Hinshaw, author of *The Mark of Shame: Stigma of Mental Illness and an Agenda for Change*. In addition, those who are suffering from mental disorders may be fearful of seeking the assistance of mental health professionals for help from the traumas that they have experienced, lest others perceive them as weak, bad, or dangerous people.

As a result, individuals who could otherwise obtain assistance for their mental issues and often become productive members of society are instead impeded from that outcome by negative social and cultural attitudes. They are likely to become dependent on their family members and society at large for shelter, food, and other basic necessities. Some become homeless, moving from place to place. Others commit crimes and are incarcerated.

According to one study of 320 incarcerated individuals at an Iowa state prison, published in the *Journal of the American Academy of Psychiatry and the Law*, the majority of prisoners had one or more psychiatric diagnoses; for example, 61 percent suffered from mood disorders and 34 percent suffered from psychotic disorders. Treatment of these mental disorders at an earlier stage may have saved society the cost of incarceration as well as saved the individuals the distress of being jailed.

Another social factor related to trauma is the concept of COMPASSION FATIGUE, a problem experienced by helping professionals, who report that they feel like they can give no more assistance to others because they are used up, benumbed, and have less (or no) empathy than the average person. This form of secondary traumatization is caused by caring for excessive numbers of severely traumatized individuals. The individual who experiences compassion fatigue can no longer share his or her knowledge and expertise toward the goal of helping others who are traumatized, because he or she has used up all emotional reserves. Returning to a normal life for some period of time and availing him or herself of the support and understanding of others in society may help the professional regain emotional steadiness.

Some social reactions are experienced by small groups within a society; for example, an extreme reaction to a traumatic event was described by Robert Jay Lifton with regard to the bombing of Hiroshima during World War II. He called the problem CONFLICTS AROUND NURTURING AND CONTAGION, a situation in which the victims of radical traumatic events believed that no one could ever truly understand what they went through or how they felt. As a result, these individuals try to hide their victimhood status and any problems they have developed as a result of the traumatic event. In addition, the victims may adopt a self-stigma, seeing themselves as less important than other individuals and as living on borrowed time.

Another type of trauma that affects some social groups is INTERGENERATIONAL TRAUMA, which refers to the actual passing of some elements of the trauma from one generation to another; for example, genetic transmission of a condition such as high levels of CORTISOL, a stress hormone, from severely traumatized individuals to their children, who are born with abnormal levels of CORTISOL. In turn this next generation are more vulnerable to PTSD, anxiety disorders, and other disorders than their peers. Trauma may also be emotionally transmitted to future generations through storytelling and exposure to people who experienced traumatic events. This is called TRANSGENERATIONAL TRAUMA.

Sometimes individuals who believe they are "burned out" by their jobs are actually affected by a trauma that may or may not be work-related. For example, in a study reported in 2006 in *Stress and Health,* researcher Gunilla Brattberg found that of individuals who were on long-term sick leave from work due to apparent stress-related poor health, screening revealed that 52 percent of them screened positively for PTSD.

Their stressful work environment and fatigue may have led to PTSD, making it impossible for these employees to continue working; however, it is alternatively possible that a traumatic event in the employee's past may have triggered the PTSD and inhibited his or her ability to cope with the demands of work. In either case, the work environment was insufficiently supportive for the employee to transcend his or her underlying problems.

One positive social aspect that affects trauma is that many people in different religious social groups obtain relief during times of trauma from their basic SPIRITUALITY and their religious beliefs. In the United States, more than 90 percent of Americans have said that they want some kind of religious education for their children, and 82 percent of adults have reported a need for spiritual growth in their lives. In times of crisis, 80 percent say that they use prayer, and 95 percent of those who pray say that they believe that those prayers are answered.

Attitudes toward the Mentally Ill

Although many people today are accepting of individuals who suffer from disorders such as depression, other mental illnesses such as POSTTRAUMATIC STRESS DISORDER (PTSD) are often *not* accepted by the general populace, who may believe that PTSD is not a valid diagnosis. Often, these people believe that will power can overcome any disorder. Some groups also believe that psychiatric medications are inherently dangerous, and they actively discourage their use. Others may believe that individuals with psychiatric diagnoses (including PTSD) are dangerous people who should be avoided. A third stigmatizing attitude toward the mentally ill is the misconception that people with mental illnesses are innocent, childlike individuals who should be protected from themselves and sometimes from others. These negative attitudes prevent individuals with PTSD and other disorders from seeking help, instead enslaving them in their mental illness. Also, taking into account the basic criteria for PTSD, difficulties in social relations usually characterize PTSD, adding to the possibility of social alienation and stigmatization.

Military veterans and the stigma of mental illness According to Thomas W. Britt in his article on the stigma of mental health problems in the military for *Military Medicine,* some groups, such as soldiers with symptoms of PTSD, may fear seeking mental health assistance for their symptoms of PTSD because of the serious stigma often associated with having mental illness among their fellow soldiers.

Says Britt, "Within a military context, service members experiencing symptoms of PTSD and considering admitting they have a problem to someone else will likely be aware of public beliefs about psychological problems, perhaps anticipating negative consequences from different individuals (e.g., fellow service members, commanders). If soldiers fear social exclusion because they have symptoms of PTSD, they may forgo seeking help due to apprehension about societal stigma."

In addition, the consequences of seeking help are important to the soldier, who does not want his or her career destroyed because of a consultation with a psychiatrist or other mental health professional. Britt pointed out that the majority of individuals in combat are men. Said Britt, "If men experience greater anxiety when seeking psychological treatment, and thus fail to seek help due to fear, then the numbers reported of individuals with a psychological problem in the military may be vastly underrepresented."

Individuals in authority are aware of this problem and believe that some military veterans with PTSD symptoms fail to seek treatment because they are concerned about possible outcomes; for example, Secretary of Defense Robert Gates has announced a change on the application for a government security clearance, which asks, "In the last seven years, have you sought mental-health counseling?" The fear of losing or not obtaining one security clearance on the basis of their answer is a major reason why many veterans do not seek mental health counseling. Gates said that this question will be eliminated. This action will hopefully facilitate the treatment of affected military veterans and speed their recovery.

Civilian trauma and the stigma of mental illness   It is not only soldiers and veterans who are stigmatized because of PTSD or of other mental illnesses. Traumatic events such as violent crimes, rape, hostage-taking, major accidents, life-threatening events, and terrorist attacks, can each affect an individual's mental health, and individuals who develop symptoms of a traumatic stress disorder may be stigmatized. Some studies have shown that, for this reason, less than 40 percent of individuals suffering from psychiatric symptoms seek help, according to Patrick Corrigan, writing for *American Psychologist*. As a result, they fail to obtain the help that they urgently need, and their recovery is thwarted.

Said Corrigan, "Stigma harms people who are publicly labeled as mentally ill in several ways. Stereotype, prejudice, and discrimination can rob people labeled mentally ill of important life opportunities that are essential for achieving life goals. People with mental illness are frequently unable to obtain good jobs or find suitable housing because of the prejudice of key members in their communities: employers and landlords. Several studies have shown that public stereotypes and prejudice about mental illness have a deleterious impact on obtaining and keeping good jobs and leasing safe housing."

Corrigan also discussed self-stigma, and he said that people may internalize inaccurate, negative societal views about those with psychiatric symptoms, seeing themselves as bad, weak, or incompetent. "Living in a culture steeped in stigmatizing images, persons with mental illness may accept these notions and suffer diminished self-esteem, self-efficacy, and confidence in one's future. Research shows that people with mental illness often internalize stigmatizing ideas that are widely endorsed within society and believe that they are less valued because of their psychiatric disorder." These attitudes of self-condemnation also serve to alienate those with disorders from the support they often need in order to begin healing.

Compassion Fatigue

Emotional exhaustion and numbness may occur after consistently providing empathy and assistance to one or more needful individuals with traumatic stress symptoms. This is called compassion fatigue, and it can be seen in mental health professionals, health care professionals, child protection workers, and members of the clergy. It may also be experienced by nonprofessionals, such as the constant caregivers of ill parents or other relatives. The term "compassion fatigue" was first coined by C. Figley in 1995 in his book, *Compassion Fatigue: Coping with Secondary Traumatic Stress Disorder in Those Who Treat the Traumatized*. Some individuals use the phrase *compassion fatigue* interchangeably with the phrases SECONDARY TRAUMATIZATION or VICARIOUS TRAUMATIZATION.

Compassion fatigue is both a cause of traumatization and an impediment to recovering from trauma. For example, the burned-out psychiatrist who cannot talk to one more widow or child who was traumatized by a disaster feels overwhelmed and "flat" from the excessive demands on his or her time and knowledge. His or her recovery, by having some "down time" away from the disaster, will facilitate the individual's ability to return to helping traumatized people. Yet others in society may press the professional to continue to work because of the extreme needs of directly traumatized people and a lack of mental health professionals to assist them. This would be an unwise course because traumatized individuals need help from others who are at their full capabilities.

A variety of studies have been done on compassion fatigue, particularly among helping professionals. In one study, the results of a survey of 236 social workers living in New York City, among whom 80 percent were involved in disaster counseling after the terrorist attacks of SEPTEMBER 11, 2001, were reported in a 2004 issue of the *International Journal of Emergency Mental Health*. The researchers considered compassion fatigue as a construct that comprised both SECONDARY TRAUMATIZATION and job burnout. The researchers also defined compassion fatigue as "the reduced capacity or interest in being empathic."

They found that social workers who had worked with traumatized victims experienced a high risk for compassion fatigue, and World Trade Center recovery involvement was the factor with the greatest risk for secondary trauma: 52 percent of those with high recovery involvement were determined to be a potential secondary trauma case, versus 25 percent of the social workers with low involvement in recovery.

It also appears that, as with traumatic experiences, compassion fatigue is more likely to develop in people with previous traumatic and psychiatric conditions.

Conflicts around Nurturing and Contagion

Conflicts around nurturing and contagion is a condition that was identified by Robert Jay Lifton in 1969 to describe the survivors of the Hiroshima bombing by the United States and their subsequent conflicted feelings, which caused them considerable difficulties in their relationships with other people. The conflict around nurturing was related to the survivors' belief that others could not truly understand their feelings and thus, any aid that was offered was not valid. The conflict around contagion referred to the belief that survivors were somehow invisibly tainted by atomic bomb radiation. They believed they had been contaminated and were not only invisible but also a danger to others. In fact, many of these victims had been burned by the blast heat and therefore had visible signs of possible contamination. People avoided contact with these victims.

Many attitudes and beliefs of these aging survivors were driven by the loss of a sense of the future, which was an outcome of the traumatic experience of shock, devastation, and the grotesqueness of the atom bomb attack. The sense of futurelessness is common in cases of severe POSTTRAUMATIC STRESS DISORDER (PTSD).

The lack of nurturance, or social support, constitutes a major risk factor for developing trauma-related disorders, according to Brewin et al. (2000) in their *Journal of Consulting and Clinical Psychology* meta-analysis of PTSD risk factors. This is particularly true with children, because abused children are usually also neglected and shunned, and thus lack social support and positive physical contact. Fear of contagion is a serious human reaction to possibly acquiring a disease or disorder by contact or exposure to the afflicted individual. This is particularly true of the mentally ill, where their psychological or emotional problems are seen as communicable to others, and therefore social distance is used as a defense by nonaffected individuals.

Intergenerational and Transgenerational Trauma

Intergenerational trauma is a subtle but pervasive source of trauma. This type of trauma occurs in children of traumatized individuals but it is usually subliminal or less obvious than trauma due to a firsthand experience. For example, second generation survivors of the Holocaust and of the Armenian genocide show significantly lowered cortisol levels, indicating a stress component in their lives. Similar effects are evident in the children of World War II veterans, tsunami victims, and the children of victims of other civilian catastrophes who suffer from *transgenerational trauma*, or trauma that transcends successive generations, but these individuals have learned about these catastrophes through hearing stories from their relatives or experiencing the social disdain of others who reviled the past behavior. For example, some Germans, even today, experience exaggerated guilt feelings, depression, and remorse for the actions of previous generations during World War II some 60 years earlier. These attitudes are shaped by others who continue to blame all Germans for wartime atrocities—or for their failure to prevent wartime atrocities.

Many survivors of cultural traumas, such as the survivors of the bombing of Hiroshima or of massive floods affecting many people, develop PTSD. Furthermore, there is considerable evidence that these cultural traumas may be passed on to subsequent generations. For example, the Jewish Holocaust during World War II was an attempt to extinguish a whole race of people. The survivors displayed PTSD symptoms, but the children of the survivors have also displayed PTSD symptoms and had levels of cortisol in their bodies consistent with PTSD, as demonstrated by Yehuda et al. in 2002. Similarly, in the case of the Armenian genocide, more than 1.5 million Armenian civilians were slaughtered. The intergenerational effects of trauma include abnormal hormone levels, a biological vulnerability toward the development of trauma symptoms, a greater life stress than seen among nontraumatized populations, relationship problems, and difficulty with making a commitment to others.

PTSD and Work Burnout

Some individuals who present with work burnout may actually be suffering from PTSD. In a study by Brattberg in Sweden, she noted that there is an association between work burnout and traumatic life events. Using the PTSD Checklist (PCL), Brattberg found that of 62 people on long-term sick leave, more than half (52 percent) had PTSD. (She also found that 24 percent had ADHD.) The research indicated a high probability that the individuals had experienced a sexual assault or another form of severe trauma. Said Brattberg, "Partially or entirely suppressed previous trauma can consume energy throughout one's life, making the individual extra vulnerable to stress."

If the traumatized individual with PTSD remains untreated, thinking erroneously that he or she was largely affected by work issues, then the underlying problem will remain unresolved. If the person then tries to return to work, the same problems will still be present. The answer is for a true diagnosis to occur followed by treatment. In such cases, individuals can often resolve their basic problems and become productive and happier workers and people.

Spiritual Psychotherapy and Trauma

Psychotherapy in general is aimed at alleviating mental, emotional, and cognitive distress in suffering people. However, a spiritual aspect also exists in these interdependent aspects of human functioning, and this refers to "meaning" or the meaning of experiences. Sufferers ask themselves "Why did this happen to me?" and try to gain lessons from these experiences. The assumption, and many people would find this debatable, is that each experience or symptom has a deeper purpose and meaning to the individual, and finding that deep inner level is a "spiritual" quest.

Religious and spiritual beliefs are traditions handed down through generations for people to develop their beliefs about the world around them and discover the purpose of life. Spirituality has become accepted by the mental health profession as a core human dimension. Coping strategies are newly defined to include spirituality as a coping resource along with social, emotional, physical, and cognitive strategies.

People often struggle to regain balance in their lives after a traumatic event. Significant changes in life priorities and the emergence of questions about the meaning of life can cause a reevaluation and shift in priorities and life goals. It can also cause a breakdown of the sense of safety and security within the affected individual. But, religious and spiritual beliefs can also become a way to cope following trauma. In the days after September 11, 2001, 90 percent of those sampled reported turning to their religious faith.

Negative religious coping reflects how the individual may believe a traumatic event is God's punishment. Studies indicate a relationship between childhood sexual abuse and negative beliefs about

God or lower levels of belief in God, such as that God is a malevolent force or God doesn't exist at all. The anger and confusion of the sexually abused person causes him or her to fail to adapt to society. However, in recovery, spirituality remains valued and important. Researchers have found that religiously committed women who are battered present with fewer posttraumatic stress disorder (PTSD) symptoms than women without a faith and commitment experience. Jewish teenagers in Israel facing imminent missile threat during the 1992 Gulf War used their religious faith and prayer to cope with traumatic stress.

Brattberg, Gunilla. "PTSD and ADHD: Underlying Factors in Many Cases of Burnout." *Stress and Health* 22 (2006): 305–313.

Britt, Thomas W. "The Stigma of Mental Health Problems in the Military." *Military Medicine* 172, no. 2 (2007): 157–161.

Corrigan, Patrick. "How Stigma Interferes with Mental Health Care." *American Psychologist* 59, no. 7 (October 2004): 614–625.

Gunter, Tracy D., M.D., et al. "Frequency of Mental and Addictive Disorders among 320 Men and Women Entering the Iowa Prison System: Use of the MINI-Plus." *Journal of the American Academy of Psychiatry and the Law* 36, no. 1 (2008): 27–34.

Hinshaw, Stephen P. *The Mark of Shame: Stigma of Mental Illness and an Agenda for Change.* New York: Oxford University Press, 2007.

soldier's heart See COMBAT-RELATED POSTTRAUMATIC STRESS DISORDER; COMBAT STRESS REACTION.

somatic experiencing (SE) therapy Therapy based on Peter Levine's substantial ideas on trauma resolution and further developed by Levine and his faculty colleagues at the Foundation for Human Enrichment. These ideas became widely known through his book (coauthored with Ann Frederick), *Waking the Tiger: Healing Trauma.* In the book, Levine describes several clinical case studies in which traumatic experience (stored in the body) is brought to awareness and processed by keeping attention on the sensations with the support and guidance of the therapist to an adaptive solution or more resolved state of being. He concludes that the body has an inherent ability to heal that, if accessed, can be used to heal traumatic experience, which is typically and chronically stored in the nervous system.

DYSREGULATION in the autonomic nervous system is seen as the core outcome of unresolved trauma, in that it interferes with the capacity to self-regulate, leading often to trauma-related health disorders, behaviors, and affect (mood).

As Levine writes,

> Traumatic events are not caused by the dangerous event itself. They arise when residual energy from the event is not discharged from the body. This energy remains trapped in the nervous system where it can wreak havoc on our bodies and minds.

The SE approach uses the capacity for a FELT SENSE or body awareness to renegotiate and heal trauma. Accessing this felt sense in ways that do not overstimulate or overactivate the stored traumatic material allows discharge or release and a healing reorganization in the nervous system.

The therapy is in general a one-on-one approach and taught in a three-year professional program offered by the Foundation for Human Enrichment in more than 15 countries all over the world. SE therapy has been successfully used with single incident trauma (and is often referred to as "shock trauma") such as car accidents, earthquakes, tsunamis, battlefield incidents, rape, and so on and has also been used with developmental traumas, such as child sexual abuse and physical abuse, neglect, and other cumulative traumatic experiences, such as attachment traumas. This therapeutic approach, with its focus on self-regulation, lends itself to use in short-term as well as long-term clinical settings for treating symptoms of traumatic stress, as well as for bringing the often-missing awareness of the body back into psychotherapy and healing modalities. It is also used in psychosocial educational approaches that are used to train individuals and groups in self-treatment and self-care strategies after traumatic events.

See also CHILD ABUSE AND NEGLECT; CHILD SEXUAL ABUSE; RESILIENCE TO STRESS; THERAPY, TYPES OF; VULNERABILITY.

Levine, Peter. *Waking the Tiger: Healing Trauma: The Innate Capacity to Transform Overwhelming Experience.* Berkeley, Calif.: North Atlantic Books, 1997.

somatization The presence of chronic painful medical symptoms for no known reason, such as headaches, heart palpitations, back pain, gastrointestinal pain, dizziness, and other symptoms that stem directly from past or recent severe emotional distress, such as POSTTRAUMATIC STRESS DISORDER (PTSD), domestic violence, past child abuse, or other severely traumatic events, such as extreme natural disasters. In addition, some medical syndromes, such as fibromyalgia or irritable bowel syndrome, are more common among those with past troubling experiences. As a result, medications such as ANTIDEPRESSANTS or other psychiatric drugs may improve some somatic conditions, and PSYCHOTHERAPY may help the person to resolve personal conflicts. Of course, medication is also needed to treat the presenting disease or disorder.

It is important to note that these symptoms are real and valid and they are not attempts of the patient to seek attention, nor are they indications of hypochondria.

In some cases, autoimmune illnesses such as thyroid disease, rheumatoid arthritis, and other disorders are more common among individuals with posttraumatic stress disorder, such as those stemming from war experiences or severe abuse.

PTSD and Somatization

Somatization is particularly prominent among patients with PTSD. According to research by Joseph Boscarino, published in the *Annals of the New York Academy of Sciences* in 2004, when 2,490 Vietnam veterans were assessed for common autoimmune disorders such as diabetes, rheumatoid arthritis, psoriasis or diabetes, PTSD was significantly associated with these conditions. The researchers also found that veterans with PTSD and other emotional disorders had a significantly higher likelihood of having clinically higher T-cell counts (indicating action of the immune system) and other markers of disease. The researchers said that this evidence "confirms the presence of biological markers consistent with a broad range of inflammatory disorders, including both cardiovascular and autoimmune diseases." They also warned that cognitive therapy alone would be insufficient to treat individuals with PTSD who may have medical disorders.

See also BODY MEMORY; BRIQUET'S SYNDROME; COGNITIVE-BEHAVIORAL THERAPY; POST-VIETNAM SYNDROME; SOMATIC EXPERIENCING; SOMATIZATION DISORDER; SOMATOFORM DISSOCIATION; SOMATOFORM DISSOCIATION QUESTIONNAIRE.

Boscarino, Joseph A. "Posttraumatic Stress Disorder and Physical Illness: Results from Clinical and Epidemiologic Studies." *Annals of New York Academy of Sciences* 1032 (2004): 141–153.

somatization disorder Longstanding complaints of physical ailments that upon examination have little or no organic or medical basis. Somatization disorder was first described by Pierre Briquet in 1859 and is often called BRIQUET'S SYNDROME.

Symptoms and Diagnostic Path

To be classified as a somatization disorder, the complainant must have symptoms of pain (such as headaches), gastrointestinal discomfort (such as diarrhea), sexual dysfunctions (erectile or menstrual difficulties), and a neurological symptom. Individuals with somatization disorder frequently go from doctor to doctor searching for a diagnosis and care and can be quite dramatic and exaggerated in describing their symptoms. Anxiety and DEPRESSION are by-products of this disorder.

Treatment Options and Outlook

People with somatization disorder express their emotions and experience through somatic experiences (hearing, seeing, feeling, moving) and, therefore, seldom seek psychotherapy. They are generally fixated on finding medical solutions to their problems and are resistant to psychotherapy of any kind. If they do seek therapy, relief is possible, often in combination with psychiatric medications. Typically, the disorder fluctuates over time but persists for a lifetime, rarely disappearing.

Risk Factors and Preventive Measures

Somatization disorder usually runs in families, and 10 to 20 percent of the close relatives of women with the disorder develop it as well, so there is some social learning phenomenon (e.g., child learns from parent or parents by modeling their

behaviors) involved in the acquisition and maintenance of this disorder. The disorder is found mainly
in women. The role of trauma in this disorder is
unknown as of this writing.

See also SOMATIZATION; SOMATOFORM DISSOCIATION.

somatoform dissociation The failure of the body
to process somatic experiences (hearing, seeing,
feeling, moving) adequately, leading to somatoform dissociative symptoms. Dissociation is a lack
of connection we have with our experiences.
Dissociative symptoms include amnesia, sense of
being detached from self, and the perception of
things appearing distorted or unreal. Somatoform
disorders are a general category that includes hysterical somatoform disorders (conversion disorder,
somatization disorder, and pain disorder associated with psychological factors) and preoccupation
somatoform disorders (Munchausen and factitious
disorder). All involve some form of dissociation
in which experience affects body perception and
functioning. The role of trauma, however, is not
clear and will emerge only with time and much
more research. However, dissociation, or disen-
gaging, or "checking out" of experience, is almost
always present, and dissociation is frequently a
marker for child abuse.

Some people have the capacity to avert the
horrible impact of traumatic experiences by using
dissociation as a coping mechanism with negative
side effects. Highly charged experiences tend to
intrude on the consciousness in the form of dissociative FLASHBACKS, NIGHTMARES, and reexperiencing the traumatic event in the mind. Dissociation
manifests itself in psychoform and somatoform
dissociative symptoms. Psychoform dissociation is
the disturbance of memory, consciousness, identity
fragmentation, and an altered sense of the environment that can involve amnesia.

Symptoms and Diagnostic Path

Visual, olfactory, auditory, affective and kinesthetic
experiences are categorized as somatoform dissociative symptoms that are reported as trauma-
related insensitivity to pain (analgesia), a lack of
body feelings (anesthesia), freezing and stilling
(motor disturbances), alternating preferences of

tastes and smells, pain, and the loss of consciousness. Somatoform dissociation is associated with
traumatization that strongly relates to a bodily
threat or a threat to life.

Mutism (inability to speak) was noted in the
battlefields of World War I when soldiers were
exposed to gas fumes, explosions, or the terror
of heavy bombardment. Nijenhuis et al. (1998)
hypothesized that somatoform dissociative symptoms evoke animallike defense reactions, from
freezing (motor inhibitions, such as difficulty in
moving), paralysis, and a lack of pain sensation to
total helplessness and emotional lack of sensitivity.

Treatment Options and Outlook

Since dissociative disorders appear to be triggered
as a response to trauma or abuse, psychotherapy is
the treatment most recommended as well as psychopharmacological mediations, especially when
patients have comorbid disorders of mood and
anxiety disorders. Clinicians may need to assess
the nature of trauma and somatoform dissociation
when there is a high level of somatic symptoms
within various psychiatric and medical disorders
that are resistant to treatment. The course of
therapy may be difficult for many people, but
many individuals with dissociative disorders learn
new ways of coping and go on to live very productive lives.

Risk Factors and Preventive Measures

One clear risk factor is physical abuse, as well as
severe CHILD SEXUAL ABUSE as reported among psychiatric patients with trauma and medical patients
with chronic pelvic pain. Other risk factors are
exposure to life-threatening traumatic events, such
as war, kidnapping, and torture.

Seeking professional help sooner rather than
later is one preventive measure to take to address
the horrendous experience and learn how to adopt
using healthy coping skills.

See also BODY MEMORY; CHILD ABUSE AND NEGLECT;
CHILD SEXUAL ABUSE; SOMATOFORM DISSOCIATION
QUESTIONNAIRE.

Naring, G., and E. R. S. Nijenhuis. "Relationships between
Self-Reported Potentially Traumatizing Events, Psychoform and Somatoform Dissociation, and Absorp-

tion, in Two Non-Clinical Populations." *Australian and New Zealand Journal of Psychiatry* 39 (2005): 982–988.
Nijenhuis, E. R. S., J. Vanderlinden, and P. Spinvoen. "Animal Defensive Reactions and Model for Trauma-Induced Dissociative Reactions." *Journal of Traumatic Stress* 11 (1998): 243–260.

Somatoform Dissociation Questionnaire (SDQ-20)

A 20-item instrument that is a screening device for dissociative processes and has good reliability and validity. The Somatoform Dissociation Questionnaire measures the severity of a range of somatoform symptoms to include analgesia (insensitivity to pain), anesthesia, motor disturbances (freezing), preferences in taste and smell, pain, and loss of consciousness. The SDQ-20 uses a five-point Likert scale to indicate to what degree a statement applies to the subject. Sample questions include, "My body, or part of it, feels numb" and "I grow stiff for awhile." The SDQ-20 has sound psychometric qualities with high reliability and good construct validity. Patients with dissociative disorder score higher than those with other psychiatric diagnoses, demonstrating criteria-related validity.

Somatoform dissociation can be understood as an adaptive response to trauma, where there is a threat of inescapable body injury resulting in post-traumatic stress disorder (PTSD) or acute stress disorder. PTSD is categorized as an anxiety disorder in the *Diagnostic and Statistic Manual-IV-TR (DSM-IV-TR)*, but other theorists, such as Naring and Nijenhuis, also support the observation that these disorders are actually dissociative in nature and describe them as dissociative imprints of the sensory and affective (feeling) elements of traumatic experiences. The visual, olfactory, affective, auditory, and kinesthetic experiences can be grouped as somatoform dissociative symptoms.

The theory behind the SDQ assumes that there is a failure of integrative process in the individual such that two or more different parts of the self emerge in experience. For example, an abused child may appear normal at school and then appear emotional and frightened at home. Emotional responses in these cases are tied to the context of the home and are isolated or unavailable at school, where the child acts in an apparently normal manner. The apparently normal part can avoid

the emotional part in order to cope with life. The normal parts, however, usually have somatoform dissociative symptoms that often represent defensive aspects of their emotional life. Pain, inhibitions of movement, a lack of body feelings (all of which can be seen in somatoform disorders) may be part of traumatic memories and experience. Trauma therapy may integrate these parts over extended time. The SDQ includes many negative and some positive dissociative symptoms.

See also BODY MEMORY; BRIQUET'S SYNDROME; COGNITIVE BEHAVIORAL THERAPY; POST-VIETNAM SYNDROME; SOMATIC EXPERIENCING THERAPY; SOMATIZATION DISORDER; SOMATOFORM DISSOCIATION; SOMATOFORM DISSOCIATION QUESTIONNAIRE.

Nijenhuis, E. R. S. et al. "The Development and Psychometric Characteristics of the Somatoform Dissociation Questionnaire (SDQ-20)." *Journal of Nervous and Mental Disease* 184 (1996): 688–694.
Naring, G. and E. R. S. Nijenhuis. "Relationships between Self-Reported Potentially Traumatizing Events, Psychoform and Somatoform Dissociation, and Absorption, in Two Clinical Populations." *Australian and New Zealand Journal of Psychiatry* 39 (2005): 982–988.

somnambulism   See PARASOMNIAS.

soul   A term that refers to the deepest aspect of an individual and that organizes much of his or her behaviors, emotions, and thoughts. The term *soul* is usually used synonymously with *spirituality*. To most observers, the soul is seen as enduring and a presence. Trauma, however, can lead to a profound compression of bodily energy that refocuses behavior toward survival instincts or survival behaviors, emotions, and cognitions. In other words, the soul is hidden or unavailable with trauma. Defensiveness protects the soul from harm.

Contact or awakening of the soul now requires healing or discharge of the trauma state. Touching into bodily sensations with awareness in a gradual way often leads to slight discharge and greater openness. An intrinsic rhythm is established between the sensations and feelings associated with trauma (dread, helplessness, rage, and so on), and experiences of expansion and openness allow pendulation. This Somatic Experiencing term means moving from arousal to nonarousal states to prevent high levels of arousal from occurring. A greater sense of curiosity, exploration, and openness develop, as body tension is discharged or released.

As healing begins to take over, the soul can emerge into awareness. Self-regulation begins, and in this state, the soul energy is more available to awareness. The body no longer defends but can be open and receptive, and relaxed but alert. Emotional regulation from higher brain functions comes through this embodiment and healing. Fragmentation gives way to wholeness. People come home to their bodies and the embodied life. The soul has a way of expressing itself.

specific phobias   There is an endless number of specific phobias. While many people have *aversions* to particular objects or situations (such as seeing snakes or insects), an aversion becomes a *phobia* when it begins to interfere with the individual's functioning. Clinical levels of phobias are always debilitating in some way to the individual and cause distress or as well as impairment. Phobias are the leading form of anxiety disorder and are found in 8.7 percent of the population, or an estimated 6.3 million adults in the United States.

Symptoms and Diagnostic Path

Specific phobias involve an intense fear of a particular triggering stimulus. The most common phobias are of heights, edges, deep water, highway driving, closed spaces, flying, small animals, snakes, and of blood and injury. There are also many other less common phobias. Essentially, any event, thing, person, or situation can become conditioned to the fear response in an individual. Fear leads to avoidance (which diminishes the fear) and avoidance produces dysfunction or diminishes one's ability to function effectively. For example, many people are afraid to fly, and they just drive to a distant destination. But if your job requires flying far distances or your family wants to travel to distant places where you cannot drive, your avoidance now adversely affects others and can compromise work, family, and social relationships.

Interestingly, most of the common fears are prepared fears, or genetically transmitted tendencies of certain stimuli to evoke fear responses in humans. Prepared fears are survival mechanisms for the species, and these fears have been passed down through the ages. This may explain why almost 90 percent of people who fear snakes have never actually seen a snake.

Many phobias go unreported because people seldom seek treatment for their phobias. In most cases, the phobic stimulus is easy enough to avoid and therefore causes little distress in the person's life.

Treatment Options and Outlook

Those who do seek treatment for their specific phobias are often in jobs or situations where they must face the phobic trigger in order to function. For example students must sit in class even though it is a confined and crowded space; telephone linemen must climb poles and may encounter snakes; many people may be required to fly as part of their jobs.

The most common forms of effective treatment for phobias are exposure-based desensitization approaches, which involve gradual exposure (approach) to the feared stimulus while working with triggering cognitions. Flooding, or extreme exposure at a full intensity, has also been used but its effect does not seem to last for long. Flooding has the added disadvantage that most people with phobias avoid these situations and therefore would not seek out such a distressing form of treatment.

Risk Factors and Preventive Measures

Phobias are sometimes called irrational fears because most people are not afraid of these situations or events. On the other hand, a careful examination of the individual's life history usually reveals precipitating events or traumas, most often from early childhood. Once avoidance (internal or external) begins to form, the specific phobia becomes more intense and chronic.

spirituality and trauma   In the United States more than 90 percent of Americans want some kind of religious education for their children, and 82 percent of adults feel a need for spiritual growth in their lives. In times of crisis, 80 percent say that they use prayer, and 95 percent of those who pray believe that those prayers are answered.

Religious and spiritual beliefs are traditions handed down through generations as people develop their beliefs about the world around them and discover what the purpose of life is. Spirituality is accepted by the mental health profession as a core human dimension. Coping strategies are now defined to include spirituality as a coping resource along with social, emotional, physical, and cognitive strategies.

People often struggle to regain balance in their lives after a traumatic event. Significant changes in life priorities and the emergence of questions as to the meaning of life can bring about a crisis of faith. But religious and spiritual beliefs can also become a way to cope following trauma. In the days after SEPTEMBER 11, 2001, 90 percent of those sampled reported turning to their religious faith for support. Religious beliefs can make individuals feel less threatened by making threatening situations more of a challenge and can help individuals derive positive outcomes even through their suffering.

Negative religious coping or blame reflects that the individual may believe that the traumatic event is God's punishment and try to cope without God's assistance. Studies indicate a relationship between childhood sexual abuse and lower levels of religious involvement and negative beliefs about God.

In recovery, spirituality remains valued and important. Researchers found that religiously committed women who are battered present with fewer POSTTRAUMATIC STRESS DISORDER (PTSD) symptoms than women without faith and commitment. Jewish teenagers in Israel facing imminent missile threat during the 1992 Gulf War used their religious faith and prayer to cope with the traumatic stress. In studies of stress on relief workers after Hurricane Hugo in South Carolina, all reported that religion was a primary positive coping strategy. Whether the trauma is war, floods, hurricanes, or abusive relationships, social support through religion and faith provides a healing way to face tragedy and facilitate recovery.

See also SOUL.

Shaw, A., S. Joseph, and A. Linley. "Religion, Spirituality, and Posttraumatic Growth: A Systematic Review." *Mental Health, Religion, & Culture* 8, no. 1 (2005): 1–11.
Weaver, A. J., L. T. Flannelly, J. Garbarino, C. R. Figley, & K. J. Flannelly. "A Systematic Review of Research on Religion and Spirituality in the *Journal of Traumatic Stress*: 1990–1999." *Mental Health, Religion & Culture* 6, no. 3 (2003): 215–225.

SSRI See SELECTIVE SEROTONIN REUPTAKE INHIBITOR.

stage-oriented treatment (phase-oriented treatment) One of the most important aspects of treatment for traumatic experience and POSTTRAUMATIC STRESS DISORDER (PTSD). Treatment is not a singular process carried out by a protocol. For trauma, treatment occurs in stages or phases, beginning with establishing a rapport and a working relationship with the client. If understanding, compassion, and trust are not present, no positive results will occur, and frequently clients will leave feeling as if therapy failed and never seeking other therapists or remedies.

Containment and resourcing are the second phase of stage-oriented treatment, in which the therapist helps the individual gain some control over arousal and frightening internal experiences. Resourcing may take months or years to establish properly.

Next is trauma work itself, and directly dealing with traumatic experiences through exposure, EYE MOVEMENT DESENSITIZATION AND REPROCESSING (EMDR), or SOMATIC EXPERIENCING. Once the individual is desensitized, it is usually necessary to build skills that were not available to the individual because of his or her past traumatic experiences. As one famous therapist likes to say, "You can't expect a woman to date successfully if the only man she has kissed is her father."

These phases are dependent on each other and the therapy may shift among them as it seems appropriate.

See also ELABORATED POSTTRAUMATIC STRESS DISORDER; THERAPY, TYPES OF.

stigmatization Attributing negative traits to a group of people because of their membership in that group. It has been known for centuries that mental illness is stigmatized by the public. The mentally ill were initially treated in asylums, then hospitals, and now in the streets. Surveys indicate that at least 80 percent of the general population is afraid of the mentally ill, and yet funding for services, structured living accommodations, and caretakers and therapists is meager.

Trauma victims see themselves as part of that stigmatization and often avoid seeking therapy and ways to relieve their distress. Often they do not connect distress and feelings of separateness with previous trauma. Therapists can misjudge, misdiagnose, and overlook the trauma base of the person's experience.

See also ATTITUDES TOWARD MENTAL ILLNESS, PUBLIC.

stimulus discrimination   The term *stimulus discrimination* comes from operant conditioning principles developed by famed psychologist B. F. Skinner. Operant conditioning teaches discrimination by reinforcing responses to one stimulus and not another. Gradually, the organism consistently responded to the "correct" or reinforced stimulus and not to the other stimuli that are extinguished. This is the simple pattern of learning to discriminate. Of course, discrimination becomes more difficult and complex as the person matures. Trauma disrupts this learning and responding because the stimulus's meaning is blurred by arousal and intense emotional expression.

Discrimination, or an ability to separate or see one part as different from another part, is built on identifying differences among stimuli; for example, red lights must be responded to differently from green lights. Dangerous situations or people must be responded to differently from safe and harmless situations and people. These are discrimination problems, and this is a skill people learn in their development.

Stockholm syndrome   A strategy for survival in which a captive bonds emotionally with his or her captor in order to stay alive. Stockholm syndrome was named after the behavior of four bank employees who were taken hostage by an escaped convict in Stockholm, Sweden, in 1973. The hostages, three women and one man, were held in a bank vault for five days with the captor's cellmate. After their release, the hostages reported no ill feelings toward their captors and said they had been more afraid of the police than of the convicts during the ordeal. The hostages supported their captors and felt they were protecting them. This behavior shocked many people and was subsequently named Stockholm syndrome.

Sometimes a kidnapped or imprisoned person becomes sympathetic to and identifies with the needs and problems of his or her captors and may become hostile or indifferent to the people to whom he or she normally closely relates. The prototype case was that of teenage heiress Patty Hearst, who was kidnapped in 1974 by members of the Symbionese Liberation Army (SLA), The SLA was a self-styled urban guerrilla warfare group that considered itself a revolutionary vanguard army. The group committed bank robberies, two murders, and other acts of violence between 1973 and 1975.

Hearst subsequently identified with and joined the SLA. International interest grew into worldwide fascination when Hearst, in audiotaped messages delivered to and broadcast by regional news media, denounced her parents and announced that she had joined the SLA. She was observed participating in their illegal activities. After her release Hearst claimed she had been held in close confinement and had been sexually assaulted and brainwashed.

The following conditions enhance this emotional attachment

- a perceived threat to the captive's physical or psychological survival, and the belief that the captor would carry out the threat
- perceived small kindnesses from the captor to the captive, such as giving them food or loosening bonds
- isolation from perspectives other than those of the captor
- a perceived inability to escape

An abuser traumatizes victims (who do not believe that they can escape, or truly cannot) by threatening their survival. The traumatized victim, isolated from others, must look to the abuser to meet his or her basic needs (food, water, shelter). If the abuser shows the victim some small kindness, the victim then must bond to the perceived positive side of the abuser, denying (or dissociating) the side of the abuser that produced the terror.

In order to keep the abuser happy, the victim begins to see the world from the abuser's perspective, to insure survival. Consequently, the victim becomes hypervigilant to the abuser's views and needs and less aware of his or her own, which seem unimportant or even counterproductive to survival. Gradually, denial of the violent side of the abuser develops and it becomes progressively harder to separate from the abuser due to the fear of losing the only positive relationship available at the time. The abuser's identity becomes the victim's own. He or she has essentially been brainwashed.

Treatment for Stockholm syndrome involves reversing the conditions that helped produce the identification and loss of self by removing isolation and helping the victim relate to others. Group therapy can be helpful but integration into friendly and understanding groups is a start toward rebuilding trust and openness with others. As with many forms of violent abuse, the victim frequently minimizes the violence through numbing and dissociation.

Recounting one's experience, keeping a journal, and talking with others and a therapist about boundaries, dangers, and acceptable behavior (for parents, male perpetrators, and so on) is essential. Exposure to kindness and reintegration into a benevolent society is important. Helping the victim integrate the dissociated sides of the abuser allows him or her to give up the hope of what the relationship with the abuser would be.

According to an article in 1999 in the *FBI Law Enforcement Bulletin,* Stockholm syndrome is much less common than believed, and most hostages are unsympathetic to their captors. According to the article, research has shown that three factors must exist in order for the syndrome to develop, including

1. The captives are held for a significant period of time (a specific length of time was not discussed).

2. The captors and the hostages significantly interact, and the hostages are not isolated from their captors.
3. The captors are kind to the hostages and do not abuse them or threaten them excessively.

Some indications that Stockholm syndrome may occur include a situation when one or more of the hostages expresses frustration, anger, or fear of the police, thinking that the police are not doing enough or that they will endanger the hostages. Another situation in which the syndrome may develop may occur when one or more of the hostages expresses sympathy toward the captors, believing that they are not so bad or that their captors will not harm them. Finally, Stockholm syndrome may develop when the captors show positive feelings toward the hostages.

See also THERAPY, TYPES OF.

Fuselier, G. Dwayne. "Placing the Stockholm Syndrome in Perspective," *FBI Law Enforcement Bulletin* (July 1999). Available online. URL: http://www.au.af/mil/au/awc/awcgate/fbi/stockholm_syndrome.pdf. Downloaded March 19, 2007.
Grahm, D., and E. Rawlings. "Bonding with Abusive Dating Partners: Dynamics of Stockholm Syndrome." *Dating Violence, Women in Danger,* edited by Barrie Levy. Seattle: Seal Press, 1991.

stress   Arousal in the body and the mind. Stress is a concept with many dimensions. It is usually a physical response in many of the sensate-action-cognitive systems of the body-mind. The term *body-mind* is used because stress affects all aspects of sensing and functioning: it is a response of the total organism in the emotional, physical, mental, and spiritual domains. Stress can vary in intensity from slight to traumatic, and it can be measured by its frequency and duration. Stress involves two components; a stressor and a response to the stressor. Most people are aware of stress in their lives and will say that they are "stressed out" or "under a lot of stress."

The person most responsible for initially developing the concept of stress was Hans Selye, a medical researcher at McGill University in Canada. Selye distinguished between stress responses that were distressful or destructive to the organism (he called these "strains" on the person) and stress responses that were less destructive or nondestructive (he called these EUSTRESS). Distress, Selye said, produces "wear and tear" on the body and can eventually lead to chronic disease and death. Eustress is also a form of arousal, but it is motivating and positive, such as an athlete's focus and drive for competition or someone who takes on a challenging project at work. Most research and clinical work has focused on the destructive effects of distress or simply "stress."

Research on the physiology of arousal has focused on BRAIN structures, hormonal responses, and nervous system reactions. The LIMBIC SYSTEM is the primary brain structure that is associated with arousal. It is here that cognitive appraisal from the prefrontal cortex is integrated with an emotional interpretation of events from the AMYGDALA and cingulated areas. Muscles tighten in preparation for action, and many stress-related responses occur in hormonal and neurological systems.

The HIPPOCAMPUS helps regulate emotional responses so that they are appropriate to the context or circumstances. In individuals with POST-TRAUMATIC STRESS DISORDER (PTSD) and DEPRESSION, abnormalities and attenuation (shrinkage of the hippocampus) have been found, so that situations are often misread as dangerous, causing a sense of insecurity in their environment. One of this century's most profound discoveries is that the body and brain respond physiologically to the environment and share this interaction. As an example, a stimulating environment for a young baby will increase body weight, and higher educational learning in adults decreases the chance of developing Alzheimer's disease. In other words, behavior shapes the brain and body, whereas we have thought that the brain controls and directs the body in some predetermined manner.

Neuroplasticity describes the fact that the brain continually changes as a result of our life experiences. Secure, supportive environments enhance regulated emotions and well-functioning physiological areas, whereas abusive environments damage the ability to regulate the emotions and the areas of the brain that are involved in interpretation and emotional processing.

The hypothalamus is a collection of tissues that make up the nerve centers that control the basic autonomic functions, or activities without conscious control. They lie at the base of the forebrain and connect down the brain stem (to the reticular formation) and up toward the cortex. The hypothalamus is the major integrator of the body's regulatory systems (heart rate, blood pressure, hunger, thirst, sex, etc.). It is the "physical" brain in the body that sends messages through the SYMPATHETIC and PARASYMPATHETIC NERVOUS SYSTEMS, the two divisions of the autonomic nervous system, to regulate body activation and calming. The hypothalamus is intimately involved with the pituitary gland, and through this connection it links the nervous system (NEUROTRANSMITTERS) to the endocrine system (neurohormones).

The pituitary gland, in turn, serves as the master gland for the endocrine system and is directly stimulated by the hypothalamus. It releases pituitary hormones into the bloodstream that support activation and arousal (by activating the adrenals). This system is called the HPA or HYPOTHALAMIC-PITUITARY-ADRENAL AXIS, and it is a major source of stress responses and physiological arousal. Activation of the adrenals produces EPINEPHRINE/ADRENALINE, CORTISOL (which increases fat mobilization, immune suppression, and increased cholesterol and glucose) and aldosterone (which increases water retention, blood pressure, and irritability).

The endocrine system works well to prepare the body and mind for action and for FIGHT OR FLIGHT RESPONSES. However, repeated, chronic, and intense activation (as seen in PTSD and other emotional disorders) tunes the physiology up to a higher level that is more easily triggered by nonthreatening or nondangerous events. Such a response is seen with PTSD, where autonomic arousal is chronically high, startle response is evident, sleep is disturbed, modulation of emotional responses is difficult, paranoia is persistent, and learning and concentration require great effort. Chronic exposure to a stressor or stressors can have a similar but less intense effect on physiology, making the individual more irritable and reactive.

A highly tuned physiology is like a car running at a high idle: it is difficult to drive, and requires the constant use of brakes. In addition, it does not function smoothly and properly and the engine gets worn out early. Likewise, a tuned-up body damages cognitive abilities, produces states of fatigue and DEPRESSION, affects the immune system, and produces wear and tear in terms of disease and failure within systems.

The cerebral cortex (or neocortex or forebrain) allows for development of analytic and verbal abilities, communication, fine motor control, rational thought, and problem solving. Voluntary control (as opposed to involuntary or sub-cortical conditioned or reflexive responsiveness) uses this area and, in many cases, can override or control involuntary responses. The frontal lobes of the cortex are particularly important in stress management because they enable humans to exert control over their emotions and to act unselfishly. This frontal lobe area does not fully develop until after 20 years of age. The frontal areas (executive functions) are also disengaged in PTSD (probably since action and not thought is required to survive in a threatening situation) and other chronic stress conditions and therefore cannot help bring the system to a normal level.

While the brain provides the structure for learning, memory, emotion, and action, the whole body participates in every event. Information is "communicated" to each cell of the body through amino acid molecules (or ligands) that circulate throughout the body and are "received" by cell receptors. In turn, the cell responds to the information from a particular ligand and corrects its functioning according to the information conveyed.

The response to chronic stress varies with different body systems. The muscle system under stress is tense. Subconscious messages keep muscles on alert. Muscle tension, in turn, keeps cognitive processes in a state of fear, anxiety, irritability, and anger. Muscle tension can lead to headaches, backaches, asthma, arthritis, and digestion and vision problems.

There is always a cardiovascular response to stress but it is a complicated one. Basically stress produces changes in blood flow pattern, blood pressure, the structure of the blood vessels, and the composition of the blood itself. The heart, the core of the cardiovascular system, can function without neurological stimulation but it does receive impulses from the brain and central nervous system.

With prolonged stress there is chronically increased heart activity, which puts a strain on blood vessels and the immune system components. Furthermore, the individual usually tries to voluntarily suppress the effects of this arousal, creating a push-pull between the voluntary and involuntary systems. Hypertension or elevated blood pressure can develop as a result of this dysregulation between the physical and voluntary aspects. Stress hormones are elevated and the immune system is depressed. Furthermore, atherosclerosis (deposits in the inner layer of the arteries) can develop and restrict blood flow in the vessels and weakening of the vessels walls, which puts the individual at risk for heart attacks, aneurysms, and strokes.

The skin also reacts to stress. Electrical activity and skin temperature rise and fall depending on activation and calming activities. In people prone to skin disorders, eczema (itchy rash) can develop and produce embarrassment and discomfort. Researchers are studying hives, psoriasis, and acne to determine if they are stress-related, but no firm conclusions are available as of this writing.

Finally, we have known for a long time that stress affects the immune system. In the short term, stress can boost the immune system. During the fight or flight stress response, the immune system adapts and readies the body for infections resulting from injuries. But if the stressor continues long term, the immune system shifts from adaptive to negative responses at the cellular level where the ability of lymphocytes (T-cells and B cells) to attack pathogens (viruses and bacteria) is compromised due to low blood count. Chronic stress that seems to be endless (abusive relationship or high-pressure job) and out of one's control results in global suppression of the immune system, which includes a decrease in humoral (antibody) immune response, the ability of antibodies to bind onto invading microbes.

People can suffer from stressors in one of three ways: (1) underactivity, which leads to diseases like cancer and susceptibility to pathogens; (2) hyperactivity, which leads to diseases like asthma and lung irritation; or (3) misguided activity, such as when the body attacks its own tissues as in rheumatoid arthritis or fibromyalgia. Misguided activity of the immune system is often called immune-deficiency disorder.

Emotions, Thoughts, Beliefs, and Stress

Emotions are energy that is experienced throughout the body-mind. Some emotions are innate or inborn and considered basic (such as compassion, and love, anger, happiness, interest, disgust, surprise, etc.). As we grow, these emotions become attached to our experiences in the world around us. Likewise, the intensity of these emotions and how we "handle" them are also products of our experience and temperament. Once conditioned (learned), internal events such as thoughts, memories, and beliefs can trigger emotional reactions. Acculturation, or cultural learning, requires some degree of inhibition of emotions. However, when emotions are blocked or inhibited consciously, or unconsciously due to stressful situations, it is more difficult to engage in the higher mental processes such as analysis, evaluation, and synthesis.

Interestingly, Davidson and colleagues have found that positive emotions are mediated by the left prefrontal area of the brain and negative emotions by the corresponding right prefrontal area. The balance between left and right activity has been termed one's "emotional set point," the place where the balance of emotion tends to settle. Of course, this set point can change with practice and conscious effort.

Our thoughts and beliefs control behavior, moods, health, and emotional responses. Beliefs are enduring patterns of thought that are usually learned in childhood. Self-image and evaluation are determined by our beliefs about ourselves. COGNITIVE BEHAVIORAL THERAPY focuses on thoughts and beliefs as a way to change emotional and behavioral patterns that are destructive and self-defeating to the individual personally, to his or her relationships and interactions with others, or to health.

Almost everyone experiences stress, many because they have a stressful lifestyle and have learned through years of conditioning to react in a stressful manner. Consciousness and practice are ways to change these automatic reaction patterns and bring a greater freedom from the ravages of distressful "stress."

See also CENTRAL NERVOUS SYSTEM; RESILIENCE TO STRESS; STRESS INOCULATION TRAINING; STRESS DAMPENING RESPONSE.

Pert, C. *The Molecules of Emotion: Why We Feel the Way We Feel.* New York: Simon and Schuster, 1999.
Pennebaker, J. W. *Opening Up; The Healing Power of Expressing Emotions.* New York: Guilford Press, 1997.

stress dampening response (SDR) SDR refers to the decrease in strength of response to stress due to alcohol use. In the 1980s several investigations were undertaken to determine if alcohol consumption reduced stress. The results were inconsistent with alcohol reducing stress in some studies but not in others. The tension-reduction hypothesis could not be confirmed unequivocally and researchers settled on the conclusion that the relationship between alcohol and stress or tension-reduction was complex. Research moved into two main areas: individual differences in alcohol effectiveness and situational factors that contribute to effectiveness.

In terms of individual differences, studies focus on family history of alcoholism, personality traits, extent of self-consciousness, level of cognitive functioning and gender. Generally, studies use people who have a family history positive for drinking (FHP) and compare them against people who have a family history negative or nonalcoholic (FHN) on SDR. In general, the FHP exhibit greater SDR on several but not all psychophysiological measures. Other studies suggest that participants with family histories of multigenerational alcoholism demonstrate an enhanced SDR. Other studies have found that FHP participants are more reactive in general to environmental stimuli. There are many questions, many confusions in these experiments and inconsistent results.

stress inoculation training (SIT) A form of COGNITIVE BEHAVIORAL THERAPY that attempts to integrate cognitive and affective factors in coping processes to deal with the aftermath of traumatic events and teaches as a preventive approach to "inoculate" against future and ongoing stressors. Stress inoculation training (SIT) is multifaceted and individually tailored to the client and his or her situation. It involves three primary phases: conceptualization, skill-building, and practice.

The first phase, conceptualization (with the therapist), uses the Socratic method of asking questions to lead the client to self-understanding to solve stressful problems and identify changeable aspects of these problems. Clients are taught how to break down stressors into short, intermediate, and long-term coping goals or strategies. In the second, skill-building phase, skills are acquired and rehearsed depending on the stressors involved. Specific coping skills might involve emotional self-regulation, self-soothing, relaxation training, cognitive restructuring, and so on. The third practice phase involves the application of learned material and follow-through in gradual steps in the real situation and also through imagery. Relapse prevention is emphasized.

SIT is conducted with individuals, couples, or small and large groups. In most instances, SIT consists of eight to 15 sessions, plus booster and follow-up sessions conducted over a three- to 12-month period.

See also EUSTRESS; RESILIENCE TO STRESS; STRESS DAMPENING RESPONSE; THERAPY, TYPES OF.

Meichenbaum, D. *A Clinical Handbook/Practical Therapist Manual for Assessing and Treating Adults with Post Traumatic Stress Disorder.* Waterloo, Ontario: Institute Press, 1994.

———. *Stress Innocation Training.* New York: Pergamon Press, 1985.

Stroop Test

Stroop Test   A test that was developed from the results of a doctoral dissertation published in 1935 by John Riley Stroop. In his study Stroop presented subjects with words printed in different colors. Since words are read more quickly and automatically than naming colors, it was easier to read the words than to identify their colors. For example, if the word *blue* is printed in the color green, the word blue is said more readily than naming the color in which it is displayed, in this case green. Interference and inhibition are both operating in this task.

The task of making an appropriate response when given two separate signals (one of which is dominant—in this case, reading the word) seems to be located in the part of the BRAIN called the

anterior cingulate. This region lies between the right and left hemispheres in the frontal portion of the brain. Its function seems to be as a conduit between the lower, more automatic brain centers and the higher, more thought-driven regions.

In the test itself, subjects are asked to name the colors of the printed word and not the word itself. This turns out to be a very difficult task. The test has been used primarily to measure attention, concentration, and memory functions and is useful in sports that require such skills, or where the lack or diminishment of these skills could be damaging to the individual as in such sports as mountaineering and boxing. In PTSD we see a diminished ability to concentrate, process intellectual information, and fully use memory. The Stroop test is useful in assessing these dimensions of functioning and has implications for measuring change in PTSD symptoms. It has been used in batteries of tests with POSTTRAUMATIC STRESS DISORDER SYNDROME (PTSD) patients and seems to have some predictive and diagnostic value.

Stroop, J. R. "Studies of Interference in Serial Verbal Reactions." *Journal of Experimental Psychology* 18 (1935): 643–662.

Structured Clinical Interview (SCID)

Structured Clinical Interview (SCID)   An assessment method for diagnosing PTSD, Acute Traumatic Stress Disorder, and Disorders of Extreme Stress Not Otherwise Specified (DESNOS). It involves a structured, branching (e.g., the interviewer has choices based on interviewee responses as to what directions to go next) interview protocol for diagnosis of Axis I (major mental illness categories) including POSTTRAUMATIC STRESS DISORDER (PTSD). The interview allows some interviewer latitude for questions and can be administered by a clinician or nurse. The SCID-I consists of nine modules, seven of which represent the major Axis I diagnostic classes. Axis I represents conditions that are treatable in some way, while Axis II represents relatively permanent conditions or personality designs that are less amenable to change. The SCID-II was developed to address Axis II disorders.

Because of this modular construction, the SCID-I is adaptable to diagnosis of a particular disorder rather than the full range of mental disorders. The structured interview has "branches" or alternative lines of questions, depending on the client responses. The SCID-I guides the administrator in testing diagnostic hypotheses during the interview itself. In this way, it represents a well-delineated objective approach to diagnosis. The final product is a presence or absence of the categories considered in terms of present behavior (current diagnosis) or lifetime occurrence.

The SCID-II was developed following the same format as SCID-I in order to diagnose Axis II disorders. It is a standardized, reliable, and accurate instrument for diagnoses of the 10 major Axis II personality disorders and, in addition, assesses depressive personality disorder, passive-aggressive personality disorder, and personality disorder not otherwise specified. This instrument provides a measure of the subject's inner experience and typical behavior and relationships. It also measures the subject's capacity for self-reflection.

Structured Interview for Disorders of Extreme Stress (SIDES)

Researchers have associated severe intrusive PTSD symptoms and functional impairment as the core pathological symptoms of Disorders of Extreme Stress Not Otherwise Specified (DESNOS). DESNOS is not formally identified as a diagnostic category in the *Diagnostic and Statistical Manual* (American Psychiatric Association, 2000) but is presented as "associated features" of PTSD linked to interpersonal trauma, such as those experienced by traumatized children, rape victims, battered wives, and military veterans who were traumatized as children. DESNOS is conceptualized as chronic problems with affect regulation, self-identity, impulse regulation, and interpersonal trust functions, as well as with pathological dissociative features.

The Structured Interview for Disorders of Extreme Stress (SIDES) consists of 48 items and was developed to define DESNOS in the following seven areas measuring lifetime and current (past six months) alterations:

1. Alteration in regulation of affect and impulses—assess modulation of anger, suicidal preoccupation or risk taking

2. Alteration in attention or consciousness, including amnesia—assess problems with information processing and dissociative episodes

3. Alteration in self-perception—assess sense of self-view or damage to self, shame

4. Alteration in perception of perpetrator (if applicable)—assess distorted view of perpetrator, attachment to perpetrator

5. Alterations in relations with others—assess sense of trust with others, being revictimized

6. Somatization—assess digestive problems, chronic pain, or unexplained physical complaints

7. Alterations in systems of meaning—assess pessimistic attitude toward the future, distorted beliefs or sense of hopelessness

Pelcovitz et al. has shown the SIDES to be a reliable and valid instrument to assess the alterations in functioning from exposure to extreme stress and provides empirical evidence to expand the current PTSD *DSM-IV-TR* diagnosis to include a new category of "Disorders of Extreme Stress."

Pelcovitz, D., B. van der Kolk, S. Roth, F. Mandel, S. Kaplan, and P. Resick, 1997. "Development of a Criteria Set and a Structured Interview for Disorders of Extreme Stress (SIDES)." *Journal of Traumatic Stress,* 10, no. 1: 3–16.

subjective units of discomfort (SUD)

A subjective number reported by the individual when asked to rate the level of anxiety in a situation that is anxiety-provoking. In order to monitor anxiety levels, psychiatrist Joseph Wolpe developed the subjective units of discomfort score as applied during SYSTEMATIC DESENSITIZATION to phobias.

The SUD score has been widely used by researchers and counselors in both clinical and research applications. The score is based on an imagined scale from 0-100, 0 representing no anxiety or extreme calm and 100 representing the greatest amount of anxiety ever experienced. The number the individual assigns to a specific situation is the SUD score. Due to the relative "quickness" to obtain a SUD score, this method has been used beyond the original application to systematic desensitization (a therapy for reducing anxiety to a particular situation, object, person or event) to measure anxiety. Its use in Eye Movement Desensitization and Reprocessing (EMDR) asks the individual to rate his or her SUD score on a scale of 1–10.

Kaplan and Smith (1995) point out that evidence to support the validity of the SUD score comes from a large body of research that indicates that systematic desensitization effectively treats a wide variety of simple phobias.

Kaplan, D., and T. Smith. "A Validity Study of the Subjective Unit of Discomfort (SUD) Score." *Measurement & Evaluation in Counseling & Development* 27, no. 4 (1995): 748–756.

substance abuse (dependence) Excessive use of or addiction to alcohol and/or illegal drugs or misused prescription medications. Substance abuse and dependence are major problems in the United States today, as well as in many countries throughout the world. Alcohol is the most commonly used drug of abuse and dependence in the United States and in the world, followed by marijuana (often known as *cannabis* in other countries). Other commonly abused drugs are opiates, particularly heroin, and stimulants such as cocaine. In cases of severe stress and trauma, adults and/or adolescents may turn to alcohol or drugs for relief from their symptoms of depression and anxiety.

According to the Department of Mental Health and Substance Abuse of the World Health Organization (WHO) in its *Global Status Report on Alcohol 2004*, the countries with the highest percentage of individuals with alcoholism in 2004 were Poland (12.2 percent), Brazil (11.2 percent), and Peru (10.6 percent). The rate for the United States was 7.7 percent.

According to the *World Drug Report 2006*, published by the United Nations, an estimated 200 million people use illegal drugs each year. In addition, WHO reported that there are an estimated 25 million people who are addicted to drugs in the world, about 0.6 percent of the global population ages 15–64 years.

Narcotic painkillers are often abused, especially by young adults, and in 2004, adults ages 18–25 years were most likely to have abused narcotic painkillers. In this age group, about 12 percent had misused narcotics in the past year, and 4 percent had abused such drugs in the past month.

Stimulants are also abused, particularly cocaine. Cocaine was abused by 13 million individuals worldwide, according to the WHO.

Other drugs of abuse in the United States and other countries are amphetamines, barbiturates and benzodiazepines. Hallucinogenic drugs are also abused by some individuals, but they have largely fallen out of favor in the United States because of the variability in their effects.

Many studies have shown that individuals who have experienced severe trauma may turn (or in some cases, return) to substance abuse or dependence in an apparent effort to self-medicate for relief from their personal anguish; for example, adults who were abused as children are more likely to abuse alcohol and/or drugs than those who were not abused. Individuals who have been physically or sexually assaulted in adulthood may turn to alcohol or drugs for relief from their emotional suffering. Kilpatrick and Acierno, 2000, reported that adolescents who had been physically or sexually assaulted, witnessed violence, or had family members who abused alcohol or drugs had a higher risk of current substance abuse. As Thomas Insel (2007), Director of National Institute of Mental Health put it recently, "The majority of those with PTSD meet the diagnostic criteria for several psychiatric disorders, especially depression and substance abuse, and many also attempt suicide."

Abuse versus Dependence

Individuals who *abuse* alcohol and/or drugs misuse the substance but usually have not developed a physical tolerance, requiring greater amounts to achieve the same desired effect, such as inebriation or euphoria. Abusers of alcohol and/or drugs may experience withdrawal symptoms (milder symptoms, such as headaches or irritability), if they suddenly stop using the substance. Individuals who are *dependent* on a substance experience physical symptoms if they suddenly stop using the substance, and these symptoms may be severe, such as seizures, hallucinations, and even death.

Those who are dependent or addicted to substances usually center their lives on seeking out and continuing to use substances despite negative

RATE PER 100,000 POPULATION OF SELECTED HEALTH CONDITIONS, AMONG ALCOHOL ABUSERS AND ALCOHOLICS, UNITED STATES, 2001–2002

	Alcohol Abuse	Alcohol Dependence
Hardening of the Arteries or Arteriosclerosis	4.65	5.47
Cirrhosis of the liver	0.75	11.07
Any other form of liver disease	3.92	12.57
Hypertension	108.65	116.69
Chest pain or angina pectoris	19.86	37.24
Rapid heart beat or tachycardia	17.00	51.54
Heart attack or myocardial infarction	3.17	6.83
Any other form of heart disease	12.75	18.47
Stomach ulcer	12.18	38.69
Gastritis	26.76	45.13
Arthritis	111.18	76.47
Schizophrenia or psychotic illness	2.38	18.46

Adapted from the National Institute on Alcohol Abuse and Alcoholism, *Alcohol Use and Alcohol Use Disorders in the United States: Main Findings from the 2001–2002 National Epidemiologic Survey on Alcohol and Related Conditions (NESARC)*, U.S. Alcohol Epidemiologic Data Reference Manual 8, number 1 (January 2006), Bethesda, Maryland: National Institutes of Health, January 2006, page 189.

consequences; obtaining the substance is the most central aspect of their lives, more important than their health, their jobs, or even their families. Their use of legal or illegal drugs becomes all-encompassing and lying, stealing, and deceiving others becomes pervasive in their relationships.

Health Issues of Substance Abusers

Substance abuse and dependence can cause major health issues in individuals. For example, alcohol abusers have a rate of 4.65 per 100,000 people for hardening of the arteries, compared to a rate of 5.47 for those who are alcohol-dependent. (SEE TABLE AT LEFT.) Both groups have a high rate of hypertension: 108.65 per 100,000 for those who are alcohol abusers and 116.69 for those who are alcohol-dependent. Alcoholics have a much higher rate of psychotic disorders than those who are alcohol abusers: 18.46 per 100,000 for alcoholics versus a rate of 2.38 for alcohol abusers.

A frequent problem for people who have experienced trauma in their lives is substance abuse. By direct evidence, trauma creates stress. Alcohol is used to numb feelings of anxiety and other distressful symptoms. Emotions are controlled by self-medicating rituals of drugs and alcohol because they do work temporarily but often lead to more serious problems of addiction. For those with PTSD, substance abuse is avoidance behavior, a way to escape the horrific memories such as terror of war as documented by the prevalence of drug use among Vietnam veterans. Avoiding problems reduces the chance of learning new and effective coping skills to deal with the effects of trauma, and with alcohol abuse, this can lead to further depression.

In considering specific psychiatric disorders, those who abuse or are dependent on alcohol have a high risk for many disorders. (SEE TABLE BELOW.) For example, about 29.2 percent of those who are

PREVALENCE OF PSYCHIATRIC DISORDERS IN PEOPLE WITH ALCOHOL ABUSE AND ALCOHOL DEPENDENCE, ONE-YEAR RATE*

	Alcohol Abuse	Alcohol Dependence
Mood disorders	12.3 percent	29.2 percent
Major depressive disorder	11.3 percent	27.9 percent
Bipolar disorder	0.3 percent	1.9 percent
Anxiety disorders	29.1 percent	36.9 percent
Generalized anxiety disorder (GAD)	1.4 percent	11.6 percent
Panic disorder	1.3 percent	3.9 percent
Post-traumatic stress disorder	5.6 percent	7.7 percent

*The one-year rate is the percentage of people who met the criteria for the disorder during the year prior to the survey.
Source: Petrakis, Ismene L., M.D., et al., "Comorbidity of Alcoholism and Psychiatric Disorders," *Alcohol Research & Health* 26, number 2 (2002): 82.

dependent on alcohol have a mood disorder, compared to 12.3 percent of those who abuse alcohol. In addition, more than a third of those who are alcoholics (36.9 percent) suffer from ANXIETY DISORDERS, compared to the also high rate of 29.1 percent among alcohol abusers. From this table, it is important to note that many individuals with anxiety and mood disorders are probably also suffering from a trauma disorder, but the mood or anxiety problem is the one diagnosed. This is a frequent problem in

categorizing mental illness and addictions because diagnosticians seldom go beyond the most obvious or main symptom and thereby neglect to look for trauma roots to those symptoms.

Among those who are drug users or addicted to drugs, the health risks depend on the type of drug that is abused. (SEE TABLE BELOW.) For example, barbiturates can be injected or taken orally, and they can lower inhibitions, slow pulse, impair coordination, memory, and judgment.

SELECTED DRUGS WITH POTENTIAL FOR ABUSE AND THEIR INTOXICATION EFFECTS/POTENTIAL HEALTH CONSEQUENCES

Substances: Category and Name	DEA Schedule/ How Administered	Intoxication Effects/Potential Health Consequences
Depressants		
barbiturates	II, III, V/injected, swallowed	Reduced pain and anxiety; feeling of well-being; lowered inhibitions; slowed pulse and breathing; lowered blood pressure; poor concentration/confusion; fatigue; impaired coordination, memory, judgment; respiratory depression and arrest, addiction
benzodiazepines	IV/swallowed	
flunitrazepam (Rohypnol)	IV/swallowed, snorted	
gamma hydroxybutyric acid (GHB)	I, oral	Also, for barbiturates: sedation, drowsiness/depression, unusual excitement, fever, irritability, poor judgment, slurred speech, dizziness
		For benzodiazepines: sedation, drowsiness/dizziness
		For flunitrazepam: visual and gastrointestinal disturbances, urinary retention, memory loss for the time under the drug's effects
		For GHB, anxiety, insomnia, tremors, delirium, convulsions, death
Dissociative anesthetic		
ketamine	III/injected, snorted, smoked	Increased heart rate and blood pressure, impaired motor function/memory loss; numbness, nausea/vomiting Also for ketamine: At high doses: delirium, depression, respiratory depression and arrest
Hallucinogens: MDMA, LSD, phencyclidine	I/Oral, smoked, snorted, injected	Increased body temperature, heightened senses; euphoria, increased pulse rate, elevated blood pressure, insomnia, loss of appetite, agitation, hallucinations, convulsions, depression, irritability, disorientation
		MDMA: Teeth grinding and dehydration, muscle aches, depression, electrolyte imbalance, cardiac arrest, kidney failure, brain damage
		LSD and phencyclidine: Inability to detect movement, feel pain or remember events. Altered perception of time and distance
Cannabis: Marijuana, hashish and hashish oil	I/smoked oral	Euphoria, relaxed inhibitions, increased appetite, disorientation, fatigue, paranoia, possible psychosis
Inhalants		
Amyl and butyl nitrates	Not scheduled/inhaled	Pearls, poppers, rush, locker room Flushing, hypotension, headache, agitation
Nitrous oxide	Not scheduled/inhaled	Impaired memory, drunken behavior, slow onset vitamin deficiency, organ damage, vomiting, respiratory depression, loss of consciousness, possible death
Other inhalants	Not scheduled/inhaled	

(table continues)

(table continued)

Substances: Category and Name	DEA Schedule/ How Administered	Intoxication Effects/Potential Health Consequences
Opioids and Morphine Derivatives (Narcotics)		
codeine	II, III, IV/injected, swallowed	Pain relief, euphoria, constricted pupils of the eyes, drowsiness/respiratory depression and arrest, slow and shallow breathing, clammy skin, nausea, confusion, constipation, sedation, unconsciousness, coma, tolerance, addiction, possible death for codeine: less analgesia, sedation and respiratory depression than morphine
fentanyl (This drug is also associated with sexual assaults)	II/injected, smoked, snorted	
heroin	I/injected, snorted, smoked	
morphine	II, III/injected, swallowed, smoked	
opium	II, III, V/swallowed, smoked	
Other opioid painkillers (oxycodone, meperidine, hydromorphone, hydrocodone, propoxyphene	II, III, IV/swallowed, injected, suppositories, chewed, crushed, snorted	
Stimulants		
amphetamines	II/injected, swallowed, smoked, snorted	Increased heart rate, blood pressure, metabolism; feelings of exhilaration, energy, increased mental alertness/rapid or irregular heart beat; reduced appetite; weight loss; heart failure
cocaine	II/injected, smoked, snorted	Also, for amphetamines: rapid breathing hallucinations/tremor, loss of coordination; irritability, anxiousness, restlessness, delirium, panic, paranoia, impulsive behavior, aggressiveness, tolerance, addiction
methamphetamine	II/injected, swallowed, smoked, snorted	For cocaine: increased temperature/chest pain, respiratory failure, nausea, abdominal pain, strokes, seizures, headaches, malnutrition
methylphenidate	II/injected, swallowed, snorted	For methamphetamine: aggression, violence, psychotic behavior/memory loss, cardiac and neurological damage; impaired memory and learning, tolerance, kidney failure, stroke, seizures, lung damage
		For methylphenidate: increase or decrease in blood pressure, psychotic episodes/digestive problems, loss of appetite, weight loss
Other compounds		
anabolic steroids	III/injected, swallowed, applied to skin	No intoxication effects.
		Hypertension, blood clotting and cholesterol changes, liver cysts and cancer, kidney cancer, hostility and aggression, acne; adolescents, premature stoppage of growth; in males, prostate cancer, reduced sperm production, shrunken testicles, breast enlargement; in female, menstrual irregularities, development of beard and other masculine characteristics

Schedule I and II drugs have a high potential for abuse. These drugs require greater storage security and there is a quota on manufacturing, among other restrictions. Schedule I drugs are available for research only and have no approved medical use; Schedule II drugs are available only by prescription (not refillable) and require a form for ordering. Schedule III and IV drugs are available by prescription, may have five refills in 6 months, and may be ordered by the doctor over the telephone. Most Schedule V drugs are available as over the counter (OTC) drugs.
Note: Taking drug by injection can increase the risk of infection through needle contamination with staphylococci, HIV, hepatitis, and other organisms.
Source: Adapted from data available from the Drug Enforcement Administration and the National Institute of Drug Abuse.

They are also addicting when misused. Opiates can be injected or taken orally, and they have many potential health consequences to substance abusers and addicts, including pain relief, euphoria, constricted pupils, drowsiness/respiratory depression and arrest, slow and shallow breathing, clammy skin, nausea, confusion, constipation, sedation, unconsciousness, coma, tolerance, addiction, and even death.

Generally, people who have a problem with substance abuse or dependence obtain treatment from rehabilitative facilities that focus essentially on "drying" them out. Frequently, trauma problems are ignored or seen as secondary to the addiction. The addiction is the focus of all interventions. Often such treatment is provided on an outpatient basis, which includes individual counseling, education, and group therapy. Many individuals also benefit from Twelve Step groups such as Alcoholics Anonymous or Cocaine Anonymous, which help them when they feel the stresses of life and may feel drawn to abuse substances again particularly if trauma is at the root of their problem.

See also ADDICTION.

Department of Mental Health and Substance Abuse, *Global Status Report on Alcohol 2004.* Geneva, Switzerland: World Health Organization, 2004. Available online. URL: http://www.who.int/substance_abuse/publications/global_status_report_2004_overview.pdf. Downloaded September 26, 2006.

Gwinnell, Esther, M.D., and Christine Adamec. *The Encyclopedia of Drug Abuse.* New York: Facts On File, 2007.

Kilpatrick, D. G., and R. Acierno, "Risk Factors for Adolescent Substance Abuse and Dependence: Data from A National Sample." *Journal of Consulting Clinical Psychology* 68, no. 1 (2000): 19–30.

National Institute on Alcohol Abuse and Alcoholism, *Alcohol Use and Alcohol Use Disorders in the United States: Main Findings from the 2001–2002 National Epidemiologic Survey on Alcohol and Related Conditions (NESARC),* U.S. Alcohol Epidemiologic Data Reference Manual 8, number 1 (January 2006), Bethesda, Md.: National Institutes of Health, January 2006.

Petrakis, Ismene L., M.D., et al., "Comorbidity of Alcoholism and Psychiatric Disorders." *Alcohol Research & Health* 26, number 2 (2002).

United Nations Office on Drugs and Crime, *World Drug Report 2006.* Vol. 1, *Analysis.* June 2006. Available online at URL: http://www.unodc.org/pdf/WDR_2006/wdr2006_volume1.pdf, downloaded on September 28, 2006.

subthreshold posttraumatic stress disorder (PTSD)

Stress after a traumatic experience that does not reach the definition of POSTTRAUMATIC STRESS DISORDER (PTSD) as it is defined by the *Diagnostic and Statistical Manual* (*DSM*) produced by the American Psychiatric Association.

One of the deficiencies in using a "categorical" diagnostic system such as the *Diagnostic and Statistical Manual* (*DSM*) is that disorders do not always neatly fall into black or white, or all-or-none, groupings but instead represent a range of intensity and frequency "symptoms" for individuals. Only those cases that fall at the extremes are actually categorized or diagnosed, leaving many people affected but not diagnosed and often unrecognized. The subthreshold posttraumatic stress disorder (PTSD) designation is an effort to try to identify people with some PTSD symptoms and to study and treat the effects these symptoms have on their lives.

Symptoms and Diagnostic Path

On the National Anxiety Disorders Screening Day (sponsored by the Anxiety Disorders Association of America) in 1997, almost one-third of the more than 9,000 individuals screened reported at least one PTSD symptom that currently affected lives. Statistic analyses showed that the more PTSD symptoms a person reported (such as flashbacks, concentration problems, sleep difficulty, etc.) the more likely he or she was to show impairment, ANXIETY DISORDERS, major DEPRESSION and suicidal ideation. These findings clearly document (1) the important role TRAUMATIC EXPERIENCE and symptoms have on development of major disorders and (2) the need to assess and address trauma experiences in treating what appear to be nontrauma-related disorders.

Treatment Options and Outlook

Traditional trauma-based therapies are difficult to recommend to people with subthreshold PTSD because they often adapt to the "symptoms" and do not see themselves in need of therapy. On the other hand, many will come to therapy for complaints other than PTSD, such as ANXIETY and depression. A skilled therapist will help uncover the traumatic roots and treat that aspect of the presenting problem.

Risk Factors and Preventive Measures

A 2003 study in the Netherlands by van Zelst et al. on prevalence and risk factors of posttraumatic stress disorder in older adults found that 13.1 percent of the population surveyed had a six-month prevalence of subthreshold PTSD. Neuroticism and adverse early childhood events were the best predictors. Furthermore, research on the elderly has barely scratched the surface on subthreshold PTSD in spite of the fact that this population is at high risk for impairment and degenerative diseases. Studies of adults find a very high incidence of suicide potential in the subthreshold population (even when major depression is factored out), greater amounts of impairment and disability than non-subthreshold people and higher rates of comorbidity. Subthreshold PTSD is seldom studied or diagnosed, and yet it appears to be a major mental problem.

See also COMBAT-RELATED POSTTRAUMATIC STRESS DISORDER ; POSTTRAUMATIC STRESS DISORDER; THERAPY, TYPES OF.

Marshall, R. D., M. Olfson, F. Hellman, C. Blanco, M. Guardino, and E. L. Struening. "Comorbidity, impairment and suicidality in subthreshold PTSD." *American Journal of Psychiatry* 158, no. 9 (2001): 1467–1473.
van Zelst, et al. "Prevalence and Risk Factors of Posttraumatic Stress Disorder in Older Adults," *Psychotherapy and Psychosomatics* 72, no. 6 (November–December 2003): 333–342.

suicide   The intentional taking of one's life, often because of a deep-seated and chronic DEPRESSION, confusion, or to gain attention or when meaning in life is lost. The depression may stem from POSTTRAUMATIC STRESS DISORDER (PTSD), another disorder, or the cause may be unknown. About 32,000 Americans die from suicide each year, which makes suicide the 11th leading cause of death in the United States. Suicide is also the leading cause of death among teenagers. Worldwide, there are about 1 million deaths per year from suicide. According to the National Institute for Mental Health (NIMH), there are between 8 and 25 attempts at suicide for every actual death that results from a suicide attempt.

Symptoms and Diagnostic Path

According to the National Mental Health Information Center, there are specific indicators of someone seriously considering suicide. Anyone who exhibits any of these symptoms should be referred to a mental health professional, significant others, or parents and/or the National Suicide Prevention Lifeline, which is available at 800-273-TALK.

Suicide warning signs include

- threatening to hurt or kill oneself or talking about wanting to hurt or kill oneself
- looking for ways to kill oneself by seeking access to guns, pills, or other means
- talking or writing about death, dying, or suicide when these actions are out of the ordinary for the person
- exhibiting feelings of hopelessness
- exhibiting feelings of rage or uncontrolled anger or seeking revenge
- acting recklessly or engaging in risky activities, seemingly without thinking
- expressing feelings of being trapped, like there is no way out
- increasing alcohol or drug use
- withdrawal from friends, family, and society
- evincing feelings of anxiety, agitation
- experiencing dramatic mood changes
- expressions of a lack of reason for living or having no sense of purpose in life

Treatment Options and Outlook

Most suicidal individuals can be treated with therapy and ANTIDEPRESSANT medications, although the risk for suicide is initially increased at the onset of the use of antidepressants, particularly among children and adolescents, and caution and vigilance should be maintained. (Some studies indicate that this risk is significantly lower among adults taking antidepressants.) Ironically, the risk of suicide is greater as the individual starts getting better, but no one knows why exactly.

Some studies have shown that cognitive therapy (also known as COGNITIVE BEHAVIORAL THERAPY or CBT) decreases the risk for suicide attempts by as much as 50 percent. For example, in a study published in the *Journal of the American Medical Association* in 2005, the researchers found that over an 18-month follow-up period, only 24 percent of the subjects in the cognitive therapy group attempted suicide, compared to 42 percent of the subjects given other services available in the community.

Risk Factors and Preventive Measures

Older individuals have the greatest risk for suicide, and individuals age 65 years or older represent about 18 percent of all deaths by suicide. According to the Centers for Disease Control and Prevention (CDC), men have a four times greater risk for suicide than women. However, women have about three times the risk of men of *attempting* (and many failing at) suicide. Men and women also vary in their means of committing suicide; for example, most men who commit suicide use firearms, while most women use poisoning. (SEE TABLE BELOW.)

Among racial groups, whites have the highest rate of suicides (a rate of 12.9 people per 100,000), followed by American Indians and Native Alaskans (12.4 per 100,000). Those with the lowest risk are non-Hispanic blacks (5.3 per 100,000) and Asian and Pacific Islanders (5.8 per 100,000).

Those with mental illnesses, such as DEPRESSION, bipolar disorder or schizophrenia, have an increased risk for suicide compared to those without these disorders. In addition, those with personality disorders have an increased risk for death by suicide. Individuals who have suffered from a past or recent trauma have an elevated risk for suicide. Part of this risk increase reflects the presence of depression, which increases suicide risks. Also, at a more complex level, traumatized individuals often lose a sense of self and have this "existential" issue to face. Individuals with a major disease such as cancer, heart disease, stroke, or Parkinson's disease also have an increased risk for suicide.

SUBSTANCE ABUSE is a major risk factor for suicide and, according to the National Strategy for Suicide Prevention, 40–60 percent of individuals who die from suicide are intoxicated at the time of their deaths.

Individuals who have attempted suicide in the past are at an increased risk for further attempts.

Other risk factors for suicide include:

- stressful life events combined with other risk factors, such as depression
- a family history of mental disorders or substance abuse
- a family history of suicide
- family violence, including physical or sexual abuse
- the presence of firearms in the home, which is the method used in more than half of all suicides
- incarceration
- exposure to the suicidal behavior of others, such as family members, peers, or even media figures

Suicide can often be prevented because those considering suicide usually exhibit signs that should be taken seriously. To prevent suicide, anyone expressing the common signs of suicide should be referred for psychiatric help immediately. In addition, those who fit into risk factors, particularly individuals who are severely depressed or who have PTSD, should be referred to mental health counselors for an assessment of their suicide risk.

If an individual believes that someone may attempt suicide, whenever possible, any firearms should be removed from that person's home. If the individual who is talking about suicide is under age 18, his or her parent or legal guardian should be

METHODS OF SUICIDE		
Suicide by:	Males (%)	Females (%)
Firearms	57	32
Suffocation	23	20
Poisoning	13	38

Source: National Institute of Mental Health, "Suicide in the U.S.: Statistics and Prevention." December 2006. Available online at URL: http://www.nimh.nih.gov/publicat/harmsway.cfm. Downloaded March 19, 2007.

contacted immediately. If the parent or legal guardian refuses to take the threat seriously and/or fails to take any action, a mental health professional should be contacted, and he or she may contact emergency personnel.

PTSD and Suicide

According to the National Center for Posttraumatic Stress Disorder, PTSD is a risk factor for suicide among military veterans, with the highest suicide risk among those who were hospitalized for a wound or who were wounded multiple times. Combat-related guilt is another risk factor for suicide among veterans with PTSD. Some experts believe that the suicide risk is greater among veterans because of the presence of PTSD alone, while others say that the suicide risk increases because of related psychiatric problems that are also present, such as depression.

Natural Disasters

Some studies have demonstrated an increased rate of suicide subsequent to a natural disaster. For example, an article by Krug and his colleagues in the *New England Journal of Medicine* in 1998 studied data from 377 counties affected by at least one disaster between 1982 and 1989. They also amassed data on suicides that occurred in the three years before and the four years after the natural disaster. For example, with regard to hurricanes, the researchers found that suicide rates increased significantly after a hurricane from 12.0 per 100,000 people before the disaster to 15.7 people per 100,000 after the hurricane. However, the authors printed a retraction some months later, indicating that they had misanalyzed the data, and the results in fact were false and inaccurate. Since this frequently quoted study of Krug et al., other researchers have attempted to assess suicidality following natural disasters on a large scale. Perhaps the best of these studies over a large area is one conducted by Shoaf and colleagues from data collected following the Northridge, California, earthquake, which shook almost all of Los Angeles County. These authors concluded that "It does not appear that suicide rates increase as a result of earthquakes in this setting [Los Angeles County]." Furthermore, cumulative disasters that followed the Northridge earthquake over a subsequent three-year period of time (such as major fires, weather, etc.) did not enhance the suicide rate. In fact, there was a "downward trend" in suicides after the Northridge earthquake and all subsequent disasters. Taken together with the retracted results from the Krug and colleague study, these results would indicate that no demonstrable increase in suicide occurs following major natural disasters.

Physicians' Rate of Suicide

According to an article by Schernhammer in a 2005 issue of the *New England Journal of Medicine*, doctors (particularly female doctors) have a significantly higher rate of suicide than others, and physicians' suicide rate is more than double that of individuals in other professions. In addition, doctors who attempt suicide are more likely to succeed than others, whether they are male or female physicians. This is presumably because of their medical knowledge and awareness of an effective means to cause death. It is also true that most doctors who commit suicide use drugs to cause their deaths. Said Schernhammer,

> There are few interventions in place to help prevent suicide among physicians. Such safeguards might include the provision of discreet and confidential access to psychotherapy and open discussion of the stress encountered in a medical career. The barriers that may prevent physicians from seeking help for mental disorders (such as the threat of losing their medical licenses) must also be addressed.

The Media and Suicide

Sometimes the popular media appears to glamorize the suicide of public figures, and some studies have shown that following the media portrayal of a suicide, the number of youth suicides subsequently increased. Media figures have been informed of the effect of glamorizing suicide and hopefully will be alert to the potential risks that can be incurred through dramatic representations of the suicides of public figures. (See MEDIA.)

Suicide-Prevention Strategies

In their article on suicide prevention strategies in the *Journal of the American Medical Association* in 2005, Mann and his colleagues reviewed numerous journal articles on suicide published between 1966 and June 2005 to evaluate the impact of specific types of recommendations on a decrease in the suicide rate. Based on these findings, they subsequently recommended that physicians receive education on recognizing and treating depression. In addition, they recommended restrictions to the means of suicide, such as barbiturates or firearms. Gatekeepers were also found to be effective. These are individuals such as members of the clergy, first responders, pharmacists, caregivers to the elderly, and individuals employed in institutional settings, such as schools, prison, and military service.

See also DEPRESSION; THERAPY, TYPES OF.

Brown, Gregory K., et al, "Cognitive Therapy for the Prevention of Suicide Attempts: A Randomized Controlled Trial." *Journal of the American Medical Association* 294, no. 5 (August 3, 2005): 563–570.

Gaynes, Bradley N., M.D., et al. "Screening for Suicide Risk in Adults: A Summary of the Evidence for the U.S. Preventive Services Task Force." *Annals of Internal Medicine* 140, no. 10 (May 18, 2004): 822–835.

Krug, Etienne G., M.D., et al. "Suicide after Natural Disasters." *New England Journal of Medicine* 338, no. 6 (February 5, 1998): 373–378.

Mann, J. John, M.D., et al. "Suicide Prevention Strategies: A Systematic Review." *Journal of the American Medical Association* 294, no. 16 (October 26, 2005): 2064–2074.

National Institute of Mental Health, "The Numbers Count: Mental Disorders in America." 2006. Available online. URL: http://www.nimh.nih.gov/publicat/numbers. cfm. Downloaded March 19, 2007.

National Institute of Mental Health, "Suicide in the U.S.: Statistics and Prevention." December 2006. Available online. URL: http://www.nimh.nih.gov/publicat/harmsway.cfm. Downloaded March 19, 2007.

Schernhammer, Eva, M.D, "Taking Their Own Lives—The High Rate of Physician Suicide." *New England Journal of Medicine* 352, no. 4 (June 16, 2005): 2373–2476.

Shoaf, K., L. B. Bourque, C. Giangreco, B. Weiss. "Suicides in Los Angeles County in Relation to the Northridge Earthquake." *Prehospital and Disaster Medicine* 19, no. 4 (2004): 307–310.

survivor guilt   Survivors of traumatic events are thankful for their survival and feel a joyous relief, yet they often begin to feel guilty for surviving while others perished. Thoughts of "I should have died too," "I could have done something to save them," or "Why did I survive?" begin to cast doubt on their survival. Sufferers feel guilty because they feel powerless and helpless at the outcome. Survivor guilt is a normal response to a traumatic event and shows how difficult it can be for some people to feel grateful for being alive following such an experience.

For example, before the collapse of the World Trade Center buildings on SEPTEMBER 11, a man climbed down 40 flights of stairs to exit the building with his coworkers and then ran a half-mile up Broadway before calling his wife with the news that he was OK. In the days that followed, his wife noticed her husband was in a daze, emotionally numb, and asking himself why *he* didn't help save more people on the stairway and why did he survive when many of his friends died. This is survivor guilt and along with helplessness, is one of the worst experiences a human being can endure.

The following are ways in which a person can manage the feelings of survivor guilt:

1. Talk to anyone who is supportive of your ordeal. Then talk some more. Acknowledge your feelings with other survivors. You are not alone in your feelings. This is the most effective way to avoid isolation and withdrawal.
2. Try not to focus on the "why did I survive" mystery. Not only is it impossible to really understand why, the most important part of the why is that you survived so your family and friends will have a future with you.
3. Forget about the "what ifs" because the what ifs did not happen. During September 11, through the uncertainty and chaos brought on by the state of war in the United States, we all did the best we could with the information available.
4. Question your irrational thoughts. If you think you could have gone back to help someone else, recount your experience with other witnesses; a broader picture may help you understand it may not have been possible. Do not blame yourself.
5. Focus on your strengths, the strategies you use to cope in times of crisis. Remind yourself of your resilience. Do not let guilt negate your positives. Do not punish yourself.

6. Channel your energies to helping others in the recovery efforts. These are activities that you can control and feel good about, not the powerlessness of the traumatic event. Taking time to meet with families of the deceased with information about their loved ones is one source of strength and control.

7. Know that your survival is significant. It is a time to reassess your life, what is valuable and meaningful to you. Make the best of your life, as it is a tribute to your survival.

8. Connect with your support network, such as support groups. You may want to turn to grief professionals or your spiritual resources in order to deal with your guilt feelings, especially if your life is in an emotional decline.

See also SURVIVOR SYNDROME.

survivor syndrome A phenomenon resulting from surviving a traumatic experience (where others have perished) or the survival from a work-related layoff (where others were let go) and similar situations. In the work situation, survivors are often highly stressed, mistrustful toward management, and insecure about their jobs. Their loyalty suffers and often they show lower productivity, DEPRESSION, resistance to change, and absenteeism.

More commonly, survivor syndrome and its behavioral and emotional characteristics refer to the effects of survival from CHILD SEXUAL ABUSE. Some mental health experts believe that childhood sexual abuse and incest lead not only to feelings of SHAME and sexual problems, but also to arthritis, low self-esteem, poor motivation, ANXIETY, and self-identity issues in adulthood. In addition, diagnosable conditions such as BORDERLINE PERSONALITY DISORDER, dissociative identity disorder, eating disorders, somatoform disorders, and SUBSTANCE ABUSE AND DEPENDENCE may also result from childhood sexual abuse.

Some experts dissent from this view and say that, while certainly some of these disorders are associated with sexual abuse in childhood, it is highly questionable whether sexual abuse is the sole cause. A review by Bower (1993) concluded that other more direct evidence must also be used to confirm past sexual abuse before it is assumed as a direct cause of a current condition.

Survivor syndrome is often marked by feelings of guilt on the survivor's part. This is common in combat situations where one's friend or colleague is killed, but another person survives. Guilt over survival can lead to self-destructive behavior patterns, such as ADDICTION, self-mutilation such as CUTTING behavior, aggressiveness, risk-taking, and depression. SURVIVOR GUILT is usually subtle, but it can have powerful effects on both behavior and mood.

Bower, B. "The Survivor Syndrome: Childhood Sexual Abuse Leaves a Controversial Trail of Aftereffects." *Science News* (September 25, 1993).

sympathetic nervous system (SNS) The SNS promotes a response of arousal and emergency energy release while depressing digestion. It is one of two systems comprising the AUTONOMIC NERVOUS SYSTEM, the other being the PARASYMPATHETIC NERVOUS SYSTEM, which acts in the opposite direction to rest and relax the body. The sympathetic nervous system consists of two paired chains of ganglia lying just to the left and right of the spinal cord, in the thoracic and lumbar areas, and connected by axons to the spinal cord. Sympathetic axons extend from the ganglia to the body's organs and activate them for emergency events. The sweat glands, the adrenal glands, the muscles that constrict blood vessels and the muscles that erect the hairs of the skin have only sympathetic input. For example, during an emergency when faced with an attacker, robber, stalker, or potential violent situation, our body readies itself for FIGHT-OR-FLIGHT RESPONSE. The SNS releases adrenaline and noradrenaline into the bloodstream, blood is diverted from digestion to the muscles, and the body is ready for a fight or to flee.

See also BRAIN; CENTRAL NERVOUS SYSTEM.

Symptom Check List-90 See INSTRUMENTS/SCALES/SURVEYS THAT EVALUATE POSTTRAUMATIC STRESS DISORDER (PTSD).

systematic desensitization (SD) A behavioral therapy technique used to treat anxiety, phobias, and excessive feeling states. Psychiatrist Joseph Wolpe developed systematic desensitization in the 1950s, when he found that anxiety symptoms could be reduced when the triggering stimulus or event was paired with a relaxation response.

The systematic desensitization (SD) process begins by having the individual learn relaxation skills, such as PROGRESSIVE RELAXATION, where the patient systematically and sequentially tightens, then relaxes, different muscle groups. Once the individual learns how it feels to relax muscles, he or she learns to recreate this sensation in various anxiety-provoking situations. Heart palpitations and hyperventilation result from autonomic arousal. These are reduced or eliminated over time with continued practice of progressive relaxation.

Next the therapist and client create a hierarchy of anxiety-provoking situations in order of least to most distressing. This is sometimes referred to as the fear hierarchy. For example, if the client is afraid of spiders, the hierarchy might begin with the lowest distressing situation as a picture of a spider and recorded as 5 on a scale of 1–100. The most distressing situation might be a spider crawling on the client and is recorded as 100.

The SD process then continues with the therapist presenting the client with the hierarchy of fear, one situation at a time starting with the least distressing scene. The client uses the relaxation skills to produce a state of relaxation, and as tolerance develops for each situation, the client moves on to the next level on the hierarchy list.

Thus, each fearful situation is faced progressively and associated with relaxation, as gradual desensitization occurs and the fear is eventually extinguished.

See also ANXIETY DISORDERS; HIERARCHY OF FEARS; THERAPY, TYPES OF.

T

terrorism The use of violence to bring extreme fear to the intended victims, usually civilians. Terrorist attacks usually involve a political or social agenda by persons too weak for open warfare and do not include actions of war by recognized countries. One terrorist organization, Al-Qaeda and its affiliates, has attacked North America, Europe, Asia, and the Middle East and takes credit for the deadliest of these attacks, that of SEPTEMBER 11. The psychological impact of terrorism on the public has intensified in recent years due to extended media coverage and Internet Web site postings by many terrorist groups predicting future attacks.

Research is showing that deliberate violence has more lasting mental health effects than do NATURAL DISASTERS and accidents. Survivors of terrorism and the community in general feel a sense of injustice, anger, and helplessness to protect themselves. A consistent finding is that most people, over time, become resilient to terrorist acts of violence, but that people who are directly exposed to the violence have a higher risk of developing posttraumatic stress disorder (PTSD).

Complex bereavement can result from terrorism, due to the sudden, unexpected, and violent nature of tragic loss of life. Recovery may be long and arduous, as it was after September 11, when the World Trade Center was destroyed in New York City, leading families and survivors to experience uncertainty about the welfare of their loved ones. Even with the widespread public support for the bereaved through public rituals and the recognition of their needs, Raphael and Wooding show in their article (2004); exposure to these attacks predicts current PTSD and DEPRESSION.

Children also display a wide range of behavioral, emotional, and physiological reactions after a terrorist attack. A minority of children will develop posttraumatic stress symptoms after a terrorist attack. Findings from the Oklahoma City bombing of the Alfred P. Murrah Federal Building in 1995 indicate that

- Children who lost a friend or relative were more likely to report immediate symptoms of PTSD than nonbereaved children.
- Arousal and fear presenting seven weeks after the bombing were significant predictors of PTSD.
- Two years after the bombing, 16 percent of the children who lived approximately 100 miles from Oklahoma City reported significant PTSD symptoms related to the event. This is an important finding because these youths were not directly exposed to the trauma and they were not related to people who had been killed or injured.
- PTSD symptomatology was predicted by media exposure and indirect interpersonal exposure, such as having a friend who knew someone who was killed or injured.
- No study specifically reported on rates of PTSD in children following the bombing. However, studies have shown that as many as 100 percent of children who witness a parental homicide or sexual assault, 90 percent of sexually abused children, 77 percent of children exposed to a school shooting, and 35 percent of urban youth exposed to community violence will develop PTSD.

See also TERROR MANAGEMENT THEORY; CHILDREN AND TRAUMA.

Raphael, B., and S. Wooding. "Early Mental Health Interventions for Traumatic Loss." In *Early Intervention for Trauma and Traumatic Loss*, edited by B. Litz, 147–178. New York: Guildford Press, 2004.

terror management theory (TMT) An area of research that studies the reactions of people when confronted with the psychological terror of their own eventual death. The theory was developed in the 1980s by Professors Sheldon Soloman, Tom Pyszcynski, and Jeff Greenberg from the theories of cultural anthropologist Ernest Becker, who argued that human awareness of death and its denial guides the major portion of human behavior.

According to terror management theory (TMT), people manage the potential terror of death through cultural values that provide meaning, security, and ways to live a meaningful life. Another anxiety buffer to death is self-esteem, the perception of living up to the standards of society, and defined roles within the culture. As cultures vary so do belief systems within different cultures, which challenge cultural beliefs about death. This in turn makes people uncomfortable enough to deny or devalue other worldviews or to try to convert others to their own worldview, which can lead to conflict.

To test terror management theory, researchers designed a mortality salient paradigm that asked people to think about their own death and to make judgments of events (such as SEPTEMBER 11) that either supported or threatened the individual's cultural worldview. Not surprisingly, after September 11, Americans avoided places and situations where terrorists might strike next, became very patriotic, and held strong American values that protected their worldviews.

See also TERRORISM.

testimony therapy A form of therapy based on the concept that giving written and/or oral testimony of traumatic experiences usually associated with torture and organized violence can serve to relieve posttraumatic symptoms. The early work with testimony therapy came from the experiences of political prisoners in Chile who gave testimony of their traumatic experiences to others. Their symptoms subsequently improved. Based on this experience, several mental health facilities and workers developed their own form of testimony therapy.

For example, van Dijk, Schoutrop, and Spinhoven developed a 12-session protocol, described in the *American Journal of Therapy,* in which victims of war or organized violence who seek asylum tell their life stories as well as their traumatic experiences and a written document is produced that can be read by the family and friends or placed in an historical archive.

Similarly, Steven Weine, a psychiatrist at the University of Illinois, Chicago campus, has reported on a testimony therapy project for survivors of the genocide or "ethnic cleansing" in Bosnia. These survivors told their story to a psychiatrist who acted as a witness and recorded their experiences through narratives. The concept of telling one's story to a supportive listening community seems to represent a deep human form of healing and placement back into the community.

In modern therapy terms, testimony could be viewed as a form of exposure therapy combined with cognitive behavioral aspects. However, it seems to be much more than survivors' simply telling someone their story of TRAUMA, TORTURE, and abuse. Instead, it is an oral history of survival, and relational in nature. Most important, however, testimony offers a way back to the community when the survivor feels alienated, alone, and devalued. It is a portal back to humanness and acceptability.

See also THERAPY, TYPES OF.

van Dijk, J. A., M. J. A. Schoutrop, P. Spinhoven. "Testimony therapy: Treatment method for traumatized victims of organized violence." *American Journal of Psychotherapy* 57 (2003): 361–373.

thalamus See BRAIN; CENTRAL NERVOUS SYSTEM; SYMPATHETIC NERVOUS SYSTEM.

therapy, types of Professional assistance that is provided to a person suffering TRAUMA, such as POSTTRAUMATIC STRESS DISORDER (PTSD), ACUTE STRESS DISORDER (ASD), or ELABORATED POSTTRAUMATIC STRESS DISORDER, as well as many other forms of traumatic stress. Therapy is provided by licensed clinical psychologists, social workers and marriage-family therapists, or psychiatrists. ANTIDEPRESSANTS or ANTIANXIETY MEDICATIONS may also be helpful to many people suffering from traumatic experiences;

however, the assistance of a mental health professional is often invaluable in helping a traumatized person resolve painful and difficult issues that were caused or triggered by the traumatic event.

There are many different forms of therapy, and some types are appropriate for many situations while others are more suitable for particular types of trauma. In addition, some individuals do well in individual therapy while others benefit from interacting in a group with others who have suffered from the same or a similar type of trauma.

Behavioral Therapies

There is a broad array of behavioral therapies used to assist trauma victims, ranging from COGNITIVE BEHAVIORAL THERAPY and COGNITIVE PROCESSING THERAPY to SYSTEMATIC DESENSITIZATION.

Cognitive Behavioral Therapy Cognitive behavioral therapy (CBT) is a proven form of treatment for many trauma disorders. The behavioral component of CBT usually involves some form of gradual exposure to the feared situation or object, while the cognitive component is aimed at changing the thinking that produces fear.

Cognitive Processing Therapy (CPT) Sexual assault victims may benefit from cognitive processing therapy (CPT), a form of therapy specifically designed to work with posttraumatic stress disorder (PTSD) in sexual assault survivors. Many people have an underlying belief that "Nice women are not raped." Therefore, in this line of thinking, if a woman is raped, she must not be a nice person. A woman with such underlying beliefs would experience shame, humiliation, and self-doubt.

Information processing therapy helps the victim incorporate what has happened to her and resolve areas that conflict with her past beliefs.

Systematic Desensitization (SD) Therapists who treat trauma with systematic desensitization (SD) may first use PROGRESSIVE RELAXATION therapy, in which the therapist teaches the client to relax muscle groups in a stepwise manner. Through repetitive practice over a period of months, the individual learns to discriminate tension from relaxation and voluntarily release tension where tension is present.

Next the therapist and client work together to create a HIERARCHY OF FEARS related to the anxiety-provoking situation, ranging from the least to the most distressing situation. For example, if the client is afraid of spiders, the hierarchy might begin with the least distressing situation, a picture of a spider, recorded as 5 on a scale of 1–100. The most distressing situation might be a spider crawling on the client and might be recorded as 100. By pairing relaxation therapy with the fear hierarchy, the client learns to desensitize and rid himself or herself of the fear.

Exposure Therapy

EXPOSURE THERAPY helps phobic individuals resolve their fear. The treatment includes a mild exposure to the feared object or experience at first, which is gradually increased to a direct exposure to it. Often exposure is combined with relaxation training and cognitive behavior therapy.

DIRECT THERAPEUTIC EXPOSURE (DTE) is a class of exposure treatments that rely on flooding or high-intensity exposure, whereas regular exposure is gradual and stepwise and used with individuals experiencing severe distress due to traumatic events. Exposure continues until the individual's anxiety peaks and eventually abates. IMAGE HABITUATION THERAPY (IHT) is a form of exposure therapy in which the patient visualizes self-evoked images of the trauma in order to produce habituation of anxiety. The patient describes the traumatic experience on an audiotape and uses the tapes in self-directed homework assignments.

During IMPLOSIVE THERAPY the individual imagines anxiety-producing situations, exaggerating them to elicit as much anxiety as possible. Anxiety toward parental figures or other anxiety-inducing sources are used. In INTEROCEPTIVE EXPOSURE THERAPY (IE), traumatized individuals are given tasks to perform to reduce their sensitivity and show them that these tasks are not harmful; for example, the person may be told to hyperventilate, which will induce an increased heart rate and dizziness but not cause any serious consequences. The individual with panic problems can benefit from IE therapy.

In IN VIVO therapy, the person recalls the clothing worn, the weapons used, and other objects present during the trauma. The client focuses on the stimuli or event fully for 30 to 45 minutes or until his or her discomfort level decreases by 50 percent.

MULTIPLE-CHANNEL EXPOSURE THERAPY (M-CET) was developed to address the high levels of physiological arousal and intense fear sensations that individuals report experiencing with PANIC ATTACK and PTSD when discussing traumatic memories. To focus in on the paniclike sensations, the individual performs such exercises as spinning in a chair, hyperventilating, or breathing through a straw. The treatment aim is to reduce fearful preoccupation with physical sensations, thereby reducing fearful reactions to trauma reminders.

TRAUMATIC INCIDENT REDUCTION (TIR) therapy can reduce the negative effects of past traumas. The client identifies a specific traumatic experience and then views the incident like a videotape, starting just prior to the traumatic incident, and watches it, without talking, until the incident is over. After the first run-through of the incident, the client is asked to view the tape again in his or her mind, from the beginning. The purpose of TIR is to help the client integrate unresolved areas of the traumatic experience.

Eye Movement Desensitization and Reprocessing (EMDR)

EYE MOVEMENT DESENSITIZATION AND REPROCESSING (EMDR) therapy is an effective form of therapy with many traumatized individuals. EMDR is an information processing therapy and uses an eight-phase treatment approach starting with a client history to identify past events that caused the pathology, as well as current situations that trigger disturbance. It also incorporates the types of experiences needed to bring the client to a full level of mental health; for example, social skills that are missing because the client was traumatized in childhood. EMDR processes both the negative experiences that cause dysfunction as well as the positive experiences that need to be incorporated. Although eye movements are the most commonly used external stimuli, the client can also use tapping and auditory tones.

Alternative Therapies

There is a broad array of alternative therapies and techniques to help the trauma-stricken. *Ayurveda*, traditional medicine within India is based on energy and balance to restore wholeness to the mind-body system. The emphasis is on the mind, body, and spirit, using such techniques as meditation, aromatherapy, yoga, nutrition, and exercise to trigger the body's own natural healing processes.

Energy therapies are based on the belief that energy fields surround and penetrate the body and that they can be manipulated by movement, meditation, prayer, or by another person who places a hand over the body, without touching it. This form of therapy is also known as *bioenergetic therapy*.

Nutritional approaches use vitamins, herbs, and other supplements that have been shown to balance moods and overcome anxieties.

Aromatherapy uses oils extracted from flowers, herbs, and plants to treat distress. The olfactory nerves send messages directly into the LIMBIC SYSTEM of the brain. Aromatherapy is used for many disorders, including stress, anxiety, and pain.

Mind-body techniques, such as yoga and deep breathing, incorporate both cognitive (mental activity) and physical (sensations) processes to relieve stress. Some examples are massage therapy, meditation, hypnosis, biofeedback, and acupuncture.

Other Therapies

TESTIMONY THERAPY assists survivors who tell their story to a psychiatrist who acts as a witness and records their experiences through narratives. Telling one's story to a supportive listening community seems to represent a deep human form of healing and placement back into the community.

ART THERAPY is another form of therapy used with trauma victims, which incorporates drawing, painting, modeling clay, and other expressive methods to help traumatized children or adults express their feelings nonverbally. Art therapy may be effective when it is difficult or impossible for individuals to talk about their feelings.

Combination Therapies

Many therapists choose to use a combination of therapies to assist their patients; for example, ANXIETY MANAGEMENT TRAINING (AMT) is a combination of relaxation therapy with cognitive awareness.

TRAUMA MANAGEMENT THERAPY is a multicomponent therapy that uses exposure therapies, desensitization, and eye movement desensitization and reprocessing (EMDR). Social skill training and anger management training are also used.

Psychoanalysis

Some mental health professionals still rely on psychoanalysis, a complex and long-term system of therapy devised by Sigmund Freud in the late 19th century. Freud believed that traumatized individuals needed to re-experience the negative experience in their minds to undergo an ABREACTION, or healing of the psychic wounds they suffered. However, many therapists today no longer share this view. In addition, psychoanalysis generally involves frequent visits with the therapist over years, a long-term approach that has fallen out of favor with many clinicians.

torture   Intentionally inflicting pain or suffering, physical or mental, as a means of punishment, to gain information, or to render the victim so traumatized he or she is unable to function. There are many forms and purposes of torture throughout history, and its practice has come under severe scrutiny and debate recently. Torture may be carried out as part of a state-sanctioned enterprise, or used by individuals or groups as a means of initiation, sadistic gratification, intimidation, or for political or criminal gain. Torture almost always produces traumatic or posttraumatic effects on the victim. Courts, governments, international tribunals, conventions, and the United Nations have all decried the use of torture. Despite these efforts to negate torture, violence, murder, and torture persist in many parts of the world.

In medieval and even modern times torture was common practice and often deemed necessary in order to extract confessions and information. In the Middle Ages, people who were accused of witchcraft were tortured for confessions. Torture was used by the U.S. against some detainees accused of terrorism following the attacks of SEPTEMBER 11, 2001. On January 22, 2009, President Barack Obama signed an Executive Order against torture by requiring the *Army Field Manual* as a guide for terror interrogations. Other government regimes use torture methods to disable or disempower dissenters by causing traumatic reactions. Sadistic individuals, often mentally ill, may use torture in the process of murdering someone.

A gross human rights violation is the severe abuse of an individual, including torture or murder. In many countries, torture is used to disable political or intellectual resistance so that individuals cannot think or take decisive action. Torture is often used in ways that do not leave visible scars.

Torture victims usually have lost their sense of personal dignity and well-being. They exhibit symptoms of traumatic stress and usually do not want to share their pain and humiliation with others, preferring to remain alone in their suffering. Political sanctuary in another country is often difficult and fears of reviving the horrors they experienced prevent many from ever seeking outside help or safer environments.

The Istanbul Protocol provides guidelines created by the United Nations regarding the documentation of torture as well as its consequences on individuals. It is also known as *The Manual on Effective Investigation and Documentation of Torture and Other Cruel, Inhuman or Degrading Treatment or Punishment*. This document is available in its full text on the Web site of the Physicians for Human Rights: http://physiciansforhumanrights.org/library/documents/reports/istanbul-protocol.pdf.

See also POST TORTURE SYNDROME; WATERBOARDING.

tranquilizers   See BENZODIAZEPINES.

transgenerational trauma   A subtle but pervasive source of trauma is called transgenerational trauma. This type of trauma occurs in children of traumatized individuals, but it is usually subliminal or less obvious than in other cases. For example, second-generation survivors of the Holocaust (Yehuda, et al., 1995) and of the Armenian genocide show significantly lowered cortisol levels, indicating a stress component in their lives. Similar effects are evident in the children of World War II veterans, tsunami victims, and the children of victims of other civilian catastrophes.

See also INTERGENERATIONAL TRAUMA; SOCIAL PERSPECTIVES ON TRAUMA.

trauma, combat versus civilian   Combat veterans as well as civilians who have never been in combat situations can be traumatized by extremely stressful situations, but there are differences among the causes and types of trauma they experience. Individuals in each group may develop POSTTRAUMATIC STRESS DISORDER (PTSD). Combat veterans are more likely to develop PTSD due to the intensity and nature of the events they experience and develop acute trauma. Sometimes the cause of their PTSD and its effects are fairly immediate, such as when a soldier sees comrades killed or maimed, but at other times it is less apparent why an individual develops PTSD, as when support personnel are traumatized. Civilians are at risk for trauma caused by many traumatic events, such as serious car crashes, major medical illnesses, assaults, and major natural disasters.

In general, estimates are that about 20 percent of women and 8 percent of men in the United States will develop POSTTRAUMATIC STRESS DISORDER (PTSD) sometime in their lifetimes, according to the National Center for Posttraumatic Stress Disorders, a branch of the Veterans Administration. About 30 percent of these people will exhibit chronic forms of the disorder throughout their lifetimes. The most common causes of PTSD in men are experiencing combat, having suffered neglect or physical abuse in childhood, being bullied, or raped, according to the National Center for Posttraumatic Stress Disorders. Among women rape, sexual molestation, physical attack, being threatened with a weapon, and childhood physical abuse are the most common causes of PTSD.

Combat-Related PTSD

Soldiers who develop COMBAT-RELATED PTSD may have such symptoms as hypervigilance, FLASHBACKS, and active avoidance of anything that reminds them of their past combat situations. Other soldiers develop symptoms of PTSD as a result of TRAUMATIC BRAIN INJURIES incurred on the battlefield.

Vietnam Veterans   Several million American soldiers served in the Vietnam War (1964–1974), and some of these individuals ultimately developed POST-VIETNAM SYNDROME, or PTSD that was specifically associated with having served in Vietnam. PTSD directly affects how individuals interact with others. Of all those who served in Vietnam, 15.2 percent of males and 8.1 percent of females have been diagnosed with PTSD, according to the National Center for Posttraumatic Stress Disorders. The lifetime prevalence of PTSD among those who served in Vietnam is 30.9 percent for men and 26.9 percent for women.

The rates of acute combat stress reactions among World War II veterans was much lower than the rates that were seen in Vietnam veterans who developed PTSD symptoms more than a year after returning from combat duties; however, it is possible that delayed PTSD was also prevalent among World War II veterans but it was not recognized or acknowledged. Some researchers such as Zahava Solomon argue that PTSD was overdiagnosed among Vietnam veterans, while others argue that DELAYED PTSD is different from the PTSD that occurs soon after a traumatic event.

In her book *Combat Stress Reaction: The Enduring Toll of War*, Zahava Solomon, professor of psychiatric epidemiology and social work at the Tel-Aviv University, states that some clinicians who treated Vietnam veterans may have mistakenly diagnosed PTSD in some soldiers. She said that some clinicians raised doubts "as to the validity of diagnoses of delayed PTSD" and pointed to "instances where malingering in pursuit of disability compensation, factitious symptoms, drug abuse and precombat psychopathology were mistakenly diagnosed as delayed PTSD."

The answer may lie not in questioning the validity of delayed PTSD, but rather in asking why a certain population that was exposed to traumatic events such as combat will initially have no apparent psychiatric disturbances and remain asymptomatic for months or years after the event—and then suddenly develop symptoms. There is little empirical research to explain why individuals who coped effectively at the time of their trauma should experience full-blown PTSD years or decades later. Delayed PTSD is still very little understood today.

Modern Troops   A Rand Corporation monograph published in 2008 describes a study of military veterans who have served in either Afghanistan or Iraq since 2001. The researchers estimated that 300,000 veterans of these wars currently suffer from either PTSD or major depression. They also estimated that 320,000 veterans had a probable traumatic brain injury that occurred during their deployment. In addition, a phone survey of 1,965 previously deployed individuals found that 14 percent screened positive for PTSD and 14 percent also screened positive for depression. Yet only about half (53 percent) of those who met the criteria for either PTSD or depression had sought any help from a doctor or mental health professional.

Combat survivors with combat-related PTSD may feel unsafe wherever they are, and they may feel particularly vulnerable when they are at home. Consequently, for self-protection, they may have dogs, guns, alarm systems, and many locks in their home. Movies, sounds, movements, smells, situational events, and reading materials can set off a maladaptive conditioned reaction; for example, the sound of a backfiring car can cause a combat veteran to plunge toward the ground, fearing a bomb. Frequently, drugs and alcohol are used to self-medicate trauma symptoms.

Avoidance represents a category of symptoms among those with PTSD, and the individual with combat-related PTSD may seek to suppress memories by using alcohol to block out unwanted thoughts. A 2008 study described in the *Journal of the American Medical Association* revealed that subsequent to their returning home from prior deployment to combat situations in Iraq or Afghanistan, among the Reserve and National Guard personnel, or citizen-soldiers, 9 percent exhibited heavy weekly drinking (for men, more than 14 drinks per week and for women, more than 7 drinks per week), 53.6 percent exhibited binge drinking (five or more drinks per day or on one occasion) and 15.2 percent had alcohol-related problems Their risk of drinking was about 60 percent higher than among Guard and Reserve troops who were not deployed to Iraq or Afghanistan, according to the Associated Press. At some points, the Guard and Reserve comprised more than half of the combat forces, which may have increased their stress levels.

The study also found among all deployed soldiers, those born after 1980 were 6.7 times more likely to exhibit new-onset binge drinking and 4.7 times more likely to show new-onset alcohol-related problems. Those with PTSD and depression were at increased odds of new-onset and continued alcohol-related problems at follow-up.

Alcohol-related problems were ascertained by asking whether the person continued to drink alcohol even though a physician had advised them to stop because of a health problem or if the person drank alcohol or was high from alcohol or hung over while working, going to school, or taking care of children, and several other criteria. Individuals who agreed to at least one item were classified as having an alcohol-related problem.

In contrast, among active duty personnel, the rates of drinking problems among individuals in combat conditions were also high, but not as high as among Reserve and Guard personnel; the rate of heavy weekly drinking was 6.0 percent, the rate of binge drinking was 26.6 percent (about half the rate seen among Reserve and Guard personnel) and the rate of alcohol-related problems was 4.8 percent, versus the 15.2 percent among the Reserve and Guard personnel.

Perhaps the greater level of drinking among the Reserve and Guard personnel compared to the active duty personnel was a consequence of the Reservists and Guardsmen not perceiving the military as their primary career, which they considered to be their full-time, civilian job. Active duty personnel did not have that perception. Being compelled to leave their full-time job could have increased stress levels among Reserve and Guard personnel. The *JAMA* researchers also suggested that the Reserve and Guard forces may not have had as strong a sense of unit cohesion or access to resources as did the active duty forces. After deployment, the active duty forces returned to work with other active duty individuals, while the individuals in the Reserve and Guard went back to their civilian jobs.

Another possible cause is that many Reserve and Guard units have been stretched thin in Iraq and Afghanistan, with some individuals serving two or more tours of duty. The explanation for younger individuals engaging in heavy drinking (whether Reserve and Guard or active duty) could also lie in the fact that, in general, young adults are more likely to be heavy drinkers than more mature adults, and many soldiers serving in Iraq and Afghanistan are young.

Said the researchers, "In conclusion, our study found that combat deployment in support of the wars in Iraq and Afghanistan was significantly associated with new-onset heavy weekly drinking, binge drinking, and other alcohol-related problems among Reserve/Guard and younger personnel after return from deployment. These results are the first to prospectively quantify changes in alcohol use in relation to recent combat deployments. Interventions should focus on at-risk groups, including Reserve/Guard personnel, younger individuals, and those with previous or existing mental health disorders."

In response to the study findings, Emanuel Pacheco, National Guard Bureau spokesman, said in 2008, "The National Guard is constantly seeking better ways to maintain and improve the behavioral health and general well-being of its warriors through synergistic programs including chaplain support, family support, employment assistance, advocacy, counseling and training. We recognize the unique needs of our citizen-soldiers and -airmen and are constantly looking for innovative ways that we can better meet those needs."

Trauma Management Trauma management therapy is proving to be the most effective treatment for chronic combat-related PTSD. This form of therapy has many components and recognizes the complex and often chronic nature of combat-related disorders. COGNITIVE BEHAVIORAL and EXPOSURE THERAPIES, desensitization, and EYE MOVEMENT DESENSITIZATION AND REPROCESSING (EMDR) are helpful with treating the individual's PTSD reactions, but social skills training and anger management are also required. To address these negative symptoms, trauma management therapy employs as its major components educational and practice experiences, exposure work, homework, and social skills training within small groups administered settings.

Military Debriefings One past means used to assist military members who have been in combat is the MARSHALL-TYPE DEBRIEFING, implemented during World War II. General George Marshall, the U.S. Army chief of staff, would gather soldiers together after combat in a warm and supportive environment where they could discuss their experiences. His focus was more on the events of the

war and less on emotion. This became known as the Marshall debriefing method of reviewing the details of the event without specifically addressing the psychological impact of combat, even though the expressions of feelings were respected. One advantage of this type of debriefing was that, during the presentation of facts and firsthand accounts of the event, soldiers were able to share their experiences and also hear different perspectives of the same experience. The goal of the Marshall-type debriefing is to promote group functioning and morale through cohesion and leadership and minimize any conflicts arising from not seeing the whole picture.

Another relevant concept with regard to military members exposed to combat is PROXIMITY, IMMEDIACY, EXPECTANCY, SIMPLICITY (PIES). This concept of psychological intervention and debriefing first came into being during the World War I for soldiers who were suffering from SHELL SHOCK or COMBAT STRESS REACTIONS. Observations made by medical officer Thomas Salmon argued for intervention as close to the front lines as possible, with sufficient rest and nutrition provided to soldiers. Salmon also advocated emphasizing to the psychologically wounded soldier that with time, he (and now *she* as well) will get better.

Here are the basic principles of combat PSYCHOLOGICAL FIRST AID:

- proximity—treatment is carried out as close to the battlefields or front lines
- immediacy—treatment as soon as possible after onset of symptoms
- expectancy—with full expectation that they will return to duty
- simplicity—food, drink and rest should be provided to the soldier

Civilian Trauma

Traumatic events such as violent crimes, rape, hostage-taking, major accidents, life-threatening events, and horrific scenes, such as terrorist attacks, can affect an individual's mental health. With regard to CIVILIAN TRAUMA, one of the best-known examples of a traumatic event occurred on SEPTEMBER 11, 2001, when terrorists seized civilian airliners and used them to bring down the World Trade Center in New York City and crash into the Pentagon in Washington, D.C., to the horror of millions of people in the United States and other countries.

In this circumstance, the individuals closest to the disaster, such as people living and working in New York City and particularly the first responder police and fire officials, were the most traumatized by this event, which probably seemed like the end of the world to them. But even individuals who had no direct contact and who watched the events on television were also extremely frightened, and some were traumatized. For example, a study of pregnant women who were near the World Trade Center at the time of the September 11 attack found that nearly half of the women developed PTSD. In addition, the examination of their babies when they were born showed the infants had altered CORTISOL (stress hormone) levels, which may have indicated that they suffered from prenatal distress.

Other Types of Trauma and Risk Factors Other examples of types of acute trauma and civilian situations include natural disasters, auto accidents, crimes (especially assaults and rape), serious medical procedures, anesthesia, bullying, and interpersonal humiliation.

Since most people do not develop acute or post-traumatic stress reactions to these events, the question becomes who is vulnerable, and is it possible to determine the risk factors for potential development of traumatic reactions. Research has shown that education (with lower education levels being equated to a higher risk for PTSD), the existence of previous trauma, and general childhood adversity predicted PTSD consistently.

In addition, elements deeper within these factors had even more predictive value, such as a past psychiatric history of disorders (particularly ANXIETY and DEPRESSION), reported childhood abuse, and a family psychiatric history, all of which are predictive for the increased risk of the development of PTSD. Additionally, the level of trauma severity, a lack of social support, and additional life stressors are all stronger predictors for disorders than are individual difference factors.

The National Violence Against Women Survey has found that physical assault commonly occurred along with rape, including for 41.4 percent of sexually assaulted men and 33.9 percent of sexually assaulted women. Epidemiological studies have suggested that the prevalence of PTSD following a sexual assault is particularly high when it is compared to other types of traumas. A study by Rothbaum et al. in 1992 found that, after 12 weeks post-assault, 47 percent of the assaulted women studied still met the criteria for PTSD.

An individual's proximity to a technological disaster (such as factory explosions, dam breaks, plane crashes, chemical spills, and train wrecks) or mass violence may have implications for mental health outcomes.

Natural Disasters Natural disasters are single-event traumas, but their impact on the individual can be very powerful. Natural disasters include earthquakes, tornadoes, tsunamis, fires, floods, hurricanes, and volcanic eruptions. Civilian populations around the world experience these traumatic events. Based on a survey of studies of PTSD subsequent to disasters, published in *Epidemiologic Reviews* in 2005, the researchers estimated that the prevalence of PTSD among direct victims of a disaster is 30 to 40 percent. They also estimated that the prevalence of PTSD among rescue workers in disasters is 10 to 20 percent and the PTSD prevalence in the general population is 5 to 10 percent.

Said the researchers, "The scope of the disaster and the group's exposure to the disaster are probably the most important factors in determining the eventual prevalence of PTSD. Simply put, some disasters are more horrifying than others, and are accompanied by more injury, property destruction, and threats to individuals. Particularly high prevalences of PTSD have been reported among victims of disasters such as the Buffalo Creek dam collapse and the Piper Alpha oil rig fire, where survivors had been in imminent danger of dying during the disaster and [they] lost colleagues and friends. In contrast, the documented prevalence of PTSD in the general population after the September 11, 2001, terrorist attacks in New York City was not disproportionately higher than in other studies of PTSD in the general population after disasters; this probably reflects the fact that while the September 11 attacks dramatically affected U.S. national discourse, exposure to the disaster for most persons in the general New York City population was relatively limited."

According to these researchers, several risk factors were identified across multiple studies. Women had a higher prevalence of PTSD after disasters than men and people with current or preexisting psychiatric problems and those who had previously experienced traumatic events had a higher risk of disaster-related PTSD. Again, however, proximity affects the proportion of those who will develop PTSD, with those who are nearer to the disaster at a higher risk.

Physical Child Abuse   More physical abuse and fatal abuse occurs with children in the first year of life than in any other one-year period of life. According to *Child Maltreatment*, published by the Department of Health and Human Services in 2008, in the year 2006, children from birth to one year old had the highest rate of victimization of any age group, at 24.4 per 1,000 children. An estimated 905,000 children were victims of maltreatment in 2006. The rate of victimization for all children was 12.1 per 1,000.

According to van der Kolk, McFarlane and Weisaeth in *Traumatic Stress,* a study of 1,245 American adolescents showed that 23 percent of the teenagers had been victims of physical or sexual assaults, as well as having been witnesses of violence against others. Twenty percent of these adolescents developed PTSD. The authors point out that 42 percent of inner-city youth reported seeing someone shot and 22 percent reported seeing someone killed.

Traumatized Helping Professionals   Rescue and emergency workers are frequently exposed to traumatic events. Firefighters who were volunteer rescue workers after the 1995 Oklahoma City bombing had a PTSD rate of 13 percent, according to an analysis by North et al. of 181 volunteer firefighters assessed about 34 months after the disaster.

Humanitarian aid workers have distress levels similar to those of emergency personnel. In a survey of PTSD symptoms in international relief personnel, researchers Eriksson et al. found that of 113 humanitarian aid staff who had recently returned to the United States from five different humanitarian agencies, the researchers found that 10 percent met the full diagnosis of PTSD in their first six months of re-entry. In addition, 30 percent

of the respondents reported significant symptoms of PTSD.

In a 1997 study by Carlier, Lamberts and Gersons, Dutch police officers who had experienced a variety of critical incidents had an overall PTSD rate of 7 percent, with 6 percent diagnosed via a structured interview at three months post-event and an additional 1 percent diagnosed at 12 months post-event.

Between 10 and 40 percent of U.S. civilians admitted to the hospital after sustaining intentional injuries (at the hands of another by physical assault) and unintentional injuries (motor vehicle accidents or job-related injuries) may go on to develop symptoms of PTSD, according to a study by Blanchard, et al. in 1996.

Trauma and Psychiatric Disorders   The majority of psychiatric inpatients have consistently been found to have histories of severe trauma, and at least 15 percent meet the diagnostic criteria of PTSD.

Depression also often accompanies PTSD. In a study of 363 trauma center injury survivors both prior to their discharge and three and 12 months post-injury, reported in the *American Journal of Psychiatry* in 2004, the researchers found that 15 percent met the full criteria for PTSD alone, depression alone, or both diagnoses at three months, compared with 14 percent at 12 months.

The researchers found that some variables were predictive for PTSD and PTSD/depression, including "event characteristics (prior psychiatric and trauma history), cognitive appraisals (anxiety about the potential impact of the injury), and acute responses (reexperiencing, arousal, and depression). With the exception of ICU admission, exactly the same combination of variables differentiated between comorbid PTSD/depression and no diagnosis." However, depression only was predicted by prior psychiatric history and prior alcohol use.

Despite the focus on the development of PTSD in the above-mentioned studies, it is clear that many people who are exposed to traumatic events will develop a spectrum of disorders including, but not limited to, PTSD. GENERALIZED ANXIETY DISORDER, SUBSTANCE ABUSE, depressive disorder, and phobia are some of the psychiatric disorders found to be significantly higher following trauma exposure. Furthermore, many psychical medical diseases are linked to trauma backgrounds and these people will be seen in the medical samples rather than psychiatric samples.

Transgenerational Trauma   A subtle but pervasive source of trauma is what is called *transgenerational trauma*. This type of trauma occurs in children of traumatized individuals, but the children's trauma is usually subliminal or less obvious. For example, the second-generation survivors of the Holocaust and of the Armenian genocide have shown significantly lowered CORTISOL levels, indicating a significant stress component is present in their lives. Similar effects have been noted in the children of World War II veterans, Vietnam war veterans, tsunami victims, and the children of the victims of other civilian catastrophes.

Eriksson, Cynthia B., et al. "Trauma Exposure and PTSD Symptoms in International Relief and Development Personnel." *Journal of Traumatic Stress* 14, no. 1 (2001): 205–212.

Galea, Sandro, Arijit Nandi, and David Vlahov. "The Epidemiology of Post-Traumatic Stress Disorder after Disasters." *Epidemiologic Reviews* 27 (2005): 78–91.

Jacobson, Isabel J., et al. "Alcohol Use and Alcohol-Related Problems Before and After Military Combat Deployment." *Journal of the American Medical Association* 200, no. 6 (August 13, 2008): 663–673.

North, Carol S., M.D., et al. "Psychiatric Disorders in Rescue Workers After the Oklahoma City Bombing." *American Journal of Psychiatry* 159, no. 5 (May 2002): 857–859.

O'Donnell, Meaghan L., Mark Creamer and Philippa Pattison. "Posttraumatic Stress Disorder and Depression Following Trauma: Understanding Comorbidity." *American Journal of Psychiatry* 161, no. 8 (August 2004): 1390–1396.

Shalev, Arieh Y., et al. "Prospective Study of Posttraumatic Stress Disorder and Depression Following Trauma." *American Journal of Psychiatry* 155, no. 5 (May 1998): 630–637.

Solomon, Zahava. *Combat Stress Reaction: The Enduring Toll of War.* New York: Plenum Publishing, 1993.

Tanielian, Terri, et al. *Invisible Wounds of War: Summary and Recommendations for Addressing Psychological and Cognitive Injuries.* Santa Monica, Calif.: The Rand Corporation, 2008.

van der Kolk, Bessel A., Alexander C. McFarlane, and Lars Weisaeth, eds. *Traumatic Stress: The Effects of Overwhelming Experience on Mind, Body, and Society.* New York: Guilford Press, 1996.

Trauma and Attachment Belief Scale (TABS)   A brief self-report and nonthreatening tool used by clinicians in 15 minutes to assess the needs and expectations of trauma survivors, based on their self-assumptions compared with others and in their relationships. The therapist uses this information to help plan a relational treatment goal for the client.

Formerly known as the Traumatic Stress Institute Belief Scale, the Trauma and Attachment Belief Scale (TABS) was designed to measure disruptions in beliefs, or cognitive schemas about the self and others from exposure to trauma or vicarious trauma. The 84-item scale assesses disruption in cognitive schema in five areas that may be psychologically affected by traumatic experiences: control, safety, esteem, intimacy, and trust.

The TABS yields a total score achieved through adding up scores on 10 subscales measuring each psychological need area in relation to the self and others, such as the Self-Trust and Others Trust. TABS items focus on relationship history and are useful in identifying psychological themes in trauma material even if the client does not meet the diagnostic criteria for posttraumatic stress disorder (PTSD). Since the TABS does not pathologize or judge the respondent, it is helpful in a therapeutic environment focused on relationship disruptions to document progress in treatment.

Pearlman, L. A., *Trauma and Attachment and Belief Scale.* Los Angeles, Calif.: Western Psychological Services, 2003.

trauma and traumatic stress disorders   Trauma and the traumatic stress disorders are conditions that arise from exposure to extraordinary life-threatening events or accumulated smaller traumas usually experienced in one's developmental years. These conditions are marked by chronic arousal, emotional numbing, avoidance of reminders of the trauma(s), and intrusive thought or dreams related to trauma events. Basic knowledge of traumatic stress disorders has been available since about the mid-1800s, but the actual existence of these disorders likely extends back to before recorded time. For example, the Neanderthal man who survived a sudden altercation with a ravenous saber-toothed tiger, either by bashing the tiger over the head with a club or darting into a cave where the tiger could not reach him, was probably traumatized for the balance of his short life.

After the encounter, the caveman (or woman) could not take an antianxiety pill, call for help on his cell phone or seek advice on the Internet. Each time the caveman ventured outside his cave thereafter, he may have feared the hot breath and ferocious hunger of the tiger, an animal intent on killing and devouring him. Instead, he proceeded with caution when venturing outside, quickly gathering berries and other food needed for survival and rushing back to his cave to avoid the tiger and the many other hungry predators that were out there.

Moving to modern times, in the past century, knowledge and understanding of trauma and traumatic stress disorders have evolved considerably, and traumatic stress disorders are better understood today than ever before.

The Basics of Traumatic Stress Disorders

The two primary traumatic stress disorders are ACUTE STRESS DISORDER and POSTTRAUMATIC STRESS DISORDER (PTSD). There are also many other subordinate types of stress disorders, such as COMPLEX PTSD, DELAYED PTSD, DISASTER SYNDROME, RAPE TRAUMA SYNDROME, and SUBTHRESHOLD PTSD, among others.

Acute stress disorder (ASD) is an intense emotional reaction that some people have to many different types of traumatic events: combat, a severe accident, an assault, a natural disaster, a very serious medical diagnosis, and other extremely distressing events. If the ASD symptoms continue for more than about a month after the traumatic event, then the individual is diagnosed with POSTTRAUMATIC STRESS DISORDER (PTSD).

No one knows how many people in the United States have suffered from ASD, but according to the National Center for Posttraumatic Stress Disorder, there is some data available on ASD caused by specific types of trauma. For example, individuals who have motor vehicle accidents have an ASD rate of from 13 to 21 percent, while victims of violent assaults have an ASD rate of 19 percent. Victims of robbery or assault have been found to have an ASD rate of about 25 percent.

The person with ASD experiences very intense emotions of anxiety and fear and may have insomnia, nightmares, and other sleep disorders. He or she may feel as if in a daze and may feel numbed or detached. Other symptoms may include depersonalization (feeling like you are not really there), derealization (feeling that this bad thing is not happening or has not really happened to you), and even amnesia (forgetting part or all of what happened surrounding the traumatic event or sometimes even greater periods of forgetfulness).

It is believed that most people recover from ASD, although some groups are at greater risk for PTSD than others, according to the *Practice Guideline for the Treatment of Patients with Acute Stress Disorder and Posttraumatic Stress Disorder*, published by the American Psychiatric Association. For example, the risk for PTSD is higher among women, among those who have undergone adverse childhood experiences, such as child abuse, and among those with other psychiatric diagnoses, such as depression or anxiety. In addition, individuals who have been sexually assaulted have a greater risk for developing PTSD than others.

Sources of Trauma

The saber-toothed tiger is no longer a threat to mankind, but despite the considerable advances of modern technology and the extended life spans enjoyed by many people, there are many other dangers in the world today. These threats often cause considerable fear and anxiety, and sometimes lead to the development of traumatic stress disorders. For example, every year thousands of children in the United States are neglected or physically or sexually abused, and the impact of this maltreatment is lifelong for most victims. In addition, thousands of children each year are emotionally and psychologically traumatized; for example, being told constantly that they are bad, useless, or unwanted, or hearing other cruel and deeply cutting statements, usually from the individuals that they trust most in the world: their own parents.

Combat is another trauma-generating experience. Countries worldwide continue to use physical power in the form of guns, tanks, and attack planes to overcome their opponents. Combat is very hard physically and emotionally on the average soldier.

Physical harm may come from a gunshot wound or an improvised explosive device (IED). Occasionally "friendly fire" occurs, when people on the same side mistakenly attack each other, sometimes causing death or severe injuries.

Civilians face many different types of dangers, including physical assaults, natural disasters, and severe medical problems, to name a few. Beatings may occur in concert with DOMESTIC VIOLENCE. A physical attack may also be perpetrated by a stranger. Some individuals and even children are sexually assaulted. Most people think of female victims when they consider sexual assault, but some men are sexually assaulted as well, particularly in prison. The sexually assaulted victim is usually at high risk for the development of POST-TRAUMATIC STRESS DISORDER (PTSD). The victim may also develop other psychological problems such as LEARNED HELPLESSNESS, a situation in which the victim believes that he or she is powerless. Depression is common among sexual and physical assault victims.

Extreme NATURAL DISASTERS can also be very traumatizing, whether it is a hurricane, blizzard, tsunami, or another event that causes serious harm and loss of lives and property. For example, Hurricane Katrina displaced an estimated 2.5 million people in 2005 when the levees in New Orleans broke. Many survivors lost the safe feeling that life is largely predictable. They initially worried about where they would receive their next meal and what would happen in the immediate present, rather than thinking about or planning for their lives next month or next year. Survivors of tsunamis and other natural disasters react similarly. Later some develop PTSD as a result of the trauma.

A serious medical issue can also be traumatizing. A diagnosis of cancer or Alzheimer's disease in one's parent, spouse, or oneself is devastating. Suddenly, the future is no longer a tale to be written but instead may seem more like a rapidly unfolding nightmare. MEDICAL STRESSORS may also occur when a beloved child is diagnosed with a life-threatening illness. Parents and children may all suffer from PEDIATRIC MEDICAL TRAUMATIC STRESS, a disorder that occurs when a child has received a serious medical diagnosis.

Another type of trauma is the fear of TERRORISM. Some of this fear has abated in the absence of further major attacks in the United States after SEPTEMBER 11, 2001. Yet people are constantly reminded of the possibility by the many rules, regulations, and requirements that were set in place because of the September 11 attacks.

It is also important to keep in mind that those who help traumatized people sometimes also need assistance. Psychological DEBRIEFINGS provide important information to police, rescue and emergency personnel. It is well known that helping professionals may themselves become burned out and devoid of empathy, a phenomenon known as COMPASSION FATIGUE or SECONDARY TRAUMATIZATION.

Child Abuse and Neglect

Sadly, thousands of children are abused and neglected each year in the United States. In 2006, the latest data available as of this writing, 905,000 children were maltreated, and of those most were neglected (423,670), while 85,324 were physically abused and 55,550 were sexually abused. Other types of abuse also occurred, such as psychological or emotional abuse, as well as cases in which children suffered multiple types of abuse.

In most cases, the children were abused or neglected by their own parents. One exception is with CHILD SEXUAL ABUSE; in such cases, the perpetrator is often a neighbor or a friend of the family rather than a parent. The effects of child maltreatment traumatize not only the child but also the adult that he or she later becomes, increasing the risk for DEPRESSION and ANXIETY DISORDERS and also for SUBSTANCE ABUSE and dependence.

Child physical abuse CHILD PHYSICAL ABUSE involves serious physical harm to the child. The physical abuse may be a chronic problem, and the child may have a history of injuries and broken bones; this is also called BATTERED CHILD SYNDROME.

When abuse comes to the attention of a state's child protective service workers, they investigate, and if the complaint appears founded, they may remove the child from the family and place him or her with a foster family or in a group home. The abusive or neglectful parent is then given a plan to follow in order to obtain their child back unless the abuse was so egregious that it would not be in the child's best interests to be returned to the family. This is the case when the child was nearly murdered or was sexually abused.

Child neglect   Neglect of a child includes failing to provide a child with the basic necessities of life, such as food, shelter, and medical care. Abandonment of a child with no plan for another person to provide for the child is also child neglect. Leaving a small child locked in a car during the hot summer months is an example of child neglect, and may result in the child's death. More children die from neglect than from abuse because infants and small children cannot provide food or shelter for themselves, nor can they seek medical care when they are ill.

Child sexual abuse   The sexual abuse of a child can cause lifelong trauma and adversely affect the child as an adult. Sexual abuse ranges from sexual touching to full intercourse between a child and an adult. A minor child cannot give consent to sexual acts, although the age of consent varies from state to state. Often the abuser orders the child to tell no one else about the abuse, and the abuser may say that he or she will harm or even kill the individuals most important to the child if the child tells anyone. It is unlikely the abuser would actually follow through on this threat, but the child does not know this.

In the case of some Catholic priests who primarily abused young boys in the late 20th century, the priests used their respected positions within the church to gain private access to the boys and also to protect themselves from the abuse being discovered. Like other abusers, some priests ordered the abused boys not to tell anyone, although some priests used God or religion to compel the child to comply with their wishes, such as by telling the child that God wanted them to participate in sexual acts or that God would be upset if they refused. The children who complied reasoned that no one would know better than a priest what God wanted. Some priests abused children for years before they were unmasked as pedophiles. The trauma this generated among the boys they abused was severe and continued into adulthood.

Emotional/psychological abuse   Sometimes the emotional or psychological abuse of a child is difficult to prove, but in general, it involves extreme belittling of the child and making him or her feel like a bad person. In fact, the child is often told that he or she *is* a bad or evil person and also may be told that he or she was born that way and/or was not a wanted child, but an "accident." There are many cruel things that a parent or other respected adult can say to a child that the child believes, to the detriment of his or her self-esteem.

Bullying   Bullying is common among preadolescents and adolescents, but it can occur to children of any age. The bully may demand money or other items from the child, who sometimes resorts to stealing from his or her own parents to give the bully what is wanted and avoid a beating. It is believed that in general most bullies who use physical force are males, but in some incidents, teenage female bullies have beaten their victims.

The bullied child is usually significantly smaller than the bully; consequently, advising the bullied child to "fight back" is bad advice because he or she could get seriously hurt. Bullies may have conduct disorder or other psychiatric problems. The bullied person may develop psychiatric problems as a result of the bullying. Rarely, a BULLYCIDE occurs, when the bullied person decides to take action and murder the bully.

Combat Conditions

Millions of individuals have experienced the physically and emotionally painful aspects of combat conditions and seeing others harmed or killed, whether in World War II, the Korean War, the Vietnam War, the Gulf War, the wars in Afghanistan and Iraq in the 21st century, or many other conflicts. Some military veterans experience SURVIVOR GUILT, wondering why they survived intact when their friends died or lost limbs or received other mutilating injuries. The results of combat are irrational, particularly in the case of suicide bombings and aimless killings, yet many people continue to seek to understand the reasons for war and death. Sometimes they find comfort in the SPIRITUALITY of religion.

Combat-related PTSD   It has been known that some people have experienced combat-related posttraumatic stress disorder since the Civil War, although it is likely that some soldiers in every war before then also suffered from this type of trauma. The full effects of the trauma may not be immediately evident and may not occur until the soldier has returned back to the normalcy of civilian life.

In Civil War times, a physician named Da Costa evaluated soldiers for symptoms of heart palpitations, shortness of breath, and burning chest pain. The patients often had other symptoms such as fatigue, diarrhea, headache, dizziness, and poor sleep. Yet Dr. Da Costa could not identify a disease or disorder that was causing these symptoms. He concluded that about half the patients were suffering from an infectious disease while in about a third of the cases the problem was caused by excessive military duties. At that time, the condition was known as *irritable heart*, although it was later named Da Costa syndrome after Da Costa himself.

Symptoms of wartime syndromes Whether the disorder is called Da Costa syndrome, COMBAT STRESS SYNDROME, or any one of many other names (including PTSD), in general, individuals with the disorder withdraw into themselves. They may also become hypervigilant about protecting their homes and their families. They may have difficulty talking about what troubles them or they may not wish to burden their loved ones with their fears. The symptoms are treatable, but many fail to seek treatment, wishing instead to pretend that all is normal.

Vietnam veterans and PTSD About 2 million men and women served in combat conditions during the Vietnam War. Most females who experienced combat at that time were nurses providing care to men wounded in combat, while men in all types of military roles experienced combat conditions during this conflict. At the time of the Vietnam War, there was an active effort to keep women out of combat, in contrast to today, when both women and men serve under actively dangerous combat situations. Experts estimate that at least 15 percent of combat veterans in the Vietnam War developed PTSD.

In a study of Vietnam veterans that compared their incidence of PTSD to various characteristics as well as death rates, published by Joseph A. Boscarino in *Combat Stress Injury: Theory, Research, and Management*, Boscarino compared 7,924 "theater" veterans (combat veterans) of Vietnam to 7,364 "era" veterans who did not serve in Vietnam. The

theater veterans had served at least one tour of duty in Vietnam while the era veterans had served at least one tour of duty in the United States, Korea, or Germany. The veterans were drawn from an earlier study that was performed in 1983.

The researchers found a PTSD rate of 10.6 percent among the theater veterans and 2.9 percent among the era veterans. About two-thirds of each group had been drafted into military service. About the same percentage of veterans had died at the time of the follow-up study, including 5.2 percent of the theater veterans and 5.5 percent of the era veterans.

In general, PTSD-positive veterans were more likely to be deceased upon follow-up. Approximately 11.8 percent of those with PTSD had died compared to 4.9 percent of the non-PTSD group who had died. However, in considering all veterans with PTSD, the researchers also found that PTSD itself was a problematic factor for both groups of veterans and particularly for the theater veterans.

The individuals with PTSD were more likely to have used drugs in the army, 8.1 percent versus 1.7 percent of those in the non-PTSD group who had used drugs during their military service.

The researchers also found that among all the Vietnam veterans who had died, 15.3 percent of those who were PTSD-positive had died from SUICIDE; however, the suicide rate was 3.4 percent among the era veterans and about eight times greater, or 26.7 percent among the theater veterans. In addition, 27.3 percent of all the PTSD-positive veterans had died from homicide; 20.0 percent of the era veterans had been murdered and 33.3 percent of the theater veterans had been killed.

In considering the cause of death among the veterans who were PTSD-positive, the researchers found that 35.1 percent of all the veterans had died from alcohol-related deaths, including 15.0 percent of the era veterans and 58.8 percent of the theater veterans, or nearly four times the rate of the era veterans. In addition, 13.0 percent of the PTSD-positive veterans died from firearm-related deaths, including 7.7 percent of the era veterans and 17.9 percent of the theater veterans.

Boscarino also noted that it was not combat exposure per se that apparently led to early deaths but it was rather PTSD exposure, whether the subjects had served in Vietnam or not. Some differences lay in some of the types of deaths; for example, as mentioned, those with PTSD who were theater veterans were more likely to die from suicide or homicide than the era veterans. In addition, the theater veterans with PTSD had an increased risk for death from cardiovascular disease and cancer, although the PTSD-positive era victims also had an increased risk for early deaths from all causes as well.

Said Boscarino, "Our study suggests that veterans with long-term PTSD are at risk for death from multiple causes. While the specific reasons for this increased mortality are unclear, these outcomes are likely related to biological, psychological, and behavioral phenomenon associated with PTSD. Although further research is warranted and issues related to barriers to care might need to be addressed, for many returning veterans today, the adverse health impact of PTSD is potentially avoidable, since effective treatments currently are available for this disorder and the sequelae related to this condition."

Afghanistan/Iraq veterans and PTSD   Some military veterans of the deployments to Afghanistan and Iraq (Operations Enduring Freedom and Iraqi Freedom, or OEF/OIF) suffer from PTSD as a result of experiencing combat conditions. PTSD is a risk for many service members, as are TRAUMATIC BRAIN INJURIES from manmade explosives. A major barrier to receiving diagnosis and treatment often lies within the combat veteran him- or herself.

According to a RAND Corporation report published in 2008, *Invisible Wounds of War,* although the military screens individuals for mental health issues post-deployment, many military members minimize or fail to reveal their mental health issues. They may fear that disclosure could delay their return home and they also have other fears related to revealing a mental health issue; for example, the RAND report listed five other barriers to receiving care:

1. The fear that medications could have too many side effects
2. The fear that revealing a need for services could harm the individual's career
3. The fear that he or she could be denied a security clearance
4. The belief that family and friends would help more than a mental health professional
5. The fear that coworkers would have less confidence if they knew about the mental health issue.

The RAND researchers performed a telephone survey of 1,965 previously deployed individuals and found that 14 percent screened positive for PTSD and also 14 percent screened positive for depression. In addition, they found that 19 percent reported a possible traumatic brain injury (concussion) that occurred during deployment. The researchers noted that depression is not considered a combat-related injury, but they believed that depression was "highly associated with combat exposure and should be considered on the spectrum of post-deployment mental health issues."

Some returning combat veterans urgently need their families to help them with physical and psychological issues, but in the past, their families have not been able to take much time off to help them. Congress addressed this issue, and on January 28, 2008, President Bush signed into law the National Defense Authorization Act (NDAA), Public Law 110-181, which included a section, Section 585(a), to amend the Family and Medical Leave Act (FMLA) to provide for up to 26 weeks' leave to allow a "spouse, son, daughter, parent, or next of kin" to care for a member of the armed forces (including members of the National Guard and Reserves) who is undergoing medical treatment, therapy, or recuperation on an outpatient basis or is on the temporary disability retired list for a serious injury or illness. In addition, the NDAA also allows an employee to take up to 12 weeks of FMLA leave if a family member is on active duty or has been called to active duty because of a contingency operation, such as the war in Iraq and Afghanistan.

Sexual and Physical Assaults

Women and men who have been sexually assaulted are usually severely traumatized by the experience. Both women and men may suffer from physical assaults at the hands of their spouses, partners, or others. Often physical assaults accompany sexual assaults, further traumatizing the victim and increasing the risk for the development of trauma disorders such as acute stress disorder or PTSD.

Sexual assaults   Sexual assaults can be very traumatizing and the victim may have trouble dealing with his or her feelings about the attack and consequently may develop a traumatic stress disorder, such as ASD, PTSD, or rape trauma syndrome. There are several common reactions to an assault; for example, if the victim knows the assailant, the victim may wonder if he or she somehow brought the assault upon himself or herself. Many victims are afraid or embarrassed to report a sexual assault, including to the police because they may think that everyone will somehow know that there is something "wrong" with them. In fact, some people do view sexually abused people as defiled or damaged individuals. To avoid this possible consequence, victims may refuse to report a sexual assault to the authorities and also refuse to receive any help from a mental health professional.

Physical attacks   Individuals may be assaulted by others whom they know and sometimes they are assaulted by strangers, as in the case of a crime such as an interrupted burglary or robbery. A physical assault can lead to the development of ASD and to PTSD. Men who are physically assaulted may feel that they are unmanly if they are unable to defend themselves, and this may be particularly true if they are unable to protect their spouses, partners, or children—even when the man is faced with overwhelming force that few men could protect against. The anxiety that the man feels as he tells himself that he *should* have protected himself or his loved ones along with the knowledge that he could *not* help himself or his family can create a cognitive dissonance that ultimately causes other serious psychological problems, such as depression.

Domestic violence   Tragically, spouse battering is common and it is also a very traumatic experience for the victims involved. Often it is the wife or female partner who is beaten (although occasionally, females assault males who live with them). She may believe that she has no power or that no one would believe her about the beatings, often because the abuser has repeatedly made such state-

ments to her and she has accepted them at face value. The battered woman may also believe that she has nowhere to go and that she cannot leave the abuser. This irrational way of thinking is common and recognized by police, shelter managers, mental health professionals, and others. It is called BATTERED WOMAN SYNDROME.

Natural Disasters

The impact of extreme natural disasters, such as severe floods, tsunamis, hurricanes, tornadoes, blizzards, and other unusual weather phenomena that harm or kill people and destroy their homes and property, can be devastating. Victims of a natural disaster may develop a DISASTER SYNDROME, a form of PTSD. The disaster challenges their normal daily sense of basic safety and puts their lives, as well as the survival of their family members at serious risk. Victims may need to depend on others and accept help from people who are complete strangers to them. The entire experience is very difficult to process for most people and often leads to PTSD symptoms. It may also lead to severe depression.

According to an article in the *Journal of the American Medical Association* in 2008, studies have shown a rate of PTSD as high as 62.5 percent in preschool children who were directly affected by Hurricane Katrina and a rate of greater than 50 percent in female caregivers and parents of children who developed new problems.

Some people develop counter-disaster syndrome when a natural disaster is predicted to occur. This is a situation in which people rush about thinking they are accomplishing important goals before a disaster strikes, but they are behaving irrationally and inefficiently. In other cases, individuals volunteer to help beyond their capabilities and in fact, their presence is counterproductive. Others may urge them to go home but they refuse to leave.

Traumatizing Medical Diagnoses

Although medical science has made amazing advances, many people still die of heart disease, cancer, and other terrible diseases each year. When individuals receive a diagnosis of such a life-threatening illness, they may feel as if they have been handed a death sentence; however, many life-extending treatments are available today. Despite this fact, the initial reactions of the diagnosed individual and his or her family members may be one of acute stress, which can develop into acute stress disorder or posttraumatic stress disorder.

PTSD: Pediatric traumatic stress For many people, diagnosis of a serious disease in their child is far more distressing than a personal medical diagnosis of a serious disease. They may develop PTSD because of this *pediatric traumatic stress,* or stress that occurs in children or their parents as a direct result of the child's medical problem. According to the Center for Pediatric Traumatic Stress at the Children's Hospital of Philadelphia, more than 11,000 children are diagnosed with cancer every year in the United States, and more than 1,000 children receive organ transplants each year, while several thousand children await an organ transplant. In addition, about 5 percent of the children in the United States are hospitalized each year for an injury or a disability or for a major acute or chronic illness.

Some issues increase the stress of the family and can lead to traumatic stress, such as the belief that the child's medical problem is life-threatening. If the child is in pain, this increases the stress levels of children and parents. Another issue is that the family often must make major medical decisions at a time of severe distress. According to one study, more than 80 percent of children and parents experienced at least one serious symptom of acute stress disorder within the first month after a child was injured in a traffic accident.

During the process of treatment, traumatic stress may develop at the time of the diagnosis or when potentially painful procedures are begun. During the course of treatment, with its ups and downs, family members may become traumatized. For example, the deaths of other children in the hospital with the same diagnosis can be traumatic to the parents and the child. Even when treatment has been completed and the child is in remission or cured, the parents and child may still worry that the problem might recur.

In a study of 97 traffic-injured children ages 5 to 17 years old and their parents, reported in *Pediatrics* in 2002, the researchers found that 88 percent of the children and 83 percent of the parents had at least one clinically significant symptom of acute stress disorder.

In this study, the most common symptom of acute stress among children was dissociation, a state within a state in which reality is altered but the person usually stays in contact with the traumatic experience. (See DISSOCIATIVE DISORDERS.) In this study, dissociation was experienced by 78 percent of the children, while the most common symptom for parents was arousal, a symptom that was experienced by 73 percent of the parents. Said the researchers, "All families require emotional support when a child is exposed to a traumatic event. As evidenced by the findings in this study, pediatric care providers can expect to see at least a few significant acute stress symptoms in most children and parents in the early aftermath of traffic-related injury. In this situation, brief education is appropriate to explain that these are typical reactions and are likely to resolve as the physical injuries heal and as the family uses its normal coping methods to deal with the immediate shock."

Adults who receive a diagnosis of severe illness When adults receive a diagnosis of cancer or learn that they or a loved one has early Alzheimer's disease, for example, the stress is enormous on both the patient and the patient's spouse or partner and family. If the person is incapacitated by illness, a spouse or other close family member may be forced to make life-affecting medical decisions for the person and must struggle to discern what the patient would have wanted at one of the most stressful times of his or her life. Many people fail to make living wills to stipulate what type of medical care they wish to have in a life or death situation, and thus the spouse or next of kin must make such extremely difficult decisions.

If the ill individual survives, the spouse or close relative may fear that the sickness will come back and may become very anxious and watchful. These individuals may place their own needs largely on "hold," trying to provide the ill person with the attention and care that is needed.

Fear of Terrorism

After the SEPTEMBER 11, 2001 attacks on the World Trade Center and the Pentagon, many people in the United States were very fearful of terrorists and possible terrorist attacks. As a result, they accepted many new limitations on their freedoms, toward the goal of catching terrorists or preventing another attack. For example, many facilities such as airports and courthouses began much more thorough screening of individuals entering the location.

In a review of the psychological impact of terrorism and disasters among children and adolescents, based on children in Australia, and published in *Prehospital and Disaster Medicine* in 2004, the researchers discussed variables that can adversely affect children. These included the severe threat to the life or survival of the child, the death of family members or close friends, a relocation or frequent moves, a previous vulnerability to stress, the presence of PTSD, and a disruption in the networks of social support. The terrorist incidents examined by the study were the attack on the World Trade Center in New York City in 2001 and the bombing of the island of Bali in 2002, which severely distressed both children and adults in Australia.

Said the authors, "In the chaos and confusion following events such as terrorism, children may be exposed to the reality of violent death, as they inadvertently become part of the acute disaster response. In the chaos following the Bali bombing, local school children were confronted with the gruesome horror of violent death as they searched for survivors who were traumatized and burned or recovered dead bodies and body parts of victims."

Caring for the Caregivers

Whether they are professional caregivers or family members who help a traumatized individual, people who provide care to others face a difficult and cumbersome task, especially when it appears to have no clear end date. Many individuals develop COMPASSION FATIGUE, as they become burned out and physically and emotionally exhausted. Compassion fatigue is also called secondary traumatization. Individuals with compassion fatigue are no longer effective at helping others.

Providing Information to Professional Helpers

Subsequent to a major disaster, police, fire, rescue, medical, and other individuals who provide help to traumatized victims need as much information about the situation as possible. The CRITICAL INCIDENT STRESS DEBRIEFING (CISD) is part of a model of CRITICAL INCIDENT STRESS MANAGEMENT (CISM), which is often used from 24 to 72 hours following a

critical incident or three to four weeks after a major disaster, such as an earthquake or a hurricane. The formal CISD process is led by a mental health professional and a peer facilitator and includes seven phases:

1. Introduction Phase: The facilitators introduce themselves and describe the rules of confidentiality, the discussion process, and expectations.
2. Fact Phase: The participants describe the critical incident event from their perspective and what activity they performed during the event.
3. Thought Phase: Participants describe their first thoughts of the event and facilitate cognitive reactions.
4. Reaction Phase: The facilitators of the debriefing ask participants questions to identify their emotional reactions.
5. Symptom Phase: Personal symptoms of stress are identified, and the participants describe how their lives have changed since the event.
6. Teaching Phase: Participants learn about stress management, coping techniques and normalizing reactions to extraordinary events.
7. Re-Entry Phase: The facilitators answer questions, re-emphasizing the importance of normalizing reactions, and provide follow-up referrals for those needing further intervention.

PSYCHOLOGICAL FIRST AID is professional assistance provided to those who are severely traumatized by a traumatic event and exhibit symptoms of an acute stress reaction, such as dissociative symptoms, detachment, and DEPERSONALIZATION. These individuals also may have a prolonged inability to sleep or eat. They may also exhibit confusion, poor concentration, and poor decision-making.

Psychological first aid is meant to counter and deflect such emotional problems in the early stages. Experts can also advise survivors when they should seek further treatment, such as when they suffer extreme sleep deprivation and frequent nightmares or exhibit symptoms of clinical depression.

Resilience to Traumatic Stress Disorders

Whether the traumatic stress has been caused by child abuse, combat, a major disaster, or another type of traumatic event, some individuals are resilient and will not develop a traumatic stress disorder. For example, according to the Administration for Children and Families in the U.S. Department of Health and Human Services, some factors that are protective against long-term negative consequences despite child abuse or neglect are individual characteristics, such as a sense of humor, optimism, creativity, intelligence, and independence. Protective factors within the environment include a caring adult in the child's life as well as neighborhood stability and access to health care.

Among military veterans who have faced traumatic events, family support is also a protective factor against the development of a traumatic stress disorder, as is the support of the community.

Types of Traumatic Stress Disorders

When an individual is severely traumatized, he or she may develop an ACUTE STRESS DISORDER, and if the symptoms continue unabated, the disorder may become a posttraumatic stress disorder (PTSD). There are various types of traumatic stress disorders.

Acute stress disorder   The initial reaction to a severe trauma may be acute stress disorder, which is characterized by symptoms similar to those of PTSD, such as re-experiencing the event (or FLASHBACKS), increased arousal (or hyperarousal), and anxiety.

The person with acute stress disorder also experiences at least three of five dissociative symptoms, including:

1. A subjective sense of numbing, detachment, or the absence of emotional responsiveness
2. A reduction in overall awareness
3. Derealization (a feeling of being detached and unaware)
4. Depersonalization (when the person has the feeling that this situation is not really happening to him or her)
5. Dissociative AMNESIA (the inability to recall important aspects of the trauma)

The distress from an acute stress disorder lasts for two or more days and up to four weeks, beyond which it is classified as PTSD.

Posttraumatic stress disorder   Posttraumatic stress disorder is a common type of anxiety disorder that may develop as a result of many different types of stressors, ranging from past child abuse to recent combat exposure to the stress of natural disasters or of life-threatening medical diagnoses to physical or sexual abuse, and many other potential stressors.

Delayed posttraumatic stress disorder   Symptoms of PTSD that occur six months or later subsequent to a traumatic event are referred to as *delayed PTSD*. Major life events or stress may trigger the development of DELAYED PTSD that stems from the feelings of helplessness that were initially experienced during the traumatic event. Delayed PTSD has occurred among Holocaust survivors as well as veterans of wars, such as World War II or the Vietnam War.

Complex posttraumatic stress disorder   Complex posttraumatic stress disorder, also known as *disorders of extreme stress not otherwise specified* (DESNOS), refers to the exposure of the individual to chronic traumas that last for months to years at a time, such as repeated physical or sexual abuse. It is also sometimes referred to as ELABORATED POSTTRAUMATIC STRESS DISORDER.

The individual with complex PTSD may experience extreme anger, persistent sadness, suicidal thoughts, and other strong emotions. He or she may also feel helpless, ashamed, and guilty, and individuals with this disorder may become convinced that they are completely different from others.

Circumscribed posttraumatic stress disorder   Circumscribed PTSD generally refers to single incident trauma, rather than to chronic problems with trauma. The traumatic event could range from a one-time incident of bullying that is extremely distressing to a severe experience, such as a kidnapping or a physical or sexual assault. Circumscribed posttraumatic disorder is different from complex PTSD, which stems from chronic abuse.

Post-torture syndrome   With post-torture syndrome, both the traumatic events and the effects of TORTURE produce posttraumatic stress symptoms in the victim. Victims are at risk for many disturbances, such as anxiety, depression, GUILT, intensive rage, memory difficulties, and psychosomatic disturbances. Torture is usually administered by another individual against the victim and human-against-human trauma is much more traumatic than impersonal trauma such as an accident or a natural disaster.

Rape trauma syndrome Initially named by Ann Wolbert Burgess and Lynda Lytle Holmstrom in their article for the *American Journal of Psychiatry* published in 1974, RAPE TRAUMA SYNDROME refers to a clustering of behaviors that occur in many victims traumatized by sexual assault, such as stomach pains and appetite loss, gynecological symptoms, and general pain throughout the body. Women also often experience emotional reactions, such as fear, humiliation, self-blame, embarrassment, anger, and a desire for revenge. Some experts consider RTS to be a subset of post-traumatic stress disorder, while others regard it as a separate disorder.

Bystander traumatization Happening upon a stranger who is experiencing trauma can also cause trauma, as with *bystander traumatization*. For example, an individual may be walking down the street when he or she sees another person being robbed or beaten, and then sees the assailant flee the scene while the victim lies moaning on the sidewalk. Witnessing the attack, as well as the realization that if he or she had been on the scene just a little earlier, it is likely that he or she would be the person lying on the pavement, can lead to a traumatic stress disorder.

Related Psychiatric Disorders

Trauma disorders, and especially posttraumatic stress disorder, are often accompanied by other psychiatric problems, such as major depressive disorder, other anxiety disorders, and sometimes even psychotic disorders that can develop as a result of severe trauma. Some studies indicate that traumatized individuals are more likely to develop BIPOLAR DISORDER than others.

Depression Clinical depression, also known as *major depressive disorder*, is a frequent accompaniment of a traumatic stress disorder. The depression may precede the traumatic stress disorder or it may be triggered by the stress disorder itself. Sometimes it may also be very difficult or impossible to determine which came first, the depression or the stress

disorder. What is important is that both psychiatric problems are treated, as well as any other psychiatric problems that the individual may have.

Anxiety disorders ANXIETY DISORDERS often develop in traumatized individuals, particularly such disorders as GENERALIZED ANXIETY DISORDER (GAD), posttraumatic stress disorder (PTSD), and PANIC ATTACKS, although other anxiety disorders such as social phobia or obsessive-compulsive disorder may develop. In most cases, individuals suffering from anxiety disorders benefit from a combination of both therapy and medication; for example, if the person has GAD, he or she may benefit from taking a BENZODIAZEPINE medication, along with receiving psychotherapy for the disorder.

Bipolar disorder In a study of 100 adults with bipolar disorder who were receiving treatment at an academic center, the researchers sought to determine whether severe childhood abuse was a factor. Reporting on their findings in the *British Journal of Psychiatry* in 2005, the researchers found that about half the subjects had suffered from severe childhood abuse. They also found that individuals who suffered from multiple types of severe childhood abuse were at risk for rapid cycling (moving rapidly back and forth from a manic or depressed state) and they were also at greater risk for suicide attempts.

Psychotic reactions Some individuals suffer psychotic reactions to extreme trauma, and this is particularly true if the trauma is an experience that is extremely severe, or it is repeatedly inflicted upon the person, as in the case of severe physical or sexual abuse. Rarely, the person may develop AMNESIA, because it is too painful to remember the circumstances of the trauma.

Some individuals may dissociate from the experience, which means that they mentally detach from their body in order to survive the markedly severe pain and humiliation. This may occur in the case of child sexual abuse, in which the child is so distressed and horrified by what is happening that he or she attempts to remove himself or herself from the scene in the only way possible: inside the mind.

DISSOCIATIVE DISORDERS sometimes stem from a traumatic event. After the abuser has finished with the victim and left the scene, the dissociation may continue and some individuals develop DISSOCIA-TIVE IDENTITY DISORDER, also known in the past as multiple personality disorder.

Sleep disorders: insomnia, nightmares, and parasomnias Many traumatized people suffer from distressing sleep disorders, such as INSOMNIA, sleepwalking and NIGHTMARES. According to Peretz Lavie in an article for the *New England Journal of Medicine,* sleep disturbances that occur directly after a traumatic event are predictive of psychiatric problems such as PTSD as well as of physical symptoms, or chronic *somatic* symptoms, such as headaches and stomach aches.

As an example, says Lavie, "Disturbed dreaming has been shown to predict a delayed onset of PTSD in veterans of the Vietnam War and in victims of crimes. Similarly, the continued presence of trauma-related sleep disturbances in female rape victims predicts future alcohol use and physical symptoms independently of other symptoms of PTSD or depression. Sleep disturbances have also been associated with a posttraumatic decline in immune function, as manifested by a decrease in the cytotoxicity [ability to kill cells] of natural killer cells."

Lavie also noted that rapid eye movement (REM) sleep, which is the period during which dreams occur, as well as the recall of dreams, have been documented as much lower among trauma victims than among those who have not suffered from traumatic events. For example, 33.7 percent of Holocaust survivors judged to be well adjusted remembered their dreams when they awakened, compared to a rate of 50.5 percent among Holocaust victims considered less well adjusted and 80 percent among non-Holocaust controls. Perhaps the "well-adjusted" Holocaust victims were blocking some dreams or they were actually dreaming less, although it is not known.

Some victims of traumatic events suffer from severe nightmares, while others may experience such PARASOMNIAS (abnormal sleep behaviors) as sleepwalking.

Assessing Trauma Disorders

Many different written instruments are available for ASSESSMENT AND DIAGNOSIS of trauma disorders.

They can be used to determine if one exists, and if one does exist, how serious it is; for example, the Harvard Trauma Questionnaire helps to measure posttraumatic stress (PTS). Other helpful instruments include the TRAUMA AND ATTACHMENT BELIEF SCALE, the TRAUMA SYMPTOM INVENTORY, the Trauma Symptom Checklist/Trauma Symptom Checklist for Children, the TRAUMATIC STRESS SCHEDULE, the Trauma-Related Guilt Inventory, and the TRAUMATIC MEMORY INVENTORY (TMI).

There are also instruments to measure the presence and severity of posttraumatic stress disorder (PTSD), such as the Davidson Trauma Scale, the Clinician-Administered Posttraumatic Stress Disorder Scale (CAPS), the PTSD Checklist, and the Posttraumatic Stress Diagnostic Scale (PSDS).

Treating Trauma Disorders

The treatment of trauma disorders usually involves a combination of psychotherapy and medications. Psychotherapy helps the individual to deal with the effects that are associated with the traumatic event (such as posttraumatic stress disorder, depression, anxiety disorders, and so forth), and medication helps resolve issues of anxiety, depression, and other disorders that may make it difficult for the individual to benefit from therapy.

Therapy There are many different types of therapies used to treat trauma victims, and the type that is used with a particular patient depends on the disorder and its severity. Many individuals are successfully treated with a COGNITIVE-BEHAVIORAL THERAPY or COGNITIVE PROCESSING THERAPY, two types of therapy that help individuals recognize their own self-destructive thoughts.

Exposure therapy is sometimes used, which involves compelling the individual to face the feared object. Some forms of exposure therapy will introduce the feared items slowly, while others start with the maximum level of exposure. EYE MOVEMENT DESENSITIZATION AND REPROCESSING (EMDR), IMPLOSIVE THERAPY, phase-oriented treatment, SOMATIC EXPERIENCING THERAPY, STRESS INOCULATION TRAINING, SYSTEMATIC DESENSITIZATION, TESTIMONY THERAPY, and TRAUMATIC INCIDENT REDUCTION therapy are all other types of therapy that have been used effectively with many traumatized victims. (For further information, see TREATMENT:

PSYCHOTHERAPY, PSYCHOPHARMACOLOGY AND ALTERNATIVE MEDICINE.)

Often individual therapy is used but sometimes therapy provided in groups can be effective by showing victims that others are suffering from the same problem and working toward mental health.

Medications Many traumatized individuals have serious problems with DEPRESSION as well as with ANXIETY DISORDERS, and these problems should be treated, if present. Antidepressants are used to treat depression, primarily selective serotonin reuptake inhibitors (SSRIs) or serotonin norepinephrine reuptake inhibitors (SNRIs). In addition, BENZODIAZEPINES are used to treat anxiety disorders. Some traumatized individuals may need two or more medications. They may also need some form of psychotherapy as well, to deal with the aftereffects of the trauma, whether they suffer from PTSD or from trauma symptoms that may not rise to the level of PTSD, as with subthreshold PTSD.

How the Body Reacts during a Traumatic Event

When an individual is living through a traumatic experience, the person's body reacts accordingly, and the brain, neurochemicals, hormones, and even the muscles and the digestive system are all dramatically affected as they respond. In fact, all of the body's nervous systems—the AUTONOMIC SYSTEM, the CENTRAL NERVOUS SYSTEM, the PARASYMPATHETIC SYSTEM, the LIMBIC SYSTEM, and the SYMPATHETIC NERVOUS SYSTEM—become actively involved.

In addition, major parts of the brain are activated, such as the AMYGDALA, the key to the processing, interpretation, and integration of emotional functioning, and command center of the brain's fear system. The amygdala receives important input from many other parts of the brain, such as the thalamus, hypothalamus, and HIPPOCAMPUS.

As with the caveman reacting to an imminent attack by a saber-toothed tiger, when an individual in the 21st century is under severe stress, the body prepares for both fighting and fleeing, otherwise known as the FIGHT OR FLIGHT RESPONSE or the *acute stress response*. This response is hard-wired into the brain, and triggers the sympathetic nervous system to release both adrenalin (epinephrine) and NOR-EPINEPHRINE from the adrenal glands, speeding up heart rate and respiration, and causing the pupils of the eyes to dilate—responses designed to make the individual acutely aware of his or her surroundings. The entire body is focused on the one goal of staying alive. (See PHYSIOLOGY OF TRAUMA for a detailed description of the process.)

Of course the days of saber-tooth tiger dangers are long past, but individuals still experience the same reactions to danger, such as car crashes, other severe accidents, or serious medical diagnoses. Even the stress of work and the demands of an unreasonable boss can trigger a fight-flight response if the demands become too extreme.

Outlook for the Future

In the future it is likely that much more information will be gained on traumatic stress disorders as well as better treatments and medications to help individuals manage these difficult problems. New research may obtain increased knowledge about the body's responses to trauma, and hopefully more knowledge will be developed to enable individuals to recover more completely and more rapidly from traumatic events that they suffer. That said, it is essentially impossible to eliminate all traumatic events and the development of subsequent traumatic disorders. Thus, diagnosis and treatment are the keys to working toward psychological and emotional health.

Administration for Children and Families. *Long-Term Consequences of Child Abuse and Neglect.* Washington, D.C.: U.S. Department of Health and Human Services. April 2006.

Boscarino, Joseph. "The Mortality Impact of Combat Stress 30 Years after Exposure: Implications for Prevention, Treatment, and Research." In Figley, Charles R. and William P. Nash, eds. *Combat Stress Injury: Theory, Research, and Management,* edited by Charles R. Figley and William P. Nash, 97–117. New York: Routledge, 2007.

Britt, Thomas W. "The Stigma of Mental Health Problems in the Military." *Military Medicine* 172, no. 2 (2007): 157–161.

Center for Pediatric Traumatic Stress and the National Child Traumatic Stress Network. *Medical Events & Traumatic Stress in Children and Families.* Available online. URL: www.nctsnet.org/nctsn_assets/pdfs/edu_materials/MedicalTraumaticStress.pdf. Accessed August 29, 2008.

Corrigan, Patrick. "How Stigma Interferes with Mental Health Care." *American Psychologist* 59, no. 7 (October 2004): 614–625.

Department of Health and Human Services, Administration on Children, Youth and Families. *Child Maltreatment 2006.* Washington, D.C.: U.S. Government Printing Office, 2008.

Galea, Sandro, Arijit Nandi, and David Vlahov. "The Epidemiology of Post-Traumatic Stress Disorder after Disasters." *Epidemiologic Reviews* 27 (2005): 78–91.

Garno, Jessica, et al. "Impact of Childhood Abuse on the Clinical Course of Bipolar Disorder." *British Journal of Psychiatry* 186 (2005): 121–125.

Helmus, Todd C., and Russell W. Glenn. *Steeling the Mind: Combat Stress Reactions and Their Implications for Urban Warfare.* Santa Monica, Calif.: RAND Corporation, 2005.

Hyams, Kenneth C., M.D., F. Stephen Wignall, M.D., and Robert Roswell, M.D. "War Syndromes and Their Evaluation: From the U.S. Civil War to the Persian Gulf War." *Annals of Internal Medicine* 125, no. 5 (1996): 398–405.

Krug, Etienne G., M.D., et al. "Suicide after Natural Disasters." *New England Journal of Medicine* 338, no. 6 (1998): 373–378.

Lamberg, Lynne. "Katrina's Mental Health Impact Lingers." *Journal of the American Medical Association* 300, no. 9 (September 3, 2008): 1,011–1,013.

Lavie, Peretz. "Sleep Disturbances in the Wake of Traumatic Events." *New England Journal of Medicine* 345, no. 25 (December 20, 2001): 1,825–1,832.

McCann, Lisa, and Laurie Anne Pearlman. "Vicarious Traumatization: A Framework for Understanding the Psychological Effects of Working with Victims." *Journal of Traumatic Stress* 3, no. 1 (1990): 131–149.

Palker-Corell, Ann, and David K. Marcus. "Partner Abuse, Learned Helplessness, and Trauma Symptoms." *Journal of Social and Clinical Psychology* 23, no. 4 (2004): 445–462.

Peterson, Alan L., Monty T. Baker, and Kelly R. McCarthy. "Combat Stress Casualties in Iraq. Prt. 1: Behavioral Health Consultation at an Expeditionary Medical Group." *Perspectives in Psychiatric Care* 44, no. 4 (July 2008): 146–158.

Tanielian, Terri, et al. *Invisible Wounds of War: Summary and Recommendations for Addressing Psychological and Cognitive Injuries.* Santa Monica, Calif.: RAND Corporation. 2008.

Ursano, Robert J., M.D., et al. *Practice Guideline for the Treatment of Patients with Acute Stress Disorder and Posttraumatic Stress Disorder.* Washington, D.C.: American Psychiatric Association, 2004.

Winston, Flaura Koplin, Nancy Kassam-Adams, Cara Vivarelli-O'Neill, et al. "Acute Stress Disorder Symptoms in Children and Their Parents after Pediatric Traffic Injury." *Pediatrics* 109, no. 6 (2002). Available online. URL: http://www.pediatrics.org/cgi/content/full/109/6/e90. Accessed August 31, 2008.

Wolbert Burgess, Ann, and Lynda Lytle Holmstrom. "Rape Trauma Syndrome." *American Journal of Psychiatry* 131, no. 9 (1974): 981–986.

Wooding, Sally, and Beverley Raphael. "Psychological Impact of Disasters and Terrorism on Children and Adolescents: Experiences from Australia." *Prehospital and Disaster Medicine* 19, no. 1 (2004): 10–20.

trauma assessment measures See ASSESSMENT AND DIAGNOSIS; INSTRUMENTS/SCALES/SURVEYS THAT EVALUATE POSTTRAUMATIC STRESS DISORDER (PTSD).

trauma bonding A concept used to explain the dynamics of abusive relationships, including the strong emotional bonds of the victim and the perpetrator as in domestic violence. The cycle of violence describes three stages in an abusive relationship: the tension building stage, the acute battery stage, and the honeymoon stage (the abuse stops with apologies).

The emotional bonds develop because of the good and bad treatment and the imbalance of power as the abuser gains more power and the victim feels worse about the perpetrator and less confident in himself or herself. The victim becomes dependent upon the perpetrator as the violence erupts, followed by the perpetrator's gifts and promises, with the perpetrator becoming the rescuer as well as the tormentor. This intermittently reinforced behavior is hard to extinguish even as the abuse ends, only for it to begin again next week, next month. Traumatic bonding is also seen in cults, and with incest, kidnapping, and other shared traumatic experiences that bond strangers.

Trauma Management Therapy or Terror Management Theory (TMT) Trauma and the subsequent development of POSTTRAUMATIC STRESS DISORDER (PTSD) is very complex, with many individual manifestations. It is usually comorbid with other psychological disorders that must be addressed. ANXIETY and DEPRESSION are common, but so too are problems in interpersonal relations, anger management issues, and negative self-concept.

TMT was developed to recognize these complexities and to provide for them in a treatment context. It is a multicomponent treatment program, developed in the Veterans Administration system, to complement the basic exposure protocol that forms the basis of the treatment program. TMT involves education, individually administered exposure, programmed practice, and group-administered social and emotional skills training. It has shown good preliminary results in open trial research and is less costly to run than "standard care" within the Veterans Administration system.

Turner, S. M., D. C. Beidel, B. C. Frueh. (2005). Multicomponent Behavior Treatment for Chronic Combat-Related Posttraumatic Stress Disorder: Trauma Management Therapy. *Behavior Modification* 29, no. 1: 39–69.

Trauma-Related Guilt Inventory (TRGI) An event-focused, self-report assessment of guilt related to trauma. Trauma-Related Guilt Inventory (TRGI) assesses cognitive and emotional guilt that is related to specific traumatic events, such as combat or physical and sexual abuse. The Trauma-Related Guilt Inventory is a 32-item inventory with three scales: Global Guilt Scale ("I experience intense guilt related to what happened"), the Distress Scale ("I am still distressed about what happened") and the Guilt Cognition Scale, which has three subscales, including Hindsight Bias/Responsibility ("I should have known better"), Wrongdoing ("I did something that went against my values") and Lack of Justification ("What I did was completely unjustified"). While the test can be self-administered, a professional testing expert needs to score and interpret the findings.

Since the TRGI assesses 22 specific trauma-related beliefs, Kubany and colleagues (1996) feel that it may have considerable utility as a treatment outcome measure in cognitive-behavioral inter-ventions for modifying survivors' beliefs about their guilty roles in trauma.

Kubany, et al. "Development and Validation of the Trauma-Related Guilt Inventory (TRGI)." *Psychological Assessment* 8, no. 4 (December 1996): 428–444.

Trauma Symptom Checklist/Trauma Symptom Checklist for Children See INSTRUMENTS/SCALES/ SURVEYS THAT EVALUATE POSTTRAUMATIC STRESS DISORDER (PTSD).

Trauma Symptom Inventory See INSTRUMENTS/ SCALES/SURVEYS THAT EVALUATE POSTTRAUMATIC STRESS DISORDER (PTSD).

traumatic brain injury (TBI) A severe injury of the BRAIN that is caused by a jolt or blow to the head or by a penetrating injury that impedes the normal functioning of the brain. Not all blows to the head result in a traumatic brain injury. TBI is also caused by violently shaking the head. Traumatic brain injuries range from mild to severe. A mild TBI may cause a brief change in consciousness and mental status. The most common type of minor TBI is known as a *concussion*. In contrast, a severe TBI may cause AMNESIA or an extended period of unconsciousness. A TBI can cause epilepsy, and it may also increase the individual's risk for other brain disorders, such as Parkinson's disease and Alzheimer's disease.

Individuals born with brain injuries or who suffer brain injuries during birth are not included under the definition of a traumatic brain injury.

The most famous patient with TBI was 25-year-old Phineas Gage, a railway construction foreman in Vermont in 1848. Gage was using explosive powder and a packing rod when a spark created an explosion that rammed a three-foot pointed rod straight through his head. The rod penetrated his skull, traversed his brain, and left the skull through his temple. In the 19th century, very little was known about the brain or TBIs, and most people who suffered them died of this type of injury. Gage was treated by a physician for 73 days, and he survived. His personality changed radically, however, and he was transformed from a mild-mannered man to an obstinate and self-absorbed person with serious behavioral and personality problems that lasted until his death in 1861. Gage's skull with its large exit hole is on display at Harvard Medical School in Cambridge, Massachusetts

Symptoms and Diagnostic Path

Individuals with TBIs may suffer from severe headaches, as well as sensitivity to light and noise, and sleep disturbances. They may also have difficulties with memory, attention, and language. Often they have psychiatric symptoms, such as DEPRESSION, ANXIETY, impulsive behavior, and inappropriate laughter. Some of the symptoms seen with TBI may resemble those of patients with POSTTRAUMATIC STRESS DISORDER (PTSD).

Other signs and symptoms of an individual with a TBI may include

- easily confused
- constant feeling of fatigue
- dizziness, lightheadedness, and loss of balance
- blurred vision or eyes that tire easily
- a ringing in the ears
- a loss of the sense of smell or taste
- slowness in speaking, thinking, acting, or reading
- nausea

In addition to medical signs and symptoms, individuals with TBI may also experience serious social and emotional problems. They may have greater difficulty relating to others than in the past, and they may experience mood changes or depression.

Some patients suffer from anterograde or retrograde POSTTRAUMATIC AMNESIA (PTA). Retrograde PTA is an impaired memory of events that occurred before the TBI. In contrast, anterograde PTA is an impaired memory of events that occurred after the TBI.

Some patients suffer from language and communication problems, such as aphasia, which is difficulty in understanding and speaking. They may have inappropriate laughter. Some individuals have very little control over their emotions.

In one study reported in the *Journal of Neuropsychiatry & Clinical Neuroscience* in 2004, the authors studied the presence of pathological laughter and crying (PLC) in 92 patients with acute symptoms after they were diagnosed with a traumatic brain injury. The researchers found a PLC prevalence of 10.9 percent in the first year. They also discovered that patients with PLC (compared to the TBI patients without PLC), displayed significantly more depressed, anxious, and aggressive behaviors and had poorer social functioning. PLC was also associated with ANXIETY DISORDERS and focal frontal lobe lesions.

Of the 10 patients with PLC, three did not receive a follow-up, so their prognosis was unknown. Five of the remaining seven patients with PLC were treated with antidepressants, and four of these patients had a complete remission of PLC within three months of beginning antidepressants, while the other patient showed a 50 percent reduction of symptoms after three months. Of the two patients who did not receive antidepressants, one patient recovered from PLC after six months and the other recovered within three months.

Said the authors, "The fact that PLC might have a deleterious effect on social interaction and functioning underscores the need for a controlled treatment trial of antidepressants in patients with PLC following TBI."

Physicians diagnose head injuries based on the patient's behavior and apparent injuries, as well as through imaging tests such as a computed tomography (CT) scan or a magnetic resonance imaging (MRI) scan. However, often emergency medical technicians (EMTs) are the first on the scene and must make a preliminary diagnosis of TBI before the physician sees the patient. The EMT seeks to stabilize the patient and prevent any further injury. EMTs work on providing sufficient oxygen flow to the patient's brain and body and controlling the blood pressure. EMTs may have to perform CPR or other emergency procedures. Many patients with probable or possible TMIs are placed on a backboard and with a neck restraint so that they are immobilized to prevent further injury to the head and spinal cord. EMTs also assess the patient by his or her response to the *Glasgow Coma Scale,* which is a 15-point test that uses three basic measures to determine the severity of the brain injury, including eye opening, best verbal response, and best motor response. According to the National Institute of Neurological Disorders and Stroke, patients are assessed as follows, using the Glasgow Coma Scale

With regard to the eye opening test, there are four scores

- 4—the patient can open the eyes spontaneously
- 3—the patient can open the eyes on a verbal command
- 2—the patient only opens the eyes in response to painful stimuli
- 1—the patient does not open the eyes in response to any stimuli

With regard to best verbal response test, there are five scores

- 5—the patient is oriented and speaking coherently
- 4—the patient is disoriented but can still speak coherently
- 3—the patient uses incoherent language or inappropriate words
- 2—the patient is making incomprehensible sounds
- 1—the patient makes no verbal responses

With regard to the best motor response test, there are six scores

- 6—the patient can move the arms and legs in response to verbal commands
- A score of 2–5—the patient shows movement in response to stimuli, including pain
- 1—the patient shows no movement in response to any stimuli

The EMTs add up the scores of the three tests to determine the severity of the TBI. A total score of 3–8 means that the patient has a severe head injury, while a score of 9–12 indicates a moderate injury. A score of 13–15 indicates a mild TBI.

Treatment Options and Outlook

An estimated half of severely injured TBI patients will need surgery, and subsequent to surgery, they will usually be placed in intensive care. Patients are also treated for the complications that may occur with TBI, such as seizures, hydrocephalus, leaks of spinal fluid, pain, and other injuries.

About half of patients with penetrating head injuries suffer from seizures, while 25 percent of patients with hematomas or brain contusions have seizures. Seizures are treated with anticonvulsant medications.

Some patients with TBIs suffer from infections within the intracranial cavity, which may occur within weeks of the original injury. Antibiotics are used and sometimes surgery is necessary to remove infected tissue.

Most patients with TBIs also suffer injuries to other parts of the body, and may have trauma to the lungs and heart, bone fractures, nerve injuries, and a variety of other injuries. In addition, often trauma victims develop an increased metabolic rate, or hypermetabolism. This can cause muscle wasting and harm to other tissues. It can also lead to hormonal and fluid imbalances. Two common results of a TBI are hypothyroidism and syndrome of inappropriate secretion of antidiuretic hormone (SIADH).

About 40 percent of patients develop postconcussion syndrome, which includes such symptoms as dizziness, vertigo, headache, problems with memory and concentration, depression irritability, apathy, and anxiety. This syndrome is more common among patients who had psychiatric problems before the TBI occurred. Treatment includes medications for pain and for the psychiatric symptoms.

Psychiatric problems are common among patients with TBIs, and families may find it extremely difficult to deal with the personality and behavioral changes that occur. Patients may exhibit problem behaviors such as aggression and violence, as well as emotional outbursts. Some patients' personalities change so much that they fit the diagnosis of BORDERLINE PERSONALITY DISORDER. Children who are injured with a TBI may fail to mature emotionally after the injury.

Medications and psychotherapy can improve many psychiatric symptoms of patients with TBIs.

However, physicians should keep in mind that patients with TBIs may be more susceptible to the side effects of medications and thus, they must be prescribed with care.

After stabilizing the patient, rehabilitation is needed by most TBI patients, who may be treated at a rehabilitation facility or the subacute unit of the hospital. Some types of rehabilitation that the patient may receive include physical therapy, speech/language therapy, occupational therapy, and psychiatry. Some patients continue to receive therapeutic treatment after they return home.

Risk Factors and Preventive Measures

Small children and elderly individuals have the greatest risk for suffering a traumatic brain injury. The Centers for Disease Control and Prevention (CDC) estimates that about 1.4 million people suffer from a traumatic brain injury each year and there are 5.3 million Americans in the United States who are disabled because of TBIs. According to a 2006 report on traumatic brain injuries in the United States, of those who suffer from a TBI each year, an estimated 50,000 die, 235,000 are hospitalized, and 1.1 million are treated and released from a hospital emergency room.

About 475,000 TBIs occur to children from birth to age 14, and 90 percent of these children are treated at emergency rooms. Although more children suffer from TBIs each year than adults ages 65 years and older (155,000), older adults are much more likely to be hospitalized or to die. An estimated 2,685 children die of TBIs per year, compared to 12,283 older adults. (SEE FIRST TABLE BELOW.)

The highest rates of TBI-hospitalizations and deaths occur among adults ages 75 years and older. In general, men suffer about 1.5 times as many TBIs as women. There are an estimated 37,000 male deaths from TBIs each year, compared to about 13,000 females who die from TBIs. (SEE SECOND TABLE BELOW.) This may be because young adult males take many more chances than young adult females, such as riding a motorcycle without a helmet, failing to use a seatbelt, and other actions.

NUMBERS OF TRAUMATIC BRAIN INJURY-RELATED EMERGENCY DEPARTMENT VISITS, HOSPITALIZATIONS, AND DEATHS, BY SEX, UNITED STATES, 2003

Sex	Emergency Department Visits	Hospitalizations	Deaths	Total
Male	710,000	184,000	37,416	931,000
Female	514,000	290,000	50,757	634,000
Total	1,224,000	290,000	50,757	1,565,000

Source: Adapted from Centers for Disease Control. "Incidence of Traumatic Brain Injury in the United States, 2002 and 2003 Updated Data Tables," Available online. URL: http://www.cdc.gov/ncipc/pub-res/TBI_in_US_04/TBI%20Tables_2003.pdf. Updated May 2007.

NUMBERS OF TRAUMATIC BRAIN INJURY-RELATED EMERGENCY DEPARTMENT VISITS, HOSPITALIZATIONS, AND DEATHS, BY AGE GROUP, UNITED STATES, 2003

Age (years)	Emergency Department Visits	Hospitalizations	Deaths	Total
0–4	216,000	18,000	1,035	235,000
5–14	188,000	24,000	1,250	213,000
15–24	313,000	56,000	9,053	378,000
25–44	254,000	58,000	13,904	326,000
45–64	163,000	50,000	11,698	225,000
≥ 65	90,000	84,000	13,796	188,000
Total	1,244,00	290,000	50,757	1,565,000

Source: Adapted from Centers for Disease Control. "Incidence of Traumatic Brain Injury in the United States, 2002 and 2003 Updated Data Tables," Available online. URL: http://www.cdc.gov/ncipc/pub-res/TBI_in_US_04/TBI%20Tables_2003.pdf. Updated May 2007.

This high death rate holds for every age category; for example, among children from birth to age four, there was an average of 1,099 deaths annually, based on data from 1995–2001. Of these deaths, 57 percent of the children were males. The highest death rate from traumatic brain injuries for males was among males age 20–24 years, accounting for 82.3 percent of all deaths from traumatic brain injuries. In averaging the numbers of deaths from TBIs at all ages, males represented 74 percent of the deaths. (SEE TABLE BELOW.)

An estimated 28 percent of all TBIs are caused by falls, according to the CDC. The TBI injury rate for falls is highest among two groups: children ages 0 to 4 years old and adults ages 75 years and older. Motor vehicle crashes cause about 20 percent of TBIs. However, individuals injured in motor vehicle and traffic accidents represent the highest number of TBI-related hospitalizations. Although falls represent the largest single category of causes of TBIs, they are not the greatest cause of hospitalizations or deaths. Instead, motor vehicle and traffic accidents represent a higher number of both hospitalizations and deaths.

TBIs in War Zones

According to Susan Okie, M.D. in her article for the *New England Journal of Medicine,* soldiers surviving wounds sustained in combat in Afghanistan and Iraq have a higher rate of TBIs than seen in other wars. Says Okie, "According to the Joint Theater Trauma Registry, compiled by the U.S. Army Institute of Surgical Research, 22 percent of the wounded soldiers from these conflicts who have passed through the military's Landstuhl Regional Medical Center in Germany had injuries to the head, face or neck." In contrast, during the Vietnam War, about 12–14 percent of the combat injuries were TBIs, and an additional 2 percent of soldiers had a fatal wound to both the head and abdomen. Says Okie,

> U.S. soldiers in Iraq and Afghanistan who have serious brain injuries receive immediate care on the battlefield and are then transported to military combat support hospitals, where they undergo brain imaging and are treated by neurosurgeons. Treatment may include the removal of foreign bodies, control of bleeding, or craniectomy to relieve pressure from swelling.

Most of the TBIs that have occurred up to 2006 in Iraq and Afghanistan were caused by improvised explosive devices (IEDs), according to experts. Protective gear and improved medical care has increased the survival rate for soldiers today.

Care should be taken by parents and other caregivers of children. Elderly individuals should be especially careful, as should any caregivers that they may have. For example, it is unwise for an elderly individual to climb on the roof to clean out the gutters, because he or she may fall. Scatter rugs can also cause individuals to trip. Often a family member can go through the house to identify potential problem areas that could cause a fall.

Individuals who take risks, such as engaging in extreme sports as well as those who fail to take

NUMBERS OF TRAUMATIC BRAIN INJURY-RELATED EMERGENCY DEPARTMENT VISITS, HOSPITALIZATIONS, AND DEATHS, BY CAUSE, UNITED STATES, 2003

Cause	Emergency Department Visits	Hospitalizations	Deaths	Total
Motor-vehicle traffic	227,000	58,000	16,357	301,000
Fall	426,000	68,000	8,949	503,000
Assault	124,000	19,000	5,871	149,000
Struck by/against	272,000	8,000	366	280,000
Other	120,000	35,000	19,124	174,000
Unknown	——	102,000	——	——
Total	1,224,000	290,000	50,757	1,565,000

Source: Adapted from Centers for Disease Control. "Incidence of Traumatic Brain Injury in the United States, 2002 and 2003 Updated Data Tables," Available online. URL: http://www.cdc.gov/ncipc/pub-res/TBI_in_US_04/TBI%20Tables_2003.pdf. Updated May 2007.

safety measures, have an increased risk of suffering from a TBI.

According to the National Institute of Neurological Disorders and Stroke, to prevent TBIs, the following actions should be taken:

- wear seatbelts in cars
- buckle children in cars in a child safety seat, booster seat, or seatbelt, depending on the child's age
- wear a helmet and make sure children wear helmets when
  - riding a motorcycle or bike
  - playing a contact sport such as ice hockey or football
  - using in-line skates or riding on a skateboard
  - batting or running bases in softball or baseball
  - riding a horse
  - skiing or snowboarding
- keep all firearms and bullets locked up when not in use.
- avoid falls by
  - using a step-stool with a grab bar to reach objects on high shelves
  - installing handrails on stairways
  - installing window guards to prevent young children from falling out of windows
  - using safety gates at the top and bottom of stairs when young children are present
- Make sure the surface of your child's playground is made of shock-absorbing material such as sand or hardwood mulch

See also ANXIETY DISORDERS; BRAIN; COMBAT-RELATED POSTTRAUMATIC STRESS DISORDER; POST-VIETNAM SYNDROME.

Langlois, Jean A., Wesley Rutland-Brown, and Karen E. Thomas. *Traumatic Brain Injury in the United States: Emergency Department Visits, Hospitalizations, and Deaths.* Atlanta, Ga.: Centers for Disease Control and Prevention, January 2006. Available online. URL: http://www.cdc.gov/ncipc/pub-res/TBI_in_US-04/TBI%20in%20the%20US_Jan_2006.pdf. Downloaded August 5, 2006.

National Institute of Neurological Disorders and Stroke. *Traumatic Brain Injury: Hope through Research. National Institutes of Health*, June 2006. Available online. URL: http://www.ninds.nih.gov/disorders/tbi/detail_tbi.htm. Downloaded August 12, 2006.

Okie, Susan, M.D., "Traumatic Brain Injury in the War Zone." *New England Journal of Medicine* 352, no. 20 (May 19, 2005): 2043–2047.

Tateno, Amane, M.D., Ricardo E. Jorge, M.D. and Robert G. Robinson, M.D., "Pathological Laughing and Crying Following Traumatic Brain Injury." *Journal of Neuropsychiatry and Clinical Neurosciences* 16 (2004): 426–434.

traumatic event It is important to note that it is not the *event* that is traumatic, it is the *effect the event has on the individual* that makes it a traumatic event. Most people seem to recover from traumatic events and do not display long-term symptoms of the experience. Only a minority will develop acute traumatic stress reactions or posttraumatic stress disorder (PTSD). The characteristics of traumatic events that produce the most trauma reactions or results are those of human against human in such situations as war, rape, torture, violent crime, and so on. Other traumatic events are NATURAL DISASTERS (hurricanes, tsunami, earthquakes) and man-made disasters (airplane crash, train derailment, factory explosion). In Vietnam, for example, at least 20 percent of the war veterans developed PTSD. Likewise, the majority of rape victims develop long-lasting PTSD.

The next most prevalent category is accidents and natural disasters. Obviously the more severe these events, the most likely and more widespread PTSD will be. Another category is attachment loss and betrayal, which can have lasting effects on relationships throughout one's lifetime. Neglect is a form of traumatization as is recurrent exposure to major stressors as seen in child abuse. Finally, lack of social support can be traumatizing to the individual.

Experience affects the biological, emotional, cognitive, and spiritual dimensions of life for the traumatized victim. Trauma leads to DYSREGULATION or dysfunction within each of these dimensions and, in turn, produces an even more pervasive and subtle problem for individuals in that their sense of self and of the world around them feels alienated, unsafe, and scary. They feel alone.

In cases of extreme or chronic traumatic stimulation, the sense of self may be so alienated from experience that several different identities or personalities may prevail and subconsciously alternate in the person's experiences. This is called DISSOCIATION or multiple personality. Most often, however, the effects are not as dramatic. Usually the traumatized person experiences a sense of alienation from others and from his or her own inner experience. They find it difficult to read people, to know how they feel emotionally, or to trust their experiences as authentic. Most trauma therapists see that awareness, integration, and restoration of the sense of self is an essential outcome of successful trauma therapy.

Peritraumatic distress is the psychiatric level of distress (intense fear, helplessness, or horror) experienced during and immediately after a traumatic event. Distress, like PERITRAUMATIC DISSOCIATION, is a coping mechanism that predicts the eventual development of POSTTRAUMATIC STRESS DISORDER (PTSD).

See also MEDICAL ILLNESS-RELATED PSYCHOLOGICAL DISTRESS; MEDICAL STRESSORS; PEDIATRIC MEDICAL TRAUMATIC STRESS; POTENTIALLY TRAUMATIZING EVENT; RAPE TRAUMA SYNDROME; THERAPY, TYPES OF; TRAUMATIC MEMORY.

McLaren, K. *Emotional Genius: Discovering the Deepest Language of the Soul.* Columbia, Calif.: Laughing Tree Press, 2001.

traumatic incident reduction (TIR)   A psychotherapeutic method used to reduce the negative effects of past traumas. Traumatic incident reduction (TIR) was developed by Frank Gerbode, M.D., as a client-centered structured procedure where the client does all the work, while the therapist/facilitator observes and facilitates the process. Proper instructions are given but no offer of interpretation or advice is provided by the therapist.

TIR therapy begins with the client identifying a specific traumatic experience. Next, the client is asked to view the experience like a videotape, with eyes closed, starting from a point just prior to the traumatic incident, and to view it, without talking, until the incident is over. The therapist then asks the client what happened and the client can reveal as much as he or she wishes to do. After the first run-through of the incident, the client is asked to view the tape again in the mind, from the beginning. This process is repeated many times during a typical 3-to-4 hour session. The purpose is to integrate, through repeated viewing, aspects of the trauma that remain unresolved. With each additional viewing, the client will begin to

- notice different things about the event, revealing things not known previously
- find different internal feelings about the trauma
- process negative emotions, allowing positive emotions to emerge
- find less discomfort and a reduction of traumatic stress symptoms

TIR's uniqueness lies in its procedure of the client "viewing" the traumatic incident repeatedly until the original target stressors are eliminated and until cognitive distortions of the original trauma are restructured.

TIR is not intended for use with clients who are

- psychotic or seriously mentally ill
- substance abusers, including those who abuse prescription medications
- not engaged in TIR of their own free choice; TIR works for clients who wish to do it
- unable to focus on TIR due to a preoccupation with personal issues that are far too painful and overwhelming at present
- unwilling to look at their past traumas

Traumatic Life Event Questionnaire (TLEQ)   The TLEQ is a brief self-report inventory or questionnaire that assesses current and prior exposure to 21 different potential traumatic events (such as natural disasters, sexual abuse, assaults, etc.). Elhai, et al., report that it is among the most widely used assessment instrument by professionals in screening for posttraumatic stress disorders. The 21 events are described in behavioral rather than emotional terms (such as "rape" or "abuse"). Respondents make their responses in a seven-point format based on frequency of occurrence. In "follow-up probes" respondents are asked if they felt fear, helplessness, or horror during any event experienced. This is consistent with the DSM definition that requires the traumatic event to be life threatening or injury threatening. The TLEQ takes only 15 minutes to complete. This inventory provides a quick screening tool for assessing trauma history and potential PTSD and can be used without requiring extensive knowledge of the respondent's life history or background. It is ideally suited for emergency rooms, mental health clinics, and victim services agencies and does not require a skills clinician or mental health worker to administer the inventory.

Elhai, J. D., M. J. Gray, T. B. Kashdan, and C. L. Franklin. "Which instruments are most commonly used to assess traumatic event exposure and posttraumatic effects? A survey of traumatic stress professionals." *Journal of Traumatic Stress* 18, no. 5 (2005): 541–545.

traumatic memory   The recall of a personal experience of a TRAUMATIC EVENT, an event that threatened death or serious injury to self or others and involved intense fear, helplessness, or horror.

Traumatic memories exist in highly distressing and sometime fragmentary psychological and physiological states associated with the traumatic experience or event. In this sense, they are "state dependent" and likely to arise when the state an individual was in when a trauma occurred is reproduced. These memories are timeless and remembered in extreme vividness and resist integration or resolution. Traumatic memories are encoded by processes such as repression and DISSOCIATION and therefore cannot be retrieved by conscious explicit memory process. They are isolated, nonverbal, highly sensory, motor and emotional fragments.

In their 1992 article van der Hart & Friedman state that a traumatic memory is reactivated by situations or stimuli such as

• sensory data
• time-related stimuli

• daily life events
• events during the therapeutic session
• emotional states
• physiological states
• stimuli recalling intimidations by perpetrators
• current trauma

Traumatic memories are more easily elicited by "right-brain" activities such as story telling, association, and imagination.

See also ECHOIC MEMORY; EXPLICIT MEMORY; IMPLICIT MEMORY; MEDICAL ILLNESS-RELATED PSYCHOLOGICAL DISTRESS; MEDICAL STRESSORS; PEDIATRIC MEDICAL TRAUMATIC STRESS; POTENTIALLY TRAUMATIZING EVENT.

van der Hart, O., and B. Friedman. "Trauma, Dissociation and Triggers: Their Role in Treatment and Emergency Psychiatry." In J. B. van Luyn et al., eds., *Emergency Psychiatry Today*. Amsterdam: Elsevier, 1992, 137–142.

Traumatic Memory Inventory (TMI)   An inventory that was developed to investigate the nature of traumatic and nontraumatic memories in detail. The Traumatic Memory Inventory (TMI) attempts to capture the complexities of how traumatic memories are retrieved by people who are experiencing a traumatic event and discover how this event differs from nontraumatic, yet highly emotional, events.

The TMI is a 60-item structured interview that collects data to assess the characteristics of traumatic memories, beginning with:

1. the nature of the trauma
2. the duration of the trauma
3. whether subjects had always remembered the trauma or when subjects were first consciously aware of the traumatic memory
4. under what circumstances the subject first experienced intrusive memories and the circumstances of how these memories presently occur
5. the sensory modalities in which memories are experienced, both past and present
   • the nature of visual images, by asking, "What did you see?"

- the nature of sounds ("What did you hear?")
- the nature of smells ("What did you smell?")
- feelings in the body ("What did you feel and where in your body?")
- emotions ("What emotional feelings did you have?")

These characteristics, along with subjects' ability to tell their experience as a narrative story, are collected to determine how the subjects remember the initial trauma, while they were most bothered by it, as well as currently. The TMI also collects clinical data on

- the nature of nightmares
- precipitants of nightmares and flashbacks
- ways that subjects gain mastery of intrusive memories (for example, eating, using drugs or alcohol, working, etc.)
- the probable confirmation of the traumatic event, as with witnesses or hospital or court records

The TMI relies on the subjects' memories of how they remembered the trauma. The strengths and weakness of this inventory are inherently built-in and threaten both the validity and reliability of the TMI due to its retrospective exploration of fragmented memory characteristics, with the potential for distortions when subjects are asked to recall how they remembered events that occurred years or even decades ago. The diverse and fragmentary nature of traumatic memories is a strength because clinicians know that over time traumatic memories may change and become incorporated into relatively normal memories, sometimes very slowly and sometimes rapidly due to treatment.

See also POSTTRAUMATIC STRESS DISORDER (PTSD).

van der Kolk, B., J. W. Hopper, and J. E. Osterman. "Exploring the Nature of Traumatic Memory: Combining Clinical Knowledge with Laboratory Methods." *Journal of Aggression, Maltreatment & Trauma* 4, no. 2 (2001): 9–31.

traumatic stress The psychological consequences that disrupt the equilibrium and homeostasis of the person exposed to a TRAUMATIC EVENT. The

traumatic event can be war, intense violence, rape, child abuse, or a natural disaster. It results in unusually strong emotional response and interferes with the person's ability to function at home and work. Most stress is seen as produced by a "stressor." When the stressor is removed, the stress response diminishes and goes away, but this is not so with traumatic stress. Here the reaction or response continues even though the stress has passed and is gone. This distinguishes traumatic from "regular" stress reactions.

Immediately following a NATURAL DISASTER or traumatic event, a person may be in shock and denial. And when the shock subsides, more intense feelings may follow with vivid memories, disruption in sleep and eating patterns, and a sense of "daze" or numbness. Other symptoms of traumatic stress include FLASHBACKS, INSOMNIA, anxiety, emotional detachment, DEPRESSION, hypervigilence, loss of memory, and excessive avoidance of trauma reminders. The symptoms normally subside within a few months. If not, a psychiatric disorder, such as POSTTRAUMATIC STRESS DISORDER (PTSD) is generally diagnosed.

See also ACUTE STRESS DISORDER; TRAUMATIC EVENT.

Traumatic Stress Institute Belief Scale See TRAUMA AND ATTACHMENT BELIEF SCALE (TABS).

Traumatic Stress Schedule (TSS) A short (30 minutes or less) screening instrument for measuring the occurrence and impact of a defined TRAUMATIC EVENT, a group of occurrences experienced by 8 percent of the U.S. adult population in any given year. The event categories assessed are: robbery, physical assault, sexual assault, tragic death of friend or family member, motor vehicle accident, military combat, loss through fire, natural disaster, hazard or danger, as well as one unspecified event. Once the respondent reports an event, there are 12 detailed closed and open-ended questions pertaining to the scope, threat to life, blame, physical injury, and range of symptoms.

A sample question from the TSS is, "In the past year did someone take something from you by force or threat of force, such as in a robbery, mugging, or hold up?" Probing questions are about persons involved, loss of property value, threat to life, blame, intrusive thoughts, avoidance behaviors, or nightmares.

The TSS functions well as a screening device for many purposes, such as epidemiological studies, and is also used for clinical and research purposes but may result in a lack of standardization if comparing to other studies using the TSS.

See also INSTRUMENTS/SCALES/SURVEYS THAT EVALUATE POSTTRAUMATIC STRESS DISORDER (PTSD).

Norris, F. "Screening for Traumatic Stress: A scale for use in the general population," *Journal of Applied Social Psychology* 20 (November 1990): 1,704–1,718.

trauma vortex   A term from SOMATIC EXPERIENCING THERAPY that refers to the power of a traumatic experience to draw or bring the person back into the trauma as they get close to the relative experience. This is much the same as being drawn into a whirlpool. The closer that a person gets to the whirlpool, the more danger there is in being drawn into the pool and pulled down under the water. It is possible to be pulled into the trauma vortex by behavior, images, sensations, affect, or meaning of an event. This is a bad thing to have happen as it can set off a widespread traumatic reaction similar to the original reaction to the traumatic event.

While the trauma vortex is a reconstruction of the trauma experience, the "healing vortex" is an opposing force that "pulls" the individual toward resolution and healing of a trauma and toward balance and self-regulation. The healing vortex lives in everyone, while the trauma vortex has been conditioned by past experience.

See also INSTRUMENTS/SCALES/SURVEYS THAT EVALUATE POSTTRAUMATIC STRESS DISORDER (PTSD); TRAUMATIC MEMORY.

treatment: psychotherapy, psychopharmacology, and alternative medicine   Traumatic stress disorders are treated by a wide range of therapies, from various forms of psychotherapy to medications that can help to ease the emotional pain of the trauma, such as antidepressants or antianxiety drugs. Some patients need a combination of therapies to recover, such as COGNITIVE BEHAVIORAL THERAPY/INTERVENTION as well as a SELECTIVE SEROTONIN REUPTAKE INHIBITOR (SSRI) antidepressant or a BENZODIAZEPINE (ANTIANXIETY MEDICATION). In some cases, one or more options available from alternative medicine, such as ART THERAPY, ayurveda from India, or another mind-body therapy, can be very helpful. In this time of instant messages and cell phones that link people on different continents, people expect life to proceed at a fast pace, so it is important to realize that recovery from a traumatic stress disorder is rarely instantaneous. Because the trauma was sufficiently threatening to make the person quite ill, recovery usually only comes with time and treatment.

Psychotherapy

Most traumatized individuals need psychotherapy, and they may benefit from individual therapy and sometimes from group therapy as well. Several key forms of therapy may provide relief for those who have been traumatized, such as BEHAVIORAL REENACTMENTS, one or more types of cognitive behavioral therapy, DIRECT THERAPEUTIC EXPOSURE, EYE MOVEMENT DESENSITIZATION AND REPROCESSING (EMDR), IMPLOSIVE THERAPY, phase-oriented treatment, SOMATIC EXPERIENCING THERAPY, STRESS INOCULATION TRAINING, SYSTEMATIC DESENSITIZATION, TESTIMONY THERAPY, and TRAUMATIC INCIDENT REDUCTION THERAPY.

Behavioral Reenactment   This technique is sometimes used with traumatized children. The child uses play therapy to help resolve anxiety about the trauma. Child psychiatrist Lenore Terr identified the value of behavioral reenactment when working with traumatized children in her pioneering study of the children who were kidnapped from a school bus and buried underground in Chowchilla, California, in 1976.

In this case, the kidnappers put 26 preschool and school-age children (ages five to 14 years) into darkened vans and then buried them alive underground in a tractor-trailer. When the trailer roof collapsed after the children had been immersed in total darkness for 28 hours, some of the children escaped, and all of them were soon rescued. The kidnappers were never able to make their $5 million ransom demand because all the phone lines in the region were busy with people frantically trying to find the children.

Despite their lack of physical injuries, the children were extremely traumatized and exhibited a sense of hopelessness about the future. In her work with these severely traumatized children, Terr noticed that many of them subsequently played games that involved burying vehicles. Although some people would consider that behavior problematic, Terr deduced that the children were actually reenacting some aspects of the original trauma to help them process their experiences and to alleviate their anxiety levels. She reasoned that behavior reenactment could be a meaningful way for children to process a horrific experience and ease their emotional pain. She wrote about her findings in *Too Scared to Cry.*

Cognitive Behavioral Therapy (CBT) With this therapy, the individual is taught to identify and to challenge irrational or unproductive thoughts, such as the thought, "I can never recover," by replacing such thoughts with more positive ones, such as, "With time, I can recover and I will recover."

The two most popular types of cognitive behavioral therapies are rational emotive behavior therapy (developed by Albert Ellis) and cognitive therapy (developed by Aaron Beck). Rational emotive behavior therapy works to identify irrational, demanding, and excessive belief patterns, such as "I must be loved by everyone" or "I have to be perfect," which are self-defeating and can produce disturbing behavior and disturbed mood. The therapist assists the client to substitute more rational and less demanding thoughts.

Cognitive therapy attacks illogical thinking processes and helps clients recognize their negative thoughts, biased interpretations, and errors in logic. "Overgeneralization," for example, is the illogical thinking that if something went wrong once it will always happen that way again. It is important to realize that isolated errors or mistakes do not predict failure every time. Clients must avoid statements such as "I always screw up."

CBT is applicable to many types of trauma. For example, people who have survived an experience in which others died often suffer from SURVIVOR GUILT. CBT can teach the individual to tell himself or herself that it was not his fault that the traumatic experience happened or that others did not survive. It does not matter if the individual initially does not believe these rational thoughts; eventually over time, many people do begin to accept them.

Phase-oriented Treatment Introduced by Pierre Janet more than a century ago, this therapy is provided in different major parts, or phases. The first phase of treatment centers on symptom management and containment. Next, the patient develops resources to help or improve affect modulation and build a sense of safety. In the next phase, the client identifies internal states and how they affect behavior. Developing these phases alone can take years.

Somatic Experiencing (SE) Therapy Somatic experiencing (SE) therapy was developed by Peter Levine and his faculty colleagues at the Foundation for Human Enrichment and described in *Waking the Tiger: Healing Trauma.* According to Levine, bodily stored traumatic experiences can be processed through awareness techniques, because of the body's inherent ability to heal. With somatic experiencing, dysregulation in the autonomic nervous system is viewed as the outcome of unresolved trauma, in that it interferes with the capacity to self-regulate, leading often to trauma-related health disorders, behaviors, and affect (mood).

The SE approach uses the capacity for a FELT SENSE or body awareness to heal the effects of the trauma. SE therapy has been successfully used with single incident traumas, such as car accidents, earthquakes, tsunamis, battlefield incidents, and rape, and also with developmental traumas, such as childhood sexual and physical abuse or neglect and other cumulative traumatic experiences such as attachment traumas.

Stage-Oriented Treatment A treatment model developed by James Chu in 1998 under the acronym SAFER, which lists the components:

S: Self-care and symptom control
A: Acknowledgement of the impact of traumatic experiences
F: Functioning and living a more normal life

E: Expression on unspeakable and intolerable feelings and learning to rid oneself of unwanted ones

R: Relationship-building that is collaborative and mutual

Stress Inoculation Training (SIT) This is a three-phased form of exposure therapy. Clients learn coping techniques such as deep muscle relaxation, thought stopping, breathing control, role playing, and other techniques that are meant to "inoculate" them against suffering from thoughts of the trauma. The client is then trained to break down his or her stressors into short, intermediate, and long-term coping goals. The third phase involves using the learned techniques and following through in gradual steps in the real situation.

According to Barbara Olasov Rothbaum and Edna B. Foa in their chapter in the book *Traumatic Stress*, some studies have found that stress inoculation training has been effective with female rape victims and significantly helped to reduce their levels of depression and fear. Although the victims in these studies were not specifically diagnosed with PTSD, they were very likely to have had PTSD because the rape had occurred within the past three months prior to the therapy, and thus, the women were still very traumatized.

Systematic Desensitization In this EXPOSURE THERAPY the client and the therapist create a mutually agreed-upon, tailored hierarchy of the client's fears from the least feared item to the most feared item, and then use relaxation that is paired with progressively increasing exposure to the trauma. For example, if the client is a combat veteran who is hypervigilant about loud noises and who is suffering from PTSD because he was present when his comrades were killed in an explosion, the hierarchy might begin with a picture of a soldier wearing full combat gear, which might be recorded as a 5 on a scale of 1 to 100. The most distressing situation on the scale might be a recording that is (or sounds like) the shelling of a camp, which would be recorded as a 100 on the scale. The client is trained to produce a state of relaxation, and as tolerance develops for each situation, the client moves on to the next level on the hierarchy list. The goal is not to make the client insensitive to extremely distress-

ing events but rather to allow him or her to learn to deal with thoughts and other reminders of them.

Psychiatrist Joseph Wolpe developed systematic desensitization as a therapy in the late 1950s in order to inhibit the anxiety symptoms of his patients. According to Wolpe, when anxiety-evoking stimuli are presented in a hierarchical order and systematically paired with a relaxation response, the individual's anxiety symptoms are reduced. This therapeutic technique has been found to be effective in working with combat veterans with posttraumatic stress disorder, according to Barbara Olasov Rothbaum and Edna B. Foa in their chapter in the book *Traumatic Stress.*

Direct Therapeutic Exposure (DTE) This is a form of therapy that, as its name sounds, exposes the traumatized person to direct reminders of the trauma. Unlike with systematic desensitization, which progressively increases the client's exposure starting with the *least* traumatic aspect of an event, DTE instead immediately exposes the client to the *most* extreme and anxiety-evoking aspects of the trauma. The theory is that over time, the fear and anxiety will abate, and as a result, the exposure continues until the client's anxiety peaks and ultimately wanes. Further research is needed, however, to determine if this form of therapy is lasting and effective.

Patrick A. Boudewyns first called this technique direct therapeutic exposure, based on his research with Vietnam veterans and patients suffering from posttraumatic stress disorder, describing it in *Flooding and Implosive Therapy: Direct Therapeutic Exposure in Clinical Practice.*

Implosive Therapy In implosive therapy the client is directed to greatly exaggerate the trauma in the mind, in order to induce as much anxiety as possible. The client is then asked to consider alternative ways to respond to the evoked anxiety in order to make it more bearable. The goal of implosive therapy is to eliminate the anxiety altogether after several sessions. This form of therapy was developed by T. C. Stampfl and D. J. Levis, and was first described by them in 1967. Research indicates that implosive therapy has short-term positive effects, but that they diminish over the long term.

Testimony Psychotherapy This is a sharing of the traumatic experience with others in a storytelling fashion. In a 1998 study, Steven Weine et al. worked with Bosnian survivors of ethnic cleansing who resettled in Chicago. After each survivor provided testimony psychotherapy as a way of relating their survival story, describing their life in war and as a refugee, Weine discovered that the rate of posttraumatic stress disorder (PTSD) diagnosis decreased from 100 percent to 74 percent immediately after testimony and then to 53 percent at six months. Sharing their story with others was clearly therapeutic.

Traumatic Incident Reduction (TIR) Therapy
This psychotherapeutic method was designed to reduce the negative effects of past traumas. This therapy, developed by Frank Gerbode, M.D., is a client-centered procedure where the client does the work while the therapist observes and facilitates the process. The client is given instructions but no interpretation or advice.

With TIR therapy, the client starts by identifying a specific traumatic experience. Next, he or she is told to watch the experience mentally like a videotape, with the eyes closed, starting from just before the traumatic incident. The person views it, without talking, until the incident is over. Next, the therapist then asks the client what happened and the client reveals as much or as little as he or she wishes. After the first run-through of the incident, the client is told to view the tape once again mentally, from the very beginning. This process is repeated many times over three to four hours. The purpose of this form of therapy is to help the client to integrate aspects of the trauma that have remained unresolved.

Eye Movement Desensitization and Reprocessing (EMDR)   This therapy was developed in 1987 by Francine Shapiro. Since its inception, hundreds of case studies and controlled empirical studies have validated the effectiveness of EMDR with trauma clients and other clients.

EMDR therapy assumes that trauma causes an overload of an information processing system that exists in all people. This processing system takes perceptions of the present and links them into already existing networks of memories in order to make sense of them. An event may be initially disturbing, but if the processing system is functioning well, the person learns from the experience and it is stored in memory with appropriate feelings, thoughts and sensations. However, if a trauma disrupts the system, the event is stored in the brain as it was originally experienced. The disturbed memory contains the image, thoughts, physical sensations, and emotions that occurred at the time. External or internal reminders can trigger that memory, and its images, thoughts, sounds, emotions, and sensations cause the symptoms of posttraumatic stress disorder (PTSD).

EMDR differs from other therapies in that it focuses on the physically stored memories in the brain with specific procedures and protocols used to process the memories to an adaptive resolution. The client is always aware of what is occurring and is not taking the suggestions of a therapist. Instead, the client's own processing mechanism activates insights and associations.

EMDR starts with a client history in phase one to identify the past events that set the groundwork for pathology, current situations that trigger disturbance, and the ability to access different types of experiences needed to bring the client to full mental health. Client preparation is the second phase of treatment to assure that the client can stay mentally focused and present with the therapist despite what is coming into consciousness internally. The client is taught self-control techniques to help return to equilibrium at any time. The assessment phase identifies the various aspects of the processing target, including the image, negative belief, emotion, physical sensation, and a preferred belief.

Three reprocessing phases use standardized procedures to guide the client through the different memory networks. These phases also include a form of bilateral stimulation (eye movements, taps, or tones) that many researchers believe stimulate an "orienting response" causing new positive associations to arise as negative ones are discarded. During the reprocessing phases, the trauma memory is transformed with new adaptive insights, emotions, sensations, and beliefs automatically arising. The rape victim can move from shame and guilt to feeling like a strong and resilient woman. These changes can occur very rapidly, often within three sessions.

EMDR sessions end with a closure phase that resolves any distress from incomplete treatment and prepares the client for continued processing between sessions. In addition to PTSD, EMDR treatment can address any clinical complaint based upon or worsened by disturbing life experiences. These more general disturbances are called small "t" trauma. That is, while humiliations in grade school may be commonplace, they can have long-lasting negative effects, having felt "traumatic" when they occurred. They also appear to be stored in the brain in a way that holds the original negative emotions, thoughts, and body sensations. Processing these types of memories can help resolve a wide range of pathologies.

Medications

Many therapists agree that psychiatric medications can help trauma victims respond better to the therapy. The most common medications prescribed to trauma victims are antidepressants and benzodiazepines (antianxiety drugs). Rarely, antipsychotic medications are also prescribed, such as when the individual is in an extremely agitated state or has lapsed into psychosis. Generally, antidepressants take weeks to become fully effective. A patient's energy levels improve first and later their mood begins to improve.

The first antidepressant approved for anxiety was clomipramine (Anafranil), a tricyclic antidepressant. Subsequently the selective serotonin reuptake inhibitors (SSRIs) were developed, and they have largely replaced the tricyclics as antidepressant agents for treating anxiety. Some examples of SSRIs include citalopram (Celexa), fluoxetine (Prozac), paroxetine (Paxil), and sertraline (Zoloft). SSRIs have been shown to influence impulse control, sleep regulation, and hyperarousal symptoms through the increased availability of serotonin to the brain. Clinical research has shown that SSRIs are very helpful in reducing core PTSD symptom clusters, such as hyperarousal, avoidance, and the re-experiencing of trauma. As a result, they are generally the first line of medication treatment for trauma.

There are also serotonin norepinephrine reuptake inhibitors (SNRIs) that inhibit the reuptake of both serotonin and norepinephrine to elevate mood, and they include such drugs as Effexor and duloxetine (Cymbalta). Sometimes atypical antidepressants are used, such as bupropion (Wellbutrin, Wellbutrin XL) that inhibit the reuptake of both norepinephrine and dopamine.

BENZODIAZEPINES (minor tranquilizers) can relieve anxiety and panic attacks, but they are controversial because of their addictive nature and the withdrawal symptoms that may occur upon discontinuation of these drugs. Although an antianxiety drug may be a logical choice for survivors following a traumatic event, more research is needed to determine their therapeutic value for the treatment of PTSD. Commonly used benzodiazepines are diazepam (Valium), alprazolam (Xanax), clonazepam (Klonopin), and lorazepam (Ativan). The benzodiazepines potentiate the effects of GABA in calming arousal and lowering norepinephrine in several areas.

The tricyclics are an older form of antidepressant that is sometimes used to treat patients suffering from trauma disorders. They help to reduce such symptoms as hyperarousal, intrusive recollections, flashbacks, and traumatic nightmares but do not necessarily decrease symptoms of depression. Another even older type of antidepressant are the monoamine oxidase inhibitors (MAOI), such as phelzine (Nardil), which can cause extreme side effects. Because of their numerous side effects and dietary constraints, however, these drugs are now seldom used.

Another type of drug is the mood stabilizer, a medication that is also prescribed to the person with bipolar disorder. Among traumatized individuals, mood stabilizers may help reduce hyperarousal and hyperreactivity symptoms such as insomnia, angry outbursts, mood swings, or irritability. Some examples of mood stabilizers are lithium carbamazepine, valproate, and lamotrigine, an anticonvulsant with mood stabilizing properties. The mood stabilizers are thought to prevent the development of sensitization and of kindling, or the arousal of the emotions surrounding the traumatic event, within the first few hours or days after exposure to such events; however, results with mood stabilizers are mixed.

Alternative Medicine

Complementary alternative medicine is extremely popular in the United States and there are several remedies that may provide some relief to the trau-matized individual.

For example, traditional Chinese medicine is based on 4,000 years of practice and looks at health as the balance of the yin and yang (negative and positive energies). Herbs, acupuncture, nutrition, and forms of exercise (such as tai chi) are used to restore balance to the diseased state, both physical and mental.

Native American Indian healing practices combine spiritual practices, herbal medicine, and purifying ceremonies that have been in use by hundreds of tribes for thousands of years for treating trauma, addictions, and medical illness.

Ayurveda, traditional medicine within India and one of the world's oldest medical systems, is based on energy and balance to restore wholeness to the mind-body system. In this system, all individuals have their own distinct bioenergetic type (*doshas*), known as Vata, Pitta, and Kapha, and it is this harmony of the three doshas that determines health and illness. The emphasis is on the mind, body, and spirit, using such techniques as meditation, aromatherapy, yoga, nutrition, and exercise to trigger the body's own natural healing processes.

Other Treatment Alternatives

There are many treatment alternatives that have few empirical studies but much anecdotal evidence of support.

- **Creative arts therapies:** The use of dance, music, drawings, and creative writing may reduce the symptoms of emotional distress. These activities address the "right brain" neurons, which can be difficult to reach using traditional behavioral talk therapy, such as COGNITIVE BEHAVIORAL THERAPY.
- **Energy therapies:** These therapies are based on the belief that energy fields surround and penetrate the body and that they can be manipulated by movement, meditation, prayer, or by another person who places a hand over the body, without touching the body. This form of therapy is also known as *bioenergetic therapy*.
- **Nutritional approaches:** The use of a broad array of vitamins, herbs, and other supplements have been shown to balance moods and overcome anxieties.
- **Aromatherapy:** In use for more than 6,000 years, since the days of ancient Rome and Egypt, aromatherapy uses oils extracted from flowers, herbs, and plants to treat distress. The olfactory nerves send messages directly into the LIMBIC SYSTEM of the brain. Research has shown that different scents can affect different brainwave patterns. Aromatherapy is used for many disorders, including stress, anxiety, and pain.
- **Mind-body techniques:** These techniques encompass both the mind and the body, and key examples include yoga, exercise, visualization, and deep breathing. Mind-body approaches have become commonplace and are often integrated into a comprehensive treatment approach for trauma survivors. Meditation, hypnosis, biofeedback, and acupuncture, along with massage and chiropractic body-touch forms of manipulations, are used extensively today in treating trauma victims.

Boudewyns, Patrick A., and Robert H. Shipley. *Flooding and Implosive Therapy: Direct Therapeutic Exposure in Clinical Practice.* New York: Plenum Press, 1983.
Olasov Rothbaum, Barbara, and Edna B. Foa. "Cognitive-Behavioral Therapy for Posttraumatic Stress Disorder." In *Traumatic Stress: The Effects of Overwhelming Experience on Mind, Body, and Society,* edited by Bessel A. van der Kolk, Alexander C. McFarlane, and Lars Weisaeth, 491–509. New York: Guilford Press, 2007.
Weine, S., et al. "Testimony Psychotherapy in Bosnian Refugees: A Pilot Study." *American Journal of Psychiatry* 155, no. 12 (December 1998): 1720–1726.

tricyclic antidepressants A specific type of prescribed medication that is sometimes used to treat DEPRESSION, whether it is caused by trauma or another cause. This category of drugs is referred to as *tricyclic* antidepressants because the chemical diagrams for these drugs resemble three connected rings. The first tricyclic, imipramine (Tofranil), was synthesized in a laboratory in the late 1940s. Other examples of commonly prescribed tricyclics are amitriptyline (Elavil), desipramine (Norpramin), and clomipramine (Anafranil).

Tricyclics are sedating and may improve sleep patterns in depressed individuals. They also increase the appetite and may cause weight gain. Other side effects include dry mouth, blurred vision, headache, excessive sweating, urinary hesitation, and constipation. Tricyclics should be used cautiously in persons with heart problems.

Tricyclic antidepressants should not be taken together with monoamine oxidase (MAO) inhibitors, another category of antidepressant. The individual who has been taking an MAO inhibitor should wait at least several weeks from when the last MAO inhibitor was taken before using a tricyclic or any other form of antidepressant.

The tricyclics have also been found to be helpful in treating pain disorders (as an analgesic), migraines, enuresis, attention-deficit hyperactivity disorder (ADHD), and ANXIETY DISORDERS. In the 1980s, considerable research was devoted to the use of tricyclics as a treatment resource for agoraphobia. Empirical studies validated its success with this population.

See also DEPRESSION; SELECTIVE SEROTONIN REUPTAKE INHIBITOR; SEROTONIN NOREPINEPHRINE REUPTAKE INHIBITOR.

Two Factor Model   See MOWRER'S TWO FACTOR THEORY

Type I, II, and III trauma   In an article published in 1991, Lenore Terr, a psychiatrist who specialized in childhood trauma, described two symptom clusters she had seen in children with traumatic reactions. She called the first symptom cluster Type I trauma, whereas types II and III were more complex, long-lasting, and difficult to treat. Type I trauma was characterized by an acute reaction to a specific event that produced detailed memories, what children called "omens" and misperceptions or distortions of the event when recalled.

Type I Trauma

Terr's research indicates that Type I trauma symptoms usually occur after a single, unexpected but traumatic experience that is difficult to forget because of persistent FLASHBACKS, avoidance

behavior, and high levels of arousal. The impairment involves one or more major areas of childhood functioning. If the child is older than three years old when the event occurs, he or she tends to retain memories of the event even in a distorted form. The Type I trauma is also known as "simple" trauma and some theorists even extended the concept to adult traumas and talked about them as "simple" or "complex" (Type II).

In Terr's original formulation, a person could have both Type I and Type II trauma simultaneously. With adults, we see that a Type II trauma in childhood puts the individual at risk for developing a Type I trauma later in life with specific events. Children with Type II trauma are usually later diagnosed with conduct disorder, attention deficit disorders, depression, or dissociative disorders.

When Type I victims meet with mental health professionals they can usually describe the critical event in great detail, along with emotional responses appropriate for the age at which the event occurred. Short-term therapies, particularly EYE MOVEMENT DESENSITIZATION AND REPROCESSING (EMDR) and SOMATIC EXPERIENCING therapy, usually prove very effective in processing the trauma and eliminating its powerful influence on present-day events.

Type II Trauma

While the Type I trauma was chronically relived as an event in one's life, the Type II traumas were seen as more "complex," involving chronic or repeated exposure to traumatic events over a period of time. Consequently, Type II traumas were more environmental in nature and extended over a period of time. Because of the chronic nature of the Type II trauma, massive denial or NUMBING, DISSOCIATION, and rage were present as coping skills. If the child is less than three years of age and declarative memory had not yet developed, the reaction would be stored as a sensory or body memory and could result later in "visions" or physical sensations. The chronic nature and intensity of the traumatic experience are major variables in the development of Type II trauma. Dissociation is almost always present as a way to cope with the ongoing abusive situation such as child abuse and sexual abuse. When Type II trauma extends into adult traumatic reactions, it is called "complex" trauma or disorders of extreme stress not otherwise specified (DESNOS).

Type II trauma victims usually come into therapy with a comorbid (coexisting) complaint such as depression, dependency and trust issues, and relationship problems. Poor self-esteem, feelings of shame, and difficulty trusting others are characteristically present. Since denial, repression, and dissociation have been both survival and coping skills, clients usually bring those to the diagnostic or therapy sessions. Clients usually also have a history of prolonged stressful conditions such as poverty, illness, physical or sexual abuse, war, or neglect.

Type III Trauma

In a published article in 1999, Eldra Solomon and Kathleen Heide proposed the introduction of a Type III trauma, which divided the Type II into two separate categories based on the severity of the intrusion or traumatic experiences. The first category was the Type II described above but the second category was based on their clinical experience with more extreme chronic situations. Said the authors, "It [Type III trauma] results from multiple and pervasive violent events beginning at an early age and continuing for years." Often there were severe boundary violations such as those seen in rituals in cult cultures with multiple perpetrators, force, and sadistic intrusions. Usually both physical and sexual abuse occurred along with torture, sadistic rituals, and violent physical and sexual acts.

The Type III trauma victims usually present themselves as feeling suicidal and hopeless for no obvious reason. Their initial evaluation of childhood is usually positive, but careful and extensive history taking will uncover patterns of prolonged severe abuse. PTSD symptoms are usually intense but memory, emotions, and body sensations are difficult to identify due to intense and automatic dissociative behaviors.

The history of clients with Type III trauma is usually littered with disappointing and abusive relationships, avoidance of intimacy, and major trust issues. The identity or self-perception of affected people is unclear and they have difficulty acknowledging and expressing their feelings. There is often clear somatization, frequent headaches, and a history of chemical dependency.

The treatment of Type III trauma clients is complex, long-term, and multiphasic, or requiring many different approaches at different times. It requires a longer period of treatment, a strong and trusting client-therapist relationship, and willingness to confront trauma experiences and issues. Since trauma, particularly early forms, affects the development of many age-appropriate behaviors, the teaching and development of adult level new behaviors, particularly social, is necessary. Self-esteem, containment, and modulation of feelings, integration of client identity, and desensitization of the effects of past events are just some of the therapeutic goals.

See also INSTRUMENTS/SCALES/SURVEYS THAT EVALUATE POSTTRAUMATIC STRESS DISORDER (PTSD); THERAPY, TYPES OF; TRAUMATIC MEMORY; TRAUMA VORTEX.

unbidden recollections of traumatic memories
See FLASHBACK.

Uniform Crime Reports (UCR) A compilation by the Federal Bureau of Investigation (FBI) of data on crimes reported in the United States by law enforcement agencies, including such crimes as murder, rape, robbery, burglary, and motor vehicle theft. This data is published annually by the FBI in its publication, *Crime in the United States*.

Police agency participation in the Uniform Crime Reports is voluntary, although many law enforcement agencies voluntarily provide the information. According to preliminary data for 2006, the rate of violent crimes (murder, forcible rape, robbery, etc.) decreased by 2.6 percent compared to the number of violent crimes that occurred in 2005.

Federal Bureau of Investigation, "Crime in the United States, 2007." Available online. URL: http://www.fbi.gov/ucr/cius2007/offenses/violent_crime/index.html. Accessed December 5, 2008.

Validity of Cognition (VoC)   A rating scale that was devised by Francine Shapiro in 1995, which is part of the procedure used in EYE MOVEMENT DESENSITIZATION AND REPROCESSING (EMDR). The scale provides seven choices to evaluate the client's intensity of beliefs about him- or herself, ranging from 1 (feels completely false) to 7 (feels totally true). The VoC is important because it provides a self-report scale of progress in desensitizing traumatic material and in shifting negative to positive self-judgment regarding the traumatic event. The SUBJECTIVE UNITS OF DISCOMFORT (SUDS) rating indicates a shift in intensity of reaction to images or senses of the traumatic event, but VoC reflects an actual cognitive belief shift from negative cognitions about oneself regarding the event (in the present) to positive cognitions regarding oneself in the present. So a rape victim, looking at the traumatic event might see herself as "stupid and naïve" as a negative cognition. After desensitization a positive cognition is "installed" or programmed in as an association to the situation. After desensitization the victim might have a positive self-evaluation of "I did the best I could" in the situation and rate the VoC as 7.

verbally accessible memories (VAMS)   See DUAL REPRESENTATION THEORY OF POSTTRAUMATIC STRESS DISORDER.

vicarious traumatization   A form of POSTTRAUMATIC STRESS DISORDER that may develop in helping professionals working with traumatized individuals as a result of directly empathizing and identifying with the issues and stressors impacting their clients. Therapists, for example, may suffer from vicarious traumatization based on severe psychological trauma as described by their patients. Sometimes there are specific events that traumatize victims and then later also traumatize their therapists, clergyman, trauma worker, or paramedic. For example, victims who were traumatized by losses suffered in Hurricane Katrina or other natural disasters often speak to support personnel about deaths of pets, friends, and relatives, loss of home and so on. Trauma workers who have had past trauma in their lives are the most susceptible to develop vicarious traumatic reactions themselves. In some cases, the MEDIA increases the traumatization of others through constant coverage of the traumatic event, such as the continuous images of the wreckage of the Twin Towers in New York on SEPTEMBER 11.

In some cases the helping professional has suffered personal losses as well as in the traumatic event, such as in a NATURAL DISASTER. If they are aware of their own experiences, they can usually put those aside to listen carefully to the other person's story.

The term *vicarious traumatization* was initially coined by McCann and Pearlman in 1990. McCann and Pearlman compared vicarious traumatization to a sort of infection and said that, eventually, the tormented recollections of the traumatized patient can "infect" the therapist. The phenomenon is also called bystander traumatization and may affect ordinary people not directly harmed by a traumatic event but who are exposed to the victims of trauma. It arises from the ability to empathize with the position of another person. Many combat experiences involve bystander traumatization in soldiers who see comrades and friends killed or injured. Children and adult bystanders who witness repeated abuse inflicted upon others have higher levels of stress than others.

Vicarious traumatization is similar to countertransference but with an important distinction:

With countertransference, the therapist responds to the client's experiences whereas with vicarious traumatization, the therapist's life (or the life of another helping professional) is significantly changed for the worse.

Many helping professionals develop vicarious traumatization; for example, physicians and emergency service personnel who are treating traumatized patients suffering from physical or sexual abuse or from wounds caused by a hurricane or natural disaster may experience vicarious traumatization.

Symptoms and Diagnostic Path

According to an article by Christian Pross, M.D., in a 2006 issue of *Torture*, some indicators of vicarious traumatization include

- an overidentification with the client
- denying the client's trauma (an unconscious mechanism to avoid traumatization)
- social withdrawal
- feelings of extreme vulnerability
- generalized hopelessness
- an increased sensitization to violence
- changes in one's sense of identity and world view

In their article on vicarious traumatization in a 2006 issue of *Pediatrics*, Paula A. Madrid and Stephanie J. Schacher said of doctors who were working with traumatized populations, "Extreme feelings of hopelessness and despair may arise, and symptoms similar to post-traumatic stress disorder such as nightmares, intrusive images, hypervigilance, exaggerated startle response, and other forms of autonomic hyperarousal, as well as transient dissociative experiences, may develop."

The authors said that pediatricians affected by vicarious traumatization may unconsciously but excessively distance themselves emotionally from their patients as a means of coping. They may also feel guilty or have a sense that they *should* have been able to do more, which may result in a professional paralysis.

Some red flags of maladaptive coping identified by Madrid and Schacher include

- preoccupation with clients' problems
- loss of interest in formerly enjoyed pleasures
- depersonalization
- weight loss or insomnia
- feelings of hopelessness and/or helplessness
- substance abuse
- violent or suicidal thoughts

Treatment Options and Outlook

Psychotherapy is often indicated for vicarious traumatization, as may be a guided form of self-assessment. If the individual becomes chronically depressed or anxious, medication (antianxiety or SSRIs) may be necessary. Affected individuals are also urged to reclaim past activities they enjoyed, which may seem unimportant in the face of severe disaster. They may fail to exercise, sleep well, or eat a healthy diet, all of which are important means to recovery.

Madrid and Schacher recommended that doctors should assess themselves to know how they behave when they are under stress. In addition, they recommended deep-breathing exercises, positive visual imagery, muscle relaxation, mediation, and other options.

Risk Factors and Preventive Measures

Helping professionals who have been traumatized themselves have an increased risk for vicarious traumatization, as do individuals who are compelled, as part of their work, to empathize with severely traumatized patients, such as those who work with abused children. Women may have a greater risk for vicarious traumatization than men.

Dr. Pross says that therapeutic self-awareness is the best way to prevent vicarious traumatization. Other means of prevention are regular examination by both colleagues and external supervisors, a limited caseload, opportunities to attend training sabbaticals, and avoiding "workaholism."

Therapists Who Counsel Sex Offenders

Often those who are vicariously traumatized are dealing with the victims of a trauma. However, in their article in *Trauma, Violence, & Abuse*, Heather M. Moulden and Philip Firestone discussed vicarious traumatization that occurs among therapists working with sex offenders. In this case, the therapist treats the predators rather than the victims and is often repelled and disgusted by the sex offenders' comments. Said the authors, "In addition to their own reactions, sexual offender therapists may also be affected by the offenders' reactions to the abuse, such as denial, arousal, victim-blame, or remorselessness." Some therapists described their feelings of anxiety, depression, isolation, vulnerability, and a decreased trust in others.

Moulden and Firestone also found that vicarious traumatization was more common among female therapists than male therapists and also that the setting for the therapy was important; for example, therapy provided in prisons or secure hospital units was more traumatic for therapists than therapy provided in a community setting.

In one study, about one-third of sexual offender therapists reported symptoms of hypervigilance with regard to their own safety. They also developed feelings of distrust toward others, especially those who worked with or volunteered with children. Said the authors, "Hypervigilance regarding one's own and others' behavior exemplifies the schematic shift described as a hallmark of VT and appears to be a commonly observed reaction to the delivery of sexual offender treatment."

Another problem with sex offenders is the high recidivism rate, which therapists may perceive as their own failure, although treatment of sex offenders is difficult and often fails. In one survey described by Moulden and Firestone, therapists responded to reoffenses of their sex-offending clients with anger (84%), disillusionment (79%), depression (74%), feelings of incompetence (73%), feelings of inadequacy (58%), and feelings of guilt (42%). In addition, the majority of male and female therapists felt personally threatened by their clients, sometimes with justifiable cause.

See also COMPASSION FATIGUE; RIPPLE EFFECT; SECONDARY TRAUMATIZATION.

Madrid, Paula A., and Stephanie J. Schacher. "A Critical Concern: Pediatrician Self-care after Disasters." *Pediatrics* 117, no. 5, Supplement Article (May 2006): S454–S457.
Moulden, Heather M., and Philip Firestone. "Vicarious Traumatization: The Impact on Therapists Who Work with Sexual Offenders." *Trauma, Violence & Abuse* 8, no. 1 (January 2007): 67–83.
Pross, Christian, M.D. "Burnout, Vicarious Traumatization and Its Prevention." *Torture* 16, no. 1 (2006): 1–9.

virtual reality exposure/virtual reality graded exposure (VRGE) Using computer-generated environments in lieu of self-generating images and powerful experiences of emotional pain. Traditional image exposure therapy re-exposes the individual to memories of traumatic events to help them reduce POSTTRAUMATIC STRESS DISORDER (PTSD) symptoms, whereas virtual reality exposure (VRE) therapy allows the individual to "re-enter" the traumatic environment through computer-generated sights and sounds. VRE facilitates the individual's emotional engagement in reducing acute PTSD.

Computer-generated environments are rich visual and auditory experiences, and they encourage individuals to pace themselves and avoid becoming overwhelmed by the re-experiencing. Virtual reality technology allows for graded exposure to increasingly fearful virtual images that can be carefully monitored throughout this process. It allows individuals to feel in control and play an active role in their experiences. Research by Difede and Hoffman (2002) has shown that VRE is effective in the treatment of anxiety disorder, PTSD, and with specific phobias, such as a fear of flying or a fear of heights.

Rothbaum (2001) used VRE to study its effectiveness on PTSD symptom reduction while working with Vietnam veterans The individual wore headgear with a display screen and stereo headphones that provided visual and audio cues from a war zone. The veteran "entered" that environment, heard the Huey helicopters fly over a virtual jungle and, over time, was able to diminish anxiety-provoking cues in a gradual and controlled manner, thus becoming desensitized to these stimuli. The clients exposed to VRE have shown encouraging results in a significant reduction from the baseline established at the beginning of therapy in symptoms associated with specific traumatic experiences six months after treatment.

See also THERAPY, TYPES OF.

Difede, J., and H. Hoffman. "Virtual Reality Exposure Therapy for World Trade Center Post-Traumatic Stress Disorder: A Case Report." *Cyber Psychology & Behavior* 5, no. 6 (2002): 529–535.

Rothbaum, Barbara O., et al. "Virtual Reality Exposure Therapy for Vietnam Veterans with Posttraumatic Stress Disorder." *Journal of Clinical Psychiatry* 62, no. 8 (August 2001): 617–622.

visual/kinesthetic dissociation (V/KD)   An exposure-based therapy approach to help trauma survivors to process traumatic memories from a more detached perspective. Visual/kinesthetic dissociation (V/KD) was first described by Erich Fromm as a procedure to separate or dissociate the "observing ego" from the "experiencing ego." In this therapy, the person is described as being "in the picture" or "not in the picture" while accessing a mental image. In the case of a person observing himself or herself in the picture, the situation is called a two-place V/K dissociation. Fromm maintained that in hypnosis, pain can be observed (observing ego) yet not felt (experiencing ego).

Bandler (1985) described a three-place V/K dissociation as having a person watch himself or herself from a third position, which allows him or her to watch himself or herself watching himself or herself go through the traumatic experience. In this way, the person can remain comfortable while still remembering the experience because the kinesthetic (feeling) portion is dissociated from the visual memory.

V/KD Procedure

The procedure in V/KD begins with the therapist establishing safety and comfort for the client and then directing the client to visualize a time just prior to the traumatic event. Next, the therapist asks the client to take on the role of observer (detachment) by imagining watching himself or herself watch himself or herself relive the traumatic experience in a movie. This detaching is achieved by asking the client to float out of themselves in order to watch themselves. The client gains comfort because he or she can control the image, making it smaller or changing colors, as well as controlling the sounds and even making the movie silent, if necessary.

After the process is repeated as many times as necessary for the traumatic memories to become less intense, the therapist has the client float back into his or her body in the present time, with feelings of strength and control.

Dietrich (2000) points out that clinical experience has shown that exposure therapy, as in the guided dissociation process in the V/KD technique, may assist traumatized individuals in distancing themselves from the emotional distress of the trauma when faced with trauma-related stimuli. Watching the "movie" can lead to cognitive reprocessing and integration.

There are many variations to V/KD, with one being the REWIND TECHNIQUE, an integrative technique that has the individuals watch themselves as in a film about the traumatic event and then replay it backwards (rewind) and re-experience the trauma as it actually happened with all sensory (sound, smell, sensations) memories intact. Once the rewind goes backwards to a starting point representing a good image, it is stopped with the individual holding onto a positive image.

See also THERAPY, TYPES OF.

Bandler, R. *Using Your Brain for a Change.* Moab, Utah: Real People Press, 1985.

Dietrich, A. "Review of Visual/Kinesthetic Disassociation in the Treatment of Posttraumatic Disorders: Theory, Efficacy and Practice Recommendations." *Traumatology* 6, no. 2 (August 2000): 85–107.

Kosiey, P., and L. McLeod. "Visual-Kinesthetic Dissociation in the Treatment of Victims of Rape," *Professional Psychology: Research and Practice* 18, no. 3 (June 1987): 276–282.

visual memory   The ability to recall sensory visual experiences from our memories such as mental images of places, objects, people, and events. Traumatic images may occur in FLASHBACKS, with the individual involuntarily recalling vivid experiences of war, child or sexual abuse, or any other horrific life-threatening event. *Iconic memory* is a brief visual memory of a visual stimulus, first proposed by George Sperling in 1960. If you were to look at an image, then close your eyes, the mental image you "see" in your mind is your iconic memory. Sperling showed that iconic memories were fragile, decayed rapidly, and were not actively maintained, hence were a temporary visual memory and not long-term.

vulnerability   The degree to which one is susceptible to developing traumatic reactions following a traumatic event. Yehuda, Flory, Southwick, and Charney developed a "translational research agenda" for studies of this resistance. RESILIENCE TO STRESS is the quality attributed to those individuals who do not develop posttraumatic stress reactions with traumatic events. The most important psychological resilience-related factors identified were "positive affectivity and optimism, cognitive flexibility, coping, social support, emotion regulation, and mastery." The authors argue that key BRAIN areas associated with TRAUMA, mainly discovered from animal studies, have been located and some of their dynamics uncovered.

Exposure to adversity or trauma does not necessarily lead to impairment and the development of psychopathology in all people. In fact, the majority of people exposed to traumatic events do not develop lasting POSTTRAUMATIC STRESS DISORDER (PTSD). Human against human abuse (violence, TORTURE, bullying, and so forth) seem to produce the highest incidence of traumatic reaction, as opposed to traumatic reaction to NATURAL DISASTERS, such as hurricanes or floods. Understanding the mechanisms of resilience will hopefully lead to prevention measures and better intervention treatments.

See also INSTRUMENTS/SCALES/SURVEYS THAT EVALUATE POSTTRAUMATIC STRESS DISORDER (PTSD); TRAUMATIC MEMORY; TRAUMA VORTEX.

Yehuda, R., J. D. Flory, S. Southwick, and D. S. Charney. "Developing an Agenda for Translational Studies of Resilience and Vulnerability following Trauma Exposure." *Annals of the New York Academy of Science* 1071, no. 1 (2006): 379–396.

war neurosis   See COMBAT STRESS REACTION.

war zone stress reaction   Commonly known as COMBAT STRESS REACTION, war zone stress reaction may be a more descriptive term to describe severe stress in war zones such as Iraq and Afghanistan.

According to the U.S. Veterans Administration, using the term *war zone stress reaction* carries more meaning and is less stigmatizing to soldiers having difficulty due to events other than direct life-threats from combat.

Symptoms and Diagnostic Path
The symptoms of war zone stress reactions include withdrawal, restlessness, psychomotor deficiencies, confusion, sweating, nausea, inactivity with fatigue, heightened sense of threat, severe suspiciousness and distrust, and nightmares.

Direct combat exposure is not the only stressor of war affecting the soldier. War zone stressors include: exposure to suffering civilians, exposure to death and destruction, guilt of personal action or inaction, anger or rage at not being prepared or trained for war experiences, nuclear or biological threats, behavior of the enemy (suicide bombers), an array of perceived threats, and the sadness of loss.

Treatment and Outlook
The military has used the BICEPS and PIES principles to treat war zone stress reactions. BICEPS' six principles to help in recovery are:

1. brevity—brief, short-term treatment (1–3 days) close to unit
2. immediacy—identify need for care immediately or as soon as possible
3. centrality—provide treatment/care not in hospital, a location for rest
4. expectancy—soldiers know they are returning to duty, not ill, and understand symptoms will pass
5. proximity—treat as close to unit as possible and have friends visit
6. simplicity—treatment is directed for return to duty, medications only when necessary

The PIES principle implies that treatment is carried out in a safe environment close to the combat area and as quickly as possible. The acronym PIES stands for

- proximity—treatment carried out close to the battlefields or front lines
- immediacy—treatment as soon as possible after onset of symptoms
- expectancy—with full expectation that they will return to duty
- simplicity—food, drink, rest

Wisely used, both BICEPS and PIES not only help soldiers recover from temporary stress reactions but may also help reduce the risk of these soldiers developing posttraumatic stress disorder (PTSD).

waterboarding   A form of interrogation in which a person is strapped to a board while water is poured over his or her face and the person feels that he or she is drowning. The purpose of this controversial form of interrogation is to obtain information, particularly from someone who is believed to be associated with terrorist activities. Proponents believe that this procedure is acceptable because the information elicited from the person being interrogated can save lives. Others believe this practice is barbaric and cruel and that it should be banned.

GLOSSARY

affective valence Negative or positive emotions that are directly associated with an event. In the case of a traumatic event, the emotions are negative.

agnosia An inability to comprehend sensory information. A condition caused by damage to the occipito-temporal area but not the sense organ itself.

blood-brain barrier An efficient filtering system that blocks infectious and large molecule agents from entering the brain. Bacterial molecules are too large to pass through the blood-brain membrane.

blood pressure/beats per minute (BPM/(BPM) Blood pressure and pulse (beats per minute) are two means to measure the level of anxiety and arousal in the body. An elevated blood pressure and pulse indicate arousal and possible anxiety.

butyrophenone Antipsychotic drugs sometimes used in the case of an acute psychotic reaction, which may be a response to a traumatic event or occur as a result of internal thought processes.

cingulate gyrus In the brain, the cingulate gyrus sits above the corpus callosum and is part of the limbic system in the brain. It has a major role in decisions regarding threats to the organism.

cognitive restructuring (CR) The identification of negative thoughts and beliefs in order to replace them with more helpful and positive thoughts.

cognitive rituals The constant and involuntary replaying in the mind of all details surrounding a traumatic event in an effort to resolve the negative reactions.

cognitive therapy for trauma related guilt (CT-TRG) A program developed by Edward Kubany in 1998 that helps survivors of trauma determine their own negative thoughts related to the trauma so that they can be trained to replace these thoughts with more constructive ones.

coherence, physiological The relationship between heart rate variability and emotional states. Physiological coherence is characterized by a high degree of order and harmony in the body.

combat severity indices Quantitative measures of events that allow leaders and others to determine the effect of combat on troops.

command rape A term used by victim's advocates to describe women in the U.S. military who are manipulated to have sex repeatedly with their superiors (which includes any military rank above theirs).

comorbid disorders Psychiatric and/or medical disorders that occur concurrently; for example, many people with posttraumatic stress disorder also have depression or anxiety disorders.

confabulation Elaborate details that are not true, provided by a person who cannot remember the facts of a situation.

contact victimization The emotional impact on a therapist of listening and responding to a client's discussion of severe trauma. It is a form of secondary traumatization, also known as bystander traumatization.

continuous traumatic stress syndrome A term coined in 1987 to refer to the situation of black residents of South African towns who were subjected to constant violence at the hands of government officials as well as from vigilantes within the black community.

counter-disaster syndrome A condition in which, subsequent to a disaster, some people attempt to accomplish actions that they believe to be important in assisting others; however, their efforts are insufficient and purposeless because they are so overwhelmed by their own emotions and the fatigue generated by the disaster.

critical incident Any negative situation that exceeds the normal experiences of an individual and that can potentially overwhelm his or her ability to cope and function effectively.

cross traumatization Severe reactions to the traumatic events experienced by others.

cumulative trauma disorder (CTD) In the field of information technology, CTD refers to injuries due to repetitive motion in the course of daily activities, such as carpal tunnel syndrome, tendonitis, and bursitis.

demobilization One key component of Everly and Mitchell's Critical Incident Stress Management model, this is an intervention provided to emergency service personnel in a large scale traumatic event where large groups of personnel are given information and rest sessions during the event.

depersonalization A feeling of being dissociated from the body, as if a person were watching him- or herself but not experiencing directly what was happening.

depressed mood A temporary feeling of sadness or low affect that commonly occurs among many people in response to daily events, illness, or other factors. A depressed mood is not the same as a clinical depression, which may last for months, during which time the individual experiences little or no elevation in mood state.

derealization A feeling, which often occurs subsequent to experiencing a traumatic event, of not being in a real environment and, instead, seeming to be on a television or movie set.

dialectic of trauma A concept developed by Judith Herman in 1992 to describe the conflict experienced by trauma survivors between their wish to deny that a traumatic event happened and the need to discuss what happened with others.

dimensions of functioning Refers to the various categories or dimensions of functioning, usually within a family. Alcoholic families, for example, tend to experience lower levels of family functioning, which invites traumatic experiences.

disorders of extreme stress not otherwise specified (DESNOS) A category in which multiple traumas have occurred that create a mixed picture of cause and symptoms. This is sometimes called complex trauma.

distal developmental disturbance Refers to the fact that trauma early in development will affect an individual's behavior far into the future.

double depression A situation in which dysthymic disorder (mild depressive symptoms) leads to major depressive disorder.

dynamic energy healing A psychic or physical healing technique that involves working in the body's energy field to promote balance and release of stored traumatic experience.

embedded trauma A traumatic experience that is unavailable to the consciousness but may exert an influence on current behavior or may be triggered into awareness by some ongoing event that is similar in nature to the trauma.

emotional contagion An empathetic reaction that causes the experiencing of similar emotions to others observed to be suffering from traumatic events.

enduring personality changes, not attributed to brain damage and disease Personality changes caused by severe trauma, such as being a victim of torture or being taken as a hostage.

formulation of meaning A survivor's search to make sense of a traumatic event and its aftermath.

full remission (FR) An oxymoron that is used in psychiatry to describe a full recovery from a disorder; however, the term *remission* implies that one is never really cured of any disorder, and that it lies in wait, ready to return.

glutamate A major excitatory neurotransmitter in the brain.

Healing from the Body Level Up (HBLU) A form of trauma therapy developed by Judith Swack, who describes herself as "a Ph.D. biochemist and immunologist and a neuro-linguistic programmer." It combines biomedical science, neurolinguistic programming, psychology, applied kinesiology, energy psychology techniques, shamanic techniques, and spiritual practices, but its effectiveness has not been scientifically proven.

heart brain A concept that was introduced by J. Andrew Armour, a neurocardiologist, to denote the fact that the heart is a complex neurophysiological system of its own, or a "heart brain."

homicide trauma syndrome Trauma experienced by family members of a murder victim that is further complicated by the anger and confusion related to the murder and which overlays the normal grief of bereavement.

hopelessness theory According to this theory, the impact of a traumatic event is related to the perceptions individuals have about the degree of negativity related to it as well as the length of the impact on the individual. The individual often does nothing to deal with or remedy a problematic situation because of the belief that any action will not resolve or cure the situation. The individual, thus, experiences a state of despair.

hyperarousal   A state of increased psychological and physiological arousal in which the following effects frequently occur: reduced pain tolerance, anxiety, exaggeration of startle responses, insomnia, fatigue, and accentuation of personality traits.

hypermnesia   The exceptional recollection of the details of events, usually related to the use of memory-enhancing drugs, hypnosis, or to the individual's response to a traumatic event.

hypocortisolemia   A condition of abnormally low levels of cortisol in the bloodstream caused by an insufficient amount of cortisol produced by the adrenal glands. It is also known as *chronic primary adrenal insufficiency* and is one extreme of cortisol production seen in trauma victims.

identity confusion   A confusion usually experienced in teenage years about one's identity as an individual. Traumatic experience during identity confusion can perpetuate the sense of confusion.

lucid memory   A memory experience that closely reproduces the original experience.

malignant memories   A term that usually refers to the recall of traumatic or unpleasant, distressing memories that are "malignant" because they have helped to form patterns of self-destructive or unproductive behavior.

negative feedback loop   The regulatory systems of the body (and probably the psychological systems as well) operate by feedback or feedback loops that signal when an action has reached a preset or accepted point and then terminate or diminish the actions.

paraesthesia/paresthesia   Feelings of pins and needles or creeping sensations in some part or all of the body. Such feelings may occur when an individual is transfixed with fear and/or anxiety and may occur with posttraumatic stress disorder (PTSD).

partial remission   Partial remission signifies a disorder that is still symptomatic but is reduced in intensity or severity.

pathogenic beliefs   Accepted ideas that are harmful to the individual, such as "I am a worthless individual."

peripheral autonomic functioning   The autonomic nervous system is part of the peripheral nervous system in the body. The peripheral nervous system consists of neurons located outside the central nervous system (brain and spinal cord).

phantom limb   A perceived itching or pain in an arm or leg that was amputated or otherwise lost, as, for example, the result of an accident.

positive and negative symptoms of posttraumatic stress disorder (PTSD)   Usually refers to coping with PTSD symptoms. Negative symptoms include avoidance, anger, social isolation, and substance abuse. Positive symptoms include seeking treatment, reestablishing a good health routine, and seeking support and social contact.

positive cognitions (PC)   Thoughts installed as part of eye movement desensitization and reprocessing (EMDR) for the treatment of trauma. Positive cognitions replace negative cognitions in viewing or remembering a traumatic event, once it is desensitized, or promote the more empowered and positive self-perception a client would desire as a result of EMDR treatment.

precipitating events   Occurrences that lead to the subsequent development of a serious trauma, such as combat experiences, a serious car accident, a sexual assault, and a severe natural disaster such as an extreme earthquake, tsunami, or hurricane.

predatory aggression   Trauma produced aggression aimed at a clearly defined target, usually based on a perceived threat.

predictors of disordered arousal   A term usually applied to sadistic rapists who associate sexual arousal with assault and violence. Generally, these perpetrators are victims of abuse and traumatic experiences.

premorbid personality   Refers to a personality that existed prior to the onset of a disorder.

psychiatric morbidity   The incidence or rate of psychiatric problems that develop within a population, usually after a traumatic event.

psychogenic amnesia   The loss of memory as a result of a severely traumatic event.

psychological impairment   A close look at the *Diagnostic and Statistical Manual* published by the American Psychiatric Association reveals that behavior becomes a "disorder" when functioning is impaired. Psychological impairment is the loss of function due to psychological factors.

repression   Burying a particularly unpleasant memory or set of memories within the mind, often memories that occurred in childhood. Such memories may include physical and/or sexual abuse or other traumatic experiences.

resourcing   The process of preparing a client for trauma therapy, which may take months or years to accomplish and usually focuses on affect modulation and control.

safety   "Do you feel safe?" is perhaps the one question a person could ask that would predict past trauma, because traumatized people almost always never feel fully safe.

secondary responses   Responses associated with emotional stress or emotional responses (primary responses). The secondary responses might include withdrawal, dependence, interpersonal mistrust, lack of self-esteem, helplessness, hopelessness, and aggression and occur as a consequence of experiencing primary stressors or dysregulating stressors.

Self-Injury Trauma Scale   This scale attempts to quantify and classify surface tissue damage caused by self-injury. Self-injurious behavior is categorized by location in the body, type of injury, number of injuries, and estimate of severity.

self-soothing   Taking deliberate steps to calm oneself in the face of emotional arousal.

sensorimotor psychotherapy   Psychotherapy that evolved out of verbal interactions with clients, usually in a one-to-one format. Sensorimotor psychotherapy utilizes the body as a form of language for communication.

sequela/sequelae   From the Latin *sequi*, meaning "to follow" in time. The term was used to describe the gradual intensification of trauma events in survivors of Nazi persecution.

Social Cognition and Object Relations Scale (SCORS)   A scale that assesses psychological functioning by using client narratives related to an array of preselected vague pictorial scenes.

spatial representation of threat   The spatial and contextual aspects of experience occur in the brain through the action of the hippocampus. Traumatic threat is generally mediated by the right hemisphere hippocampus.

spiritual psychotherapy   Psychotherapy is aimed at alleviating mental, emotional, and cognitive distress; spiritual psychotherapy incorporates a spiritual aspect, which also exists in trauma and is usually expressed as a lack or loss of meaning in life and a sense of alientation or separateness. The spiritual quest, which is often a goal of therapy, is to reconnect with others and with life itself.

stress-induced analgesia (SIA)   Relief from pain that is brought on by severe stress.

transient situational disturbance   An early *Diagnostic and Statistical Manual (DSM)* category thought to be a temporary stress reaction that would abate with time. It is one of the precursors to PTSD categorization.

trauma membrane   Subsequent to a traumatic event, some survivors begin to withdraw and envelop themselves in a protective membrane that reduces the chance of encountering stimuli that might trigger or reactivate the original trauma. Also called psychic defense, this membrane often is provided by a network of trusted friends and family members in a compassionate effort to protect the survivor. This membrane could be functional or dysfunctional, depending on how long it stays intact.

trauma neurosis   An older term, mainly used in Freudian psychology, to denote a neurosis that was caused by outside factors rather than by unconscious material.

trauma reconstruction   Refers to the surgical techniques used to rebuild traumatic bodily injuries sustained mostly in motor vehicle accidents. It can also refer to detailing a trauma with a client.

APPENDIX I
IMPORTANT NATIONAL ORGANIZATIONS

This appendix includes major organizations that provide information, resources, or therapy to individuals who have been traumatized or their families and colleagues.

Adult Children of Alcoholics World Service Organization
P.O. Box 3216
Torrance, CA 90510
(310) 534-1815
http://www.adultchildren.org

Adult Survivors of Child Abuse
Morris Center for eHealing from Child Abuse
P.O. Box 14477
San Francisco, CA 94114
(415) 928-4576
http://www.ascasupport.org

Al-Anon
1600 Corporate Landing Parkway
Virginia Beach, VA 23454
(757) 563-1600
http://www.al-anon.org

Alateen
1600 Corporate Landing Parkway
Virginia Beach, VA 23454
(888) 425-2666
http://www.ai-anon.alateen.org

Alcoholics Anonymous World Services, Inc.
Grand Central Station
P.O. Box 459
New York, NY 10163
(212) 870-3400
http://www.alcoholics-anonymous.org

Alliance for Children and Families
11700 West Lake Park Drive

Milwaukee, WI 53244
(414) 359-1040
http://www.alliance1.org

American Academy of Addiction Psychiatry
1010 Vermont Avenue NW
Suite 710
Washington, DC 20005
(202) 393-4484
http://www.aaap.org

American Academy of Child and Adolescent Psychiatry
3615 Wisconsin Avenue NW
Washington, DC 20016
(202) 966-7300
http://www.aacap.org

American Academy of Pediatrics
National Headquarters
141 Northwest Point Boulevard
P.O. Box 927
Elk Gove Village, IL 60007
(847) 434-4000
http://www.aap.org

American Art Therapy Asociation, Inc.
5999 Stevenson Avenue
Alexandria, VA 22304
(888) 290-0878
http://www.arttherapy.org

American Association of Suicidology
5221 Wisconsin Avenue NW
Washington, DC 20015
(202) 237-2280
http://www.suicidology.org

American Council on Alcoholism
1000 East Indian School Road
Phoenix, AZ 85014

(703) 248-9005
http://www.aca-usa.org

American Foundation for Suicide Prevention
120 Wall Street
22nd Floor
New York, NY 10005
(888) 333-2377
http://www.asfsp.org

American Medical Association
515 North State Street
Chicago, IL 60610
(312) 464-5000
http://www.ama-assn.org

American Nurses Association
600 Maryland Avenue SW
Suite 100 West
Washington, DC 20024
(202) 554-4444
http://www.nursingworld.org

American Professional Society on the Abuse of Children
P.O. Box 30669
Charleston, SC 29417
(843) 764-2905
http://www.apsac.com

American Psychiatric Association
1400 K Street NW
Washington, DC 20005
(202) 682-6000
http://www.psych.org

American Psychological Association
750 First Street NE
Washington, DC 20002
(202) 336-5500
http://www.apa.org

American Public Human Services Association
810 First Street NE
Suite 500
Washington, DC 20002
(202) 682-0100
http://www.aphsa.org

Anxiety Disorders Association of America
8730 Georgia Avenue

Suite 600
Silver Spring, MD 20910
(240) 485-1001
http://www.adaa.org

Association for Behavioral and Cognitive Therapies
305 7th Avenue
New York, NY 10001
(212) 647-1890
http://www.aabt.org

Association of State and Territorial Health Officials
2231 Crystal Drive
Suite 450
Arlington, VA 22202
(202) 371-9090
http://www.astho.org/

Brain Injury Association of America, Inc.
8201 Greensboro Drive
Suite 611
McLean, VA 22102
(703) 761-0750
http://www.biausa.org

Brain Resources and Information Network (BRAIN)
P.O. Box 5801
Bethesda, MD 20824
(800) 352-9424
http://www.ninds.nih.gov

Brain Trauma Foundation
523 East 72nd Street
8th Floor
New York, NY 10021
(212) 772-0608
http://www.braintrauma.org

Center for Mental Health Services
Emergency Services and Disaster Relief Branch
5600 Fishers Lane
Room 17C-20
Rockville, MD 20857
http://www.mentalhelath.org/cmhs/emergency-
services/index.htm

Center for Pediatric Traumatic Stress
The Children's Hospital of Philadelphia

3535 Market
34th Street and Civic Center Boulevard
Room 1492
Philadelphia, PA 19105
(267) 426-5205
http://www.chop.edu/consumer/jsp/microsite/
    microsite.jsp?id=77744

**Center for Substance Abuse Prevention
    (CSAP)**
Substance Abuse and Mental Health Services
    Administration
1 Choke Cherry Road
Rockville, MD 20857
(240) 276-2000
http://prevention.samhsa.gov/

**Center for Substance Abuse Treatment
    (CSAT)**
Substance Abuse and Mental Health Services
    Administration
1 Choke Cherry Road
Room 2-1075
Rockville, MD 20857
(240) 276-2700
http://csat.samhsa.gov/

**Centers for Disease Control and Prevention
    (CDC)**
1600 Clifton Road NE
Atlanta, GA 30333
(404) 639-3311
http://www.cdc.gov

Child Welfare Information Gateway
Children's Bureau
1250 Maryland Avenue SW
8th Floor
Washington, DC 20024
(703) 385-7565
http://www.childwelfare.gov

Child Welfare League of America
Headquarters
440 First Street NW
3rd Floor
Washington, DC 20001
(202) 638-2952
http://www.cwla.org

Dart Center for Journalism & Trauma
University of Washington
102 Communications Building
Box 353740
Seattle, WA 98195
http://www.dartcenter.org

Depression and Bipolar Support Alliance
730 North Franklin
Suite 501
Chicago, IL 60610
(800) 826-3632
http://dbsalliance.org

**Depression and Related Affective Disorders
    Association**
8201 Greensboro Drive
Suite 300
McLean, VA 22102
(703) 610-9026
http://www.drada.org

Disaster Psychiatry Outreach
50 Broad Street
#1714
New York, NY 10004
(212) 598-9995
http://www.disasterpsych.org

EMDR International Association
5806 Mesa Drive
Suite 360
Austin, TX 78731
(512) 451-5200
http://www.emdria.org

FaithTrust Institute
2400 North 45th Street
Number 10
Seattle, WA 98193
(206) 634-1903
http://www.faithtrustinstitute.org

Family Research Laboratory
126 Horton Social Science Center
University of New Hampshire
Durham, NH 03824
(603) 862-1888
http://www.unh.edu/frl/

Family Violence Prevention Fund
383 Rhode Island Street
Suite 304
San Francisco, CA 94103
(415) 252-8900
http://endabuse.org

Federal Emergency Management Agency
(information for children and adolescents)
P.O. Box 2012
Jessup, MD 20794
(800) 480-2520
http://www.fema.gov/kids

Food and Drug Administration (FDA)
5600 Fishers Lane
Rockville, MD 20857
(888) 463-6332
http://www.fda.org

Group for the Advancement of Psychiatry
P.O. Box 570218
Dallas, TX 75357
(972) 613-3044
http://www.groupadpsych.org

**The Higher Education Center for Alcohol
and Other Drug Prevention**
Education Development Center, Inc.
55 Chapel Street
Newton, MA 02458
(800) 676-1730
http://www.higheredcenter.org

Institute on Violence, Abuse and Trauma
6160 Cornerstone Court East
San Diego, CA 92121
(858) 623-2777
http://www.ivatcenters.org

**International Critical Incident Stress
Foundation**
3290 Pine Orchard Lane
Suite 106
Ellicott City, MD 21042
(410) 750-9600
http://www.icisf.org

**International Foundation for Research &
Education on Depression (iFRED)**
7040 Bembe Beach Road

Suite 100
Annapolis, MD 21403
(410) 268-0044
http://www.ifred.org

**International Society for Prevention of Child
Abuse and Neglect**
245 West Roosevelt Road
Building 6, Suite 39
West Chicago, IL 60185
(630) 876-6913
http://www.ispcan.org

**International Society for the Study of
Dissociation**
8201 Greensboro Drive
McLean, VA 22102
(703) 610-9037
http://www.issd.org

**International Society for Traumatic Stress
Studies**
60 Revere Drive
Suite 500
Northbrook, IL 60062
(847) 480-9028
http://www.istss.org

Kempe Children's Center
1825 Marion Street
Denver, CO 80218
(303) 864-5300
http://www.kempecenter.org

**Minnesota Center Against Violence and
Abuse**
School of Social Work
University of Minnesota
105 Peters Hall
1404 Gortner Avenue
St. Paul, MN 55108
(612) 624-0721
http://www.mincava.umn.edu/

**Mood and Anxiety Disorder Programs
(MAP)**
National Institute of Mental Health
9000 Rockville Pike
Bethesda, MD 20892
(866) 627-6464
http://intramural.nimh.nih.gov/mood

Mothers Against Drunk Driving (MADD)
511 East John Carpenter Freeway
Suite 700
Irving, TX 75062
(800) GET-MADD (438-6233)
http://www.madd.org

National Association for Children of Alcoholics
11426 Rockville Pike
Suite 100
Rockville, MD 20852
(888) 554-2627
http://www.nacoa.net

National Association for Native American Children of Alcoholics
P.O. Box 2708
Seattle, WA 98111
(206) 903-6574

National Association of Local Boards of Health
1840 East Gypsy Lane Road
Bowling Green, OH 43402
(419) 353-7714
http://www.nalboh.org

National Association of School Psychologists
National Emergency Assistance Team
4340 East West Highway
Suite 402
Bethesda, MD 20814
(301) 657-0270
http://www.nasponline.org/NEAT

National Association of Social Workers
750 First Street NE
Suite 700
Washington, DC 20002-4241
(202) 408-8600
http://www.socialworkers.org

National Association of State Controlled Substances Authorities
72 Brook Street
Quincy, MA 02170
(617) 472-0520
http://www.nascsa.org

National Center for Children Exposed to Violence
Yale Child Study Center
230 South Frontage Road
P.O. Box 207900
New Haven, CT 06520
(203) 785-7047
http://www.nccev.org/violence/children_terrorism.
htm

National Center for Child Traumatic Stress
University of California, Los Angeles
11150 West Olympic Boulevard
Suite 650
Los Angeles, CA 90064
(310) 235-2633
http://www.nctsnet.org

National Center for Posttraumatic Stress Disorder (PTSD)
Department of Veterans Affairs
(802) 296-6300
http://www.ncptsd.va.gov
ncptsd@va.gov

National Center for Victims of Crime
2000 M Street NW
Suite 480
Washington, DC 20036
(202) 467-8700
http://www.ncvc.org

National Center on Addiction and Substance Abuse at Columbia University
633 Third Avenue
New York, NY 10017
(212) 841-5200
http://www.casacolumbia.org

National Center on Substance Abuse and Child Welfare
4940 Irvine Boulevard
Suite 202
Irvine, CA 92612
(714) 505-3525
http://www.ncsacw.samhsa.gov

National Clearinghouse for Alcohol and Drug Information (NCADI)
11426-28 Rockville Pike
Rockville, MD 20852

(800) 729-6686
http://www.health.org

National Clearinghouse on Child Abuse and Neglect Information
330 C Street SW
Washington, DC 20447
(703) 385-3206
http://nccanch.acf.hhs.gov

National Conference of State Legislatures
7700 East First Place
Denver, CO 80230
(303) 364-7700
http://www.ncsl.org

National Council on Child Abuse and Family Violence
1025 Connecticut Avenue NW
Suite 1000
Washington, DC 20036
(202) 429-6695
http://www.nccafv.org

National Eating Disorders Association
Informational and Referral Program
603 Stewart Street
Suite 803
Seattle, WA 98101
(800) 931-2237
http://www.nationaleatingdisorders.org/

National Institute of Mental Health
6001 Executive Boulevard
Room 8184, MSC 9663
Bethesda, MD 20892
(301) 443-4513
http://www.nimh.nih.gov

National Institute on Alcohol Abuse and Alcoholism
5635 Fishers Lane
MSC 9304
Bethesda, MD 20892
(301) 443-0595
http://www.niaaa.nih.gov

National Mental Health Association
2001 North Beauregard Street
12th Floor
Alexandria, VA 22311

(703) 684-7722
http://www.nmha.org

National Mental Health Information Center
P.O. Box 42577
Washington, DC 20015
(800) 789-2647
http://www.mentalhealth.samhsa.gov

National Organization for Victim Assistance (NOVA)
Courthouse Square
510 King Street
Suite 424
Alexandria, VA 22314
(703) 535-NOVA
http://www.trynova.org/

National Rehabilitation Information Center (NARIC)
4200 Forbes Boulevard
Suite 202
Lanham, MD 20706
(301) 459-5900
http://www.naric.com

National Resource Center for Child Traumatic Stress
Duke University
905 West Main Street
Suite 25-B
Durham, NC 27701
(919) 682-1552
http://www.nctsnet.org/nccts/nav.do?pid=ctr_main

National Self-Help Clearinghouse
365 Fifth Avenue
Suite 3300
New York, NY 10016
(212) 817-1822
http://www.selfhelpweb.org

National Stroke Association
9707 East Easter Lane
Englewood, CO 80112
(303) 649-9299
http://www.stroke.org/site/PageNavigator/HOME

National Voluntary Organizations Active in Disaster (NVOAD)
1720 I Street NW

Suite 700
Washington, DC 20006
(202) 955-8396
http://www.nvoad.org

National Women's Health Network
514 10th Street NW
Suite 400
Washington, DC 20004
(202) 347-1140
http://www.womenshealthnetwork.org

Office for Victims of Crime
810 7th Street NW
Washington, DC 20531
(800) 851-3420
http://www.ojp.usdoj.gov/ovc

Office on Violence Against Women
810 7th Street NW
Washignton, DC 20531
(202) 307-6026
http://www.ojp.usdoj.gov/vawo/

Rape, Abuse & Incest National Network (RAINN)
2000 L Street NW
Suite 406
Washington, DC 20036
(202) 544-1034
http://www.rainn.org

Sidran Institute
200 East Joppa Road
Suite 207
Towson, MD 21286
(410) 825-8888

http://www.sidran.org

Social Security Administration (SSA)
Office of Public Inquiries
6401 Security Boulevard
Baltimore, MD 21235
(800) 772-1213
http://www.ssa.gov

Substance Abuse and Mental Health Services Administration (SAMSHA)
Department of Health and Human Services
1 Choke Cherry Road
Rockville, MD 20857
(240) 276-2000
http://www.samhsa.gov

United States Association for Body Psychotherapy
7831 Woodmont Avenue
Bethesda, MD 20814
http://www.usabp.org

U.S. Department of Education
400 Maryland Avenue SW
Washington, DC 20202
(800) USA-LEARN
https://www.ed.gov

U.S. Department of Health and Human Services
Administration for Children and Families
200 Independence Avenue SW
Washington, DC 20201
(202) 619-0257
http://www.acf.hhs.gov/

APPENDIX II
DIVISIONS OF THE NATIONAL CENTER FOR PTSD

The National Center for PTSD is an organization run by the Veterans Administration, with 7 offices throughout the United States.

Behavioral Science Division
VA Boston Healthcare System
150 South Huntington Avenue
Boston, MA 02130
(857) 364-4124

Clinical Neurosciences Division
VA Medical Center
950 Campbell Avenue
West Haven, CT 06516
(203) 932-5711, extension 2464

Education Division
VA Palo Alto Health Care System
3801 Miranda Avenue
Palo Alto, CA 94304
(650) 493-5000, extension 27314

Evaluation Division
VA Connecticut Healthcare System
950 Campbell Avenue
West Haven, CT 06516
(203) 937-3851

Executive Division
VA Medical Center
215 North Main Street
White River Junction, VT 05009
(802) 296-5132

Pacific Islands Division
1132 Bishop Street
Suite 307
Honolulu, HI 96813
(808) 566-1546

Women's Health Science Division
VA Boston Healthcare System
150 South Huntington Street
Boston, MA 02130
(857) 364-4145

APPENDIX III
FEDERAL EMERGENCY AND TRAUMA AGENCIES

This appendix lists agencies involved in federal emergencies and disasters.

National Center for Injury Prevention and Control
4770 Buford Highway NE
Atlanta, GA 30341
(800) 232-4636
http://www.cdc.gov/ncipc

National Center for Posttraumatic Stress Disorder (PTSD)
Department of Veterans Affairs
(802) 296-6300
http://www.ncptsd.va.gov

Rural Emergency Medical Services & Trauma Technical Assistance Center
300 North Wilson Avenue
Suite 802-H
Bozeman, MT 59715
(406) 587-6370
http://ruralhealth.hrsa.gov

U.S. Department of Homeland Security Federal Emergency Management Agency (FEMA)
500 C Street SW
Washington, DC 20472
(800) 621-FEMA (Disaster assistance)
http://www.fema.gov

U.S. Fire Administration
16825 South Seton Avenue
Emmitsburg, MD 21727
(301) 447-1000
http://www.usfa.dhs.gov

APPENDIX IV
STATE OFFICES OF EMERGENCY MEDICAL SERVICES AND TRAUMA ASSISTANCE

Alabama

EMS Division
Alabama Department of Health
The RSA Tower
201 Monroe Street
Suite 750
Montgomery, AL 36130-3017
(334) 206-5383
(334) 206-5260 (fax)
http://www.alapubhealth.org

Alaska

**Injury Prevention & Emergency Medical
Services**
P.O. Box 240249
Anchorage, AK 99524
(907) 269-8078
http://www.chems.alaska.gov/

Arizona

Bureau of Emergency Medical Services
150 North 19th Avenue
Suite 540
Phoenix, AZ 85007
(602) 364-3150
http://www.azdhs.gov/berns/

Arkansas

Division of EMS and Trauma Systems
Arkansas Department of Health
4815 West Markham Street
Slot 38
Little Rock, AR 72205-3867

(501) 661-2262
(501) 280-4901 (fax)
http://www.healthyarkansas.com/ems/

California

Emergency Medical Services Authority
1930 9th Street
Suite 100
Sacramento, CA 95814
(916) 322-4336
(916) 324-2875 (fax)
http://www.emsa.ca.gov/

Colorado

Colorado Department of Health
EMS Division, EMSD-ADM-A3
4300 Cherry Creek Drive South
Denver, CO 80222
(303) 692-2980
(303) 782-0904 (fax)
http://www.cdphe.state.co.us/em/index.html

Connecticut

Office of EMS
Department of Public Health
410 Capital Avenue
MS#12
P.O. Box 340308
Hartford, CT 06134-0308
(860) 509-7406
(860) 509-7539 (fax)
http://www.ct.gov/dph/cwp/view.
    asp?a=3127&q=387362

Delaware

Blue Hen Corporate Center
655 South Bay Road
Suite 4-H
Dover, DE 19901
(302) 739-6637
(302) 739-2352 (fax)
http://www.dhss.delaware.gov/dhss/main/maps/
    other/bluhenml.htm

District of Columbia

Emergency Health & Medical Services
800 9th Street SW
3rd Floor
Washington, DC 20024
(202) 645-5628
(202) 645-0526 (fax)
http://app.doh.dc.gov/about/index_ehms.shtm

Florida

Emergency Medical Services
Florida Department of Health
2002-D Old St. Augustine Road
Tallahassee, FL 32301-4881
(904) 487-1911
(904) 487-2911 (fax)
http://www.doh.state.fl.us/demo/ems/index.html

Georgia

Emergency Medical Services
47 Trinity Avenue SW
Suite 104-LOB
Atlanta, GA 30334-5600
(404) 657-6700
(404) 657-4255 (fax)
http://health.state.ga.us/programs/ems/

Hawaii

EMS System
State Department of Health
3627 Kilauea Avenue
Room 102

Honolulu, HI 96816
(808) 733-9210
(808) 733-8332 (fax)
http://hawaii.gov/health/family-child-health/ems/
    index.html

Idaho

Emergency Medical Services Bureau
Department of Health and Welfare
3092 Elder Street
Boise, ID 83705
(208) 334-4000
(208) 334-4015 (fax)
http://www.healthandwelfare.idaho.gov/portal/
    alias__Rainbow/lang__en-US/tabID__3344/
    DesktopDefault.aspx

Illinois

Division of Emergency Medical Services
Illinois Department of Public Health
535 W. Jefferson Street
Springfield, IL 62761
(217) 785-2080
(217) 785-0253 (fax)
http://www.idph.state.il.us/home.htm

Indiana

Indiana EMS Commission
302 W. Washington
Room E208 IGCS
Indianapolis, IN 46204-2258
(317) 232-3980
(317) 232-3895 (fax)

Iowa

Emergency Medical Services
Iowa Department of Public Health
Lucas State Office Building
Des Moines, IA 50319-0075
(515) 281-3239
(515) 281-4958 (fax)
http://www.idph.state.ia.us/ems/

Kansas

Board of Emergency Medical Services
Landon State Office Building
900 SW Jackson Street
Suite 1031
Topeka, KS 66612-1228
(785) 296-7296
(785) 296-6212 (fax)
http://www.ksbems.org/

Kentucky

**Kentucky Board of Emergency Medical
    Services**
2545 Lawrenceburg Road
Frankfort, KY 40601
(859) 256-3565
http://kbems.ky.gov

Louisiana

Bureau of Emergency Medical Services
P.O. Box 94215
Baton Rouge, LA 70804
(504) 342-4881
(504) 342-4876 (fax)
http://www.dhh.louisiana.gov/

Maine

Maine Emergency Medical Services
16 Edison Drive
Augusta, ME 04330
(207) 287-3953
(207) 287-6251 (fax)
http://www.state.me.us/dps/ems/

Maryland

Emergency Medical Services
MIEMSS
636 W. Lombard Street
Baltimore, MD 21201-1528
(410) 706-5074
(410) 706-4768 (fax)
http://www.miemss.org/

Massachusetts

Office of EMS
Department of Public Health
Two Boylston Street
3rd Floor
Boston, MA 02116
(617) 753-7300
(617) 753-7320 (fax)
http://mass.gov/dph/oems/

Michigan

Division of EMS
Michigan Dept. of Consumer & Industry Affairs
P.O. Box 30664
Lansing, MI 48909
(517) 335-8547
(517) 335-8582 (fax)
http://www.michigan.gov/mdch/0,1607,7-132-
    2946_5093_28508---,00.html

Minnesota

Minnesota EMS Regulatory Board
2829 University Avenue SE
Suite 310
Minneapolis, MN 55414-3222
(612) 627-5424
(612) 627-5442 (fax)
http://www.emsrb.state.mn.us/

Mississippi

Office of Health Protection
EMS/Trauma Care System
P.O. Box 1700
Jackson, MS 39215
(601) 576-7380
http://www.ems.doh.ms.gov/

Missouri

Bureau of Emergency Medical Services
Missouri Department of Health
P.O. Box 570
Jefferson City, MO, 65101

(573) 751-6356
(573) 751-6348 (fax)
http://www.dhss.mo.gov/EMS/

Montana

EMS & Trauma Systems Section
Emergency Medical Services and Injury
  Prevention Section
Department of Public Health & Human Services
Cogswell Building
P.O. Box 202951
Helena, MT 59620-2951
(406) 444-4458
(406) 444-1814 (fax)
http://www.dphhs.mt.gov/ems/

Nebraska

Division of Emergency Medical Services
301 Centennial Mall South
3rd Floor
P.O. Box 95026
Lincoln, NE 68509-5007
(402) 471-0124
(402) 471-0169 (fax)
http://www.hhs.state.ne.us/ems/emsindex.htm

Nevada

Emergency Medical Services Office
Nevada State Health Division
4150 Technology Way
Suite 300
Carson City, NV 89706
(775) 684-4200
(775) 684-5313 (fax)

New Hampshire

Bureau of Emergency Medical Services
Department of Safety
33 Hazen Drive
Concord, NH 03305
(603) 271-4568
http://www.nh.gov/safety/ems/

New Jersey

**NJ Department of Health & Senior Services,
  Office of EMS**
P.O. Box 360
Trenton, NJ 08625-0360
(609) 292-7837
http://www.state.nj.us/health/ems/

New Mexico

EMS Bureau, Department of Health
1301 Siler Road
Building F
Santa Fe, NM 87507
(505) 476-8200
(505) 476-8201 (fax)
http://www.nmems.org/

New York

Bureau of EMS
New York State Health Department
433 River Street
Suite 303
Troy, NY 12180-2299
(518) 402-0996
(518) 402-0985 (fax)
http://www.health.state.ny.us/nysdoh/ems/main.
  htm

North Carolina

Office of EMS
701 Barbour Drive
P.O. Box 29530
Raleigh, NC 27603
(919) 733-2285
(919) 733-7021 (fax)
http://www.ncems.org/

North Dakota

Division of Emergency Health Services
ND Department of Health
600 E. Boulevard Avenue
Bismarck, ND 58505-0200
(701) 328-2388

(701) 328-1890 (fax)
http://www.ndhealth.gov/ems/

Ohio

Emergency Medical Services Division
Ohio Department of Public Safety
P.O. Box 182073
1970 West Broad Street
Columbus, OH 43218
(614) 466-9447
http://www.ems.ohio.gov/general

Oklahoma

Emergency Medical Services Division
1000 Northeast Tenth
Room 1104
Oklahoma City, OK 73117
(405) 271-4027
http://www.health.state.ok/us/programs/ems/

Oregon

**Emergency Medical Services & Trauma
   Systems**
800 NE Oregon Street
Suite 607
Portland, OR 97232
(971) 673-0520
http://www.oregon.gov/DHS/ph/ems

Pennsylvania

Pennsylvania EMS Office
Health and Welfare Building
7th and Forster Streets
Room 1032
Harrisburg, PA 17120
(717) 787-8740
(717) 772-0910 (fax)
http://www.dsf.health.state.pa.us/health/cwp/
   view.asp?Q=237548

Rhode Island

Emergency Medical Services Division
Department of Health

3 Capitol Hill
Room 404
Providence, RI 02908-5097
(401) 222-2401
(401) 222-1250 (fax)
http://www.health.state.ri.us/hsr/professions/
   ems/index.php

South Carolina

Division of EMS
DHEC
2600 Bull Street
Columbia, SC 29201
(803) 737-7204
(803) 737-7212 (fax)
http://www.scdhec.net/health/ems/

South Dakota

Emergency Medical Services Program
Department of Health
600 East Capitol
Pierre, SD 57501
(605) 773-4031
(605) 773-5904 (fax)
http://www.state.sd.us/dps/ems/

Tennessee

Division of Emergency Medical Services
227 French Landing
Suite 303
Heritage Place, Metro Center
Nashville, TN 37243
(615) 741-2584
(615) 741-4217 (fax)
http://health.state.tn.us/ems/

Texas

EMS Trauma System
Texas Department of State Health Services
1100 West 49th Street
Austin, TX 78756
(512) 834-6700
http://www.tdh.state.tx.us/hcqs.ems

Utah

Bureau of EMS, Department of Health
P.O. Box 142004
Salt Lake City, UT 84114-2004
(801) 273-6666
http://health.utah.gov/ems/

Vermont

Office of EMS and Injury Prevention
Department of Health
P.O. Box 70
108 Cherry Street
Burlington, VT 05402
(802) 863-7310
(802) 863-7577 (fax)
http://healthvermont.gov/hc/ems/ems_index.aspx

Virginia

Office of Emergency Medical Services
Virginia Department of Health
1538 East Parham Road
Richmond, VA 23228
(804) 371-3500
(804) 371-3543 (fax)
http://www.vdh.state.va.us/oems/

Washington

**Office of Emergency Medical Services and
    Trauma System**
P.O. Box 47853
Olympia, WA 98504
(360) 236-2828
http://www.doh.wa.gov/hsqa.emstrauma/
OEMSTS.htm

West Virginia

**West Virginia Office of Emergency Medical
    Services**
350 Capitol Street
Room 425
Charleston, WV 25301
(304) 558-3956
(304) 558-1437 (fax)
http://www.wvoems.org/

Wisconsin

**Emergency Medical Services, Division of
    Health**
P.O. Box 309
Madison, WI 53701-0309
(608) 266-9781
(608) 261-6392 (fax)
http://dhs.wisconsin.gov/ems/

Wyoming

**Wyoming Office of Emergency Medical
    Services**
Hathaway Building
4th Floor
Cheyenne, WY 82002
(307) 777-7955
http://wdhfs.state.wy.us/ems

APPENDIX V
STATE MENTAL HEALTH AGENCIES

Alabama

Department of Mental Health and Mental Retardation
RSA Union Building
100 North Union Street
Montgomery, AL 36130-3417
(334) 242-3454
(800) 367-0955 (toll-free)
http://www.mh.state.al.us

Alaska

Division of Mental Health and Developmental Disabilities
Department of Health and Social Services
P.O. Box 110620
Juneau, AK 99811-0620
(907) 465-3370
(800) 465-4828 (toll-free)
(907) 465-2225 (TDD)
http://www.hss.state.ak.us/dbh/

Arizona

Department of Health Services
Division of Behavioral Health Services
150 North 18th Avenue
#200
Phoenix, AZ 85007
(602) 364-4558
http://www.hs.state.az.us/bhs/index.htm

Arkansas

Division of Mental Health Services
Department of Human Services
4313 West Markham Street
Little Rock, AR 72205-4096
(501) 686-9164
(501) 686-9176 (TDD)
http://www.state.ar.us/dhs/dmhs/

California

Department of Mental Health
Health and Welfare Agency
1600 Ninth Street
Room 151
Sacramento, CA 95814
(916) 654-3565
(800) 896-4042 (toll-free)
(800) 896-2512 (TDD)
http://www.dmh.cahwnet.gov

Colorado

Colorado Mental Health Services
3824 West Princeton Circle
Denver, CO 80236
(303) 866-7400
http://www.cdhs.state.co.us/ohr/mhs/

Connecticut

Department of Mental Health and Addictions Services
410 Capitol Avenue
Hartford, CT 06106
(860) 418-6700
(800) 446-7348 (toll-free)
(888) 621-3551 (TDD)
http://www.dmhas.state.ct.us

Delaware

Division of Substance Abuse and Mental Health
Department of Health and Social Services
1901 N. DuPont Highway
Main Building
New Castle, DE 19720
(302) 255-9427
http://www.state.de.us/dhss/dsamh/dmhhome.htm

District of Columbia

Department of Mental Health Services
77 P Street NE
4th Floor
Washington, DC 20002
(202) 673-7440
(888) 793-4357 (7WE-HELP)
http://dmh.dc.gov/dmh/site/default.asp

Florida

Department of Children and Families
1317 Winewood Boulevard
Building 1, Room 202
Tallahassee, FL 32399-0700
(850) 487-1111
http://www.state.fl.us/cf_web/

Georgia

Division of Mental Health, Mental Retardation and Substance Abuse
Department of Human Resources
2 Peachtree Street, NW
Suite 22-224
Atlanta, GA 30303
(404) 657-2168
http://www2.state.ga.us/departments/dhr/mhmrsa/index.html

Hawaii

Behavioral Health Services Administration
Department of Health
P.O. Box 3378
Honolulu, HI 96801
(808) 586-4419
http://www.state.hi.us/doh/about/behavior.html

Idaho

Department of Health and Welfare
450 West State Street
Boise, ID 83720-0036
(208) 334-5500
http://www2.state.id.us/dhw/index.htm

Illinois

Office of Mental Health
Department of Human Services
319 East Madison Street, Centrum Building, Third Floor
Springfield, IL 62701
(217) 785-6023
http://www.dhs.state.il.us

Indiana

Division of Mental Health
Department of Family and Social Services Administration
402 West Washington Street
Room W-353
Indianapolis, IN 46204-2739
(317) 232-7844

Iowa

Division of Mental Health and Developmental Disabilities
Hoover State Office Building
1305 East Walnut Street
Des Moines, IA 50319-0114
(515) 281-3573

Kansas

Department of Social and Rehabilitation Services
Docking State Office Building
915 SW Harrison Street
Topeka, KS 66612
(785) 296-3959
http://www.srskansas.org

Kentucky

Department for Mental Health and Mental Retardation Services
Cabinet for Human Resources
100 Fair Oaks Lane
Frankfort, KY 40621-0001
(502) 564-4527
http://mhmr.chs.ky.gov/Default.asp

Office of Mental Health
P.O. Box 4049
Bin #12
Baton Rouge, LA 70821-4049
(225) 342-2540
http://www.dhh.state.la.us/OMH/index.htm

Maine

Adult Mental Health Services
Department of Behavioral and Developmental
   Services
40 State House Station
Augusta, ME 04333
(207) 287-4200
(888) 568-1112 (toll-free)
http://www.state.me.us/dmhmrsa

Maryland

Department of Health and Mental Hygiene
201 West Preston Street
Baltimore, MD 21201
(410) 767-6860
(800) 735-2258 (TDD)
(877) 463-3464 (toll-free)
http://www.dhmh.state.md.us

Massachusetts

Department of Mental Health
25 Staniford Street
Boston, MA 02114
(617) 626-8000
(617) 727-9842 (TDD)
http://www.state.ma.us/dmh/_MainLine/Mission-
   Statement.HTM

Michigan

Department of Community Health
Lewis-Cass Building
320 South Walnut Street
Sixth Floor
Lansing, MI 48913
(517) 373-3500
(517) 373-3573 (TDD)
http://www.michigan.gov/mdch

Minnesota

Department of Human Services
Mental Health Program Division
Human Services Building
444 Lafayette Road
Saint Paul, MN 55155-3828
(651) 297-3510
http://www.dhs.state.mn.us/Contcare/mental-
   health/default.htm

Mississippi

Department of Mental Health
Robert E. Lee Building
Suite 1101
239 North Lamar Street
Jackson, MS 39201
(601) 359-1288
601-359-6230 (TDD)
http://www.dmh.state.ms.us

Missouri

Department of Mental Health
P.O. Box 687
Jefferson City, MO 65102
(800) 364-9687 (toll-free)
(573) 526-1201 (TDD)
http://www.dmh.missouri.gov

Montana

Addictive and Mental Disorders Division
Department of Public Health and Human Services

555 Fuller
Helena, MT 59620
(406) 444-4928
http://www.dphhs.state.mt.us

Nebraska

Office of Mental Health, Substance Abuse and Addictions Services
P.O. Box 98925
Lincoln, NE 68509
(402) 479-5166
http://www.hhs.state.ne.us/beh/mhsa.htm

Nevada

Mental Health & Developmental Services Division
Department of Human Resources
Kinkead Building
Room 602
505 East King Street
Carson City, NV 89701
(775) 684-5943
http://www.mhds.state.nv.us

New Hampshire

Division of Behavioral Health
Department of Health and Human Services
State Office Park South
105 Pleasant Street
Concord, NH 03301
(603) 271-8140
(800) 735-2964 (TDD)
(800) 852-3345 (toll-free, statewide)
http://www.dhhs.state.nh.us

New Jersey

Division of Mental Health Services
50 East State Street
Capitol Center
Post Office 727
Trenton, NJ 08625-0727
(609) 777-0702
http://www.state.nj.us/humanservices/dmhs

New Mexico

Behavioral Health Services Division
Harold Runnels Building
1190 Saint Francis Drive
Room North 3300
Santa Fe, NM 87505-6110
(505) 827-2601
(800) 362-2013 (consumer hotline)
http://www.nmcares.org

New York

Office of Mental Health
44 Holland Avenue
Albany, NY 12229
(518) 474-4403
(800) 597-8481 (toll-free)
http://www.omh.state.ny.us

North Carolina

Division of Mental Health, Developmental Disabilities, and Substance Abuse Services
Department of Health & Human Resources
3001 Mail Service Center
Raleigh, NC 27699-3001
(919) 733-7011
(919) 733-1221 (fax)
http://www.dhhs.state.nc.us/mhddsas

North Dakota

Division of Mental Health & Substance Abuse Services
600 South Second Street
Suite 1D
Bismarck, ND 58504-5729
(701) 328-8940
(800) 755-2719 (toll-free, statewide)

Ohio

Department of Mental Health
30 East Broad Street
8th Floor
Columbus, OH 43215

(614) 466-2337
http://www.mh.state.oh.us

Oklahoma

Department of Mental Health and Substance Abuse Services
P.O. Box 53277
Capitol Station
Oklahoma City, OK 73152
(405) 522-3908
(800) 522-9054 (toll-free)
(800) 522-7233 (toll-free, Domestic Violence Safeline)
http://www.odmhsas.org

Oregon

Oregon Department of Human Services
Mental Health and Addiction Services
500 Summer Street NE
E86
Salem, OR 97301
(503) 945-5763
(503) 947-5330 (TDD)
http://www.dhs.state.or.us/mentalhealth/

Pennsylvania

Office of Mental Health and Substance Abuse Services
P.O. Box 2675
Harrisburg, PA 17105-2675
(717) 787-6443
(877) 356-5355 (toll-free)
http://www.dpw.state.pa.us/omhsas/dpwmh.asp

Rhode Island

Department of Mental Health, Mental Retardation and Hospitals
14 Harrington Road
Cranston, RI 02920
(401) 462-3201
http://www.mhrh.state.ri.us

South Carolina

Department of Mental Health
P.O. Box 485
2414 Bull Street
Columbia, SC 29202
(803) 898-8581
http://www.state.sc.us/dmh

South Dakota

Division of Mental Health
Department of Human Services
Hillsview Plaza
East Highway 34
c/o 500 East Capitol
Pierre, SD 57501-5070
(605) 773-5991
(800) 265-9684 (toll-free)
http://www.state.sd.us/dhs/dmh

Tennessee

Department of Mental Health and Developmental Disabilities
Cordell Hull Building
425 Fifth Avenue North
Third Floor
Nashville, TN 37243
(615) 532-6500
http://www.state.tn.us/mental/

Texas

Texas Department of Mental Health and Mental Retardation
Central Office
909 West Forty Fifth Street
Austin, TX 78751
(512) 454-3761
(800) 252-8154 (toll-free, statewide)
http://www.mhmr.state.tx.us

Utah

Division of Mental Health
Department of Human Services
120 North 200 West

Fourth Floor, Suite 415
Salt Lake City, UT 84103
(801) 538-4270
http://www.hsmh.state.ut.us

Vermont

**Department of Developmental and Mental
    Health Services**
Weeks Building
103 South Main Street
Waterbury, VT 05671-1601
(802) 241-2610
http://www.state.vt.us/dmh

Virginia

**Department of Mental Health, Mental
    Retardation and Substance Abuse
    Services**
P.O. Box 1797
Richmond, VA 23218
(804) 786-3921
(804) 371-8977 (TDD)
(800) 451-554 (toll-free)
http://www.dmhmrsas.state.va.us/

Washington

Mental Health Division
Department of Social and Health Services
P.O. Box 45320
Olympia, WA 98504-5320
(360) 902-0790
(800) 446-0259 (toll-free, statewide)
http://www.wa.gov/dshs/

West Virginia

**Bureau for Behavioral Health and Health
    Facilities**
Department of Health and Human Resources
350 Capitol Street
Room 350
Charleston, WV 25301-3702
(304) 558-0627
http://www.wvdhhr.org/

Wisconsin

Bureau of Community Mental Health
Department of Health and Family Services
P.O. Box 7851
1 West Wilson Street
Room 433
Madison, WI 53702-7851
(608) 267-7792
http://www.dhfs.state.wi.us/mentalhealth

Wyoming

Mental Health Division
Department of Health
6101 Yellowstone Road
Room 259-B
Cheyenne, WY 82002
(307) 777-7094
http://mhd.state.wy.us/

APPENDIX VI
STATE HEALTH DEPARTMENTS

Alabama

Alabama Department of Public Health
The RSA Tower
201 Monroe Street
Montgomery, AL 36104
(334) 206-5300
http://www.adph.org

Alaska

Office of the Commissioner
Health and Social Services
350 Main Street
Room 404
P.O. Box 110601
Juneau, AK 99811
(907) 465-3030
http://health.hss.state.ak.us/commissioner

Arizona

Arizona Department of Health Services
150 North 18th Avenue
Phoenix, AZ 85007
(602) 542-1000
http://www.azdhs.gov

Arkansas

Department of Health
4815 West Markham
Little Rock, AR 72203
(501) 661-2000
http://www.healthyarkansas.com/health.html

California

California Department of Health
714 P Street
Room 1253
Sacramento, CA 95899
(916) 440-7400
http://www.dhs.ca.gov

Colorado

**Colorado Department of Public Health and
  Environment**
4300 Cherry Creek Drive South
Denver, CO 80246
(303) 692-2000
http://www.cdphe.state.co.us/ic/infohom.html

Connecticut

**Connecticut Department of Public
  Health**
410 Capitol Avenue
P.O. Box 340308
Hartford, CT 06134
(860) 509-8000
http://www.ct.gov/dph/site/default.asp

Delaware

Delaware Health and Social Services
1901 North DuPont Highway
New Castle, DE 19720
(302) 255-9040
http://www.state.de.us/dhss

District of Columbia

Department of Health
825 North Capitol Street NE
Washington, DC 20002
(202) 671-5000
http://doh.dc/gov/doh/site/default.asp

Florida

Department of Health
4052 Bald Cypress Way
Tallahassee, FL 32399
(850) 245-4147
http://esetappsdoh.doh.state.fl.us

Georgia

Georgia Department of Community Health
2 Peachtree Street
40th Floor
Atlanta, GA 30303
(404) 656-4507
http://dch.georgia.gov

Hawaii

Hawaii State Department of Health
1250 Punchbowl Street
Honolulu, HI 96813
(808) 586-4400
http://www.hawaii.gov/health

Idaho

Idaho Department of Health and Welfare
450 West State Street
Boise, ID 83720
(208) 334-5500
http://www.healthandwelfare.idaho.gov

Illinois

Illinois Department of Public Health
535 West Jefferson Street
Springfield, IL 62761
(217) 782-4977
http://www.idph.state.il.us

Indiana

Indiana State Department of Health
2 North Meridian Street
Indianapolis, IN 46204
(317) 233-1325
http://www.in.gov/isdh

Iowa

Iowa Department of Public Health
321 East 12th Street
Des Moines, IA 50319
(515) 281-7689
http://www.idph.state.is.us/

Kansas

Kansas Department of Health and Environment
Curtis State Office Building
1000 SW Jackson
Topeka, KS 66612
(785) 296-1500
http://www.kdheks.gov

Kentucky

Cabinet for Health and Family Services
Office of the Secretary
275 East Main Street
Frankfort, KY 40621
(800) 372-2973 (toll-free)
http://chfs.ky.gov

Louisiana

Louisiana Department of Health & Hospitals
628 North 4th Street
P.O. Box 629
Baton Rouge, LA 70821
(225) 342-5568
http://www.dhh.louisiana.gov

Maine

Maine Center for Disease Control and Prevention
286 Water Street

State House Station 11
Augusta, ME 04333
(207) 287-8016
http://www.maine.gov/dhhs.boh

Maryland

Maryland Department of Health & Mental Hygiene
201 West Preston Street
Baltimore, MD 21201
(410) 767-8500
http://www.dhmh.state.md.us/

Massachusetts

Massachusetts Department of Public Health
250 Washington Street
Boston, MA 02108
(617) 624-6000
http://www.mass.gov/dph/dphhome.htm

Michigan

Michigan Department of Community Health
Capitol View Building
201 Townsend Street
Lansing, MI 48913
(517) 373-3740
http://www.michigan.gov/mdch

Minnesota

Minnesota Department of Health
P.O. Box 64975
St. Paul, MN 55164
(651) 201-5000
http://www.health.state.mn.us

Mississippi

Mississippi Department of Health
570 East Woodrow Wilson Drive
Jackson, MS 39216
(601) 576-7400
http://www.msdh.state.ms.us

Missouri

Missouri Department of Health & Senior Services
P.O. Box 570
Jefferson City, MO 65102
(573) 751-6400
http://www.dhss.mo.gov

Montana

Montana Department of Public Health and Human Services
1400 Broadway
Helena, MT 59620
(406) 444-1861
http://www.dphhs.mt.gov/

Nebraska

Nebraska Department of Health and Human Services
P.O. Box 95944
Lincoln, NE 68509
(402) 471-2306
http://www.hhs.state.ne.us

Nevada

Nevada Department of Health and Human Services
505 East King Street
Room 600
Carson City, NV 89710
(775) 684-4000
http://www.hr.state.nv.us/

New Hampshire

New Hampshire Department of Health and Human Services
State Office Park South
129 Pleasant Street
Concord, NH 03301
(603) 271-4688
http://www.dhhs.state.nh.us

New Jersey

Department of Health and Senior Services
P.O. Box 360
Trenton, NJ 08625
(609) 292-7837
http://www.state.nj.us/health/

New Mexico

New Mexico Department of Health
1190 South St. Francis Drive
Santa Fe, NM 87502
(505) 827-2613
http://www.health.state.nm.us

New York

New York State Department of Health
Corning Tower
Empire State Plaza
Albany, NY 12237
http://www.health.state.ny.us

North Carolina

**North Carolina Department of Health and
    Human Services**
2001 Mail Service Center
Raleigh, NC 27699
(919) 733-4534
http://www.dhhs.state.nc.us

North Dakota

North Dakota Department of Health
600 East Boulevard Avenue
Bismarck, ND 58505
(701) 328-2372
http://www.ndhan.gov

Ohio

Ohio Department of Health
246 North High Street
Columbus, OH 43126
(614) 644-8562
http://www.odh.ohio.gov

Oklahoma

Oklahoma Health Care Authority
4545 North Lincoln Boulevard
Suite 124
Oklahoma City, OK 73105
(405) 522-7300
http://www.ohca.state.ok.us

Oregon

Oregon Public Health Division
800 NE Oregon Street
Portland, OR 97232
(503) 731-4000
http://oregon.gov/DHS/ph

Pennsylvania

Pennsylvania Department of Health
Health and Welfare Building
7th and Forster Streets
Harrisburg, PA 17120
(717) 787-6436
http://www.dsf.health.state.pa.us/health/site/
    default.asp

Rhode Island

Rhode Island Department of Health
3 Capitol Hill
Providence, RI 02908
(401) 222-2231
http://www.health.state.ri.us

South Carolina

**South Carolina Department of Health and
    Human Services**
P.O. Box 8206
Columbia, SC 29202
(803) 898-2500
http://www.dhhs.state.sc.us

South Dakota

South Dakota Department of Health
600 East Capitol Avenue

Pierre, SD 57501
(605) 773-3361
http://www.state.sd.us/doh

Tennessee

Tennessee Department of Health
Cordell Hull Building
3rd Floor
Nashville, TN 37247
(615) 741-3111
http://state.tn.us/health

Texas

Texas Department of State Health Services
1100 West 49th Street
Austin, TX 78756
(512) 458-7111
http://www.dshs.state.tx.us

Utah

Utah Department of Health
288 North 1460 West
Salt Lake City, UT 84114
(801) 538-6101
http://www.health.utah.gov

Vermont

Vermont Department of Health
108 Cherry Street
Burlington, VT 05402
(802) 863-7200
http://healthvermont.gov

Virginia

Virginia Department of Health
P.O. Box 2448
Richmond, VA 23218
(804) 864-7600
http://www.vdh.state.va.us

Washington

**Washington Department of Social and
   Health Services**
P.O. Box 45010
Olympia, WA 98504
(360) 902-7800
http://www1.dshs.wa.gov

West Virginia

Office of Community Health Systems
350 Capitol Street
Room 515
Charleston, WV 25301
(304) 558-3210
http://www.wvochs.org

Wisconsin

Department of Health and Family Services
1 West Wilson Street
Madison, WI 53702
(608) 266-1865
http://www.shfs.state.wi.us

Wyoming

Wyoming Department of Health
117 Hathaway Building
2300 Capitol Avenue
Cheyenne, WY 82002
(307) 777-7656
http://wdh.state.wy.us

BIBLIOGRAPHY

Abramson, Lyn Y., and Martin E. P. Seligman. "Learned Helplessness in Humans: Critique and Reformulation." *Journal of Abnormal Psychology* 87, no. 1 (1978): 49–74.

Administration on Children, Youth, and Families. *Child Maltreatment 2004.* Children's Bureau, U.S. Department of Health and Human Services, Washington, D.C., 2006.

Albucher, R. C., and I. Liberszon. "Psychopharmacological Treatment in PTSD: A Critical Review." *Journal of Psychiatry Research* 36 (2002): 355–367.

Al-Chalabi, Ammar, Martin R. Turner, and R. Shane Delamont. *The Brain.* Oxford, England: One World Publications, 2006

Alexander, David A. "Early Mental Health Intervention After Disasters." *Advances in Psychiatric Treatment* 11 (2005): 12–18.

Ancharoff, Michelle R., James F. Munroe, and Lisa M. Fisher. "The Legacy of Combat Trauma: Clinical Implications of Intergenerational Transmission," In *International Handbook of Multigenerational Legacies of Trauma,* edited by Yael Danieli. New York: Plenum Press, 1998.

Anderson, Mark, M.D., et al. "School-Associated Violent Deaths in the United States, 1994–1999." *Journal of the American Medical Association* 286, no. 21 (December 5, 2001): 2,595–2,702.

Antonovsky A. *Health Stress and Coping.* San Francisco: Jossey-Bass, 1979.

———. *Unraveling the Mystery of Health. How People Manage Stress and Stay Well.* San Francisco: Jossey-Bass, 1987.

———. "The Structure and Properties of the Sense of Coherence Scale." *Social Science & Medicine* 36 (March 1993): 725–733.

Armour, J. A., "Anatomy and Function of the Intrathoracic Neurons Regulating the Mammalian Heart." In *Reflex Control of the Circulation,* edited by I. H. Zucker and J. P. Gilmore. Boca Raton, Florida: CRC Press, 1991.

Armstrong, K. R., P. E. Lund, L. T. McWright, and V. Tichenor. "Multiple Stressor Debriefing and the American Red Cross: The East Bay Hills Fire Experience." *Social Work,* 40 (1995): 83–90.

Arnow, B. A., "Relationship between Childhood Maltreatment, Adult Health and Psychiatric Outcomes, and Medical Utilization." *Journal Clinical Psychiatry* 6, Supplement 12 (2004): 10–15.

Bandler, R. *Using Your Brain for a Change.* Moab, Utah: Real People Press, 1985.

Bass, C. "Hyperventilation Syndrome, 'A Chimera, editorial.'" *Journal of Psychosomatic Research* 42, no. 5 (1997): 421–426.

Baumert, J., H. Simon, H. Gundel, G. Schmitt, and K. H. Ladwig. "The Impact of Event Scale-Revised: Evaluation of the Subscales and Correlations to Psychophysiological Startle Response Patterns in Survivors of a Life-Threatening Cardiac Event: An Analysis of 129 Patients with an Implanted Cardioverter Defibrillator." *Journal of Affective Disorder* 82(1) (October 1, 2004): 29–41.

Beck Aaron T., M.D., and Gary Emery. *Anxiety Disorders and Phobias: A Cognitive Perspective.* New York: Basic Books, 2005.

Begić, Dražen, Ljubomir Hotujac, and Nataša Jokić-Begić. "Electroencephalographic Comparison of Veterans with Combat-Related Post-Traumatic Stress Disorder and Health Subjects." *International Journal of Psychophysiology* 40 (2001): 167–172.

Bell, Holly, Shanti Kulkarni, and Lisa Dalton. "Organizational Prevention of Vicarious Trauma." *Families in Society: The Journal of Contemporary Human Services* 84, no. 4 (2003): 463–470.

Berkowitz, Nancy F. "Wendy Wall: In the Wake of Childhood Trauma." *Brief Treatment and Crisis Intervention* 4, no. 4 (2004): 377–387.

Birmes, P., L. Hatton, A. Brunet, and L. Schmitt. "Early Historical Literature for Post-Traumatic Symptomatology." *Stress and Health* 19 (1): 17–26, 2003.

Blake, D. D., F. W. Weathers, L. M. Nagy, D. G. Kaloupek, G. Klauminzer, D. S. Charney, and T. M. Keane. "A Clinical Rating Scale for Assessing Current and Lifetime PTSD: The CAPS-1." *Behavior Therapist* 18: 187–188.

Blanchard, E. G., D. Rowell, E. Kuhn, R. Rogers, and D. Wittrock. "Posttraumatic Stress and Depressive Symptoms in a College Population One Year after the September 11 Attacks: The Effect of Proximity." *Behavior Research and Therapy* 43 (2005): 143–150.

Blanchard, E. B., et al. "Who Develops PTSD from Motor Vehicle Accidents?" *Behaviour Research and Therapy* 34, no. 1 (1996): 1–10.

Boscarino, Joseph A., Charles R. Figley, and Richard E. Adams. "Compassion Fatigue following the September 11 Terrorist Attacks: A Study of Secondary Trauma among New York City Social Workers." *International Journal of Emergency Mental Health*, 6, no. 2 (2004): 1–9.

Boscarino, Joseph A. "Posttraumatic Stress Disorder and Physical Illness: Results from Clinical and Epidemiologic Studies." *Annals of New York Academy of Sciences* 1032 (2004): 141–153.

Boudewyns, Patrick A., and Robert H. Shipley. *Flooding and Implosive Therapy: Direct Therapeutic Exposure in Clinical Practice.* New York: Plenum Press, 1983.

Bower, B. "The Survivor Syndrome: Childhood Sexual Abuse Leaves a Controversial Trail of Aftereffects." *Science News* (September 25, 1993).

Bowlby, John. *Maternal Care and Mental Health.* Geneva Switzerland: World Health Organization, 1951.

Bremner, J. Douglas, et al. "Measurement of Dissociative States with the Clinician-Administered Dissociative States Scale (CADSS)" *Journal of Traumatic Stress* 11, no. 1 (1998): 125–136.

Breslau, N., and G. C. Davis. "Posttraumatic Stress Disorder: The Stressor Criterion," *Journal of Nervous and Mental Disorder* 75, no. 1 (1987): 255–264.

Brewin, C. R., B. Andrew, and J. D. Valentine. "Meta-analysis of Risk Factors for Posttraumatic Stress in Trauma Exposed Adults." *Journal of Consulting and Clinical Psychology* 68, no. 5 (2000): 748–766.

Brewin, C., T. Dalgleish, and S. Joseph. "A Dual Representation Theory of Posttraumatic Stress Disorder." *Psychological Review* 103, no. 4 (1996): 670–686.

Brewin, C. R., B. Andrews, and J. D. Valentine. "Meta-analysis of Risk Factors for Posttraumatic Stress Disorder." *Journal of Consult. & Clinical* 68, no. 5 (2000): 748–766.

Brewin, C. "Implications for Psychological Intervention." In *Neurophysiology of PTSD: Biological, Cognitive, and Clinical Perspectives*, edited by J. Vasterling and C. Brewin. New York: Guilford Press, 2005.

Briere, J. *Child Abuse Trauma: Theory and Treatment of the Lasting Effects.* Newbury Park, Calif.: Sage, 1992.

Briere, John, and Catherine Scott, M.D. *Principles of Trauma Therapy: A Guide to Symptoms, Evaluation, and Treatment.* Thousand Oaks, Calif.: Sage Publications, 2006.

Briere, J. *Trauma Symptoms Inventory Professional Manual.* Odessa, Florida: Psychological Assessment Resources, 1995.

Brown, E. S., et al. "The Psychiatric Sequelae of Civilian Trauma." *Comprehensive Psychiatry* 41 (2000): 19–23.

Brown, Gregory K., et al. "Cognitive Therapy for the Prevention of Suicide Attempts: A Randomized Controlled Trial." *Journal of the American Medical Association* 294, no. 5 (August 3, 2005): 563–570.

Burba, Benjaminas, M.D., et al. "A Controlled Study of Alexithymia in Adolescent Patients with Persistent Somatoform Pain Disorder." *Canadian Journal of Psychiatry* 51, no. 7 (June 2006): 468–471.

Bureau of Justice Statistics. "National Crime Victimization Survey: Criminal Victimization, 2005." *Bureau of Justice Statistics Bulletin* (September 2006).

Burton, L. A. "Social Adjustment Scale Assessments in Traumatic Brain Injury." *Journal of Rehabilitation* (October–December 1993).

Butler, C., and A. Z. J. Zeman. "Neurological Syndromes Which Can Be Mistaken for Psychiatric Conditions." *Journal of Neurology, Neurosurgery, and Psychiatry* 76 (2005): 31–38.

Cardeña, Etzel, and Kristin Croyle, eds. *Acute Reactions to Trauma and Psychotherapy: A Multidisciplinary and International Perspective.* Binghamton, New York: Haworth Medical Press, 2005.

Carlier, I. V. E., R. D. Lamberts, and B. P. Gersons. "Risk Factors for Posttraumatic Symptomatology in Police Officers: A Perspective Analysis." *Journal of Nervous and Mental Disease* 185, no. 8 (1997): 498–506.

Carlson, E. B., et al. "Validity of the Dissociative Experiences Scale in Screening for Multiple Personality Disorder: A Multicenter Study." *American Journal of Psychiatry* 150 (1993): 1,030–1,036.

Cartwright, Rosalind. "Sleepwalking Violence: A Sleep Disorder, a Legal Dilemma, and a Psychological Challenge." *American Journal of Psychiatry* 161, no. 7 (July 2004): 1,149–1,158.

Carver, Charles S., Michael F. Scheier, and Jagdish Kumari Weintraub. "Assessing Coping Strategies: A Theoretically Based Approach." *Journal of Personality and Social Psychology* 56, no. 2 (1989): 267–283.

Carver, C. S. "You Want to Measure Coping But Your Protocol's Too Large: Consider the Brief COPE." *International Journal of Behavioral Medicine* 4, no. 1 (1997): 92–99.

Centers for Disease Control and Prevention. "Births, Marriages, Divorces, and Deaths: Provisional Data for 2005." *National Vital Statistics Reports* 54, no. 20 (July 21, 2006): 1–7.

Child Welfare Information Gateway. "Recognizing Child Abuse and Neglect: Signs and Symptoms." Washington, D.C.: Children's Bureau, Administration on

Children, Youth and Families (April 2006). Available online. URL: http://www.childwelfare.gov/pubs/factsheets/signs.cfm. Downloaded July 15, 2006.

Choe, Injae. "The Debate Over Psychological Debriefing for PTSD." *The New School Psychology Bulletin* 3 no. 2 (2005): 71–82.

Clark, Robin E., Judith Freeman Clark, and Christine Adamec. *The Encyclopedia of Child Abuse. Third Edition.* New York: Facts On File, Inc., 2007.

Cohen, Judith A., Anthony P. Mannarino, and Esther Deblinger. *Treating Trauma and Traumatic Grief in Children and Adolescents.* New York: Guilford Press, 2006.

Cosgray, R. E. and R. W. Fawley. "Could It Be Ganser's Syndrome." *Archives of Psychiatric Nursing* 3, no. 4 (August 1989): 241–245.

Damlouji, Namir F., M.D., and James M. Ferguson, M.D. "Three Cases of Posttraumatic Anorexia Nervosa." *American Journal of Psychiatry* 142, no. 3 (March 1985): 362–363.

Davidson, Jonathan R. T., M.D. "Recognition and Treatment of Posttraumatic Stress Disorder." *Journal of the American Medical Association* 286, no. 5 (August 1, 2001): 584–588.

Davidson, J., R. Smith, and H. Kudler. "Validity and Reliability of the DSM-III Criteria for Posttraumatic Stress Disorder: Experience with a Structured Interview." *Journal of Nervous and Mental Disease.* 177 (1989): 336–341.

De-Bellis, M.D., et al. "Urinary Catecholamine Excretion in Sexually Abused Girls." *Journal of the American Academy of Child and Adolescent Psychiatry* 33 (3) (1994): 320–327.

De Jong, Joop T. V. M., M.D., et al. "Lifetime Events and Posttraumatic Stress Disorder in 4 Postconflict Settings." *Journal of the American Medical Association* 286, no. 5 (August 1, 2001): 555–562.

Department of Mental Health and Substance Abuse, *Global Status Report on Alcohol 2004.* Geneva, Switzerland: World Health Organization (2004). Available online. URL: http://www.who.int/substance_abuse/publications/global_status_report_2004_overview.pdf. Downloaded September 26, 2006.

DeVoe, J. F., et al. *Indicators of School Crime and Safety: 2005.* Washington, D.C.: U.S. Government Printing Office, 2005.

Dietrich, A. "Review of Visual/Kinesthetic Disassociation in the Treatment of Posttraumatic Disorders: Theory, Efficacy and Practice Recommendations. *Traumatology* 6, no. 2 (August 2000): 85–107.

Difede, J., and H. Hoffman. "Virtual Reality Exposure Therapy for World Trade Center Post-Traumatic Stress Disorder: A Case Report." *Cyber Psychology & Behavior* 5, no. 6 (2002).

Doctor, Ronald. *The Complex/Relational Trauma Syndrome in Children and Adults.* Unpublished paper, 2002.

———, and Ada P. Kahn, with Christine Adamec. *The Encyclopedia of Phobias, Fears, and Anxieties. Third Edition.* New York: Facts On File, Inc., 2007.

Driessen, Martin, et al. "Magnetic Resonance Imaging Volumes of the Hippocampus and the Amygdala in Women with Borderline Personality Disorder and Early Traumatization." *Archives of General Psychiatry* 57 (2000): 1,115–1,122.

Dube, Shanta R., et al. "Childhood Abuse, Household Dysfunction, and the Risk of Attempted Suicide Throughout the Life Span: Findings from the Adverse Childhood Experiences Study." *Journal of the American Medical Association* 286, 24 (December 26, 2001): 3,089–3,096.

———. "Long-Term Consequences of Childhood Sexual Abuse by Gender of Victim." *American Journal of Preventive Medicine* 28, 5 (2005): 430–438.

Dumond, Robert W. "Confronting America's Most Ignored Crime Problem: The Prison Rape Elimination Act of 2003." *Journal of the American Academy of Psychiatry and the Law* 31, no. 3 (2003): 354–360.

Elhai, J. D., M. G. Gray, T. B. Dashdan, and C. L. Franklin. "Which Instruments Are Most Commonly Used to Assess Traumatic Event Exposure and Posttraumatic Effects?: A Survey of Traumatic Stress Professionals. *Journal of Traumatic Stress* 18, no. 5 (October 2005): P541–545.

Elser, A. S., and C. H. Schenck. "Dreaming: A Psychiatric View and Insights from the Study of Parasomnias." *Schweizer Archives für Neurologie und Psychiatrie* 156 (2005): 440–470.

Eriksson, C. B., et al. "Trauma Exposure and PTSD Symptoms in International Relief and Development Personnel." *Journal of Traumatic Stress* 14, no. 1 (2001): 205–212.

Everly, G. S., S. H. Boyle, and J. M. Lating. "The Effectiveness of Psychological Debriefing with Vicarious Trauma: A Meta-Analysis." *Stress Medicine* 15, no. 4 (1999): 229–233.

Everly, G., et al. In *Personality Psychology,* edited by Everly G. and J. Lating, 33–51. Washington, D.C.: American Psychologist.

Falsett, S. A., H. S. Resnick, J. Davis, and N. G. Gallagher. "Treatment of Posttraumatic Stress Disorder with Comorbid Panic Attacks: Combining Cognitive Processing Therapy with Panic Control Treatment Techniques." *Group Dynamics: Theory, Research, and Practice* 5, no. 4 (2001): 252–260.

Figley, Charles R., ed. *Compassion Fatigue: Coping with Secondary Traumatic Stress Disorder in Those Who Treat the Traumatized.* New York: Brunnzer/Mazel, 1995, 1–8.

Figley, Charles R., and Rolf J. Kleber. "Beyond the 'Victim': Secondary Traumatic Stress." In *Beyond Trauma: Cultural and Societal Dynamics,* edited by Rolf J. Kleber, Charles R. Figley, and Berthold P. R. Gersons, 75–98. New York: Plenum Press, 1995.

Finkelhor, D., and A. Browne. "The Traumatic Impact of Child Sexual Abuse: A Conceptualization." *American Journal of Orthopsychiatry* 55, no. 4 (1985): 530–541.

Foa, E. B., L. Cashman, L. Jaycox, and K. Perry. "The Validation of a Self-Report Measure of Posttraumatic Stress Disorder: The Posttraumatic Diagnostic Scale." *Psychological Assessment* 9 (1997): 445–451.

Foa, E. B., D. S. Riggs, C. V. Dancu, and B. O. Rothbaum. "Reliability and Validity of a Brief Instrument for Assessing Post-traumatic Stress Disorder." *Journal of Traumatic Stress* 6 (1993): 459–473.

Freud, Sigmund. *An Outline of Psycho-Analysis.* New York: Norton, 1949.

———. *On the History of the Psycho-Analytic Movement.* New York: Norton, 1966.

Freyd, Jennifer. *Betrayal: The Logic of Forgetting Childhood Abuse.* Cambridge, Mass.: Harvard University Press, 1996.

———. "II. Violations of Power, Adaptive Blindness and Betrayal Trauma Theory." *Feminism & Psychology* 7, no. 1 (1997): 22–32.

Fullerton, C. S., R. J. Ursano, K. Vance, and L. Wang. "Debriefing following Trauma." *Psychiatric Quarterly* 71, no. 3 (2000): 259–276.

Fuselier, G. Dwayne. "Placing the Stockholm Syndrome in Perspective." *FBI Law Enforcement Bulletin* (July 1999). Available online. URL: http://www.au.af/mil/au/awc/awcgate/fbi/stockholm_syndrome.pdf. Downloaded March 19, 2007.

Gaensbauer, T. J. "Trauma in the Preverbal Period." *Psychoanalytic Study of the Child* 50 (1995): 122–149.

Garno, Jessica L., Joseph F. Goldberg, Paul Michael Ramirez, and Barry A. Ritzler. "Impact of Childhood Abuse on the Clinical Course of Bipolar Disorder." *British Journal of Psychiatry* 186 (2005): 121–125.

Gaynes, Bradley N., M.D., et al. "Screening for Suicide Risk in Adults: A Summary of the Evidence for the U.S. Preventive Services Task Force." *Annals of Internal Medicine* 140, no. 10 (May 18, 2004): 822–835.

Gendlin, Eugene T. *Focusing.* New York: Bantam, 1982.

George, C., M. West, and O. Petterm. "The Adult Attachment Projective: Disorganization of Adult Attachment at the Level of Representation." In *Attachment Disorganization,* edited by Solomon, J. and C. George, 462–507. New York: Guilford Press, 1999.

Girdano, D. A., D. E. Dusek, D. E. Everly and G. S. Everly. *Controlling Stress and Tension,* Seventh edition. New York: Pearson Books, 2005.

Goldberg, L. R., and J. J. Freyd. "Self-Reports of Potentially Traumatic Experiences in an Adult Community Sample: Gender Differences & Test-Retest Stability of the Items in a Brief Betrayal-Trauma Survey." *Journal of Trauma & Dissociation* 7, no. 3 (2006): 39–63.

Golier, J., et al. "The Relationship of Borderline Personality Disorder to Posttraumatic Stress Disorder and Traumatic Events." *American Journal of Psychiatry* 160 (November 2003): 2,018–2,024.

Gottesman, R., R. Komotar, and A. Hillis. "Neurologic Aspects of Traumatic Brain Injury." *International Review of Psychiatry* 15, no. 4 (2003): 302–309.

Gurvits, T. V., et al. "Neurologic Soft Signs in Chronic Posttraumatic Stress Disorder." *Archives of General Psychiatry* 57, no. 2 (2000): 181–186.

Gwinnell, Esther, M.D., and Christine Adamec. *The Encyclopedia of Addictions and Addictive Disorders.* New York: Facts On File, Inc., 2005.

———. *The Encyclopedia of Drug Abuse.* New York: Facts On File, Inc., 2007.

Hageman, I. M., H. S. Anderson, and M. B. Jergensen. "Posttraumatic Stress Disorder: A Review of Psychobiology and Pharmacotherapy." *Acta Psychiatric Scandinavica* 104 (2001): 411–422.

Hamblen, Jessica. *PTSD in Children and Adolescent, A National Center for PTSD Fact Sheet.* Washington, D.C.: U.S. Department of Veterans Affairs, 2005.

Hammerberg, M. "Penn Inventory for Posttraumatic Stress Disorder: Psychometric Properties." *Psychological Assessment* 4 (1992): 67–76.

Harris, William W., Frank W. Putnam, M.D., and John A. Fairbank. "Mobilizing Trauma Resources for Children." In *Interventions for Children Exposed to Violence.* Johnson & Johnson Pediatric Institute, 2006. Available online at http://www.nctsn.org/nctsn_assets/pdfs/reports/HarrisManuscript.pdf. Downloaded July 15, 2006.

Harvey, A. G., and R. A. Bryant. "The Relationship between Acute Stress Disorder and Posttraumatic Stress Disorder: A Prospective Evaluation of Motor Vehicle Accident Survivors." *Journal of Consulting and Clinical Psychology* 66, no. 3 (1998): 507–512.

Healy, David. *Images of Trauma: From Hysteria to Post-Traumatic Stress Disorder.* London: Faber and Faber, 1993.

Helmus, Todd C., and Russell W. Glenn. *Steeling the Mind: Combat Stress Reactions and Their Implications for Urban Welfare.* Santa Monica, Calif.: Rand Corporation,

2005. Available online. URL: http://www.rand.org/pubs/monographs/2005/RAND_MG191.pdf. Downloaded August 15, 2006.

Henkel, Linda, Nancy Franklin, and Marcia K. Johnson. "Cross-Modal Source Monitoring Confusings between Perceived and Imagined Events." *Journal of Experimental Psychology: Learning, Memory and Cognition* 26, no. 2 (March 2000): 321–335.

Hentz, Patricia. "The Body Remembers: Grieving and a Circle of Time." *Qualitative Health Research* 12, no. 2 (February 2002): 161–172.

Herman, Judith Lewis. "Complex PTSD: A Syndrome in Survivors of Prolonged and Repeated Trauma." *Journal of Traumatic Stress* 5, no. 3 (1992): 377–391.

Herman, Judith, M.D. *Trauma and Recovery.* New York: Basic Books, 1997.

Hilton, Jeanne M., and Karen Kopera-Frye. "Patterns of Psychological Adjustment among Divorced Custodial Parents." *Journal of Divorce & Remarriage* 41, no. 3/4 (2004): 1–30.

Hodas, Gordon R., M.D. Responding to Childhood Trauma: The Promise and Practice of Trauma Informed Care. Paper published by the Pennsylvania Office of Mental Health and Substance Abuse Services (February 2006). Available online. URL: http://www.nasmhpd.org/general_files/publications/ntac_pubs/Responding%20to%20Childhood%20Trauma%20%20Hodas.pdf#search=%22(%22childhood%29trauma%22)%20journal %20pdf%22. Downloaded October 4, 2006.

Hoffman, S. G., and Spiegal, D. A. (1999). "Panic control treatment and its application." *Journal of Psychotherapy Practice and Research* 8, no. 1: 3–11.

Hoge, Charles W., M.D., et al. "Combat Duty in Iraq and Afghanistan, Mental Health Problems, and Barriers to Care." *New England Journal of Medicine* 351, no. 1 (July 1, 2004): 13–22.

Holmes, E., C. R. Brewin, and R. Hennessy. "Trauma Films, Information Processing, and Intrusive Memory Development." *Journal of Experimental Psychology* 133, no. 1 (2004): 3–22.

Holmes, T. H., and R. H. Rahe. "The Social Readjustment Rating Scale." *J. Psychosom. Res.* 11 (1967): 213–218.

Howe, David. *Child Abuse and Neglect: Attachment, Development and Intervention.* New York: Palgrave Macmillan, 2005.

Horowitz, M. J., N. Wilner, and W. Alvarez. "Impact of Event Scale: A Measure of Subjective Distress." *Psychosomatic Medicine* 41 (1979): 209–218.

Huang, G., et al. "Prevalence and Characteristics of Trauma and Posttraumatic Stress Disorder in Female Prisoners in China." *Comprehensive Psychiatry* 47, no. 1 (January–February 2006): 20–29.

Husum, H., and G. Strada. "Injury Severity Score versus New Injury Severity Score for Penetrating Injuries." *Prehospital and Disaster Medicine* 17, no. 1 (2002): 27–32.

Hyams, Kenneth C., M.D., F. Stephen Wignall, M.D., and Robert Roswell, M.D. "War Syndromes and Their Evaluation: From the U.S. Civil War to the Persian Gulf War." *Annals of Internal Medicine* 125, no. 5 (September 1, 1996): 398–405.

Iribarren, Javier, et al. "Post-Traumatic Stress Disorder: Evidence-Based Research for the Third Millennium." *eCAM* 2, no. 4 (2005): 503–512.

Ito, Y., et al. "Increased Prevalence of Electrophysiological Abnormalities in Children with Psychological, Physical and Sexual Abuse." *Journal of Neuropsychiatry and Clinical Neurosciences* 5, no. 4 (1993): 401–408.

Iwata, B. A., G. M. Pace, R. C. Kissel, P. A. Nau, and J. M. Farber. "The Self-Injury Trauma (SIT) Scale: A Method for Quantifying Surface Tissue Damage Caused by Self-Injurious Behavior." *Applied Behavioral Analysis* 23, no. 1 (1990): 99–110.

Janet, P. *Psychological Healing.* Vols 1, 2. New York: Macmillan, 1925. (Originally published as *Les medications psychologiques.* Vols 1–3. Paris, Felix Alcan, 1919).

Janson, Gregory R., and Richard J. Hazler. "Trauma Reactions of Bystanders and Victims to Repetitive Abuse Experiences." *Violence and Victims* 19, no. 2 (April 2004): 239–255.

Johnson, D. M., C. Zlotnick, and M. Zimmerman. "The Clinical Relevance of a Partial Remission Specifier for Posttraumatic Stress Disorder." *Journal of Traumatic Stress* 16, no. 5 (October 2005): 515–518.

Johnston, Lloyd D., et al. *Monitoring the Future: National Survey Results on Drug Use, 1975–2004.* Vol. 2, *College Students & Adults Ages 19–45.* Bethesda, Md.: National Institute on Drug Abuse, National Institutes of Health, 2005.

Jones, Edgar, and Simon Wessely. "War Syndromes: The Impact of Culture on Medically Unexplained Symptoms." *Medical History* 49 (2005): 55–78.

Kang, Han K., and Kenneth C. Hyams, M.D. "Mental Health Care Needs among Recent War Veterans." *New England Journal of Medicine* 352, no. 13 (March 31, 2005): 1,289.

Kaplan, D., and Smith, T. "A Validity Study of the Subjective Unit of Discomfort (SUD) Score." *Measurement & Evaluation in Counseling & Development* 27, no. 4 (1995): 748–756.

Katon, Wayne J., M.D. "Panic Disorder." *New England Journal of Medicine* 354, no. 22 (June 1, 2006): 2,360–2,367.

Kazak, Anne E., et al. "Posttraumatic Stress Disorder (PTSD) and Posttraumatic Stress Symptoms (PTS) in

Families of Adolescent Childhood Cancer Survivors." *Journal of Pediatric Psychology* 29, no. 3 (2004): 211–219.

Keane, T. M., J. M. Caddell, and K. L. Taylor. Mississippi Scale for Combat-Related PTSD: Three studies in reliability and validity. *Journal of Consulting and Clinical Psychology* 56 (1988): 85–90.

Kempe, C. H., et al. "The Battered Child Syndrome." *Journal of the American Medical Association* 181 (1962): 107–112.

Kendall-Tackett, Kathleen A. "Chronic Pain Syndromes as Sequelae of Childhood Abuse." In *Child Maltreatment*. Kingston, N.J.: Civic Research Institute, 2005.

Kessler, R. C., A. Sonnega, E. Bromet and C. B. Nelson. "Posttraumatic Stress Disorder in the National Comorbidity Survey." *Archives of General Psychiatry* 52, no. 12 (1995): 1,048–1,060.

Kilcommons, A., and A. Morrison. "Relationships between Trauma and Psychosis: An Exploration of Cognitive and Dissociative Factors." *Acta Psychiatric Scandinavica* 112 (2005): 351–359.

Kilpatrick, D. G., et al. *The National Survey of Adolescents: Preliminary Findings on Lifetime Prevalence of Traumatic Events and Mental Health Correlates.* Charleston, S.C.: Medical University of South National and National Crime Victims Research and Trauma Center, 1995.

King, D., D. Vogt, and L. King. "Risk and Resilience Factor in the Etiology of Chronic Posttraumatic Stress Disorder. In *Early Intervention for Trauma & Traumatic Loss,* edited by B. T. Litz. New York: Guilford Press, 2004.

Klorer, P. Gussie. "Expressive Therapy with Severely Maltreated Children: Neuroscience Contributions." *Art Therapy: Journal of the American Art Therapy Association* 22, no. 4 (2005): 213–220.

Kolb, J. E., and J. G. Gunderson. "Diagnosing Borderline Patients with a Semistructured Interview." *Archives of General Psychiatry* 37, no. 1 (1980): 37–41.

Kosiey, P., and L. McLeod. "Visual-Kinesthetic Dissociation in the Treatment of Victims of Rape." *Professional Psychology: Research and Practice* 18, no. 3 (June 1987): 276–282.

Kounin, J. S. *Discipline and Group Management in Classrooms.* New York: Holt, Rinehart and Winston Inc., 1970.

Krakow, B., et al. "A Controlled Study of Imagery Rehearsal for Chronic Nightmares in Sexual Assault Survivors with PTSD." *Journal of the American Medical Association* 286, no. 5 (2001): 537–545.

Krakow, Barry, M.D., et al. "Imagery Rehearsal Therapy for Chronic Nightmares in Sexual Assault Survivors with Posttraumatic Stress Disorder: A Randomized Controlled Trial." *New England Journal of Medicine* 286, no. 5 (August 1, 2001): 537–545.

Krug, Etienne G., M.D., et al. "Suicide after Natural Disasters." *New England Journal of Medicine* 338, no. 6 (February 5, 1998): 373–378.

Kubany, E. S., et al. "Development and Validation of the Trauma-Related Guilt Inventory (TRGI)." *Psychological Assessment* 8, no. 4 (December 1996): 428–444.

Kubany, E. S., S. N. Haynes, M. B. Leisen, J. A. Owens, A. S. Kaplan, S. B. Watson, and K. Burns. "Development and Preliminary Validation of a Brief Broad-Spectrum Measure of Trauma Exposure: The Traumatic Life Events Questionnaire. *Psychological Assessment* 12 (2000): 210–224.

Lamberg, Lynne. "Katrina Survivors Strive to Reclaim Their Lives." *Journal of the American Medical Association* 296, no. 5 (August 2, 2006): 499–502.

Langlois, Jean A., Wesley Rutland-Brown, and Karen E. Thomas, National Center for Injury Prevention and Control. *Traumatic Brain Injury in the United States: Emergency Department Visits, Hospitalizations, and Deaths.* Atlanta, Georgia: Centers for Disease Control and Prevention (January 2006). Available online. URL: http://www.cdc.gov/ncipc/pub-res/TBI_in_US-04/TBI%20in%20the%20US_Jan_2006.pdf. Downloaded August 5, 2006.

Lasiuk, G. C., and K. M. Hegadoren. "Posttraumatic Stress Disorder Part I: Historical Development of the Concept." *Perspectives in Psychiatric Care* 42, no. 1 (February 2006): 13–20.

Lavie, Peretz. "Sleep Disturbances in the Wake of Traumatic Events." *New England Journal of Medicine* 345, no. 25 (December 20, 2001): 1,825–1,832.

Lee, Royce, M.D., et al. "Childhood Trauma and Personality Disorder: Positive Correlation with Adult CSF Corticotropin-Releasing Factor Concentrations." *American Journal of Psychiatry* 162, no. 5 (May 2005): 995–997.

Leskeda, J., M. Dieperink, and P. Thuras. "Shame and Posttraumatic Stress Disorder." *Journal of Traumatic Stress* 15, no. 3 (2002): 223–226.

Leventhal, John M. "Test of Time: 'The Battered-Child Syndrome' 40 Years Later." *Clinical Child Psychology and Psychiatry* 8, no. 4 (2003): 543–545.

Levine, Peter. *Waking the Tiger: Healing Trauma: The Innate Capacity to Transform Overwhelming Experience.* Berkeley, Calif.: North Atlantic Books, 1997.

Lifton, Robert J. "Beyond Psychic Numbing: A Call to Awareness." *American Journal of Orthopsychiatry* 52, no. 4 (October 1982): 619–629.

Linden M., B. Schippan, K. Baumann, and R. Spielberg. "Posttraumatic Embitterment Disorder (PTED). Differentiation of a Specific Form of Adjustment Disorders." *Nevenartz* 75, no. 1 (2004): 51–57.

Linehan, M. *Cognitive-Behavioral Treatment of Borderline Personality Disorder.* New York: Guilford Press, 1993.

London, Kamala, et al., "Disclosure of Child Sexual Abuse: What Does the Research Tell Us about the Ways That Children Tell?" *Psychology, Public Policy, and Law* 11, no. 1 (2005): 194–226.

Lyons, M. J., et al. "Do Genes Influence Exposure to Trauma?" *American Journal of Medical Genetics* 48 (1993): 22–27.

Lyons, Judith A., and Joseph R. Scotti. "Behavioral Treatment of a Motor Vehicle Accident Survivor: An Illustrative Case of Direct Therapeutic Exposure." *Cognitive and Behavioral Practice* 2, no. 2 (Winter 1995): 343–364.

Madariaga, C. "Psychosocial Trauma." In *Posttraumatic Stress Disorder, and Torture.* Santiago, Chile: Ediciones Cintras, 2002.

Mann, J. John, M.D., et al. "Suicide Prevention Strategies: A Systematic Review." *Journal of the American Medical Association* 294, no. 16 (October 26, 2005): 2,064–2,074.

Madrid, Paula A., and Stephanie J. Schacher. "A Critical Concern: Pediatrician Self-Care after Disasters." *Pediatrics* 117, no. 5, Suppl. (May 2006): S454–S457.

Magarian, Gregory J., M.D., Deborah A. Middaugh, M.D., and Douglas H. Linz, M.D. "Hyperventilation Syndrome: A Diagnosis Begging for Recognition." *Western Journal of Medicine* 138 (May 1983): 733–736.

Matthews, Karen A., and Brooks B. Gump. "Chronic Work Stress and Marital Dissolution Increase Risk of Posttrial Mortality in Men from the Multiple Risk Factor Intervention Trial." *Archives of Internal Medicine* 162 (February 11, 2002): 309–315.

McAllister, T., and R. Ferrell. "Evaluation and Treatment of Psychosis after Traumatic Brain Injury." *NeuroRehabilitation* 17 (202): 357–368.

McClaskey, Thomas R. "Decoding Traumatic Memory Patterns at the Cellular Level." American Academy of Experts in Traumatic Stress (1998). Available online. URL: http://www.aaets.org/article30htm. Downloaded March 7, 2008.

McLaren, K. *Emotional Genius: Discovering the Deepest Language of the Soul.* Columbia, Calif.: Laughing Tree Press, 2001.

Meichenbaum, D. *A Clinical Handbook/Practical Therapist Manual for Assessing and Treating Adults with Post Traumatic Stress Disorder.* Waterloo, Ontario: Institute Press, 1994.

———. *Stress Innovation Training.* New York: Pergamon Press, 1985.

Mikulincer, Mario. "Causal Attribution, Coping Strategies, and Learned Helplessness." *Cognitive Therapy and Research* 13, no. 6 (1989): 565–582.

Miller, Laurie, M.D., with Christine Adamec. *The Encyclopedia of Adoption. Third Edition.* New York: Facts On File, Inc., 2007.

Mitchell, J. T., and G. S. Everly, Jr. *Critical Incident Stress Debriefing: CISD, An Operations Manual for the Prevention of Traumatic Stress among Emergency Service and Disaster Workers. Second Edition.* Ellicott City, Md.: Chevron Publishing Corporation, 1996.

Moulden, Heather M., and Philip Firestone. "Vicarious Traumatization: The Impact on Therapists Who Work with Sexual Offenders." *Trauma, Violence & Abuse* 8, no. 1 (January 2007): 67–83.

Moulds, M. L., and R. D. Nixon. "In Vivo Flooding for Anxiety Disorders: Proposing Its Utility for the Treatment of Post Traumatic Stress Disorder." *Journal of Anxiety Disorder* 20 (2006): 498–509.

Muller, Rený J. "When a Patient Has No Story to Tell: Alexithymia." *Psychiatric Times* 17, no. 7 (July 2000). Available online. URL: http://psychiatrictimes.com/p000771.html. Downloaded September 12, 2006.

Mullings, Janet L., James W. Marquart, and Deborah J. Hartley. *The Victimization of Children: Emerging Issues.* Binghamton, N.Y.: Haworth Press, 2003.

Mundy, E., and A. Baum. "Medical Disorders as a Cause of Psychological Trauma and Posttraumatic Stress Disorder." *Current Opinion Psychiatry* 17, no. 2 (2004): 123–128.

Muss, D. A. "A New Technique for Treating Post-Traumatic Stress Disorder." *British Journal of Clinical Psychology* 30 (1991): 91–92.

Naring G., and E. R. S. Nijenhous. "Relationships between Self-Reported Potentially Traumatizing Events, Psychoform and Somatoform Dissociation, and Absorption, in Two Clinical Populations." *Australian and New Zealand Journal of Psychiatry* 39 (2005): 982–988.

National Institute of Mental Health. "The Numbers Count: Mental Disorders in America." 2006. Available online. URL: http: www.nimh.nih.gov/publicat/numbers.cfm. Downloaded March 19, 2007.

———. "Suicide in the U.S.: Statistics and Prevention" (December 2006). Available online. URL: http://www.nimh.nih.gov/publicat/harmsway.cfm. Downloaded March 19, 2007.

National Institute of Neurological Disorders and Stroke. *Traumatic Brain Injury: Hope through Research. National Institutes of Health* (June 2006). Available online. URL: http://www.ninds.nih.gov/disorders/tbi/detail_tbi.htm. Downloaded August 12, 2006.

National Institute on Alcohol Abuse and Alcoholism. *Alcohol Use and Alcohol Use Disorders in the United States: Main Findings from the 2001–2002 National Epidemiologic Survey on Alcohol and Related Conditions (NESARC).* U.S.

Alcohol Epidemiologic Data Reference Manual 8, no. 1 (January 2006). Bethesda, Md.: National Institutes of Health, January 2006.

National Institute on Drug Abuse. "Childhood Sexual Abuse Increases Risk for Drug Dependence in Adult Women." Available online. URL: http://www.nida.nih.gov/NIDA_Notes/NNVol17N1/childhood.html. Downloaded August 2, 2006.

Newman, E., D. Kaloupek, and T. Keane. "Assessment of Posttraumatic Stress Disorder in Clinical and Research Settings." In Traumatic Stress, edited by B. Van der Kolk, A. McFarlane, and L. Weisaeth. New York: Guilford Press, 1996.

Newman, Matthew L., George W. Holden, and Yvon Delville. "Isolation and the Stress of Being Bullied." Journal of Adolescence 28 (2005): 343–357.

Newman, Tony. Promoting Resilience: A Review of Effective Strategies for Child Care Services, prepared for the Centre for Evidence-Based Special Services. University of Exeter, United Kingdom, 2002.

Nijenhuis, E. R. S., J. Vanderlinden, and P. Spinvoen. "Animal Defensive Reactions and Model for Trauma-Induced Dissociative Reactions." Journal of Traumatic Stress 11 (1998): 243–260.

Nijenhuis, E. R. S., et al. "The Development and Psychometric Characteristics of the Somatoform Dissociation Questionnaire (SDQ-20)." Journal of Nervous and Mental Disease 184 (1996): 688–694.

9/11 Commission Report. Washington, D.C.: Government Printing Office, 2004.

Norris, F. "Screening for Traumatic Stress: A Scale for Use in the Genera Population." Journal of Applied Social Psychology 20 (November 1990): 1,704–1,718.

North, C. S., et al. "Psychiatric Disorders in Rescue Workers after the Oklahoma City Bombing." American Journal of Psychiatry 159, no. 5 (2002): 857–859.

North, Carol S. "Somatization in Survivors of Catastrophic Trauma: A Methodological Review." Environmental Health Perspectives 110, Suppl. 4 (August 2002): 637–640.

Noy, Shabtai. "Gradations of Stress as Determinants of the Clinical Picture Immediately After Traumatic Events." Traumatology 6, no. 3 (2001): 1–9.

Noy, Shabtai. "The Traumatic Process: Conceptualization and Treatment." Prehospital and Disaster Medicine 19, no. 1 (January–March 2004): 37–45.

O'Keefe, Maura. "Incarcerated Battered Women: A Comparison of Battered Women Who Killed Their Abusers and Those Incarcerated for Other Offenses." Journal of Family Violence 12, no. 1 (1997): 1–19.

Office of the Assistant Secretary for Planning and Evaluation. Male Perpetrators of Child Maltreatment: Findings from NCANDS. Washington, D.C.: U.S. Department of Health and Human Services, January 2005.

Office on Women's Health. "Bulimia Nervosa." Available online. URL: http://womenshealth.gov/faq/Easyread/bulnervosa-etr.htm. Downloaded March 7, 2008.

Office on Women's Health. "Anorexia Nervosa." Available online. URL: http://womenshealth.gov/faq/Easyread/anorexia-etr.htm. Downloaded March 7, 2008.

Oppenheimer, B. S., and M. A. Rothschild. "The Psychoneurotic Factor in the Irritable Heart of Soldiers." Journal of the American Medical Association 70 (1918): 1,919–1,922.

Orenstein, Herbert, M.D. "Briquet's Syndrome in Association with Depression and Panic: A Reconceptualization of Briquet's Syndrome." American Journal of Psychiatry 146, no. 3 (March 1989): 334–338.

Orr, S., R. Pitman, N. Lasko, and L. Herz. "Psychophysiological Assessment of Posttraumatic Stress Disorder Imagery in World War II and Korean Combat Veterans." Journal of Abnormal Psychology 102, no. 1 (1993): 152–159.

Otto, M. W., et al. "Posttraumatic Stress Disorder Symptoms Following Media Exposure to Tragic Events: Impact of 9/11 on Children at Risk for Anxiety Disorders." Journal of Anxiety Disorders 21, no. 7 (2007): 888–902.

Palm, Kathleen M., Melissa A. Polusny, and Victoria M. Follette. "Vicarious Traumatization: Potential Hazards and Interventions for Disaster and Trauma Workers." Prehospital and Disaster Medicine 19, no. 1 (January–March 2004): 73–78.

Parker-Corell, Ann, and David K. Marcus. "Partner Abuse, Learned Helplessness, and Trauma Symptoms." Journal of Social and Clinical Psychology 23, no. 4 (2004): 445–462.

Pearlman, L. A. Trauma and Attachment and Belief Scale. Los Angeles: Western Psychological Services, 2003.

Pelcovitz, D., B. van der Kolk, S. Roth, F. Mandel, S. Kaplan, and P. Resick. "Development of a Criteria Set and a Structured Interview for Disorders of Extreme Stress (SIDES)." Journal of Traumatic Stress 10, no. 1: 3–16.

Pennebaker, J. W. Opening Up: The healing power of expressing emotions. New York: Guilford Press, 1997.

Pert, C. Molecules of Emotion. New York: Simon and Schuster, 1999.

Petit, William A., Jr., M.D., and Christine Adamec. The Encyclopedia of Endocrine Diseases and Disorders. New York: Facts On File, Inc., 2005.

Petrakis, Ismene, L., M.D., et al. "Comorbidity of Alcoholism and Psychiatric Disorders." Alcohol Research & Health 26, no. 2 (2002): 81–89.

Pizarro, Judith. "The Efficacy of Art and Writing Therapy: Increasing Positive Mental Health Outcomes and Participant Retention after Exposure to Traumatic Experience." *Art Therapy: Journal of the American Art Therapy Association* 21, no. 1 (2004): 5–12.

Pribor, E. F., et al. "Briquet's Syndrome, Dissociation, and Abuse." *American Journal of Psychiatry* 150 (1993): 1,507–1,511.

Pross, Christian, M.D. "Burnout, Vicarious Traumatization and Its Prevention." *Torture* 16, no. 1 (2006): 1–9.

Pynoos, R. S., A. M. Steinberg, and A. Goenjian. "Traumatic Stress in Childhood and Adolescence, Recent Developments and Current Controversies." In *Traumatic Stress,* edited by B. A. van der Kolk, A. C. McFarlane, and L. Weisaeth. New York: Guilford Press, 1996.

Raphael, B., and S. Wooding. "Early Mental Health Interventions for Traumatic Loss." In *Early Intervention for Trauma and Traumatic Loss,* edited by B. Litz. New York: The Guilford Press, 2004.

Rauch, S. L., B. A. van der Kolk, R. E. Fisher, N. M. Alpert, S. P. Orr, C. R. Savage, A. J. Fischman, M. A. Jenike, and R. K. Pitman. "A Symptom Provocation Study of Posttraumatic Stress Disorder Using Positron Emission Tomography and Script-Driven Imagery." *Archives of General Psychiatry* 53, no. 5 (May 1996): 380–387.

Renner, W., I. Salem, and K. Ottomeyer. "Cross-Cultural Validation of Measures of Traumatic Symptoms in Groups of Asylum Seekers from Chechnya, Afghanistan, and West Africa." *Social Behavior and Personality* 34, no. 9 (2006): 1,101–1,114.

Resnick, H. S., S. A. Falsetti, D. G. Kilpatrick, and J. R. Freedy. "Assessment of Rape and Other Civilian Trauma-Related Post-Traumatic Stress Disorder: Emphasis on Assessment of Potentially Traumatic Events." In *Stressful Life Events,* edited by T. W. Miller. Madison, Wis.: International Universities Press, 1996, 231–266.

Rothbaum, B. O., E. B. Foa, D. S. Riggs, T. Murdock, and W. Walsh. "A Prospective Examination of Posttraumatic Stress Disorder in Rape Victims." *Journal of Traumatic Stress* 5 (1992): 455–475.

Rothbaum, Barbara O., et al. "Virtual Reality Exposure Therapy for Vietnam Veterans with Posttraumatic Stress Disorder." *Journal of Clinical Psychiatry* 62, no. 8 (August 2001): 617–622.

Rothschild, Babette, with Marjorie Rand. *Help for the Helper: The Psychophysiology of Compassion Fatigue and Vicarious Trauma.* New York: Norton, 2006.

Ruggiero, K., K. Del Ben, J. Scotti, and A. Rabalais. "Psychometric Properties of the PTSD Checklist-Civilian Version." *Journal of Traumatic Stress* 16, no. 5 (October 2003): 495–502.

Rusch, M., and B. Grunert. "Imagery Rescripting for Recurrent, Distressing Images." *Cognitive and Behavioral Practice* 7 (2000): 173–182.

Ruzek, Josef, and Patricia Watson. "Early Intervention to Prevent PTSD and Other Trauma-Related Problems." *PTSD Research Quarterly* 12, no. 4 (Fall 2001): 1–3.

Rynerson, E., J. Favell, and M. Saindon. "Group Intervention for Bereavement after Violent Death." *Psychiatric Services* 53 (October 2002): 1,340.

Saakvitne, K., H. Tennen, and G. Affleck. "Exploring Thriving in the Context of Clinical Trauma Theory: Constructivist Self Development Theory." *Journal of Social Issues* 54, no. 2 (1998): 279–299.

Saigh, P. A., and J. D. Bremmer. *Posttraumatic Stress Disorder: A Comprehensive Text.* Needham Heights, Mass.: Allyn & Bacon, 1999.

Saxe, G. N., et al. "Dissociative Disorders in Psychiatric Inpatients." *American Journal of Psychiatry* 50 (1993): 1,037–1,042.

Scaer, Robert. *Trauma Spectrum.* New York: Norton, 2005.

Schenck, Carlos H., M.D., and Mark W. Mahowald, M.D. "Parasomnias." *Postgraduate Medicine* 107, no. 3 (2000): 145–156.

Schernhammer, Eva, M.D. "Taking Their Own Lives—The High Rate of Physician Suicide." *New England Journal of Medicine* 352, no. 4 (June 16, 2005): 2,373–2,476.

Schlenger, S. J., et al. "Psychological Reactions to Terrorist Attacks: Findings from the National Study of Americans' Reactions to September 11." *Journal of the American Medical Association* 288, no. 1 (2002): 581–588.

Schore, A. N. "The Effects of Early Relational Trauma on Right Brain Development, Affect Regulation, and Infant Mental Health." *Infant Journal of Mental Health,* 22 (2001): 201–269.

Schreuder, B. J. N., V. Igreja, J. van Dijk, and W. Kleijn. "Intrusive Re-Experiencing of Chronic Strife or War." *Advances in Psychiatric Treatment* 7 (2001): 102–108.

Schubinger, H., R. Scott, and A. Tzelepis. "Exposure to Violence among Inner-City Youth." *Journal of Adolescent Health* 14, no. 3 (1993): 214–219.

Shalev, A. Y. "Acute Stress Reactions in Adults." *Biological Psychiatry* 51 (2002): 532–543.

Shapiro, F. *Eye Movement Desensitization and Reprocessing.* 2nd ed. New York, Guilford Press, 2001.

Shaw, A., S. Joseph, and A. Linley. "Religion, Spirituality, and Posttraumatic Growth: A Systematic Review." *Mental Health, Religion, & Culture* 8, no. 1 (2005): 1–11.

Shear, K., et al. "Reliability and Validity of a Structured Interview Guide for the Hamilton Anxiety Rating Scale (SIGH-A)." *Depression and Anxiety* 13 (2001): 166–178.

Sherman, Michelle D., Dona K. Zanotti, and Dan E. Jones. "Key Elements in Couples Therapy with Veterans with Combat-Related Posttraumatic Stress Disorder." *Professional Psychology Research and Practice* 36, no. 6 (2005): 626–633.

Siegel, D. "Toward an Interpersonal Neurobiology of the Developing Mind: Attachment Relationships, 'Mindsight,' and neural integration." *Infant Mental Health Journal* (Special Edition on Contributions of the Decade of the Brain to Infant Psychiatry) 22 (2001): 67–94.

Sifneos, Peter E., "Alexithymia, Clinical Issues, Politics and Crime." *Psychotherapy and Psychosomatics* 69 (2000): 113–116.

Smucker, M. R., and J. Niederee. "Treating Incest-Related PTSD & Pathogenic Schemas through Imaginal Exposure & Rescripting." *Cognitive and Behavioral Practice* 2, no. 1 (1995): 63–92.

Solomon, Z. *Combat Stress Reaction: The Enduring Toll of War.* New York: Plenum Publishing, 1993.

Stampfl, T. C., and D. J. Levis. "Essentials of Implosive Therapy: A Learning-Theory Based Psychodynamic Behavioral Therapy." *Journal of Abnormal Psychology* 72 (1967): 496–503.

States, James H., M.D., and Clarke D. St. Dennis. "Chronic Sleep Disruption and the Reexperiencing of Posttraumatic Stress Disorder Symptoms Are Improved by Olanzapine: Brief Review of the Literature and a Case-Based Series." *Primary Care Companion Journal of Clinical Psychiatry* 5, no. 2 (2003): 74–79.

Stein, M. G. "Genetic and Environmental Influences on Trauma Exposure and Posttraumatic Disorder Symptoms." *American Journal of Psychiatry* 159 (2002): 1,675–1,681.

Stores, Gregory. "Dramatic Parasomnias." *Journal of the Royal Society of Medicine* 94 (April 2001): 173–176.

Substance Abuse and Mental Health Services Administration. *Take Action against Bullying.* Washington D.C.: U.S. Department of Health and Human Services, 2003.

Summit, Roland C. "Abuse of the Child Sexual Abuse Accommodation Syndrome." *Journal of Child Sexual Abuse* 1, no. 4 (1992): 153–163.

Summit, Roland C., M.D. "The Child Abuse Accommodation Syndrome." *Child Abuse & Neglect* 7 (1983): 177–193.

Sundin, Eva C., and Mardi J. Horowitz. "Harowitz' Impact of Event Scale Evaluation of 20 Years of Use." *Psychosomatic Medicine* 65, no. 5 (September–October 2003): 870–876.

Sundin, Eva C., and Mardi J. Horowitz. "Impact of Event Scale: Psychometric Properties." *British Journal of Psychiatry* 180 (2002): 205–209.

Tateno, Amane, M.D., Richard E. Jorge, M.D., and Robert G. Robinson, M.D. "Pathological Laughing and Crying Following Traumatic Brain Injury." *Journal of Neuropsychiatry and Clinical Neurosciences* 16 (2004): 426–434.

Taylor, Bonita E., et al. "Compassion Fatigue and Burnout among Rabbis Working as Chaplains." *Journal of Pastoral Care & Counseling* 60, nos. 1–2 (Spring–Summer 2006): 35–42.

Tedeschi, R. G., C. L. Park, and L. G. Calhoun. "Posttraumatic Growth: Conceptual Issues." In *Posttraumatic Growth: Positive Changes in the Aftermath of Crisis,* edited by R. G. Tedeschi, C. L. Park, and L. G. Calhoun, 1–22. Mahwah, N.J.: Lawrence Erbaum.

Teicher, Martin H., et al. "Childhood Neglect Is Associated with Reduced Corpus Callosum Area." *Biological Psychiatry* 56, no. 1 (July 2004): 80–85.

Terr, L. *Unchained Memories: True Stories of Traumatic Memories Lost and Found.* Basic Books, New York, 1994.

Tjaden, P., and N. Thoennes. *Full Report of the Prevalence, Incidence, and Consequences of Violence Against Women: Findings from the National Violence against Women Survey.* Washington, D.C.: National Institute of Justice and Centers for Disease Control and Prevention, 2000.

Topdjian, V. "Post-Generational Trauma in First, Second and Third Generational Children of Armenian Genocide Survivors." Master thesis, California State University at Northridge, 2007.

Turner, S. M., D. C. Beidel, and B. C. Frueh. "Multicomponent Behavior Treatment for Chronic Combat-Related Posttraumatic Stress Disorder. Trauma Management Therapy." *Behavior Modification* 29, no. 1 (2005): 39–69.

United Nations Office on Drugs and Crime. *World Drug Report 2006.* Vol. 1, *Analysis.* United Nations (June 2006). Available online. URL: http://www.unodc.org/pdf/WDR_2006/wdr2006_volume1.pdf. Downloaded September 28, 2006.

Ursano, R. J., et al. "Peritraumatic Dissociation and Posttraumatic Stress Disorder following Motor Vehicle Accidents." *American Journal of Psychiatry* 15 (1999): 1,808–1,810.

U.S. Army. "Combat Operational Stress Reaction (COSR) ('Battle Fatigue')." Available online from http://chppm-www.apgea.army.mil/documents/TG/TECHGUID/TG241.pdf#search=%22battele%20fatigue%20normal

%20common%20signs%20self%20buddy%20army %22. Downloaded August 17, 2006.

Vaiva, G., et al. "Relationship between Posttrauma GABA Plasma Levels & PTSD at 1 Year Follow-Up." *American Journal of Psychiatry* 163 (August 2006): 1,446–1,448.

Van der Hart, O., and B. Friedman. "Trauma, Dissociation and Triggers: Their Role in Treatment and Emergency Psychiatry." In *Emergency Psychiatry Today,* edited by J. B. van Luyn et al., 137–142. Amsterdam: Elsevier.

van der Kolk, B. A. "The Body, Memory, and the Psychobiology of Trauma." In *Sexual Abuse Recalled: Treating Trauma in the Erta of the Recovered Memory Debate,* edited by Judith L. Alpert, 29–60. Northvale, N.J.: Jason Aronson (1995).

———. "The Body Keeps the Score: Memory and the Evolving Psychobiology of Post Traumatic Stress." *Harvard Review of Psychiatry* 1, no. 5 (1994): 253–265.

van der Kolk, Bessel A., M.D. "The Neurobiology of Childhood Trauma and Abuse." *Child and Adolescent Psychiatric Clinics* 12 (2003): 293–317.

van der Kolk, Bessel A., Onno van der Hart, and Jennifer Burbridge. "Approaches to the Treatment of PTSD." In *Extreme Stress and Communities: Impact and Intervention,* edited by S. Hobfoll, and M. de Vries. Norwell, Massachusetts: Kluwer Academic, 1995.

van der Kolk, B. A., S. Roth, D. Pelcovitz, and F. Mandel. *Complex PTSD: Results of the PTSD Field Trials for DSM-IV.* Washington, D.C., American Psychiatric Association, 1993.

van der Kolk, B. A., et al. "Disorders of Extreme Stress: The Empirical Foundation of a Complex Adaptation to Trauma." *Journal of Traumatic Stress* 18, no. 5 (October 2005): 389–399.

van der Kolk, et al. "Dissociation, affect dysregulation and somatization: The complex nature of adaptation to trauma." *American Journal of Psychiatry 153,* no. 7 (1996), pgs. Festschrift Supplement: 83–93.

van der Kolk, B. A., and R. Fisler. "Dissociation & the Fragmentary Nature of Traumatic Memories: Overview & Exploratory Study." *Journal of Traumatic Stress* 8, no. 4 (1995): 505–525.

van der Kolk, B. A., M. S. Greenberg, S. P. Orr, and R. K. Pitman. "Endogenous Opioids and Stress-Induced Analgesia in Post Traumatic Stress Disorder." *Psychopharmacology Bulletin,* 25 (1989): 108–112.

van der Kolk, B., J. W. Hopper, and J. E. Osterman. "Exploring the Nature of Traumatic Memory: Combining Clinical Knowledge with Laboratory Methods." *Journal of Aggression, Maltreatment & Trauma* 4, no. 2 (2001): 9–31.

van der Kolk, Bessel A., Alexander McFarlane, and Lars Weisaeth, eds. *Traumatic Stress.* New York: Guilford Press, 1996.

van Griensven, Frits, et al. "Mental Health Problems among Adults in Tsunami-Affected Areas in Southern Thailand." *Journal of the American Medical Association* 296, no. 5 (August 2, 2006): 537–548.

van Dijk, J. A., M. J. A. Schoutrop, and P. Spinhoven. "Testimony Therapy: Treatment Method for Traumatized Victims of Organized Violence." *American Journal of Psychotherapy* 57 (2003): 361–373.

van Zelst, W. H., et al. "Prevalence and Risk Factors of Posttraumatic Stress Disorder in Older Adults." *Psychotherapy and Psychosomatics* 72, no. 6 (November–December 2003): 333–342.

Vaughan, K., and N. Tarrier. "The Use of Image Habituation Therapy." *British Journal of Psychiatry* 161 (1992): 658–664.

Violante, J., C. Castellano, J. O'Rourke, and D. Paton. "Proximity to the 9/11 Terrorist Attack and Suicide Ideation in Police Officers." *Traumatology* 12, no. 3 (2006): 248–254.

Watson, C., M. P. Juba, V. Manifold, T. Kuccala, and P. E. Anderson. "The PTSD Interview: Rationale, Description, Reliability and Current Validity of a *DSM-III*-Based Technique." *Journal of Clinical Psychology* 47 (1991): 179–188.

Wax Deiber, Marla, et al. "Ganser's Syndrome in a Man with AIDS." *Psychosomatics* 44, no. 4 (July–August 2003): 342–345.

Weaver, A. J., L. T. Flannelly, J. Garbarino, C. R. Figley, and K. J. Flannelly. "A Systematic Review of Research on Religion and Spirituality in the *Journal of Traumatic Stress*: 1990–1999." *Mental Health, Religion & Culture* 6, no. 3 (2003): 215–225.

Weine, S., et al. "Testimony Psychotherapy in Bosnian Refuges: A Pilot Study." *American Journal of Psychiatry* 155, no. 12 (December 1998): 1,720–1,726.

Wetzel, Richard D., et al. "Briquet's Syndrome (Hysteria) Is Both a Somatoform and a 'Psychoform' Illness: A Minnesota Multiphasic Personality Inventory Study." *Psychosomatic Medicine* 56 (1994): 564–569.

Wilson, John P. "PTSD and Complex PTSD: Symptoms, Syndromes, and Diagnoses." In *Assessing Psychological Trauma and PTSD.* 2nd ed., edited by John P. Wilson and Terence M. Keane. New York: Guilford Publications, 2004.

Winston, Flaura K., M.D., et al. "Screening for Risk of Persistent Posttraumatic Stress in Injured Children and Their Parents." *Journal of the American Medical Association* 290, no. 5 (August 6, 2003): 643–649.

Wolbert Burgess, Ann, and Lynda Lytle Holmstrom. "Rape Trauma Syndrome." *American Journal of Psychiatry* 131, no. 9 (September 1974): 981–986.

Wolchik, Sharlena A., et al. "Six-Year Follow-up of Preventive Interventions for Children of Divorce: A Randomized Controlled Trial." *Journal of the American Medical Association* 288, no. 15 (October 16, 2002): 1,874–1,881.

Yehuda, R., S. L. Halligan, and L. M. Bierer. "Cortisol Levels in Adult Offspring of Holocaust Survivors: Relation to PTSD Symptoms Severity in the Parent and Child." *Psychoneuroendocrinology* 27 (2001): 171–180.

Yehuda, R., J. D. Flory, S. Southwick, and D. S. Charney. "Developing an Agenda for Translational Studies of Resilience and Vulnerability Following Trauma Exposure." *Annals of the New York Academy of Science* 1071, no. 1 (2006): 379–396.

Yehuda, Rachel, et al. "Enhanced Suppression of Cortisol Following Dexamethasone in Posttraumatic Stress Disorder." *American Journal of Psychiatry* 150 (1993): 83–86.

Yehuda, R., et al. "Impact of Cumulative Lifetime Trauma and Recent Stress on Current Posttraumatic Stress Disorder Symptoms in Holocaust Survivors." *American Journal of Psychiatry* 152, no. 12 (1995): 1,815–1,818.

Yehuda, R., et al. "Low Cortisol & Risk for PTSD in Adult Offspring of Holocaust Survivors." *The American Journal of Psychiatry* 157, no. 8 (2000): 1,252–1,259.

Yehuda, Rachel. "Post-Traumatic Stress Disorder." *New England Journal of Medicine* 346, no. 2 (January 10, 2002): 108–114.

Young, Bruce H. "The Immediate Response to Disaster: Guidelines for Adult Psychological First Aid." In *Interventions Following Mass Violence and Disasters: Strategies for Mental Health Practice.* New York: Guilford Publications, 2006.

Zeanah, C., and M. Sheeringa Zeanah. "The Experience and Effects of Violence in Infancy." In *Children in a Violent Society,* edited by J. D. Osofsky. New York: Guilford Press, 1997.

Zucker, Marla, et al. "Dissociative Symptomatology in Posttraumatic Stress Disorder and Disorders of Extreme Stress." *Journal of Trauma & Dissociation* 7, no. 1 (2006): 19–31.

INDEX

in memory 45, 57, 83, 137–
138, 149, 172–173, 196
neuroplasticity of 250
in resilience 223
right hemisphere of 83
as social organ 43–44
stress response in. *See*
biological factors related to
the stress response
brain electroencephalogram
107, 116
brainstem 44, 57
Brattberg, Gunilla 238, 241
breathing retraining **46**
for anxiety disorders 190,
191
for hyperventilation
syndrome 46, 145, 199
Breslau, N. 205, 206
brevity, immediacy, centrality,
expectancy, proximity, and
simplicity (BICEPS) 144, 313
Brewin, C. R. 206, 240
Brief Betrayal Trauma Survey
(BBTS) 18, 20
Brief COPE 18–19, 22, 23,
81–82
Briere, John 19, 155, 156, 231
Briquet, Paul 46, 141, 243
Briquet's syndrome **46–48,** 141,
243
Britt, Thomas W. 238–239
Broken Mirror (Phillips) 39
Brown, J. 166
Bryant, R. A. 2
BTT. *See* betrayal trauma theory
bulimia nervosa 39
"bullycide" **48–50,** 65–66, 102,
279
bullying **48–50,** 63, 65–66, 279
buprenorphine 3
bupropion 128, 168, 192, 303
Burba, Benjaminas 7
Bureau of Justice Statistics 178
burnout 238, 241. *See also*
compassion fatigue
Burton, L. A. 236
Bush, George W. 281

BuSpar 13
buspirone 13
butyl nitrate 257
butyrophenone 314
BWS. *See* battered woman
syndrome
bystander traumatization 286,
308

C

Caddell, J. M. 157
Callahan, Roger 10
Cambodian refugees 19, 153,
158
Campral 3
CAN. *See* child abuse and
neglect
cannabis 257
Cannon, Walter 124
CAPS. *See* Clinician-
Administered PTSD Scale
CAPTA. *See* Child Abuse
Prevention and Treatment Act
car accident. *See* motor vehicle
crash/accident
carbamazepine 39, 172
cardiovascular system, stress
and 251
caregivers. *See* compassion
fatigue
Carlier, I. V. E. 275
Carlson, Eve Bernstein 20–21,
107
Carver, Charles S. 22, 81
Cashman, L. 157
catecholamine **51,** 197
causes/risk factors of traumatic
stress disorders **51–56**
CBC. *See* complete blood count
CBT/CBI. *See* cognitive
behavioral therapy/
interventions
Celexa 2, 171, 230, 303
cellular memory **56–57**
Census Bureau 178
Centers for Disease Control and
Prevention 109, 261, 293–294

central nervous system (CNS)
31, 56, **57**
cerebellum 57
cerebral cortex 44, 45, 46, 57,
195–196, 251
cerebrum 57
Charcot, Jean-Martin xii–xiii
Charney, D. S. 312
checking, in OCD 188
child abuse and neglect (CAN)
51, **58–61,** 64–65, 278–279
and addiction 3, 26, 52, 60,
66, 67, 255
and altered pain perception
52, 64
and amnesia 11, 36–37, 142
and anxiety disorders 53,
60–61, 67
and attachment disorders 26,
29, 64
battered child syndrome xiv,
33–34, 63, 185, 278
betrayal trauma theory on
36–37, 142
and bipolar disorder 286
and body memories 199
and borderline personality
disorder 43
and brain development 58,
84, 196
and bullying 48, 64
categories of 58, 64–65
and chronic pain 60–61
and cortisol levels 198
and cutting and self-
mutilation 52, 64, 88
cycle of 34, 35, 58, 185
and delayed PTSD 93, 102
and dissociative disorders
27–28, 52, 64, 194
false memories of 63, 123,
221
federal guidelines on 58–59
and fibromyalgia 41, 199
identifying 34, 63
as non-accidental trauma 185
and numbing 37, 142, 186,
212

cycle of 289
domestic. *See* battered woman syndrome; battering
FBI reports on 307
national survey on 178–180
in schools 49, 50
virtual reality exposure/virtual reality graded exposure (VRGE) 120, **310–311**
visual/kinesthetic dissociation (V/KD) 10, **311**
visual memory **311–312**
Vlahov, David 72
VoC. *See* Validity of Cognition
volcano 181
vulnerability **312**

W

Waking the Tiger (Levine) 232, 242, 300
Wald, J. 160
Walker, Leonore 34
walking the labyrinth 9–10
Wallace, Andrew 99
war neurosis xiii, 139, 235. *See also* combat stress reaction
war zone stress reaction 212, **313**. *See also* combat stress reaction
waterboarding **313**
Watson, C. 156
Watson, J. B. 81
Watson, Patricia 91
Weine, Steven 130, 267, 302
Weintraub, Jagdish Kumari 22, 81

Weisaeth, Lars 275
Weiss, Daniel S. 21, 154, 155
Wellbutrin 128, 168, 192, 303
West, Malcolm 4
white matter 57
wildfire 181–182
Willauger, R. 161
Wilner, Nancy 21, 154, 157
Wilson, John P. 139, 212
withdrawal symptoms 3, 12, 35, 255
Wolbert Burgess, Ann 102–103, 219, 286
Wolpe, Joseph 136, 210–211, 254, 265, 301
women. *See also* battered woman syndrome; rape trauma syndrome
body memories in 41
Briquet's syndrome in 46, 47, 141
as bullies 48, 279
cutting and self-mutilation in 64, 89
depression in 168
effects of divorce on 110
generalized anxiety disorder in 128
insomnia in 152
panic disorder in 14, 191
PTSD in xii, 205, 275
risk of suicide in 261
Wooding, S. 266
work burnout 238, 241. *See also* compassion fatigue
World Health Organization (WHO) 11, 159, 221, 255

World War I 76, 91–92, 138, 212, 235, 244. *See also* shell shock
World War II. *See* Hiroshima bombing; Holocaust
World War II veterans
convoy fatigue in 77–78, 139
debriefings for 169, 273
delayed PTSD in 93
gross stress reaction in 132
military psychiatrists for 76, 143
risk of combat stress reactions in 77
somatic symptoms in 138
writing therapy 17, 67

X

Xanax 2, 13, 35, 172, 303

Y

Yehuda, Rachel 88, 96, 205, 241, 312
yellow bile 117
Young, Bruce H. 213–214

Z

zaleplon 151
Zoloft 171, 230, 234, 303
zolpidem 151
Zyprexa 151